Fetal Cardiovascular Imaging

Fetal Cardiovascular Imaging
A Disease-Based Approach

Jack Rychik, MD
Director, Fetal Heart Program
Robert S. and Delores Harrington Endowed Chair in Pediatric Cardiology
The Children's Hospital of Philadelphia
Professor of Pediatrics
University of Pennsylvania School of Medicine
Philadelphia, Pennsylvania

Zhiyun Tian, MD
Chief, Fetal Cardiovascular Imaging
Fetal Heart Program, Cardiac Center
The Children's Hospital of Philadelphia
Clinical Associate of the University of Pennsylvania School of Medicine
Philadelphia, Pennsylvania

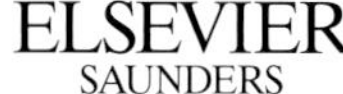

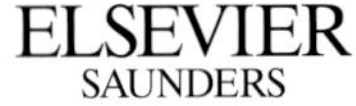

SAUNDERS

1600 John F. Kennedy Blvd.
Ste 1800
Philadelphia, PA 19103-2899

FETAL CARDIOVASCULAR IMAGING: A DISEASE-BASED APPROACH ISBN: 978-1-4160-3172-7

Library of Congress Cataloging-in-Publication Data

Fetal cardiovascular imaging : a disease based approach / editors, Jack Rychik, Zhiyun Tian.
p. ; cm.
Includes bibliographical references and index.
ISBN 978-1-4160-3172-7 (hardcover: alk. paper)
1. Fetal heart–Ultrasonic imaging. 2. Congenital heart disease–Diagnosis. I. Rychik, Jack, 1959- II. Tian, Zhiyun.
[DNLM: 1. Fetal Heart–anatomy & histology. 2. Fetal Heart–ultrasonography. 3. Heart Defects, Congenital–ultrasonography. 4. Image Processing, Computer-Assisted–methods. 5. Ultrasonography, Prenatal–methods. WQ 209]
RG628.3.E34F47 2011
618.3'261–dc23 2011023509

Editor: Natasha Andjelkovic
Developmental Editor: Julia Bartz
Editorial Assistant: Brad McIlwain
Publishing Services Manager: Pat Joiner-Myers
Designer: Steven Stave
Marketing Manager: Cara Jespersen

Printed in China

Last digit is the print number: 9 8 7 6 5 4 3 2 1

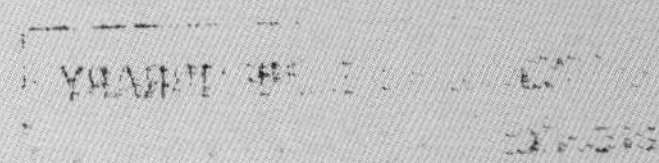

Contributors

Meryl S. Cohen, MD
Associate Professor of Pediatrics, University of Pennsylvania School of Medicine; Medical Director, Echocardiography Laboratory, and Associate Director, Cardiology Fellowship Program, The Children's Hospital of Philadelphia, Philadelphia, Pennsylvania
Atrioventricular Canal Defects; Heterotaxy Syndrome and Complex Single Ventricle

Sarah M. Cohen, MPH
Department of Obstetrics and Gynaecology, Hadassah-Hebrew University Medical Centers, Mount Scopus, Jerusalem, Israel
Three- and Four-Dimensional Imaging in Fetal Echocardiography

Karl Degenhardt, MD, PhD
Clinical Associate, University of Pennsylvania School of Medicine; Pediatric Cardiologist, Division of Cardiology, The Children's Hospital of Philadelphia, Philadelphia, Pennsylvania
Embryology of the Cardiovascular System

Denise Donaghue, RN, MSN
Coordinator, Fetal Heart Program, The Children's Hospital of Philadelphia, Philadelphia, Pennsylvania
Counseling and Support for the Family Carrying a Fetus with Cardiovascular Disease

Mark A. Fogel, MD
Professor of Cardiology and Radiology, University of Pennsylvania School of Medicine; Director of Cardiac Magnetic Resonance, Division of Cardiology, The Children's Hospital of Philadelphia, Philadelphia, Pennsylvania
Anatomical and Functional Fetal Cardiac Magnetic Resonance Imaging: An Emerging Technology

Jennifer Glatz, MD
Clinical Associate, University of Pennsylvania School of Medicine; Pediatric Cardiologist, Division of Cardiology, The Children's Hospital of Philadelphia, Philadelphia, Pennsylvania
Aortopulmonary Window; Double-Inlet Left Ventricle

Max Godfrey, BSc (Hons), MBBS
Fellow in Pediatric Cardiology, Schneider Children's Medical Center of Israel, Petach Tikvah, Israel
The Fetal Circulation

Donna A. Goff, MD, MS
Instructor, University of Pennsylvania; Senior Imaging Fellow, Fetal Heart Program, The Children's Hospital of Philadelphia, Philadelphia, Pennsylvania
Cardiac Masses and Tumors; Twin Reverse Arterial Perfusion

David J. Goldberg, MD
Assistant Professor of Pediatrics, Perelman School of Medicine at the University of Pennsylvania; Attending, Division of Pediatric Cardiology, The Children's Hospital of Philadelphia, Philadelphia, Pennsylvania
Ventricular Septal Defects; Atrial Septal Defects; Aortic Stenosis

Shobha Natarajan, MD
Assistant Clinical Professor, University of Pennsylvania School of Medicine; Attending Cardiologist, The Children's Hospital of Philadelphia, Philadelphia, Pennsylvania
Malalignment of Conal Septum with Arch Obstruction; Corrected Transposition of the Great Arteries

Matthew J. O'Connor, MD
Fellow, Pediatric Cardiology, University of Pennsylvania School of Medicine; Fellow, Pediatric Cardiology, The Children's Hospital of Philadelphia, Philadelphia, Pennsylvania
Arrhythmias in the Fetus

Michael D. Quartermain, MD
Assistant Professor of Pediatrics, University of Pennsylvania School of Medicine; Assistant Professor of Pediatrics, Division of Cardiology, The Children's Hospital of Philadelphia, Philadelphia, Pennsylvania
Transposition of the Great Arteries; Double-Outlet Right Ventricle; Coarctation of the Aorta

Lindsay Rogers, MD
Instructor in Pediatrics, University of Pennsylvania School of Medicine; Fellow, Pediatric Cardiology, The Children's Hospital of Philadelphia, Philadelphia, Pennsylvania
Aortic Stenosis and Mitral Valve Dysplasia Syndrome

Jack Rychik, MD
Director, Fetal Heart Program, Robert S. and Delores Harrington Endowed Chair in Pediatric Cardiology, The Children's Hospital of Philadelphia; Professor of Pediatrics, University of Pennsylvania School of Medicine, Philadelphia, Pennsylvania
The Fetal Circulation; The Fetal Cardiovascular Examination; Prenatal Practice Care Model and Delivery of the Fetus with Cardiovascular Disease; Counseling and Support for the Family Carrying a Fetus with Cardiovascular Disease; Congenital Absence of Aortic Valve Leaflets; Hypoplastic Left Heart Syndrome; Aortic Stenosis and Mitral Valve Dysplasia Syndrome; Echo "Bright" Spot in the Heart; Ectopia Cordis; Diverticulum or Aneurysm of the Ventricle; Conjoined Twins; Fetal Cardiomyopathy; Abnormalities of the Ductus Arteriosus; Agenesis of the Ductus Venosus; Twin-Twin Transfusion Syndrome; Sacrococcygeal Teratoma; Cerebral Arteriovenous Malformation; Pulmonary Arteriovenous Malformation; Congenital Cystic Adenomatoid Malformation; Congenital Diaphragmatic Hernia

Maully J. Shah, MBBS
Associate Professor of Pediatrics, University of Pennsylvania School of Medicine; Director, Cardiac Electrophysiology, The Children's Hospital of Philadelphia, Philadelphia, Pennsylvania
Arrhythmias in the Fetus

Ori Shen, MD
Obstetric Ultrasound Unit, Department of Obstetrics and Gynaecology, Shaare Zedek Medical Center, Jerusalem, Israel
Three- and Four-Dimensional Imaging in Fetal Echocardiography

Amanda Shillingford, MD
Assistant Professor of Pediatrics—Cardiology, Medical College of Wisconsin; Staff Physician, Children's Hospital of Wisconsin, Milwaukee, Wisconsin
Tetralogy of Fallot; Tetralogy of Fallot with Pulmonary Atresia; Tetralogy of Fallot with Absent Pulmonary Valve Syndrome; Truncus Arteriosus

Anita Szwast, MD
Division of Cardiology, Department of Pediatrics, University of Pennsylvania School of Medicine; Assistant Professor of Pediatrics, Division of Cardiology, The Children's Hospital of Philadelphia, Philadelphia, Pennsylvania
Pulmonary Stenosis; Pulmonary Atresia with Intact Ventricular Septum; Ebstein's Anomaly and Other Abnormalities of the Tricuspid Valve; Tricuspid Atresia

Deepika Thacker, MBBS, MD
Assistant Professor, Thomas Jefferson University Hospital, Philadelphia, Pennsylvania; Pediatric Cardiologist, Nemours Cardiac Center, Alfred I. duPont Hospital for Children, Wilmington, Delaware
Ventricular Septal Defects; Aortic Stenosis

Simcha Yagel, MD
Head, Department of Obstetrics and Gynaecology, Hadassah-Hebrew University Medical Centers, Mount Scopus, Jerusalem, Israel
Three- and Four-Dimensional Imaging in Fetal Echocardiography

Preface

Fetal Cardiovascular Imaging: A Disease-Based Approach is a combination textbook with still images and an accompanying library of videos. Whereas a number of texts exist on the "how-to" and technical aspects of fetal echocardiography, our goals were to adequately cover these areas, but focus more so on the variety of disorders and conditions that affect the fetal cardiovascular system, with emphasis on the imaging specifics particular to the condition of interest.

How can the printed pages of a book adequately inform on a complex diagnostic process that involves the imaging of a moving, beating structure, that of the fetal heart? The answer is simply that a book of text alone is inadequate to achieve this task. In the year 2011, technologies for imparting knowledge allow for the combination of visual media in order to best convey the optimal informative and educational experience. This book was therefore created as an equal partner and complement to an imaging library with an array of imaging videos available for your review. The chapters are organized as individual anomalies, with broad coverage of primary congenital heart defects and other conditions that secondarily affect the fetal cardiovascular system. Each chapter is further divided into sections on genetics, prenatal diagnosis, prenatal pathophysiology, prenatal management, postnatal pathophysiology and management, and finally, prognosis and outcome. In this manner a comprehensive overview from diagnosis, to care, to outcome, can be gleaned for a variety of fetal cardiovascular conditions.

This book and video library was initiated by the realization that over the past few years, we had collected a wealth and breadth of fetal cardiovascular images covering a wide range of anomalies. Sharing this library of images beyond our walls was of utmost importance. Each of our chapters includes a number of case examples of real patients we have seen, with demonstration of various points of importance and interest. The ideal experience for this educational encounter is an initial reading of the text and then a visit to the images to witness the heart in motion. Each of the conditions can be systematically studied in this manner. Alternatively, the image library can act as a reference with which to compare unknowns in the real clinical world, in order to help identify and correctly diagnose challenging patients. When faced with a set of unknown images in the clinic setting, a look at our image library may confirm a particular diagnosis or send the practitioner off to the next anomaly on the differential diagnosis list. If the images match up, then a look back to the text can inform on the physiology, management and counseling appropriate for the condition at hand.

Although derived from our pediatric cardiology based practice, this book and imaging library is designed with a multidisciplinary audience in mind. Practitioners of maternal fetal medicine, obstetrics, pediatric cardiology, medical sonography, perinatology, neonatology and radiology all have a growing interest in fetal medicine with focus on the fetal heart and vasculature. We hope this book will be of use to the greater community at large sharing in the care for the unborn child.

Jack Rychik
Zhiyun Tian

Acknowledgments

This project was born of an idea to fill a void and provide a reliable source of imaging knowledge in the developing discipline of cardiovascular care before birth. Dr. Tian and I first discussed the notion of a book and took up this challenge a while back, longer than either of us would like to admit. Finally, here it is. No endeavor, certainly not a book and video imaging project of this scope, can come to fruition by the energies of the creators and editors alone, no matter how motivated. There are a number of people to thank who have encouraged and supported this project along the way, facilitating its completion.

My wife Susan and my daughters Jordana, Leora, and Natali have tolerated countless hours, nights, weekends and then weeks of separation from me as I worked on this project. Words cannot express how grateful I am for your sacrifices and steadfast love. You are my facilitators, my enablers, and without your support this endeavor would never be possible.

I have had the unique opportunity to learn about congenital heart disease from an incredible group of brilliant and provocative thinkers. Alvin Chin, John Murphy, William Norwood, and Marshall Jacobs provided me with a strong foundation of knowledge. I thank them for instilling in me an appreciation for the importance of rigorous logic as the source for all good clinical care.

Natasha Andjelkovic and Julia Bartz of Elsevier were instrumental in encouraging me to keep moving forward, and I thank them for their advice and patience. My Division of Cardiology Chief, Dr. Robert Shaddy, and Department of Pediatrics Chair, Dr. Alan Cohen, saw in me the potential to complete this task, if only I could focus more fully on the project. I am forever indebted for their support of my taking a brief sabbatical in Israel, which allowed me to re-energize and complete this task. While in Israel, I also had the fortunate opportunity to develop a professional relationship with Dr. Simcha Yagel of Hadassah Hospital, an endlessly energetic maternal fetal medicine specialist whose brilliance and gracious hospitality were instrumental at a critical time of writing.

I am fortunate to work with an amazingly talented and dedicated group of individuals. In addition to Dr. Zhiyun Tian, co-editor of this project, Peggy McCann, RCDS, and Debra Soffer, RCDS, are personally responsible for the high-quality echocardiograms that comprise this effort. It is primarily their three pairs of incredibly gifted hands at the echo machine that fashioned these images. Denise Donaghue, RN, and I have dedicated the past 10 years of our careers to building the Fetal Heart Program at The Children's Hospital of Philadelphia, a task of which we are immensely proud. Without Denise's vision, dedication, and incredible skill, we would not have had the program and clinical experiences with which to generate the knowledge for this book. Nurse coordinator Jill Combs, RN, and social workers Lucia Figueroa and Jennifer Diem-Inglis have been steadfastly amazing at coordinating compassionate care for our pregnant mothers, this at what can be considered one of the most traumatic of life experiences—uncovering the presence of a serious fetal anomaly. It is this synthesis of skilled imaging, coordination of care, and compassionate family centered counseling that has created our unique service. To all of the members of the Fetal Heart Program, thank you for your work—you make me proud to be a part of your team.

Finally, I must thank the countless patients and families who have sought our opinions and advice over the years and have entrusted us with their care. I have learned from each and every one of you.

Jack Rychik

Acknowledgments

For the past 2 decades, I have had the privilege of working in the Fetal Heart Program at The Children's Hospital of Philadelphia. Over the years, we have carefully accumulated a large number of cases and always knew we would someday share this image collection with our medical community. Thus, it is extremely gratifying that Dr. Jack Rychik and I, with the support of our many colleagues and Elsevier, have produced this book and imaging library.

I am indebted to many for helping this dream come true.

First, I would like to thank my family: My parents raised me to be a strong and giving person and always told me "love what you do and be the best." My four brothers have unconditionally supported and encouraged me to set and achieve higher standards.

I would like to thank my birth country, China, where I received an excellent education, enabling me to lay a firm foundation for my career today.

I wish to express my gratitude to my teachers and mentors in China and the United States. Your guidance and support for me, with your knowledge and experience, has made it possible for me to be successful in this field.

I would also like to thank The Children's Hospital of Philadelphia, an amazing organization that has given me a most incredible opportunity to grow and advance my skills. I want to thank the hospital leadership and colleagues for their dedicated support during the past 2 decades. I deeply love my work environment and my office family members, who have always provided me with a nurturing environment.

To my students, the young physicians from China, you have given your unselfish support to this effort. I will always remember those evenings and weekends you dedicated to helping me edit our images, and all of the happy times we spent together.

Most important, my grateful thanks to all of the patients, mothers, and babies (before you were born) that I have served for the last 20 years. Each of you gave me the privilege to help you through the use of ultrasound, to learn from your imaging, to understand your heart and to find answers to difficult questions before you were born. Without you, this book would not be possible.

Finally, I thank my husband Michael, for his love and support, and my son Steven, who followed me into medicine and has made me proud and happy every day.

Zhiyun Tian

Foreword

During the past 2 decades, we have witnessed significant developments in the diagnosis and treatment of fetal anatomic and genetic abnormalities. The prenatal detection and serial sonographic, echocardiographic, and MRI study of fetuses with anatomic malformations has permitted delineation of the natural history of these lesions, definition of the pathophysiologic features that affect clinical outcome, and formulation of management based on prognosis. This is true for fetuses with cardiac and non-cardiac disease. The diagnosis and treatment of human fetal defects has also evolved rapidly as a result of a better understanding of fetal pathophysiology derived from animal models. Most fetal anomalies that are correctable and can be diagnosed in utero are best managed by appropriate medical and surgical therapy after maternal transport and planned delivery at term. Prenatal diagnosis may also influence the timing or mode of delivery and in some cases may lead to elective termination of the pregnancy. In some highly selected circumstances, various forms of in utero therapy are now available. The crucial concept in this burgeoning field is that accurate diagnosis is imperative for effective family counseling, pregnancy management, and therapy. This textbook entitled *Fetal Cardiovascular Imaging: A Disease-Based Approach* beautifully describes all of the hallmarks of prenatally diagnosed cardiovascular disease.

Since the most severely affected fetuses often die in utero or shortly after birth, a fetal surgical approach has been defined for highly selected fetuses with thoracic masses or sacrococcygeal teratoma associated with fetal hydrops. Fetal cardiovascular pathophysiology is paramount in these conditions. The fetal surgical approach to in utero myelomeningocele repair has been developed as an approach to a potentially devastating but non-life-threatening malformation. The field has evolved to the point where an NIH-sponsored prospective randomized clinical trial is now comparing fetal repair to postnatal repair of myelomeningocele. This trial provides the groundwork for future critical testing of fetal therapeutic procedures.

Much work is being performed on the perioperative anesthetic management of the fetal surgery patient. Anesthetic considerations include the physiologic changes of pregnancy, preterm labor, the effects of tocolytic drugs, maternal and fetal anesthesia, and postoperative analgesia. The effect of these changes on the cardiovascular status of the fetus is important and is the principal reason why fetal echocardiographic monitoring is now used on a routine basis for all of our fetal surgical procedures.

Minimally invasive or fetoscopic approaches will have an increasing therapeutic role in the future as indications, instrumentation, and techniques are refined. Fetoscopic laser ablation of abnormal shared placental vessels in Twin-Twin Transfusion Syndrome (TTTS) is now established therapy, although patient selection criteria—particularly related to the cardiovascular status in TTTS—need further study. There is now a very large clinical experience with percutaneous shunt procedures for lower urinary tract obstruction and for thoracic diseases associated with fetal hydrops such as congenital cystic adenomatoid malformation of the lung and fetal hydrothorax. Percutaneous approaches in utero are now being evaluated in cases of critical aortic stenosis with evolving hypoplastic left heart syndrome in an effort to maintain two ventricle physiology. Percutaneous approaches are also being used to perform an atrial septostomy in cases of hypoplastic heart syndrome with intact atrial septum in an attempt to avert the pulmonary vasculopathy seen in this condition.

The Ex Utero Intrapartum Therapy (EXIT) procedure for intrinsic and extrinsic causes of fetal airway obstruction is now well established and has been used at many medical centers by multidisciplinary teams. This approach provides time to perform procedures such as direct laryngoscopy, bronchoscopy, or tracheostomy to secure the fetal airway, thereby converting an emergent airway crisis into a controlled situation during birth. Similarly, we now use the Immediate Postpartum Access to Cardiac Therapy (IMPACT) procedure to specially deliver prenatally diagnosed cardiac patients who need immediate postnatal therapy.

In the future, in utero hematopoietic stem cell transplantation will be a promising approach for treatment of a potentially large number of fetuses affected by congenital hematologic and immunologic disorders. Advances in gene transfer technology and prenatal diagnosis prompt consideration of a fetal gene therapy approach to correct genetic disease. For many genetic diseases, the fetal period may be the only time in which genetic intervention can prevent disease manifestations. It is conceivable that these approaches may be used to benefit fetuses with cardiovascular disease.

The contributors to this book, under the editorial leadership of Doctors Rychik and Tian, are mostly current members of the Cardiac Center faculty at The Children's Hospital of Philadelphia. Thus, the presentations reflect the philosophy of one center, gleaned from more than 2 decades of experience. This book is directed toward fetal and pediatric cardiologists, pediatric cardiac surgeons, pediatric cardiac anesthesiologists, perinatologists, echocardiographers, neonatologists, geneticists, pediatricians, and nurses who are vital components of a multidisciplinary team that manages the fetus with a cardiac defect. With continuing research efforts and clinical application, the care of the fetal cardiac patient will continue to improve.

N. Scott Adzick, MD
Surgeon-in-Chief
The Children's Hospital of Philadelphia
Director, Center for Fetal Diagnosis and Treatment
Philadelphia, Pennsylvania

Contents

I Introduction

1 The Fetal Circulation

Max Godfrey and Jack Rychik

Introduction

We begin our examination of the normal fetal circulation with a description of the anatomical pathways involved (Figure 1-1).

Oxygenated blood leaves the placenta via the umbilical vein (UV). From the UV, between 20% and 50% of the blood flows into the ductus venosus (DV), which joins the inferior vena cava (IVC) shortly before it enters the floor of the right atrium (RA). The rest of the UV blood perfuses the liver, and then rejoins the IVC circulation via the hepatic veins. Blood within the IVC that originated from the DV is mainly streamed preferentially through the foramen ovale (FO) into the left atrium (LA), through the mitral valve (MV) into the left ventricle (LV), and then out through the aortic valve (AoV) and into the ascending aorta (AAo). This blood then flows across the aortic arch, where it provides relatively oxygenated blood to the head, myocardium, and upper body via the coronary, carotid, and subclavian arteries, with a small portion continuing on via the aortic isthmus to the descending aorta (DAo).

Deoxygenated blood from the superior vena cava (SVC), together with the majority of non–DV-originating blood in the IVC flows into the RA, through the tricuspid valve (TV) into the right ventricle (RV) and out through the pulmonic valve (PV) into the pulmonary artery (PA). From the PA, approximately 20% of the blood flows to the lungs, with the remainder flowing through the ductus arteriosus (DA) to join the DAo, where it makes up the majority of the flow. The blood flowing through the DAo supplies the internal organs and the lower body, as well

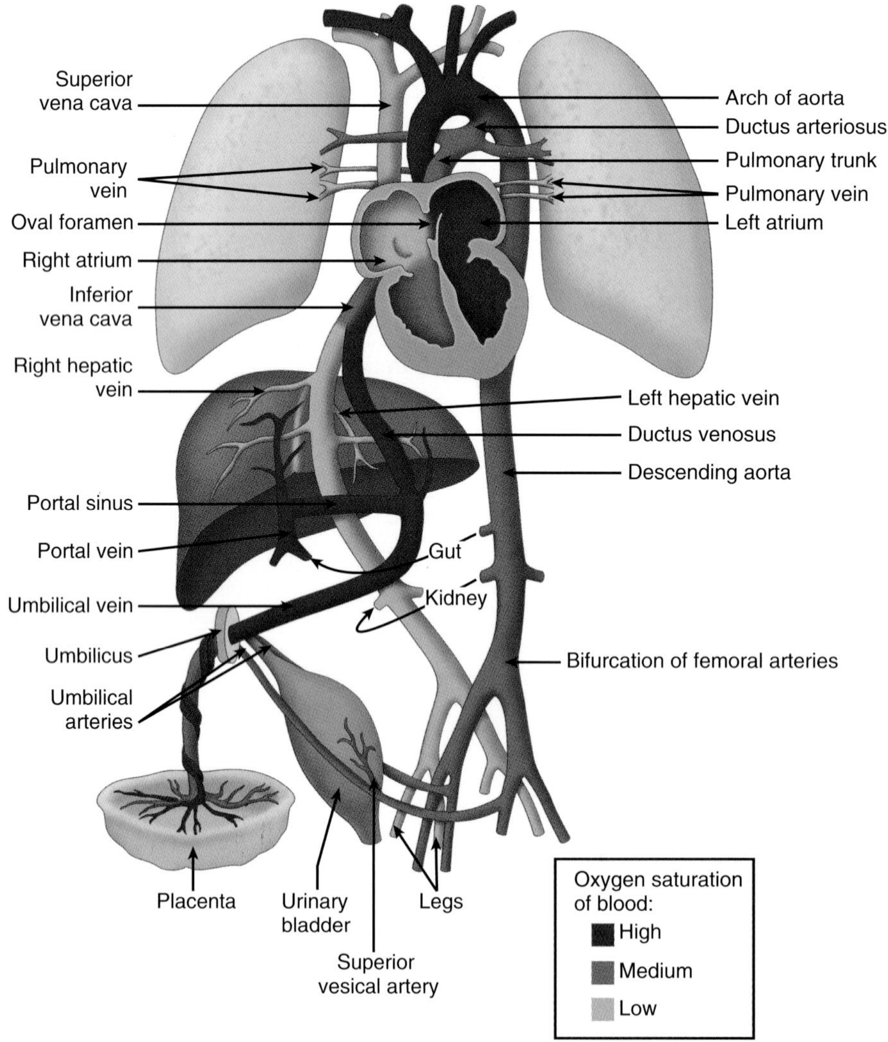

Figure 1-1. The fetal circulation demonstrating flow pathways from placenta to fetus. *Shadings* indicate the various oxygen saturations. The most highly oxygenated blood returns via the umbilical vein and is preferentially directed across the foramen ovale to the left atrium and left ventricle. Relatively deoxygenated blood mixes in the right atrium and moderately saturated blood is then ejected out of the right ventricle across the ductus arteriosus to the descending aorta. The umbilical arteries arise from the internal iliac arteries and deliver blood to the placenta to replenish oxygen supplies.

as the two umbilical arteries that return blood to the placental circulation. Thus, the fetal circulation is essentially a parallel circulation with three circulatory "shunts": the DV, the FO, and the DA. This circulatory design has a targeted goal—the brain, coronary circulation, and upper body are essentially supplied with relatively oxygenated blood via the LV, whereas the lower body receives mainly deoxygenated blood via the RV.

The majority of foundational research into the fetal circulation has been carried out on fetal sheep, which have the advantage of being large mammals, yet with a gestational duration about half the length of humans. More recent research based on ultrasonographic and Doppler studies has highlighted important differences between humans and sheep. This is perhaps not surprising because sheep fetuses have two UVs, a faster growth rate, a higher body temperature, a lower hemoglobin, a smaller brain, a differently positioned liver, and a longer intrathoracic IVC.[1]

Ductus Venosus, Hepatic Circulation, and Inferior Vena Cava

The DV is a small vessel that has been variously described as being shaped like a trumpet or an hourglass. It connects the UV to the IVC as it enters the RA, at the confluence with the hepatic veins (Figure 1-2). Early animal studies indicated that 50% of UV blood flow was channeled into the DV,[2] with the amount of shunt through the DV proportional to the UV flow,[3] implying a significant physiological role for this pathway. However, more recent studies of human fetuses using noninvasive ultrasonographic techniques have shown that the amount shunted through the DV is less and, moreover, that there is a decrease in shunting throughout gestation (i.e., more UV blood traversing the liver with later gestation). Kiserud and coworkers[4] demonstrated that the percentage of blood shunted through the DV decreases from approximately 30% at 18 to 19 weeks' gestation to approximately 20% at week 30, although with wide variations between subjects. Bellotti and colleagues[5] found that the percentage shunted was approximately 40% at 20 weeks, decreasing to approximately 15% at term. Work based on mathematical impedance modeling of the hepatic venous network suggests that the shunt decreases from 50% at 20 weeks to 20% at term.[6] Interestingly, the data suggesting a shunt of 50% from the original seminal study of Rudolph and Heymann in 1967[2] do not appear to be controlled for gestational age. Thus, there may be less conflict between the animal and the human data than has been suggested. As a greater percentage of UV return is directed through the liver with later gestation, it raises the speculation of the liver playing an important role in third-trimester fetal maturation and growth through the release of proteins and mediators. The role of the liver as "gate-keeper" to placental venous return in the growing fetus is a fascinating one, and still poorly understood.

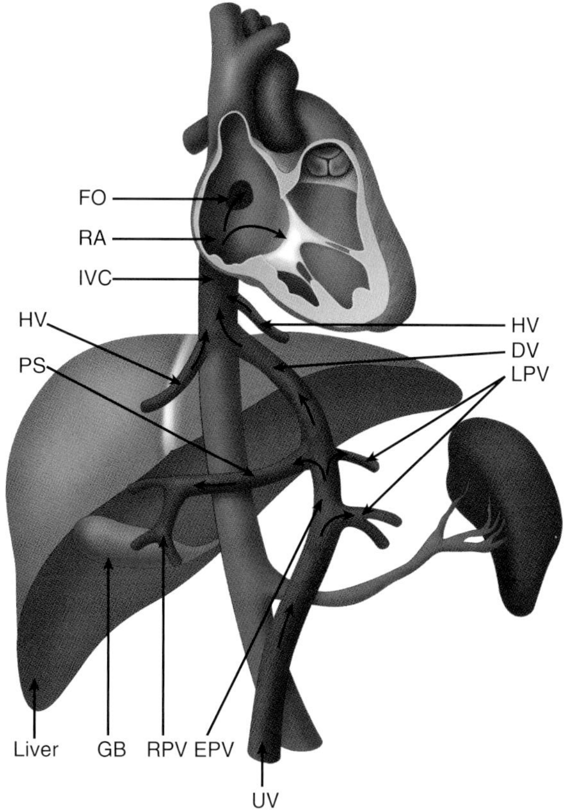

Figure 1-2. Schematic representation of the fetal umbilical, portal, and hepatic circulations. The *arrows* indicate the direction of blood flow and the *color* shows the degree of oxygen content (*red* = high; *blue* = low). DV, ductus venosus; EPV, extrahepatic portal vein; FO, foramen ovale; GB, gallbladder; HV, hepatic vein; IVC, inferior vena cava; LPV, left portal vein; PS, portal sinus; RA, right atrium; RPV, right portal vein; UV, umbilical vein.

Within the IVC entry site at the floor of the RA, the column of blood originating from the DV is preferentially streamed across the FO into the LA,[7] and the remainder enters the RA and crosses the TV. The mechanism by which this occurs is likely related to the complex geometry of the vessels as they enter the RA floor; the phenomenon can be demonstrated on Doppler color flow mapping.[8] In sheep, there are valvelike structures at the opening of the DV and left hepatic vein that may physically direct the different flows from within the IVC.[8] However, these structures do not appear to exist in the same way in the human fetus.[9] Kiserud and Acharya[10] suggest that the rapid increase in velocity of the blood within the DV, caused by the pressure gradient, means that the blood column originating from the DV has the highest kinetic energy; thus, it is this blood that opens the FO valve and enters the LA.

A related controversy concerns the presence of a sphincter mechanism within the DV by which flow may be increased or decreased.[11] It has been demonstrated, in both animal and human models, that the flow through the DV is increased in certain conditions such as hypovolemia[12] and hypoxemia.[13] Some studies have favored the presence of a discrete sphincter mechanism that controls the caliber of the DV,[8,14] whereas others propose that the entire vessel is tonically controlled by neurohumoral mechanisms.[15,16] Alternatively, a drop in resistance to flow through a relaxation of the portal vascular system may direct blood away from the DV. This notion is supported by the finding of a greater degree of smooth muscle in the walls of the fetal portal venous system than in the DV.

Blood from the left hepatic vein is also shunted preferentially through the FO, owing to the position of its entry into the IVC just under the eustachian valve.[17] In fact, the liver, despite its high metabolic activity in the fetus, extracts relatively little oxygen (10–15%[18]), such that hepatic venous blood is fairly well oxygenated and, thus, potentially contributes to the highly oxygenated blood-streaming phenomenon within the fetal heart.

Foramen Ovale

In the postnatal human infant, the FO is commonly thought of as being a connection between the two atria, causing shunts from one side to the other. It has also been described as such in the fetus.[19] However, it is contended that in the fetus, the anatomical and functional arrangement is different. The FO flap and the crista dividens of the interatrial septum act as a "valve," directing the stream of blood from the IVC, which enters essentially between the two atria from below. The stream of blood is divided due to position, direction, and velocity, with DV and left hepatic venous blood directed to the left atrium, while abdominal IVC blood is directed to the RA.[17] Changes in pressure on either side will change the balance of flow, and this can have far-reaching consequences for the development of the fetal heart. For example, in aortic stenosis, left atrial pressure is elevated thereby increasing shunting of blood to the RA, which by neglecting the LA, may eventually leading to left-sided hypoplasia,[20,21] although the causal chain of events is very much controversial.[22] Experimental models have shown that normal flow distributions within the developing heart may be critical for normal cardiac morphogenesis.[23,24]

Ductus Arteriosus

The DA is a large vessel with muscular walls, which connects the pulmonary trunk and aorta. The systolic flow within the DA has the highest velocity of all the fetal cardiovascular system, and the velocity increases with increasing gestational age.[25] The human DA shunts an estimated 78% of the right ventricular output, or 46% of the combined cardiac output (CCO),[26] away from the lungs to join the DAo and perfuse the lower body. These figures are slightly lower than in sheep models, which suggest that the DA carries 88% of the right ventricular output and 58% of the CCO.[9] The patency of the DA depends on levels of circulating prostaglandin E_2 (PGE_2),[27] but the flow through the DA is dependent on the resistance of the pulmonary vasculature. The pulmonary vasculature undergoes changes during the third trimester of gestation such that increases in partial pressure of oxygen (PO_2) cause resistance to decrease and, therefore, flow through the DA to change accordingly.[28] This mimics the physiological processes that take place after birth with the onset of breathing and can theoretically be used as an in utero test for fetal pulmonary vascular development such as in conditions of congenital heart disease or pulmonary hypoplasia.

The sensitivity of the DA to PGE_2 in utero has clinical significance, because maternal administration of PGE_2 inhibitors such as indomethacin can cause the DA to close with catastrophic consequences.[29] The response to indomethacin is thought to be potentiated by stress, and intraoperative echocardiography demonstrates that indomethacin used in fetal surgery induces more potent constriction of the DA.[30] Interestingly, there seems to be some "physiological" constriction of the DA as gestation proceeds toward term, which may explain the increased velocity that is seen in the DA relative to the PA.[25] Because the lungs represent a major site of PGE_2 metabolism,[31] it would seem plausible that this constriction of the DA is due to increased prostaglandin degradation because pulmonary perfusion increases toward the end of gestation.[32]

Aortic Isthmus

The isthmus of the aorta (the section of the aortic arch between the take-off of the left subclavian artery and the insertion of the DA) represents a watershed region between the aortic arch, which transmits relatively well oxygenated blood to the head and upper body, and the DA, which transmits relatively deoxygenated blood to the lower body.[33] The isthmus may also represent a functional division between these two arterial circuits, because noradrenaline and acetylcholine injected into either side of the isthmus in the fetal lamb can be demonstrated to affect only that side for at least a few heartbeats.[34] Animal studies have shown that, under physiological conditions, only 10% to 15% of the CCO is transmitted through the isthmus[34] because the majority of blood in the ascending aorta is distributed to the myocardium, head, and upper limbs via the coronary, carotid, and subclavian arteries. One of the most important hemodynamic factors influencing the direction of flow through the isthmus is the relative resistances of the cerebral and placental circulations. If the placental resistance (which is normally very low) increases sufficiently, the two circuits (upper and lower body) can be separated, with blood ejected from the LV perfusing the heart and upper body only, with negligible forward flow (because the placenta is no longer the site of lowest vascular resistance). Meanwhile, the RV perfuses the lower body exclusively. As placental resistance progressively increases, retrograde flow can be detected in the isthmus.[33] Indeed, the isthmus represents an example of the plasticity of the fetal circulation to adapt to varying circumstances. For example, as in cases of reduced left ventricular output, DA blood flows retrograde through the isthmus to supply the AAo and aortic arch.[10]

Pulmonary Trunk and Right-sided Dominance

Experiments in fetal lambs have shown that of the CCO, 60% to 65% is ejected from the RV and 35% to 40% from the LV,[34] while of the blood ejected from the RV, approximately 90% is shunted through the DA, with only approximately 10% (i.e., ~3.5% of CCO) reaching the lungs. The proportion ejected through the branch pulmonary arteries has been demonstrated to increase throughout gestation, almost doubling from the second third of pregnancy to near term.[35]

Studies on human fetuses, using echocardiographic techniques to measure flow volumes, have found a wide variety of values for these ratios. Rasanen and associates[32] found that the proportion of CCO perfusing the lungs in the human fetus at 20 weeks' gestation was 13%, increasing to 25% at 30 weeks, and remaining fairly constant from then on. That study, using echocardiography, found that the ratio of proportion of CCO ejected by each ventricle (RV:LV) was 53:47 at 20 weeks, increasing to a maximum of 60:40 at term—that is, slightly less than the results from animal studies. Conversely, St. John Sutton and coworkers[36] reported a mean pulmonary blood flow that comprised 22% of CCO, with a RV:LV ratio of 52:48, which remained unchanged throughout the second half of gestation. Mielke and Benda[26] reported that the RV:LV ratio was 59:41, the proportion of RV flow reaching the branch PAs was approximately 20%, and the pulmonary flow represented 11% of CCO. None of these values was found to change significantly throughout gestation. Table 1-1 summarizes these results.

Researchers have consistently found that there is a significant right ventricular dominance in human fetuses and that this dominance is less prominent than in animal models.[37] There are a number of plausible explanations; however, the reason for this right-sided dominance in cardiac output is unclear. Rudolph[34] hypothesizes that it is due to the increased afterload faced by the LV. This afterload is caused by the narrowing of the aorta at its isthmus, which causes the cross-sectional area to be reduced by half. Alternatively, the RV preferentially perfuses the placenta, which is an organ in demand of significant flow throughout gestation. These demands upon the RV lead to a particular ventricular geometry, which is abandoned once the RV transitions to the role of a low-pressure pulmonary ventricle after birth.

The reduced right ventricular dominance found in human fetuses relative to animals is suggested to be due to an increased brain volume, which necessitates increased blood flow. The blood flow to the brain is supplied by the LV, which therefore needs to provide a relatively higher proportion of CCO.[38]

Placental Development and Physiology

The placenta, apart from being the site of gaseous and nutrient exchange in the fetomaternal unit, is also of great importance from a cardiovascular perspective. The placenta begins to develop from as early as 6 to 7 days postconception, when the blastocyst first attaches to the uterine epithelium, having hatched from the zona pellucida.[39] The development of the placenta is effected by the formation of successive generations of branching villi, finger-like projections of trophoblast, which extend into the maternal blood surrounding them. This process starts between days 12 and 18 postconception[40] with the appearance of the primary villi. The appearance of connective tissue within the villi marks the transition to secondary villi, and the formation of capillaries within the villous stroma defines the transition to tertiary villi. These represent the first unit capable of providing surface area for the exchange of substances between the fetal and the maternal circulations.[41] Subsequently, the trophoblast undergoes differentiation into two major lineages, the syncytiotrophoblast and the invasive trophoblast. The syncytiotrophoblast is the cell lineage responsible for the fetomaternal transfer of substances and is also the site of the endocrine functions of the placenta.[42,43] The

Table 1-1 Study Data Regarding Percentage Distribution of Blood Flow in the Fetal Circulation

	RUDOLPH AND HEYMANN (ANIMAL STUDIES)[34,35]	ST. JOHN SUTTON ET AL[36]	RASANEN ET AL[32]	MIELKE AND BENDA[26]
Number of subjects	44*	38	63	Various (85-197)
RV/LV	65%	52%	53%*	59%
PBF/CCO	3.7%†	22%	13%*	11%
DA/RV	90%	47%	75.5%‡	78%

*Reference is to study by Rudolph and Heymann,[35] which provides the data on PBF/CCO in animal studies.
†Increases with gestational age.
‡Decreases with gestational age.
CCO, combined cardiac output; DA, ductus arteriosus; LV, left ventricle; PBF = pulmonary blood flow; RV, right ventricle.

invasive trophoblast further differentiates into interstitial and endovascular subtypes. The interstitial invasive trophoblasts are responsible for anchoring the placenta within the uterine wall, and the endovascular invasive trophoblasts invade the maternal spiral arteries, transforming them into distensible, dilated vessels, capable of delivering the increased blood flow that will be required as gestation progresses. Failure of the normal development of the invasive process has been implicated in the etiology of preeclampsia, intrauterine growth retardation, and intrauterine fetal death, although there is some controversy as to which stage of the process is responsible for which condition.[44] Nutrient and gaseous exchange takes place at the level of the chorionic villi, which contain fetal capillary loops and which are bathed in maternal blood, supplied by the spiral arteries and drained by uterine veins. Vascular endothelial growth factor (VEGF) and fibroblast growth factor (FGF) are thought to play crucial roles in promoting placental angiogenesis as well as regulating placental blood flow.[45]

As has been mentioned, the development of an effective placental circulation requires that the spiral arteries transform to low-resistance vessels. Under normal circumstances, the placenta is the site of the lowest resistance in the fetal circulation.[33] Studies of the pulsatility index (PI = difference between the peak systolic velocity and the minimum diastolic velocity, divided by the mean velocity) of the umbilical artery have shown that it falls at the end of the first trimester. This is thought to be due to decreasing placental resistance caused by the increased placental angiogenesis and endovascular invasive trophoblast action occurring at this time.[46] The umbilical artery PI seems to be mainly influenced by the development of trophoblastic villous structures.[47] Similarly, some fetuses with chromosomal abnormalities show increased resistance to blood flow in the umbilical artery during early pregnancy; this has been suggested to be caused by abnormal villous vascularization.[48]

Animal studies have shown that the placental circulation makes up approximately 40% of CCO,[34] whereas noninvasive human studies estimate that the figure is slightly lower at approximately 33% and that this remains constant throughout the majority of gestation.[49] Interestingly, a study using methodology similar to that the sheep studies, performed in exteriorized human fetuses, arrived at a similar figure, approximately 30%.[50]

Variability in placental anatomy and functionality are suspected in congenital heart disease, but this fascinating topic has not been extensively studied. The placenta remains a "black box" with much yet to be learned about its role in programming the cardiovascular state of its developing human partner for the remainder of life, for those with a normal, as well as a malformed heart.

References

1. Kiserud T. Physiology of the fetal circulation. *Semin Fetal Neonatal Med*. 2005;19:493-503.
2. Edelstone DI, Rudolph AM, Heymann MA. Liver and ductus venosus blood flows in fetal lambs in utero. *Circ Res*. 1978;42: 426-433.
3. Rudolph AM, Heymann MA. The circulation of the fetus in utero: methods for studying distribution of blood flow, cardiac output and organ blood flow. *Circ Res*. 1967;21:163-184.
4. Kiserud T, Rasmussen S, Skulstad SM. Blood flow and degree of shunting through the ductus venosus in the human fetus. *Am J Obstet Gynecol*. 2000;182:147-153.
5. Bellotti M, Pennati G, De Gasperi C, Battaglia FC, Ferrazzi E. Role of ductus venosus in distribution of umbilical flow in human fetuses during second half of pregnancy. *Am J Physiol*. 2000;279: 1256-1263.
6. Pennati G, Corno C, Costantino ML, Bellotti M. Umbilical flow distribution to the liver and the ductus venosus in human fetuses during gestation: an anatomy-based mathematical modeling. *Med Eng Phys*. 2003;25:229-238.
7. Edelstone DI, Rudolph AM. Preferential streaming of ductus venosus blood to the brain and heart in fetal lambs. *Am J Physiol*. 1979;237:H724-H729.
8. Schmidt KG, Silverman NH, Rudolph AM. Assessment of flow events at the ductus venosus inferior vena cava junction and at the foramen ovale in fetal sheep by use of multimodal ultrasound. *Circulation*. 1996;93:826-833.
9. Rudolph AM. Circulation in the normal fetus and cardiovascular adaptations to birth. In Yagel S, Silverman NH, Gembruch U, eds. *Fetal Cardiology*. 2nd ed. New York: Informa Healthcare; 2009: 131-152.
10. Kiserud T, Acharya G. The fetal circulation. *Prenat Diagn*. 2004;24: 1049-1059.
11. Fasouliotis SJ, Achiron R, Kivilevitch Z, Yagel S. The human fetal venous system. *J Ultrasound Med*. 2002;21:1145-1158.
12. Meyers RL, Paukick RP, Rudolph CD, Rudolph AM. Cardiovascular responses to acute, severe haemorrhage in fetal sheep. *J Dev Physiol*. 1991;15:189-197.
13. Kiserud T, Ozaki T, Nishina H, Rodeck C, Hanson MA. Effect of NO, phenylephrine, and hypoxemia on ductus venosus diameter in fetal sheep. *Am J Physiol Heart Circ Physiol*. 2000;279:1166-1171.
14. Drose JA. Embryology and physiology of the fetal heart. In Drose JA, ed. *Fetal Echocardiography*. 2nd ed. St. Louis: Elsevier; 2009:1-14.
15. Mavrides E, Moscoso G, Carvalho JS, Campbell S, Thilaganathan B. The human ductus venosus between 13 and 17 weeks of gestation: histological and morphometric studies. *Ultrasound Obstet Gynecol*. 2002;19:39-46
16. Tchirikov M, Kertschanska S, Schröder HJ. Differential effects of catecholamines on vascular rings from ductus venosus and intrahepatic veins of fetal sheep. *J Physiol*. 2003;548:519-526.
17. Kiserud T, Eik-Nes SH, Blaas HG, Hellevik LR. Foramen ovale: an ultrasonographic study of its relation to the inferior vena cava, ductus venosus and hepatic veins. *Ultrasound Obstet Gynecol*. 1992;2: 389-396.
18. Bristow J, Rudolph AM, Itskovitz J, Barnes R. Hepatic oxygen and glucose metabolism in the fetal lamb. Response to hypoxia. *J Clin Invest*. 1983;71:1047-1061.
19. Atkins DL, Clark EB, Marvin, WJ Jr. Foramen ovale/atrial septum area ratio: a marker of transatrial blood flow. *Circulation*. 1982; 66:281-283.
20. Fishman NH, Hof RB, Rudolph AM, Heymann MA. Models of congenital heart disease in fetal lambs. *Circulation*. 1978;58: 354-364.
21. Hornberger LK, Sanders SP, Rein AJJT, Spevak PJ, Parness IA, Colan SD. Left heart obstructive lesions and left ventricular growth in the midtrimester fetus: a longitudinal study. *Circulation*. 1995;92: 1531-1538.
22. Eghtesady P, Michelfelder E, Altaye M, Ballard E, Hirsh R, Beekman RH III. Revisiting animal models of aortic stenosis in the early gestation fetus. *Ann Thorac Surg* 2007;83:631-639.
23. Gruber PJ, Epstein JA. Development gone awry: congenital heart disease. *Circ Res*. 2004;94:273-283.
24. Hove JR, Köster RW, Forouhar AS, Acevedo-Bolton G, Fraser SE, Gharib M. Intracardiac fluid forces are an essential epigenetic factor for embryonic cardiogenesis. *Nature*. 2003;421:172-177 .
25. Huhta JC, Moise KJ, Fisher DJ, Sharif DS, Wasserstrum N, Martin C. Detection and quantitation of constriction of the fetal ductus arteriosus by Doppler echocardiography. *Circulation*. 1987;75: 406-412.

26. Mielke G, Benda N. Cardiac output and central distribution of blood flow in the human fetus. *Circulation*. 2001;103:1662.
27. Clyman RI, Mauray F, Roman C, Rudolph AM. PGE_2 is a more potent vasodilator of the lamb ductus arteriosus than is either PGI_2 or 6 keto PGFα. *Prostaglandins*. 1978;16:259-264.
28. Rasanen J, Wood DC, Debbs RH, Cohen J, Weiner S, Huhta JC.; Reactivity of the human fetal pulmonary circulation to maternal hyperoxygenation increases during the second half of pregnancy: a randomized study. *Circulation*. 1998;97:257-262.
29. Moise KJ, Huhta JC, Sharif DS, et al. Indomethacin in the treatment of premature labor. Effects on the fetal ductus arteriosus. *N Engl J Med*. 1988;319:327-331.
30. Rychik J, Tian Z, Cohen MS, et al. Acute cardiovascular effects of fetal surgery in the human. *Circulation*. 2004;110:1549-1556.
31. Shaw JO, Moser KM. The current status of prostaglandins and the lungs. *Chest*. 1975;68:75-80.
32. Rasanen J, Wood DC, Weiner S, Ludomirski A, Huhta JC. Role of the pulmonary circulation in the distribution of human fetal cardiac output during the second half of pregnancy. *Circulation*. 1996;94:1068-1073.
33. Bonnin P, Fouron JC, Teyssier G, Sonesson SE, Skoll A. Quantitative assessment of circulatory changes in the fetal aortic isthmus during progressive increase of resistance to umbilical blood flow. *Circulation*. 1993;88;216-222.
34. Rudolph AM. Distribution and regulation of blood flow in the fetal and neonatal lamb. *Circ Res*. 1985;57:811-821.
35. Rudolph AM, Heymann MA. Circulatory changes during growth in the fetal lamb. *Circ Res*. 1970;26:289-299.
36. St. John Sutton M, Groves A, MacNeill A, Sharland G, Allan L. Assessment of changes in blood flow through the lungs and foramen ovale in the normal human fetus with gestational age: a prospective Doppler echocardiographic study. *Br Heart J*. 1994;71:232-237.
37. Oberhoffer R, Högel J, Lang D. Normal characteristics of cardiac dimensions and function in the fetus. *Eur J Ultrasound*. 1995;2:93-106.
38. De Smedt MCH, Visser GHA, Meijboom EJ. Fetal cardiac output estimated by Doppler echocardiography during mid- and late gestation. *Am J Cardiol*. 1987;80:338-342.
39. Huppertz B. The anatomy of the normal placenta. *J Clin Pathol*. 2008;61:1296-1302.
40. Castellucci M, Kosanke G, Verdenelli F, et al. Villous sprouting: fundamental mechanisms of human placental development. *Hum Reprod Update*. 2000;6:485-494.
41. Yagel S, Goldman-Wohl DS. Placental implantation and development. In Yagel S, Silverman NH, Gembruch U, eds. *Fetal Cardiology*. 2nd ed. New York: Informa Healthcare; 2009:27-40.
42. Fournet-Dulguerov N, MacLusky NJ, Leranth CZ, et al. Immunohistochemical localization of aromatase cytochrome P-450 and estradiol dehydrogenase in the syncytiotrophoblast of the human placenta. *J Clin Endocrinol Metab*. 1987;65:757-764.
43. Murphy VE, Smith R, Giles WB, Clifton VL. Endocrine regulation of human fetal growth: the role of the mother, placenta, and fetus. *Endocr Rev*. 2006;27:141-169.
44. Huppertz B. Placental origins of preeclampsia challenging the current hypothesis. *Hypertension*. 2008;51:970.
45. Reynolds LP, Redmer DA. Angiogenesis in the placenta. *Biol Reprod*. 2001;64:1033-1040.
46. Matias A, Montenegro N, Areias JC, Leite LP. Haemodynamic evaluation of the first trimester fetus with special emphasis on venous return. *Hum Reprod Update*. 2000;6:177-189.
47. Makikallio K, Jouppila P, Rasanen J. Human fetal cardiac function during the first trimester of pregnancy. *Heart*. 2005;91:334-338.
48. Jauniaux E, Gavrill P, Khun P, Kurdi W, Hyett J, Nicolaides KH. Fetal heart rate and umbilico-placental Doppler flow velocity waveforms in early pregnancies with a chromosomal abnormality and/or an increased nuchal translucency thickness. *Hum Reprod*. 1996;11:435-439.
49. St. John Sutton MG, Plappert T, Doubilet P. Relationship between placental blood flow and combined ventricular output with gestational age in normal human fetus. *Cardiovasc Res*. 1991;25:603-608.
50. Rudolph AM, Heymann MA, Teramo KAW, Barrett CT, Räihä NCR. Studies on the circulation of the previable human fetus. *Pediatr Res*. 1971;5:452.

2

Embryology of the Cardiovascular System

Karl Degenhardt

Congenital heart disease (CHD) can broadly be thought of as what happens when normal heart development goes awry. Although the range of defects may seem endless, there are limitations. Pathologists, cardiologists, and cardiothoracic surgeons have successfully developed systems for the nomenclature, definition, and classification of CHD. Accordingly, the chapters of this book are organized by cardiac lesions. This systematic approach is possible only because there are two significant restraints on what leads to CHD. One is the progression of cardiac development. The heart forms through a sequential series of embryological events. The effects of certain events going wrong will not be observed unless prior events were successfully completed. For example, you cannot have abnormal looping of the heart tube without the tube itself first forming. The second constraint is viability. Defects that are incompatible with intrauterine life do not get the attention of the cardiac surgeon or cardiologist and may provide only cardiac pathologists with topics of academic discussions. As imaging technologies have improved, a greater range of disease has been seen by fetal cardiologists and sonographers. Now, fetal echocardiography may be performed at earlier stages of gestation and can reveal structural defects that would not prove viable later in development. In addition, new insights continue to be made about the progression of CHD during development. This adds increased onus on those diagnosing and treating patients prenatally to understand normal cardiac developmental biology and how the embryological processes may be perturbed. Many key events in cardiac development are complete before imaging can be performed, but advancing technology brings us ever closer to being able to observe these events in patients (Figure 2-1).

Early Cardiogenesis

The earliest steps in the formation of the heart start at the time of gastrulation, which is the formation of the three germ layers—ectoderm, endoderm, and mesoderm. A subset of cells from the mesoderm layer will give rise to the bulk of the heart, and these cells make up the cardiogenic fields. They arise on the two sides of the midline and meet in the middle at the anterior part of the embryo to form the cardiac crescent (Figure 2-2). Recent work has shown that the cardiogenic fields can be subdivided into two groups—the first heart field and the second heart field (sometimes referred to as the *posterior* and *anterior heart fields*), which, in turn, will form the left and right myocardium, respectively. Thus, before the ventricles

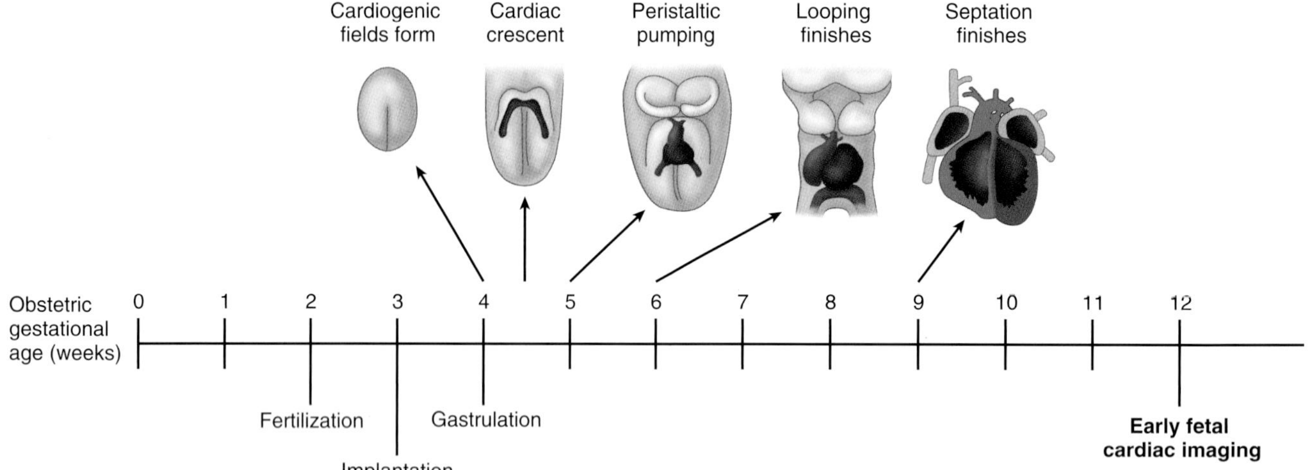

Figure 2-1. Approximate timeline of events in cardiac development relative to gestational age. Note that fetal echocardiography is possible shortly after ventricular and outflow tract septation is complete.

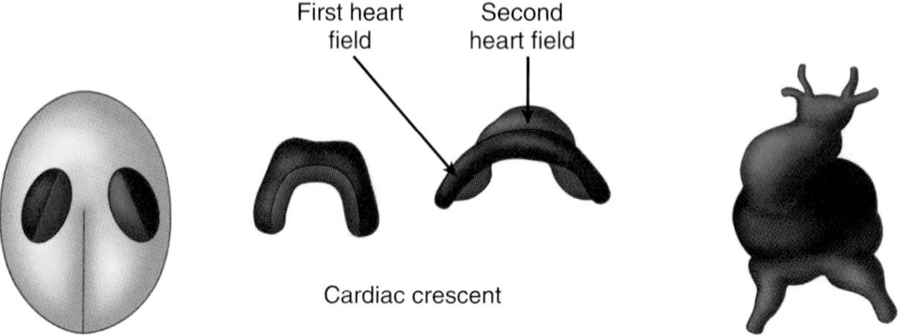

Figure 2-2. Shortly after gastrulation, the cardiogenic fields are specified including the first *(red)* and second *(blue)* heart fields. They form separate parts of the cardiac crescent and give rise to the left ventricle (first heart field) and right ventricle and outflow tract (second heart field).

themselves form, there is already a molecular basis for differences between the right and the left ventricular myocardium. The two sides of the cardiac crescent fuse along the midline to form the primitive heart tube. The primitive heart tube can itself be subdivided into regions along the caudal to rostral axis: sinus venosus, primitive atria, primitive ventricle, bulbus cordis (conus), and truncus arteriosus. The primitive heart tube begins to contract in a peristaltic manner at approximately 5 weeks' gestation.

Cardiac Looping

As the primitive heart tube develops, it folds on itself and twists in a process called *looping* (Figure 2-3). The mechanism that underlies this process continues to be debated, but one recent hypothesis that has gained favor is that looping results from differential ballooning out of the chambers, rather than rotational movement of the cells. Normally, the looping occurs to the right and results in a D-looped heart. In some cases of CHD, looping may occur to the left (L-looped). The process of looping is the first visible sign of left-right asymmetry apparent in the developing embryo, although genes involved in this process have been shown to be differentially expressed before this process occurs. Looping sets up the relationship between the inflow tract, the outflow tract, and the ventricular septum of the right ventricle, which is important in the nomenclature of CHD.

Septation

In mammals and birds, the pulmonary and systemic circulations are separate; they are in series with one another in adults. In order for this to occur, the atria, atrioventricular (AV) valves, the ventricles, and the outflow tract must be divided during development.

Atrial and Canal Septation

Because atrial and canal septation are linked, they are discussed together. The atria are the first structures to begin to septate, and the last to finish, with the foramen ovale not closing under normal conditions until after birth (and then remaining probe patent for some time). At the beginning of the sixth week of gestation, the pulmonary venous confluence (see later) evaginates into the roof of the embryonic atrium between the two growing atrial appendages (Figure 2-4). Cranial to this, the septum primum (primary atrial septum) forms as a muscular septum in the shape of a crescent. It grows from the dorsal wall of the atrium toward the AV canal. It has been described as completely dividing the atria first (hence, *primum*) and then later becoming perforated to form the foramen ovale. However, it likely never fully closes, because blood needs to flow from the right atrium to the left throughout development. The septum secundum arises along the rim of the pulmonary vein as a structure called the *dorsal mesenchymal protusion* (also called the *atrial spine, spina vestibule,* or *vestibular spine*). It has been

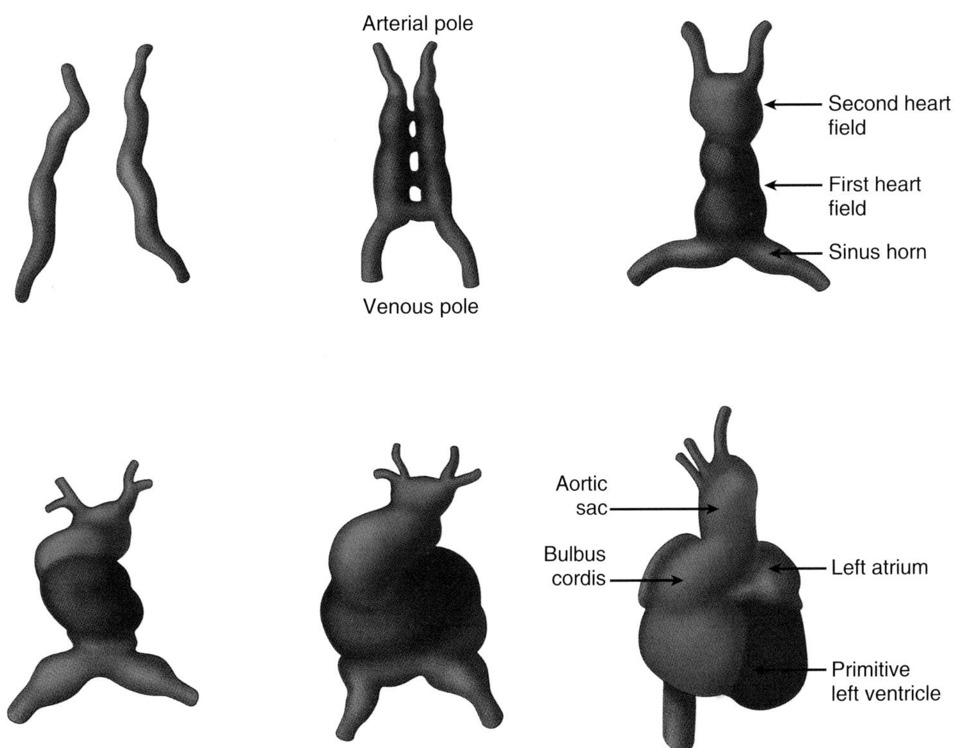

Figure 2-3. Fusion of the heart tubes and looping. Cells from either side of the midline begin to form tubes, which fuse together. The arterial pole is anterior, and the venous pole is posterior. During looping, the arterial pole comes anterior and somewhat rightward as the chambers balloon out.

appreciated that this consists of both atrial cells as well as "extracardiac mesenchyme" that migrates in from the dorsal attachment of the heart to the body. The septum secundum contributes to the division of the AV valve to allow formation of separate tricuspid and mitral valves. Defects in the formation of the dorsal mesenchymal protrusion lead to the formation of a common AV canal in the most extreme cases and to an atrial septal defect in more mild cases. Confusingly, defects in the septum secundum result in "primum" atrial septal defects.

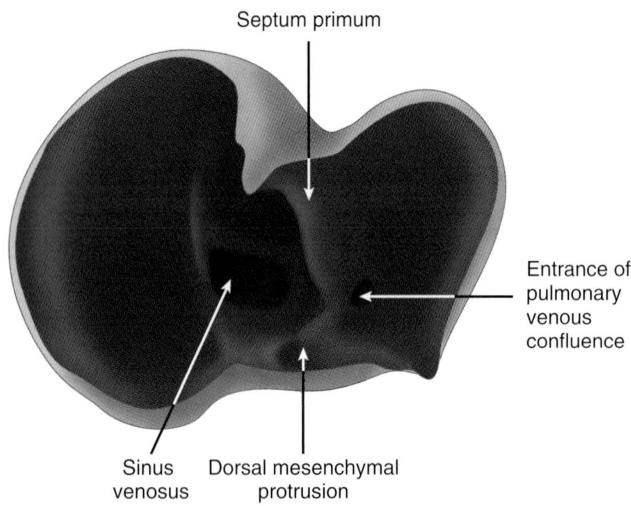

Figure 2-4. Ventral view of the atria during the initial stages of septation.

Conversely, defects of the septum primum are called "secundum" atrial septal defects. The thin, membranous septum primum forms to the left of the more muscular septum secundum and functions as a flap valve allowing right-to-left flow. Postnatally, when the pressure in the left atrium becomes higher than that of the right, the flap closes the foramen ovale to complete the septation of the atria.

Ventricular Septation

Following normal looping, the primitive right and left ventricles are positioned relatively rightward and leftward to each other (Figure 2-5). It is important to remember that they are not at the same level in the anteroposterior plane. The primitive right ventricle is more anterior. The flow of blood comes into the left ventricle, then goes across the bulboventricular foramen to the right ventricle and out the as-yet-undivided outflow tract. As development progresses, inflow becomes more directed toward both ventricles. (Failure of this process can result in a double-inflow left ventricle [DILV]—a situation much more common than double-inflow right ventricle). The ventricular septum begins to grow toward the AV canal and outflow tract from the apical and inferior portion of the junction between the primitive right and left ventricle. This forms the muscular part of the interventricular septum. Incomplete growth during this stage can result in muscular septal defects. Septation of the ventricle is complete when the muscular septum meets the canal septum between the AV valves and the conal septum just

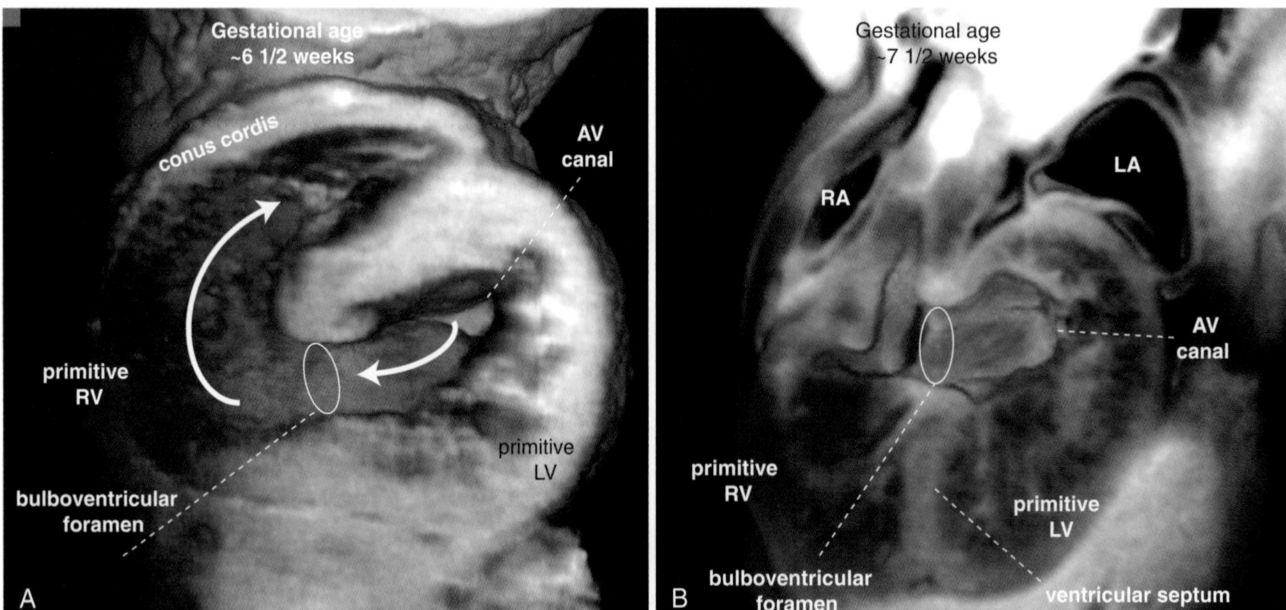

Figure 2-5. Three-dimensional volume-rendered images of human embryonic hearts. **(A)** Frontal view of a normal (D-loop) heart shows that the atrioventricular (AV) canal is initially aligned over the primitive left ventricle (LV). Blood flows (shown by the *arrows*) from the forming atria through the AV canal to the LV. The blood then leaves the LV via the bulboventricular foramen to the primitive right ventricle (RV). The blood then goes through the conus cordis to the truncus arteriosus (not in the plane of this picture). **(B)** After another week further in development, the AV canal (highlighted in *yellow*) is aligned over both ventricles and the ventricular septum is forming. The outflow tract is not fully septated at this point. (**A** and **B**, Based on EFIC data from the online Human Embryo Atlas: Dhanantwari P, Lee E, Krishnan A, et al. Human cardiac development in the first trimester: a high-resolution magnetic resonance imaging and episcopic fluorescence image capture atlas. *Circulation.* 2009;120:343-351.)

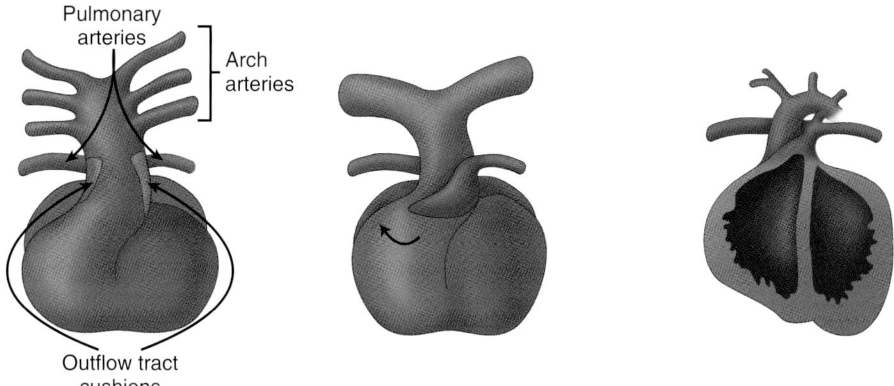

Figure 2-6. Prongs of neural crest cells migrate into the truncus to separate the pulmonary and aortic arteries. Rotation of the outflow tract myocardium plays a key role in proper ventriculoarterial alignment as septation progresses.

below the now separate outflow tracts. If the canal septum has not formed properly, a canal type ventricular septal defect may be left. Similarly, if the conal septum forms to far anterior or posterior, the muscular septum may not fuse with the conal septum, causing a septal malalignment defect. Finally, if the conal septum forms normally but there is incomplete fusion between it and the muscular septum, a conoventricular defect results. In the area at which these structures meet, there is the thinner membranous septum.

Outflow Tract Septation

Critical to the separation of the pulmonary and systemic circulation are a population of cells known as the *cardiac neural crest*. These cells migrate from the dorsal neural tube and surround the forming pharyngeal arch arteries (where they also play a critical role in the remodeling of the arch). Two prongs of neural crest cells continue to migrate toward the outflow tract on opposite sides of the truncus (Figure 2-6). The junction between the fourth arch artery (forming the pulmonary artery) and the sixth arch arteries grows into the truncus, following the prongs of neural crest cells to divide the arteries. Coincident with this septation is the rotation of the outflow tract, which may contribute to the apparent spiraling of the truncus. Interference with the neural crest results in truncus arteriosus in a number of animal models. Indeed, disruption of the gene *Tbx1* leads to defects in neural crest migration in a mouse model of DiGeorge's syndrome with conotruncal defects. In addition, failure of the rotation of the outflow tract has been implicated as contributing to transposition of the great arteries and double-outlet right ventricle.

Arch Artery Formation and Maturation

The arch arteries are initially formed as a set of bilateral, paired vessels in the pharyngeal (or branchial) arches arising from the aortic sac. In the early embryo, they resemble the gill arteries of a fish. The pharyngeal arch arteries surround the forming trachea and esophagus and connect to paired dorsal aortas (Figure 2-7). During normal development, specific vessels regress while others persist. Failure of this regression can lead to vascular rings, a right-sided arch and other vascular anomalies. For instance, normally, the left fourth arch artery persists and the right fourth arch artery regresses, leaving behind the left-sided aortic arch. Similarly, when the right fourth arch persists, and the left regresses, a right-sided aortic arch results. If neither fourth arch artery regresses, there will be a double aortic arch, which forms a ring around the trachea and esophagus. Conversely, if both regress, an interrupted aortic arch results. The ductus arteriosus arises from the sixth arch artery, and it too undergoes unilateral regression normally, leaving behind the left-sided ductus. Additional combinations of failed regression exist that result in encircling of the trachea and esophagus—in particular, persistence of the origin of the right subclavian from the right dorsal aorta. Knowledge of the anatomy of the arch artery primordia allows for understanding of the various arch abnormalities that are possible.

Venous Development

Similar to the development of the arch arteries, the systemic venous return to the heart begins with a number of paired, evolutionarily conserved structures that undergo patterned, asymmetrical regression to leave behind the normal connections to the heart (Figure 2-8). The head region of the embryo drains to the heart through the anterior cardinal veins, which connect to a common cardinal vein. In humans, a connecting vessel (the thymicothyroid anastamosis) must form between the anterior cardinal veins to allow the regression the left anterior cardinal vein. This bridging vein becomes the innominate vein and allows drainage from both the left and the right through the right anterior cardinal vein, which becomes the right superior vena cava. Failure of this bridging vein to form results in bilateral superior venae cavae. The posterior drainage from the embryo is through three sets of paired structures into the sinus venous, a part of the developing atria. The blood returns from the placenta via

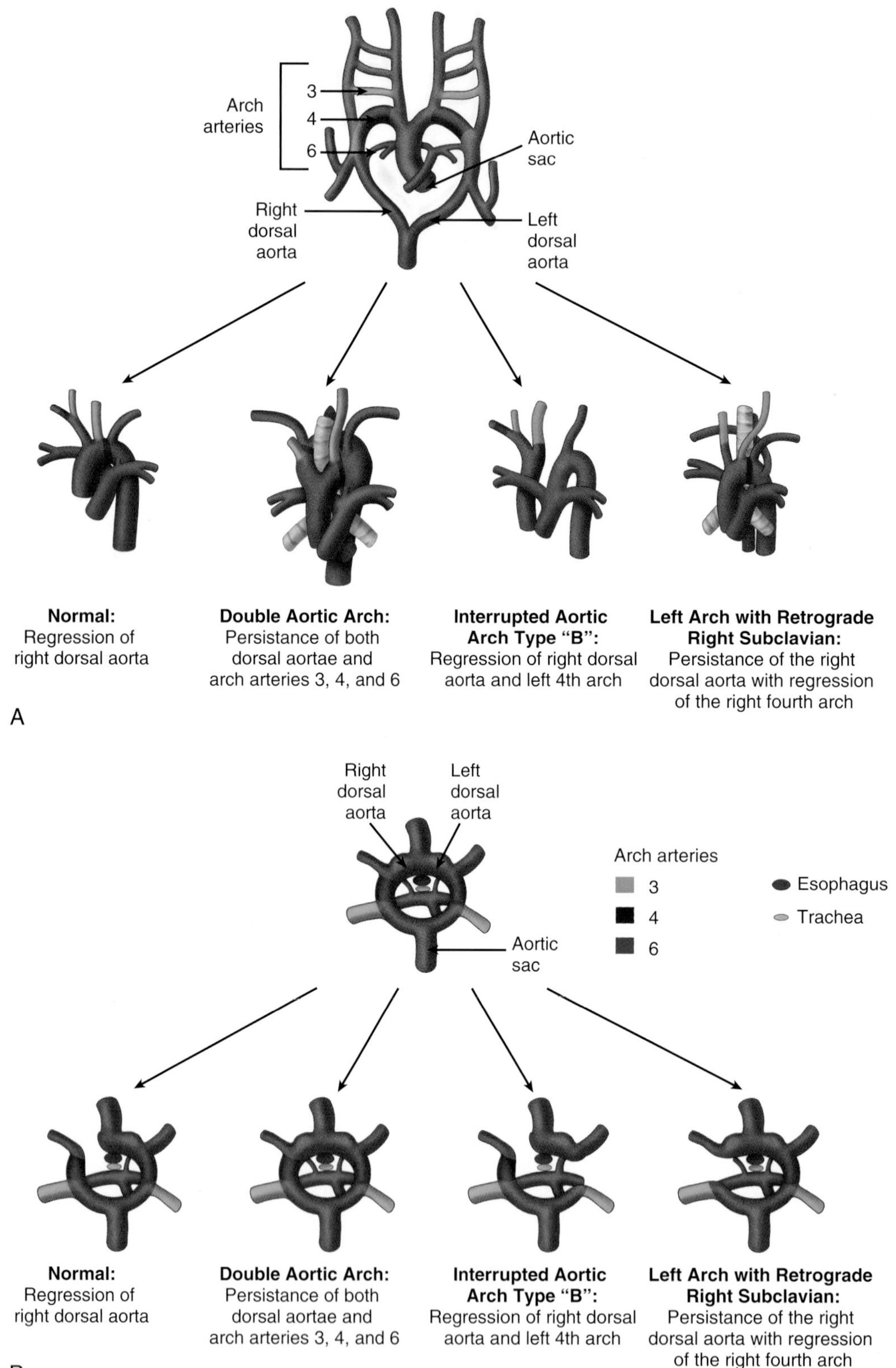

Figure 2-7. The aortic sac initially connects to the paired dorsal aortas through a series of paired arch arteries. Regression of specific arch arteries results in the normal left arch or common arch anomalies as illustrated. In **A**, the vascular remodeling is shown as viewed from the anterior perspective. **B** shows the same processes in a more schematized diagram (sometimes called the "totipotent arch"), as viewed from the cranial perspective. The color code of the structures is the same in both **A** and **B**.

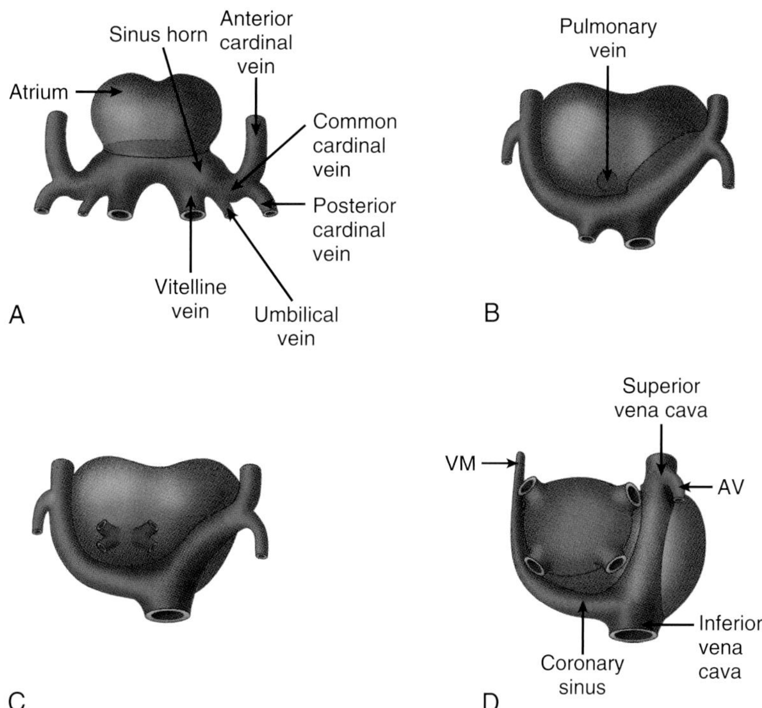

Figure 2-8. Posterior views of the atria show the relationship between the developing systemic and pulmonary veins (**A** to **D** show earlier to later points in development respectively). The anterior and posterior cardinal veins come together to form the common cardinal vein, which drains into the sinus horn. The umbilical vein and vitelline vein also enter the sinus horn. The sinus horn drainage becomes right-sided and the left umbilical vein and vitelline vein regress, leaving the coronary sinus. The pulmonary vein enters the atria to the left of the septum primum initially as a single vessel. As this vessel becomes progressively incorporated into the back wall of the atria, four pulmonary veins come to have separate entrances. AV, azygous vein; VM, vein of Marshall.

the umbilical veins, which course through the liver as the ductus venosus. Early on, the left side regresses, leaving a single umbilical vein that returns oxygenated blood to the right atrium. When the umbilical cord is clamped, the ductus venosus constricts, like the ductus arteriosus, leaving behind the ligamentum venosus. The embryonic liver and yolk sac drain to the heart via the vitelline veins, and the rest of the posterior embryo proper drains via the posterior cardinal veins to the common cardinal vein. Normally, the left side of each of these paired structures regresses. The right vitelline vein becomes the hepatic segment of the inferior vena cava. Failure of this structure to merge with the posterior cardinal vein results in interruption of the inferior vena cava with the azygous vein becoming the avenue of return for the inferior part of the body. This structure runs posteriorly, connecting to the superior vena cava in the chest. In this situation, the liver drains separately into the right atrium.

The anlage of the pulmonary vein exists from the earliest time in heart looping as the "midpharyngeal endothelial strand," which is connected to the back wall of the common atrium. With the formation of the lungs, the midpharyngeal endothelial strand lumenizes to form the common pulmonary vein. Septation of the atria must occur to the right of its entrance in order for the pulmonary veins to drain to the left atrium. Thus, abnormal atrial septation can lead to anomalous pulmonary return. The common pulmonary vein is subsequently incorporated into the atrium, forming the bulk of the posterior left atrial wall. Only after this has occurred can the four individual veins be seen to have separate entrances into the atrium. If the common pulmonary vein does not develop properly, other connections between the pulmonary vasculature and the systemic veins will form and/or persist, resulting in anomalous pulmonary venous connections with total anomalous venous return. Partial anomalous venous return occurs when one or more of the individual pulmonary veins do not connect to the common pulmonary vein but, rather, make separate connections to systemic venous structures.

Later Cardiovascular Development

The developmental processes described above are generally completed by the 8th week after conception (10th week of gestation), and the fetal circulatory pattern that is established persists until birth. However, continued growth and development of the structures depends on maintenance of normal physiology. For instance, as in the postnatal heart, the myocardial wall thickness depends on the force that the ventricle generates. Similarly, the volume load, or flow, through various structures will greatly influence the size of chambers, valves, and vessels. This is a familiar concept to pediatric cardiologists because they monitor growth of structures in patients with CHD and abnormal physiology. The effects of altered flow, however, are much more dramatic in the embryo, because most structures must increase many times their size in the 30 weeks between the establishment of the structures and birth. Indeed, models of CHD have been established by surgical alterations of circulation in the fetal lamb. Such experiments have shown that disruption of blood flow leads to hypoplasia and/or atresia of downstream structures. This concept is sometimes referred to as "no flow, no grow."

For a number of reasons, the fetal cardiologist must bear in mind the potential for growth of a structure in response to the flow through it. First, it must be remembered that a small abnormality early in cardiac development will lead to dramatic, and to some degree, predictable defects in cardiovascular structure. For instance, aortic stenosis may lead to aortic arch hypoplasia, coarctation, and in some cases, hypoplastic left heart syndrome. Second, despite normal early cardiac development, structural defects can develop in a fetus with the abnormal physiology that can arise in twin-twin transfusion syndrome. Finally, as our collective experience with fetal echocardiography has grown, we have been able to witness the progression of heart disease through development. As we better understand this new aspect of the natural history of CHD, the opportunities to intervene in utero to improve outcomes and possibly prevent disease have arisen. Early successes have been seen in treatment of twin-twin transfusion and hypoplastic left heart syndrome. In the latter, therapy is directed toward relief of aortic obstruction, thus allowing improved flow through the left ventricle and aortic arch, which in turn, lessens the degree of hypoplasia of the left-sided structures. The high risk of such procedures, as well as our relative inability to predict the progression of disease, limits the utility of in utero interventions at this time. However, with improvements in techniques and the identification of better echocardiographic predictors of heart disease, fetal interventions will likely increase in their efficacy and will be performed with greater frequency.

Suggested Readings

Anderson RH, Baker EJ, Redington A, Rigby ML, Penny D, Wernovsky G. *Paediatric Cardiology*. 3rd ed. Edinburgh: Churchill Livingstone; 2009.

Anderson RH, Brown NA, Moorman AF. Development and structures of the venous pole of the heart. *Dev Dyn*. 2006;235:2-9.

Anderson RH, Brown NA, Webb S. Development and structure of the atrial septum. *Heart*. 2002;88:104-110.

Bajolle F, Zaffran S, Kelly RG, et al. Rotation of the myocardial wall of the outflow tract is implicated in the normal positioning of the great arteries. *Circ Res*. 2006;98:421-428.

Bajolle F, Zaffran S, Meilhac SM, et al. Myocardium at the base of the aorta and pulmonary trunk is prefigured in the outflow tract of the heart and in subdomains of the second heart field. *Dev Biol*. 2008;313:25-34.

Christoffels VM, Mommersteeg MT, Trowe MO, et al. Formation of the venous pole of the heart from an Nkx2-5-negative precursor population requires Tbx18. *Circ Res*. 2006;98:1555-1563.

Dhanantwari P, Lee E, Krishnan A, et al. Human cardiac development in the first trimester: a high-resolution magnetic resonance imaging and episcopic fluorescence image capture atlas. *Circulation*. 2009; 120:343-351.

Gruber PJ, Epstein JA. Development gone awry: congenital heart disease. *Circ Res*. 2004;94:273-283.

Hurst JW, O'Rourke RA, Walsh RA, Fuster V. *Hurst's the Heart Manual of Cardiology*. New York: McGraw-Hill Medical; 2009.

Kelly RG, Buckingham ME. The anterior heart-forming field: voyage to the arterial pole of the heart. *Trends Genet*. 2002;18:210-216.

Kirby ML. *Cardiac development*. Oxford and New York: Oxford University Press; 2007.

Moorman AF, Christoffels VM. Cardiac chamber formation: development, genes, and evolution. *Physiol Rev*. 2003;83:1223-1267.

Moss AJ, Allen HD. *Moss and Adams' Heart Disease in Infants, Children, and Adolescents: Including the Fetus and Young Adult*. Philadelphia: Lippincott Williams & Wilkins; 2008.

Sadler TW, Langman J. *Langman's Medical Embryology*. Baltimore and Philadelphia: Lippincott Williams & Wilkins; 2006.

Srivastava D. Making or breaking the heart: from lineage determination to morphogenesis. *Cell*. 2006;126:1037-1048.

Stoller JZ, Epstein JA. Cardiac neural crest. *Semin Cell Dev Biol*. 2005; 16:704-715.

Webb S, Brown NA, Wessels A, Anderson RH. Development of the murine pulmonary vein and its relationship to the embryonic venous sinus. *Anat Rec*. 1998;250:325-334.

Webb S, Brown NA, Anderson RH. Formation of the atrioventricular septal structures in the normal mouse. *Circ Res*. 1998;82:645-656.

Webb S, Kanani M, Anderson RH, Richardson MK, Brown NA. Development of the human pulmonary vein and its incorporation in the morphologically left atrium. *Cardiol Young*. 2001;11:632-642.

Zaffran S, Kelly RG, Meilhac SM, Buckingham ME, Brown NA. Right ventricular myocardium derives from the anterior heart field. *Circ Res*. 2004;95:261-268.

3

The Fetal Cardiovascular Examination

Jack Rychik

Ultrasound assessment of the fetal cardiovascular system is a challenging but very rewarding process. Although the term *fetal echocardiography* may imply assessment of the fetal heart alone, much information is to be gleamed from a comprehensive look at vascular structures outside of the heart. Hence, in this chapter, the term *fetal echocardiography* refers to a comprehensive ultrasound assessment of the fetal cardiovascular system. Technical advances and operator skill have improved substantially with an explosion of new knowledge gained in this field. Fetal cardiovascular ultrasonic imaging is currently an excellent means to detect and understand congenital structural defects and complex diseases and observe the course of normal or abnormal human cardiovascular development throughout gestation. As such, it has contributed greatly to the burgeoning field of care and treatment for the human before birth.

How does one wield this powerful tool? In this chapter, we review the current modalities of fetal echocardiography, discuss the conceptual approach to imaging, review the tools used to evaluate functional aspects of the fetal heart and key vascular structures, and discuss the timing of fetal cardiovascular imaging.

What Is Needed, Indications, and Modalities of Fetal Echocardiography

In order to perform fetal echocardiography, a number of technical items, system processes, and knowledge-based skills are required (Box 3-1). Dedicated equipment with an appropriate imaging system and transducers is necessary. Curvilinear transducer probes are optimal in order to provide a wide range of view; however, conventional pediatric imaging probes may be adopted as well. Because the heart is a moving structure, image acquisition must be made over the passage of time. Frame rates of 80 to 100 Hz are frequently needed to view important events occurring at heart rates in excess of 140 bpm. Cardiac structures should be evaluated as they move through the cardiac cycle as well as over multiple cardiac cycles. Still-frame image assessment is appropriate for static structures such as the fetal brain or abdomen, but it is not appropriate when assessing the fetal cardiovascular system. The capacity for cine loop or video review of image change over time is necessary. The capacity for Doppler evaluation of blood flow through pulsed wave techniques as well as color flow imaging is important. Capture and storage of cine loops or video images for analysis and review is essential and can ideally be achieved through digital means, with many good systems currently on the market.

A number of excellent ultrasound systems are commercially available on the market today. Vendors have responded to input from the medical community, leading

Box 3-1 Requirements Necessary to Perform Fetal Echocardiography

Technical and Programmatic Requirements

- Dedicated ultrasound system outfitted for fetal cardiovascular imaging.
- Appropriate transducer probes, preferably curvilinear at frequency range 5-8 MHz.
- Equipment that allows the capacity to assess cardiac motion over time (still frame assessment is not sufficient).
- Capacity for Doppler echocardiography (pulsed wave and color flow imaging).
- Record and store system for cine loops or video.
- Dedicated sonographer and physician group with specialized knowledge base and skills.
- Quality assurance system with regular meetings in place to review imaging and interpretation skills.

Knowledge-based Requirements

- Be able to recognize the full spectrum of simple and complex, acquired and congenital, heart disease and its manifestations throughout gestation.
- Have the skill and ability to apply all modalities of echocardiography including two-dimensional, M-mode, pulsed wave, continuous wave, and Doppler color flow mapping imaging in recognizing and evaluating both the normal and the abnormal fetal cardiovascular state.
- Have knowledge of the anatomy and physiology of the developing cardiovascular system throughout the stages of human development.
- Have a thorough understanding of the spectrum of fetal arrhythmias and the ability to utilize the spectrum of echocardiographic modalities for their assessment.
- Be knowledgeable in the principles of biological ultrasound instrumentation and its application in human pregnancy.
- Have a thorough understanding of maternal-fetal physiology as well as maternal diseases that may affect the developing fetus.
- Be familiar with the latest developments in obstetrical diagnostics, which include invasive and noninvasive tests available throughout pregnancy.
- Have knowledge of the growing field of invasive fetal intervention and its possible effects on the fetal cardiovascular system.

to the evolution of a series of systems that provide superb quality imaging. One of the challenges has been optimizing a system for the hybrid needs of the fetal cardiovascular imager. System production has developed into two camps—those dedicated specifically to (1) cardiological assessment primarily targeted toward the adult and child and (2) general body radiological or obstetrical imaging. The needs of the fetal echocardiographer are a combination of these two systems—hardware and software technology that focuses on optimizing obstetrical targets at a distance from the transducer, but yet provides for high frame rates necessary for cardiovascular assessment. Today, these goals can be met by the purchase of an obstetrical ultrasound system outfitted specifically for fetal cardiovascular assessment or a cardiology system outfitted for obstetrical scanning.

Fetal echocardiography is typically performed using ultrasound at frequencies ranging from 4 to 8 MHz. Lower frequencies provide for greater tissue penetration, however, at lower resolution, whereas higher frequencies provide greater resolution but have greater dissipation of energy as the ultrasound beam travels through tissue. Furthermore, lower frequencies provide for optimal Doppler echocardiography and color flow imaging. The 4- to 8-MHz range of frequency used in fetal echocardiography provides for an appropriate balance between ultrasound tissue propagation and image resolution.

In addition to specialized equipment, dedicated operator skills are necessary. Sonographers and physicians who perform fetal echocardiography should be trained specifically to undertake this task. The operator skills necessary are above and beyond those required for pediatric echocardiography or obstetrical imaging alone. Guidelines have been developed by various societies and professional organizations. Fetal echocardiography is of interest to both pediatric cardiologists and maternal-fetal medicine and perinatology specialists and can be performed by highly qualified and skilled professionals from either field. Maintenance of knowledge and specialized skills is required through continuing medical education efforts in order to keep up with rapid developments in the field. The knowledge base to perform fetal echocardiography must include not only information on how to image and diagnose but also a basic understanding of the physiological implications of fetal cardiovascular disease and its impact on the pregnancy. A regular quality assurance system should be in place in order to review image quality and interpretation accuracy. Review sessions are of most benefit if held in a multidisciplinary manner with experts in obstetrical care, maternal-fetal medicine, imaging, and pediatric cardiology in attendance. If counseling is to be performed, additional skills and knowledge are necessary—in particular, knowledge concerning the most recent management strategies, medical or surgical treatments, and outcomes for the disease at hand.

Table 3-1 Maternal and Fetal Indications for Fetal Echocardiography

MATERNAL INDICATIONS	FETAL INDICATIONS
Family history of CHD	Abnormal obstetrical ultrasound screen
Metabolic disorders (e.g., diabetes, phenylketonuria)	Extracardiac abnormality
Exposure to teratogens	Chromosomal or genetic abnormality
Exposure to prostaglandin synthetase inhibitors (e.g., ibuprofen, salicylic acid)	Irregular heart rhythm
Rubella infection	Hydrops
Autoimmune disease (e.g., Sjögren's syndrome, systemic lupus erythematosus)	Increased first-trimester nuchal translucency
Familial inherited disorders (Ellis van Creveld, Marfan's syndrome, Noonan's syndrome)	Multiple gestation and suspicion of twin-twin transfusion syndrome
In vitro fertilization	

CHD, congenital heart disease.

Indications for Fetal Echocardiography

Most forms of fetal congenital heart disease occur in mothers who have no specific identifiable risk factors. Nevertheless, several maternal risk factors as well as fetal risk factors are considered indications for a high-level evaluation of the cardiovascular system through fetal echocardiography (Table 3-1). No doubt, additional risk factors and markers will emerge in the future as work toward understanding the basis for congenital heart disease and its genetic origins continues to progress.

Modalities of Fetal Echocardiography

Ultrasound energy can be transmitted through biological tissue with a wealth of information provided utilizing a variety of different echocardiographic modalities.

Two-dimensional Imaging

Two-dimensional tomographic cuts through structures are displayed in real time. This is the primary modality of fetal echocardiography and allows for identification of fine structures in motion. Myocardial and valvar tissues can be analyzed, dimensions assessed, and their functional aspects evaluated. Through a series of high-resolution two-dimensional sweeps and views, a mental reconstruction of three-dimensional of anatomy takes place.

In general, many factors influence two-dimensional image resolution; however, it is important to recall an essential principle: an ultrasonic beam cannot resolve between two structures in space that are less than the distance of a wavelength of the frequency applied. The relationship between wavelength and frequency is defined as follows: c = f × w, where c = speed of ultrasound in biological tissue, which is 1540 m/sec; f = frequency in cycles/sec (Hz); and w = wavelength. If, for example, one were to apply a frequency of 5 MHz (5,000,000 cycles/sec) in looking at a structure, the wavelength through biological tissue would be 1,540,000 mm/sec divided by 5,000,000 cycles/sec, which is equal to 0.3 mm. Hence, this ultrasound beam would not be able to distinguish structures that are less than 0.3 mm apart from each other, a fundamental limitation based on the ultrasound physics. This is important because operators need to keep in mind the frequency used when very small structures are measured in early gestation, structures that may be only a few millimeters in size.

Two-dimensional resolution is both temporal and spatial. In order to capture events that are occurring over very brief periods of time, rapid sampling and image creation, or fast frame rates, improve temporal resolution. Frame rates are optimized when assessing structures as close as possible to the transducer and when the region of interest is limited in scope. Hence, maneuvering the patient and probe to bring the fetus as close as possible to the transducer is important, as is keeping the sector of imaging limited and focused only on the structures of interest. As the ultrasound beam penetrates tissues, it will best assess structures that are in line with the beam and not lateral to it. Hence, *axial resolution*, the imaging of structures parallel to the axis of the ultrasound beam, is superior to *radial resolution*, the imaging of structures that are perpendicular or horizontal to the beam. This principle becomes important when attempting to visualize and measure structures such as the left ventricular outflow tract or the size of a ventricular septal defect. Positioning the structures such that they lie parallel to the beam of ultrasound will improve the accuracy of assessment.

DOPPLER PRINCIPLE

Frequency shift (Fs) = 2 Fi V Cos X/c

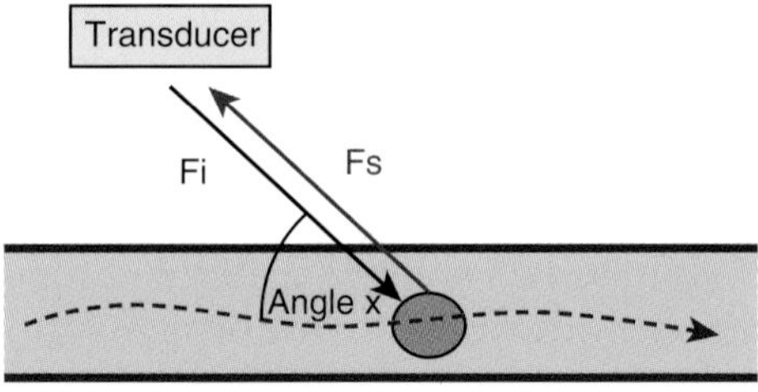

Figure 3-1. The Doppler principle states that the frequency of ultrasound energy (frequency shift [Fs]) reflected by moving blood is related to the initial frequency emitted (Fi) and the velocity of the moving blood and inversely related to the speed of ultrasound in biological tissue.

Doppler Echocardiography

Application of the Doppler principle allows for assessment of *velocity* and *direction* of blood flow through the heart and vasculature (Figure 3-1). Transmission of ultrasound at a set known frequency can be directed at a moving target such as blood moving through a vessel. The reflected ultrasound energy will have a different frequency (frequency shift) based on the angle of insonation and the velocity of movement of the blood. Utilizing this relationship, the velocity of blood movement can be identified. Pulsed wave Doppler echocardiography is the process in which packets of ultrasound energy are emitted into a biological field, with transducer piezoelectric crystals alternatively firing and "listening" for a reflective acoustic response. This technique allows for the determination of blood flow *direction* as well as *velocity*; however, it is limited in its ability to assess relatively high velocities at a distance from the transducer. Continuous wave Doppler echocardiography is the process in which some piezoelectric crystals are continuously firing sound energy and others are continuously listening. This technique allows for assessment of high velocities at a distance, but one loses the capacity to identify position and location because all velocities within the line of firing will be measured. For purposes of fetal echocardiography, pulsed wave Doppler is most commonly used because velocities are generally low. A region of interest or *gate* is placed within a cavity or vessel and velocity information is obtained. However, if a high velocity is noted, one may need to switch to continuous wave Doppler to complete the analysis.

Doppler velocity information is portrayed in a "spectral" manner, with velocity displayed on the y axis and time on the x axis. This provides for a means of assessing the behavior of blood flow within a set region over a cardiac cycle. Normal anticipated patterns of flow have been described for the various structures of the heart and vasculature. Blood flow within a region can be *laminar*, in which case, blood cells are all moving at the relative same velocity at any one point in time within the cardiac cycle. Laminar flow suggests a normal pattern with no disturbance of blood velocities and is portrayed as a smooth curve on spectral Doppler display. Alternatively, blood flow can be *turbulent*, in which case, the blood cells within a region of interest are moving at different velocities at any one given point in time. Turbulence occurs when there is a disturbance in blood flow such as in the presence of a valvar stenosis or vascular narrowing. This is portrayed as a filled-in curve on the spectral Doppler display, with varying velocities plotted at any one point in time (Figure 3-2).

Velocity information is of value for a variety of reasons. First, normal velocities of flow through fetal cardiovascular structures are described; hence, velocity measurements noted to be out of the normal range provide insight into a disease state. Second, velocity information can be converted into pressure data. The Bernoulli principle describes the relationship between velocity and pressure differences across a region of interest (Figure 3-3). This principle is of clinical use in many settings. For example, it allows for

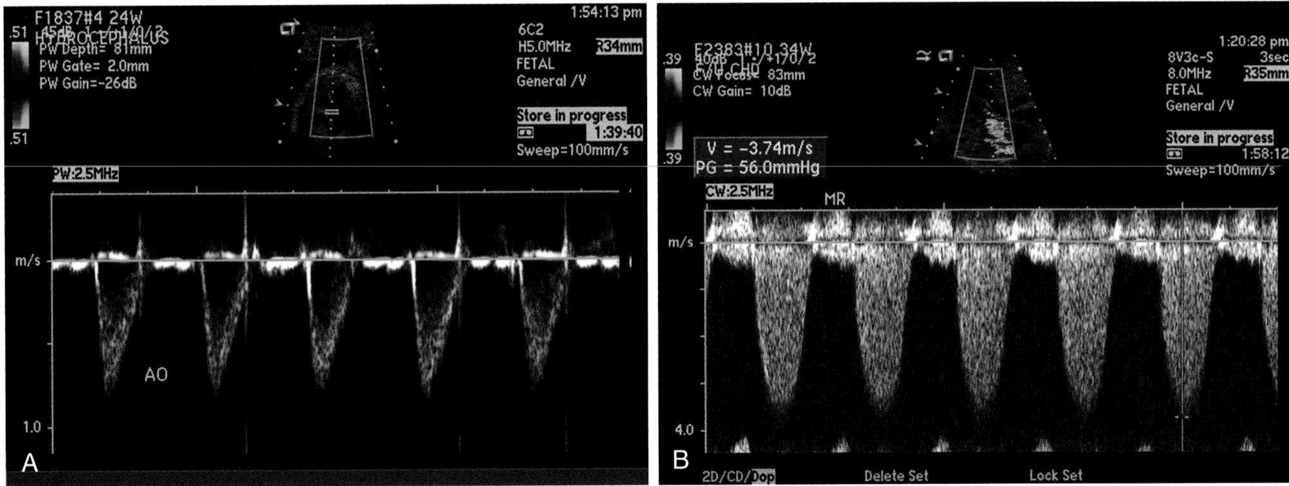

Figure 3-2. (**A**) Spectral Doppler display of laminar blood flow. Note the central clearing of the waveform, which implies that the blood cells in the region of interest are moving at a common velocity at any one point of time in the cardiac cycle. AO, aorta. (**B**) Spectral Doppler display of turbulent blood flow with an elevated peak velocity. Note that the waveform appearance is filled in, suggesting that at any one time point in systole, blood cells in the region of interrogation are moving at various velocities—some at low velocity, and some at high velocity. This is consistent with a stenosis and disturbance of blood flow. MR, mitral regurgitation.

BERNOULLI'S PRINCIPLE

$$P_1 - P_2 = 4x\,(V_2^2 - V_1^2)$$

if $V_1 < 1$ meter/sec, then

Change in pressure = 4x $Vmax^2$

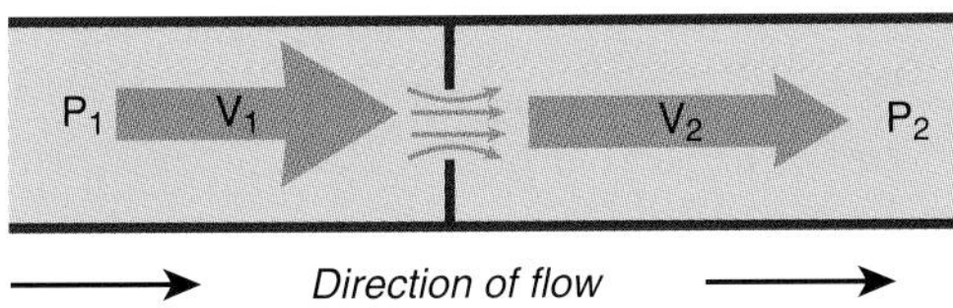

Direction of flow

Figure 3-3. The Bernoulli principle describes the relationship between the pressure (P) drop across an area of stenosis and the difference in velocity (V) of blood flow across the stenosis. The pressure drop is equal to four times the peak velocity (Vmax) squared across the narrowing, assuming that the velocity proximal to the narrowing is less than 1 m/sec. An important assumption of this formula is that the narrowing is discrete and not of a long segment, such that viscous forces and frictional forces can be ignored.

an estimate of ventricular pressures from the peak velocity of atrioventricular (AV) regurgitant jets. For example, if there is tricuspid regurgitation and the peak velocity of the regurgitant jet is 3 m/sec, by application of the modified Bernoulli equation, the difference between the right ventricular cavity and the right atrium is 4×3^2, or 36 mm Hg. Note that this is not the right ventricular pressure itself, but rather the difference between the ventricle and the atrium. In order to estimate the ventricular pressure, one needs to add an estimate of the right atrial pressure, which in the fetus is approximately 3 to 5 mm Hg. Another example is in the estimation of valvar gradients. A peak velocity of 2.5 m/sec across the aortic valve indicates a 25 mm Hg peak gradient across the valve.

Pulsatile waveforms can be derived from Doppler echocardiography interrogation of vascular structures. Such waveform analysis provides information concerning distal vascular bed impedance or, alternatively, vessel constriction. Arterial waveforms such as those derived from the umbilical artery (UA), renal artery, or ductus arteriosus (DA) typically have both systolic and diastolic components and can be analyzed by a comparison of the relative amounts of diastolic flow to systolic flow. An increased diastolic flow to systolic flow may reflect either (1) a distal low-resistance vascular bed or (2) vessel constriction causing continued persistence of systolic flow into diastole. Examples of increased diastolic flow relative to systolic flow due to low distal impedance include tracings obtained from the UA (due to low placental resistance) or from a vessel leading to an arteriovenous malformation. An example of increased diastolic flow relative to systolic flow due to vessel constriction includes the Doppler signal obtained when sampling a constricted DA. The relative degree of diastolic flow to systolic flow can be characterized and the distal vascular bed impedance can be quantified using a variety of indices (Figure 3-4).

1. The peak-systolic–to–end-diastolic velocity ratio (S/D ratio) is a simple ratio of the highest systolic velocity of the waveform to the end-diastolic velocity.
2. The *resistance index (RI)* is the peak systolic velocity (S) minus the end-diastolic velocity (D) divided by the systolic velocity [(S – D)/S]. An RI value = 1.0 reflects the highest resistance possible, with no evidence for diastolic flow.
3. The *pulsatility index (PI)* is the peak systolic velocity (S) minus the end-diastolic velocity (D) divided by the mean velocity (MV) [(S – D)/MV], acquired through a tracing of the waveform. The pulsatility index is one of the more commonly used indices because it is reported to be the least sensitive to variations in angle of Doppler interrogation. Whereas the absolute velocity measures will certainly vary based on angle of

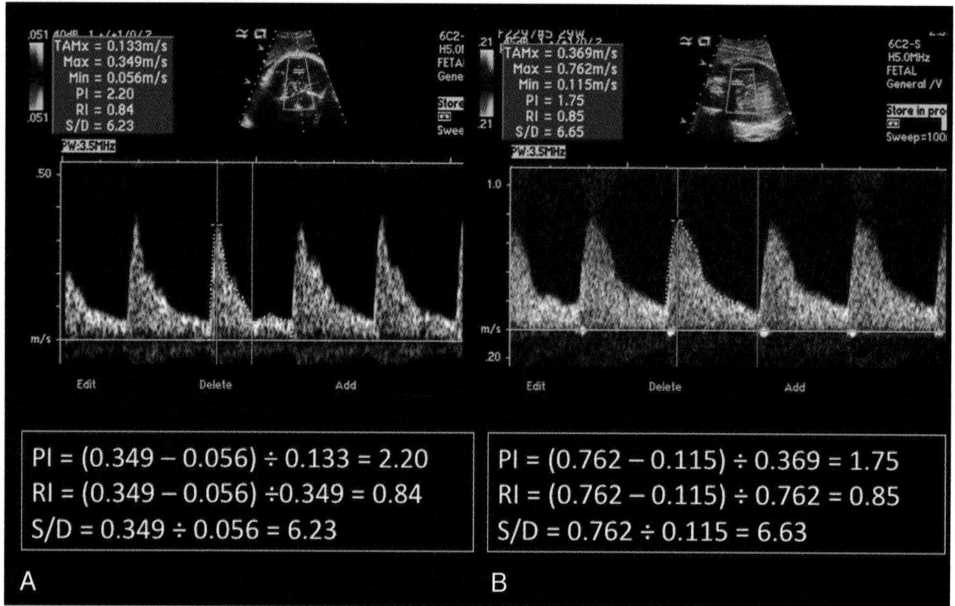

Figure 3-4. Pulsatile waveform analysis from two different samples of the middle cerebral artery. Calculations of the pulsatilty index (PI), resistance index (RI), and systolic-to-diastolic (S/D) velocity flow ratio. The waveform appearance and contours are different in example **A** and **B**, yet the RI and S/D ratio values are not markedly different. The PI values, however, are different (**A**, 2.20; **B**, 1.75). This demonstrates the value of the PI calculation over the other indices because the PI is better at characterizing the complete waveform over the cardiac cycle because it incorporates the area under the curve of flow.

interrogation, the ratio of values as calculated through the PI should be the same regardless of the angle.

Color Flow Imaging

Color flow imaging is a form of Doppler echocardiography in which pixels within a region of interest are assigned a color based on the direction and the velocity of blood flow. Shades of red are assigned to blood moving toward the direction of the transducer (maternal abdomen) and shades of blue are assigned to blood moving away from the transducer; the brighter the shade of color, the higher the velocity of blood flow. Laminar, or undisturbed, flow within a region will appear as a single color or a smooth color transition, and turbulent flow will appear as a variety of different colors within a defined region, reflecting the heterogeneity of velocities. Color flow imaging is limited in that it can portray only relatively low velocities with accuracy; high velocities will undergo *aliasing* in which colors wrap around the spectrum from blue to red or vice versa. When aliasing occurs, pulsed wave or continuous wave Doppler can help identify the peak velocity with greater accuracy.

The Strategy and Approach to Fetal Cardiovascular Imaging

In the child or adult undergoing echocardiography, the position of the subject relative to the imager is known and the approach is sequential, regimented, and standardized. The patient to be examined is lying supine on a table with the chest always facing upward and the spine down. However, in a fetal examination, the position of the subject is variable from patient to patient and, in fact, can change during the course of an individual study. Evaluation of form and function is the goal; however, the order in which structures are assessed will vary from patient to patient. A mental checklist, therefore, is of utmost importance for the operator, so as not to miss important elements of the examination. This is what makes fetal cardiovascular imaging so much fun! Each patient is a challenge, and each is approached in a slightly different manner with the objective of mentally reconstructing the various pieces of imaging data into a comprehensive, logical picture that portrays the cardiovascular state.

The American Society of Echocardiography has established key elements of the fetal heart examination.[1] The order of acquisition of these elements may vary based on fetal position; however, in each study, we strive to obtain a standard set of views and sweeps through tomographic planes that provides for creation of an accurate three-dimensional paradigm of the cardiovascular anatomy. The information from these views/sweeps is incorporated into a cognitive framework referred to as the *segmental approach* (Box 3-2). Image acquisition itself is not necessarily performed in a segmental manner, but the operator must make certain all of the segments have been inspected and evaluated with confidence before the examination can be considered complete.

Essential components of the fetal examination provide for an assessment of the segments from multiple planes and angles. These essential components are listed in Table 3-2. Two-dimensional imaging is always performed first.

Box 3-2 Segmental Analysis of the Fetal Cardiovascular System

Segments to be identified and evaluated:

- Systemic veins
- Pulmonary veins
- Atria
- Atrioventricular connections
- Ventricles
- Outflow tracts
- Great vessels
- Ductal and aortic arches
- Vascular beds (middle cerebral artery and umbilical artery)

Table 3-2 Essential Components of the Fetal Echocardiogram

FEATURE	ESSENTIAL COMPONENT
Anatomic overview	Fetal number and position in the uterus Establish position of stomach, liver, descending aorta and inferior vena cava Establish cardiac position and cardiothoracic ratio
Biometric examination	Biparietal diameter Head circumference Femur length
Cardiac imaging views/sweeps	Four-chamber apical view Apical view angled toward great arteries (five-chamber view) Long-axis view (left ventricular outflow) Long-axis view (right ventricular outflow) Short axis sweep Caval long axis view Ductal arch view Aortic arch view
Doppler examination	Umbilical artery Umbilical vein Ductus venosus Inferior vena cava/hepatic veins Pulmonary veins Foramen ovale Atrioventricular valves Semilunar valves Ductus arteriosus Aortic arch
Examination of rhythm and rate	M-mode of atrial and ventricular wall motion Doppler examination of atrial and ventricular flow patterns

Once a structure is well delineated, color flow imaging may be applied to ascertain a visual sense of the flow characteristics across the structure. Doppler echocardiography is then utilized for interrogation of specific regions of interest and spectral flow patterns are determined, as needed.

There are a variety of approaches to performance of the fetal echocardiogram.[2] The following is our strategy for the approach (Figure 3-5). These descriptions relate to the anticipated normal position of the cardiac structures, with views and sweeps that will vary based on the findings at hand.

Umbilical Cord, Fetal Biometry, Position of Fetus, Abdominal Situs, Cardiac Position, and Heart Size

Before assessment of the heart, an evaluation of the number of vessels in the umbilical cord should be performed with confirmation of the normal presence of two arteries and a single umbilical vein (Figure 3-6). Doppler assessment of UA and umbilical vein flow patterns are then performed (Figure 3-7). Measures of fetal biometry (e.g., biparietal diameter, head circumference, femur length) are obtained (Figure 3-8) and incorporated into a commercially available algorithm that provides for an estimated fetal weight and gestational age based on weight. This is then compared with the gestational age based on dates of conception in order to determine whether there is appropriate fetal growth. The position of the fetus as either breech, or head down, spine anterior or posterior, should be ascertained such that fetal left and right side relative to maternal left and right can be confirmed. The use of a handheld model such as a doll may be helpful in understanding the position of the fetus. Once fetal left and right are confirmed, the abdominal situs is determined. A transverse view of the abdomen just beneath the level of the diaphragm is obtained. The positions of the stomach (normally on the left), liver (normally on the right), descending aorta (normally to the left of the spine), and inferior vena cava (normally anterior and to the right of the spine) are then identified (Figure 3-9). From the transverse abdominal view, a sweep cephalad is performed. The position of the heart within the chest (normally in the left chest, with apex pointing to the left) is confirmed. The size of the heart in relation to the chest cavity is measured (Figure 3-10). From a quick visual sense of the image, one should normally be able to fit three hearts into the chest cavity in a transverse view. Quantitatively, the cardiothoracic area ratio should be less than 0.4. These elements of the examination are to be determined at the outset of the scan before proceeding any further.

Four-chamber Apical View

In the four-chamber apical view, the longitudinal axis of the heart is displayed with the apex either up or down. The atria, position of the atrial septum (normally bowing right to left), ventricles, and AV valves can be assessed (Figure 3-11). The conotruncus is not seen in the four-chamber apical view. A normal four-chamber view does not rule out the presence of a conotruncal anomaly, an anomaly of the great arteries, or an abnormality of the outflow tracts. From the standard four-chamber view, a sweep posteriorly will demonstrate the coronary sinus and a sweep anteriorly will demonstrate the left ventricular outflow tract and the proximal aorta (Figure 3-12). Posterior and slight superior angulation will provide an image of the entry of the pulmonary veins to the left atrium (Figure 3-13).

Establishment of each ventricle as being either of *right* or *left* morphology should be undertaken in this view. The right and left ventricles each have distinctive features, regardless of their spatial position. A ventricle should, therefore, be considered of *right* morphology even if it is positioned on the left side of the heart or vice versa, as in the anomaly known as corrected transposition of the great arteries (see Chapter 15). The morphological right and left ventricles are distinguished from each other by specific features, which are listed in Table 3-3. The two AV valves, tricuspid and mitral, also have distinctive features. The AV valve's architecture and anatomy offers clues as to the morphological nature of the ventricle associated. As a rule, the morphological tricuspid valve will drain into a morphological right ventricle, and the morphological mitral valve will drain into a morphological left ventricle.

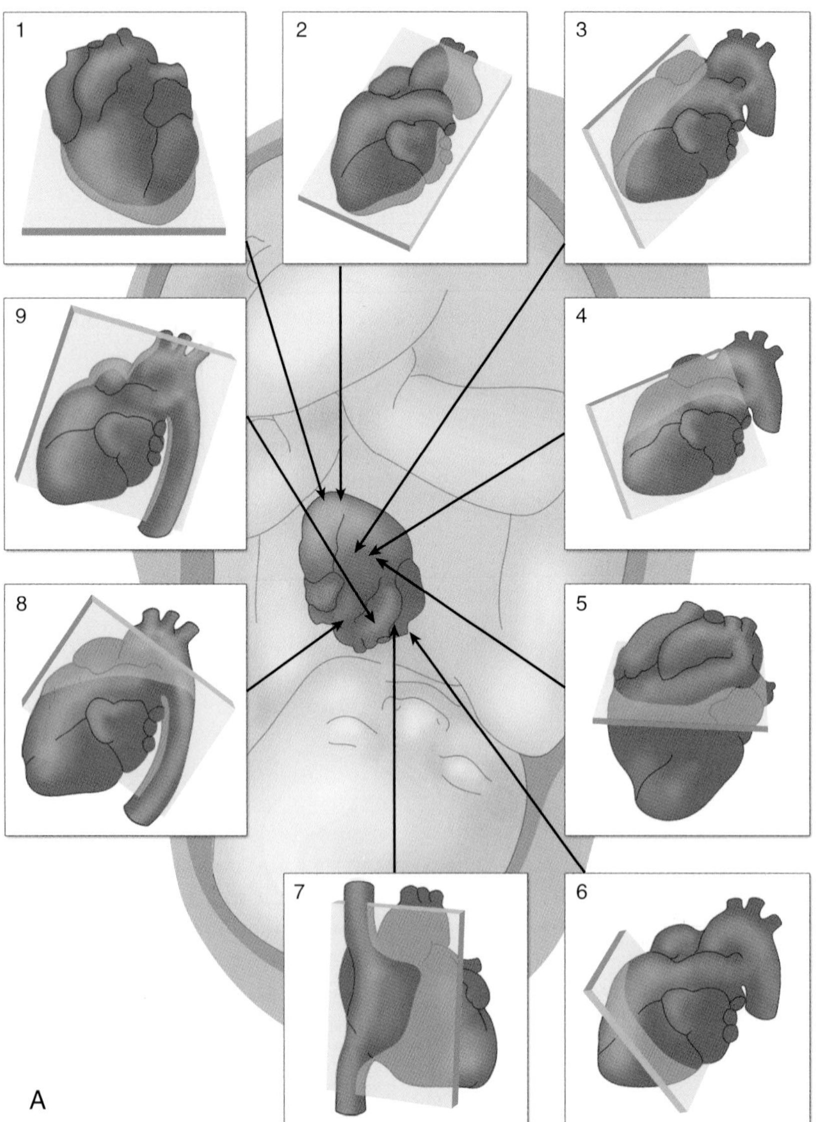

Figure 3-5. (A) The tomographic planes used to image the fetal cardiovascular system. Starting at the **top left,** the following views are demonstrated in a clockwise manner: (1) apical (four-chamber) view; (2) apical five-chamber view angled toward the left ventricular outflow tract and aorta; (3) long-axis view of the left ventricular outflow tract; (4) long-axis view of the right ventricular outflow tract; (5) short-axis view at the level of the great vessels; (6) short-axis view with caudad angling at the level of the ventricles; (7) caval long-axis view; (8) ductal arch view; and (9) aortic arch view.

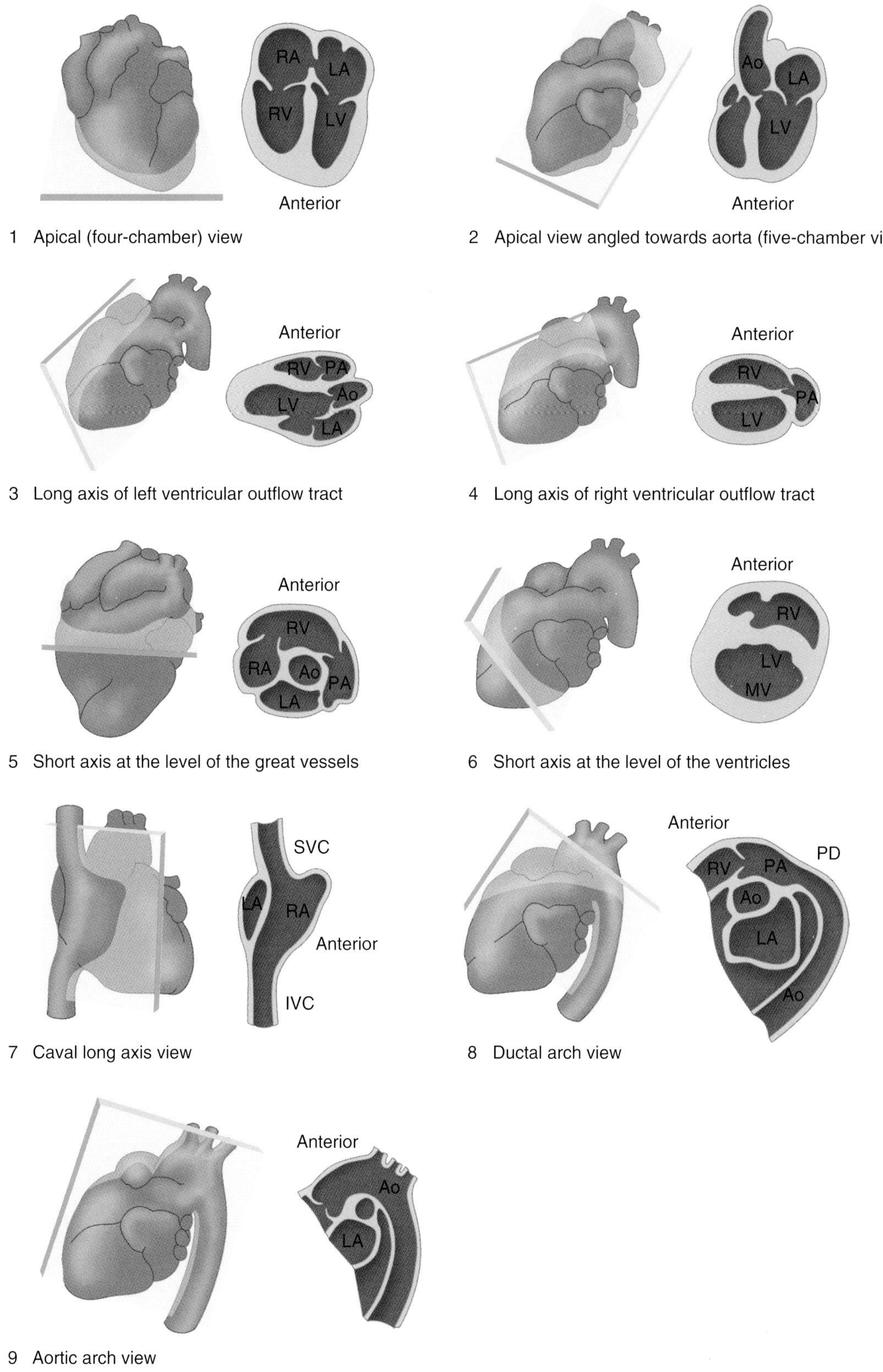

Figure 3-5, cont'd (**B**) The anatomical correlates for each of the designated tomographic imaging planes used for imaging of the fetal cardiovascular system. Each numbered view relates to the clockwise illustration of the fetal heart in **A.** Ao, aorta; IVC, inferior vena cava; LA, left atrium; LV, left ventricle; MV, mitral valve; PA, pulmonary artery; PD, patent ductus arteriosus; RA, right atrium; RV, right ventricle; SVC, superior vena cava. (**A** and **B**, With permission from the American Society of Echocardiography guidelines and standards for performance of the fetal echocardiogram. *J Am Soc Echocardiogr.* 2004;17:803-810.)

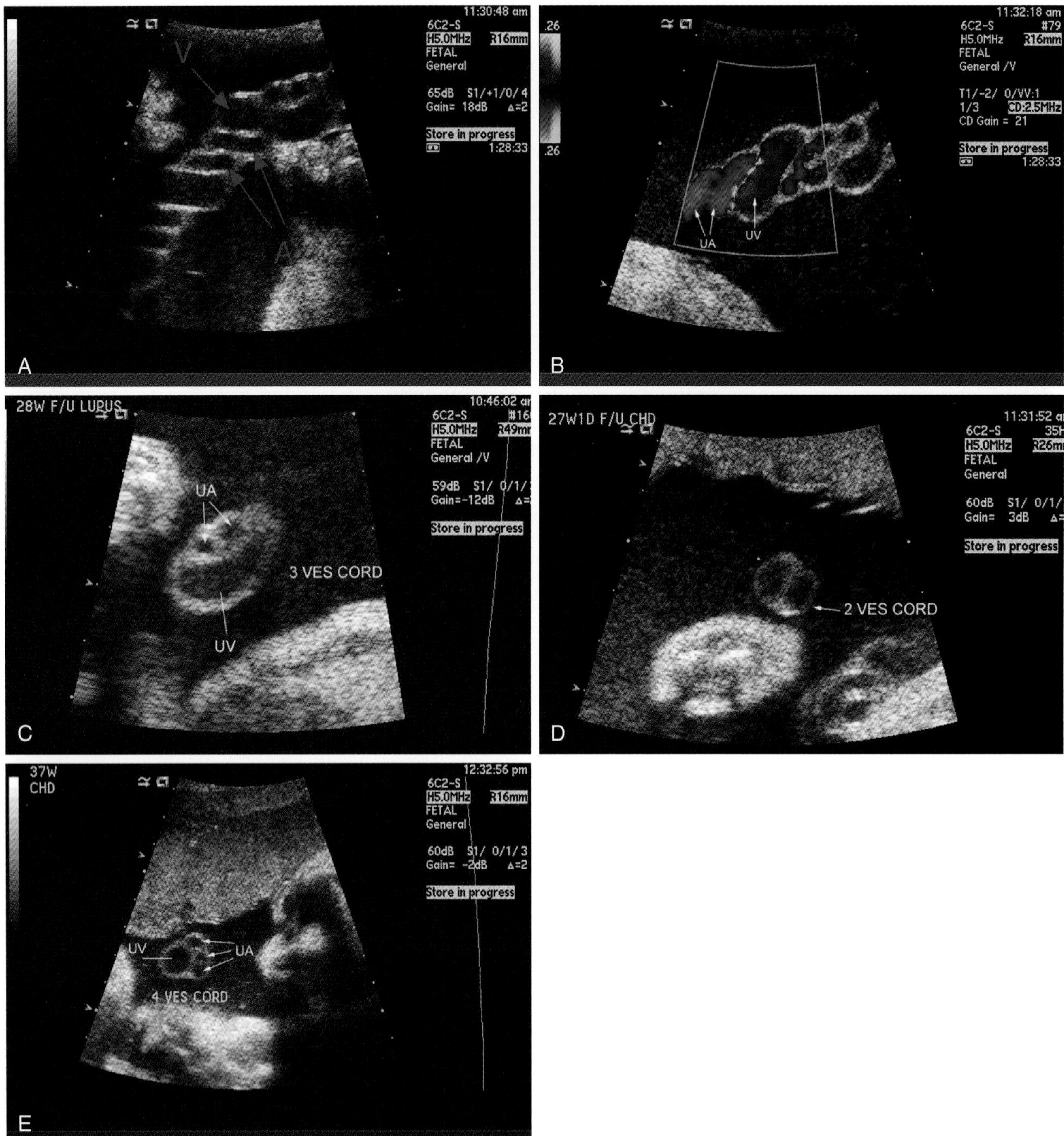

Figure 3-6. (A) Two-dimensional image of the umbilical cord. There are two arteries (A) and one vein (V). The arteries are smaller than the vein, with vessel walls that are slightly thicker and more echo bright than the vein wall. (B) Color flow image demonstrates opposing directions of flow between the two umbilical arteries (UAs; *blue)* and the umbilical vein (UV; *red).* (C) Short-axis cut through the umbilical cord demonstrates a normal three-vessel cord with two arteries and one vein. (D) Short-axis cut through the umbilical cord demonstrates a two-vessel cord, with one artery and one vein. (E) Image of a very rare anomaly of a four-vessel cord. There are three UAs and one UV.

Ventricular Long-axis View and Sweep

Aligning the transducer with the left ventricular outflow tract will provide an image of the long axis of the heart. Assessment of the normal mitral valve–to–aortic valve fibrous continuity can be made as well as an evaluation for any left ventricular outflow tract obstruction. The proximal ascending aorta can also be seen. The ventricular septum is well delineated in this plane and can be inspected for any defects. Sweeping slightly superior allows for visualization of the long axis of the right ventricle outflow with focus on the right ventricular outflow tract and proximal main pulmonary artery with

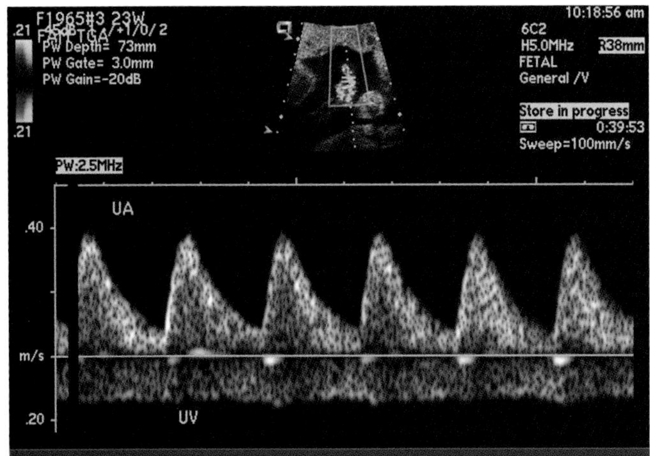

Figure 3-7. Doppler sample of the umbilical cord incorporating flow from the umbilical artery (UA), which is pulsatile and above the baseline, and the umbilical vein (UV), which is continuous and below the baseline.

bifurcation into the branch pulmonary arteries (Figure 3-14). This view is helpful in confirming the normal origin of the two great vessels. The larger of the two vessels and one that bifurcates early into branches is the pulmonary artery, which normally arises from the right ventricle; the smaller of the two vessels, which courses for a distance, does not immediately branch and provides the origin for head/upper limb arteries is the aorta, which normally arises from the left ventricle.

Cardiac Short-axis View and Sweep

The short-axis view is obtained at a right angle to the long-axis view of the heart. The landmark for the starting position is the right ventricular outflow tract as it normally wraps around the aorta and left ventricular outflow tract seen arising from the center of the heart (Figure 3-15). The portion of the ventricular septum between the aorta and the pulmonary artery is the conus

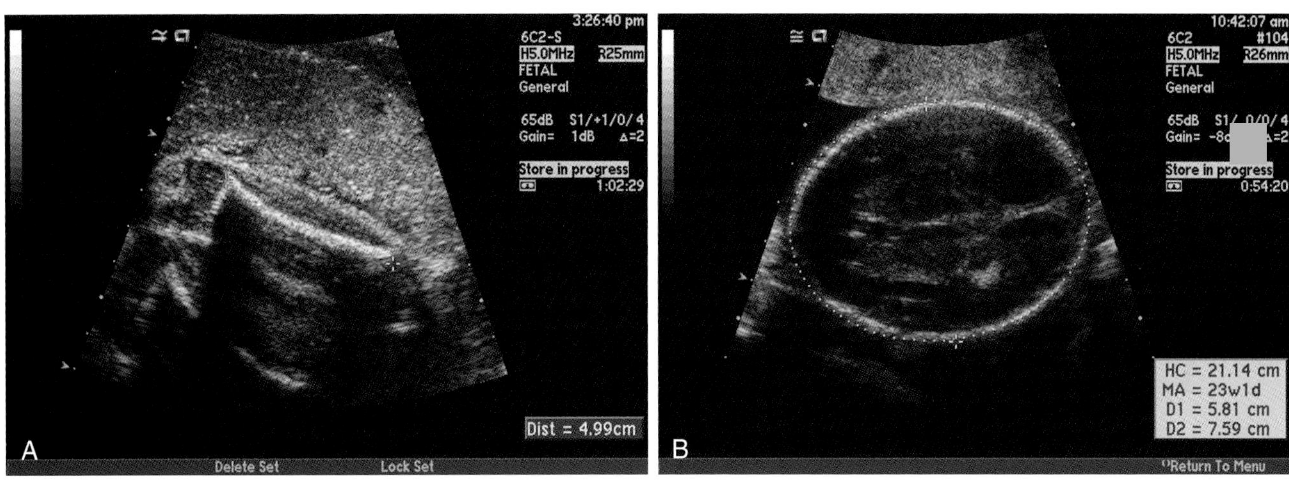

Figure 3-8. (**A**) Measurement of the femur length for biometry assessment. (**B**) Measurement of head circumference for biometry assessment.

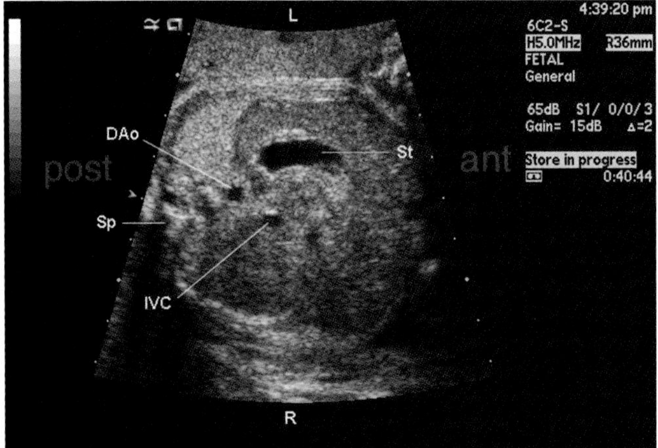

Figure 3-9. Transverse abdominal view. Top is left (L) of the fetus, bottom is right (R) of the fetus; the left of the image is posterior (post) and the right of the image is anterior (ant). There is normal situs solitus. The stomach (St) and the descending aorta (DAo) are to the left side of the spine (Sp), and the inferior vena cava (IVC) is to the right of the spine.

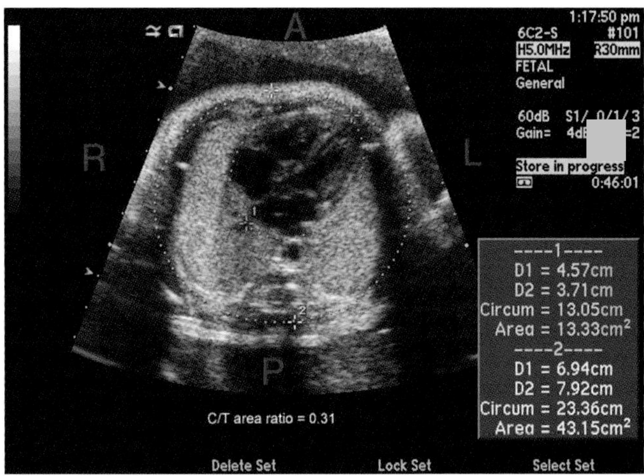

Figure 3-10. The heart is in the normal position in the chest with the apex pointing to the left (L). The cardiothoracic (C/T) area ratio is 13.33/43.15 = 0.31, which is normal. A, anterior; P, posterior; R, right.

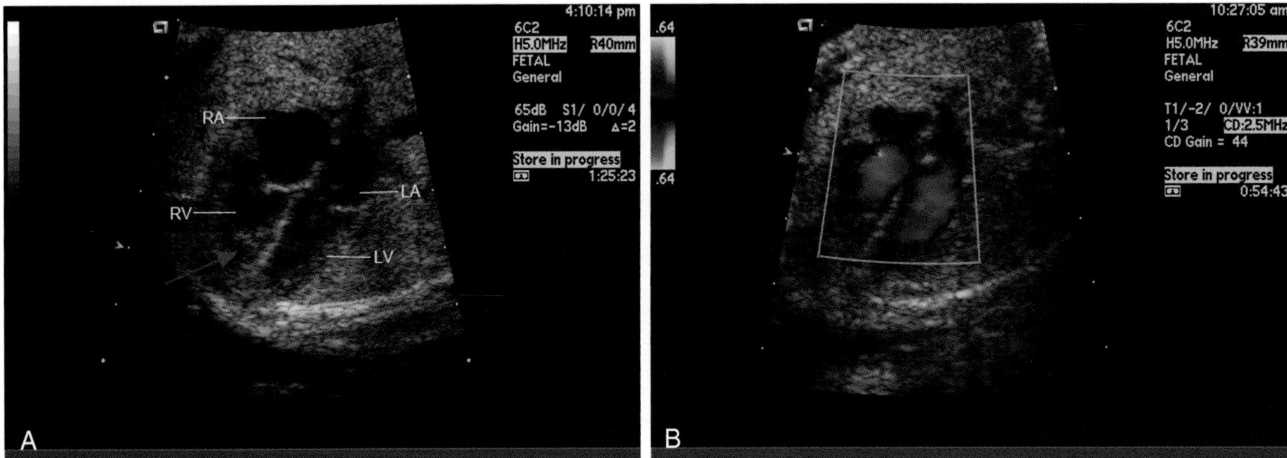

Figure 3-11. (A) Apical four-chamber view of a normal heart. The RA is slightly larger than the LA. The LV cavity is slipper-shaped with a smooth septal surface. The RV cavity is more globular in shape and rounded than the LV. There is a prominent moderator band of muscle in the RV with heavy trabeculation of the right ventricular side of the ventricular septum. (B) Apical four-chamber view of a normal heart with color flow across the atrioventricular valves in diastole. The color flow outlines the extent of the ventricular cavities. Color fills the LV cavity close to the apex, whereas it does not fill close to the apex on the RV cavity. This in part defines the RV in that the RV cavity apex is occupied by muscle to a greater degree than the LV.

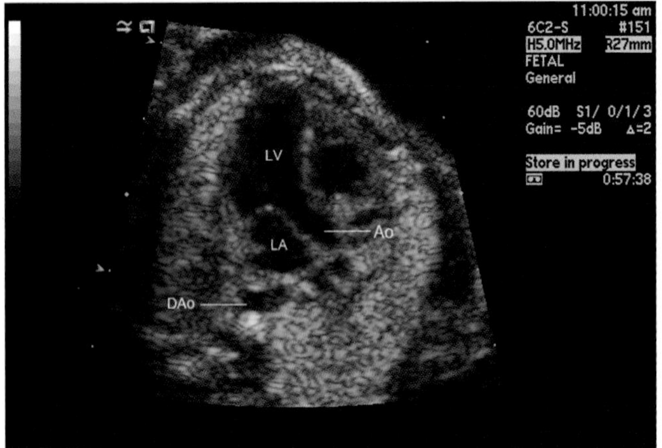

Figure 3-12. Anterior angulation from the starting position of the four-chamber apical view demonstrates the left ventricular outflow tract and the aorta arising from the LV.

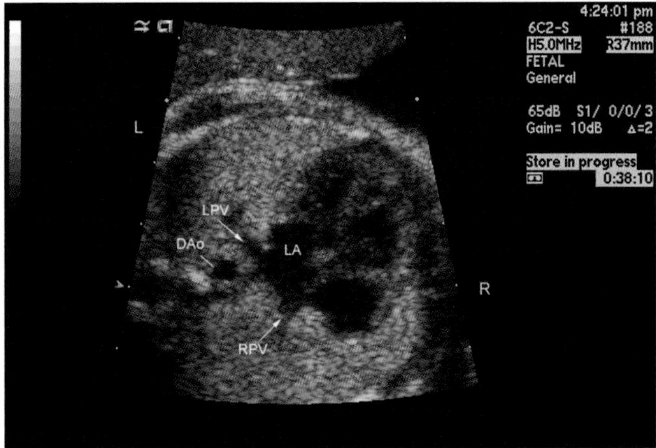

Figure 3-13. Posterior angulation from the starting position of the four-chamber apical view demonstrates the right (RPV) and left (LPV) pulmonary veins entering into the LA.

Table 3-3 Morphological Distinguishing Features of the Right and Left Ventricles

PARAMETER	RIGHT VENTRICLE	LEFT VENTRICLE
Cavity shape and appearance	Triangular.	Bullet shaped.
Cavity extension to the cardiac apex	Falls short of the cardiac apex.	Extends to the apex.
Ventricular septal surface	Heavily trabeculated with a prominent muscle bundle known as the *moderator band.*	Smooth-walled, fine trabeculations, no moderator band.
Myocardial appearance	Relatively thick and irregularly hypertrophied free wall and septum with variable muscle bundles.	Relatively thin and homogeneous-appearing free wall, no muscle bundles.
Atrioventricular valve position	Tricuspid valve annulus plane is slightly offset from center crux of the heart and more apically positioned.	Mitral valve annulus is not offset and is in fibrous continuity with the aortic valve annulus.
Atrioventricular valve attachments	Tricuspid valve will have attachments to the ventricular septum.	Mitral valve is free of any attachments to the septum.
Atrioventricular valve appearance in cross-section	Tricuspid valve has three leaflets and a single large papillary muscle.	Mitral valve has two leaflets and attaches to two papillary muscles.

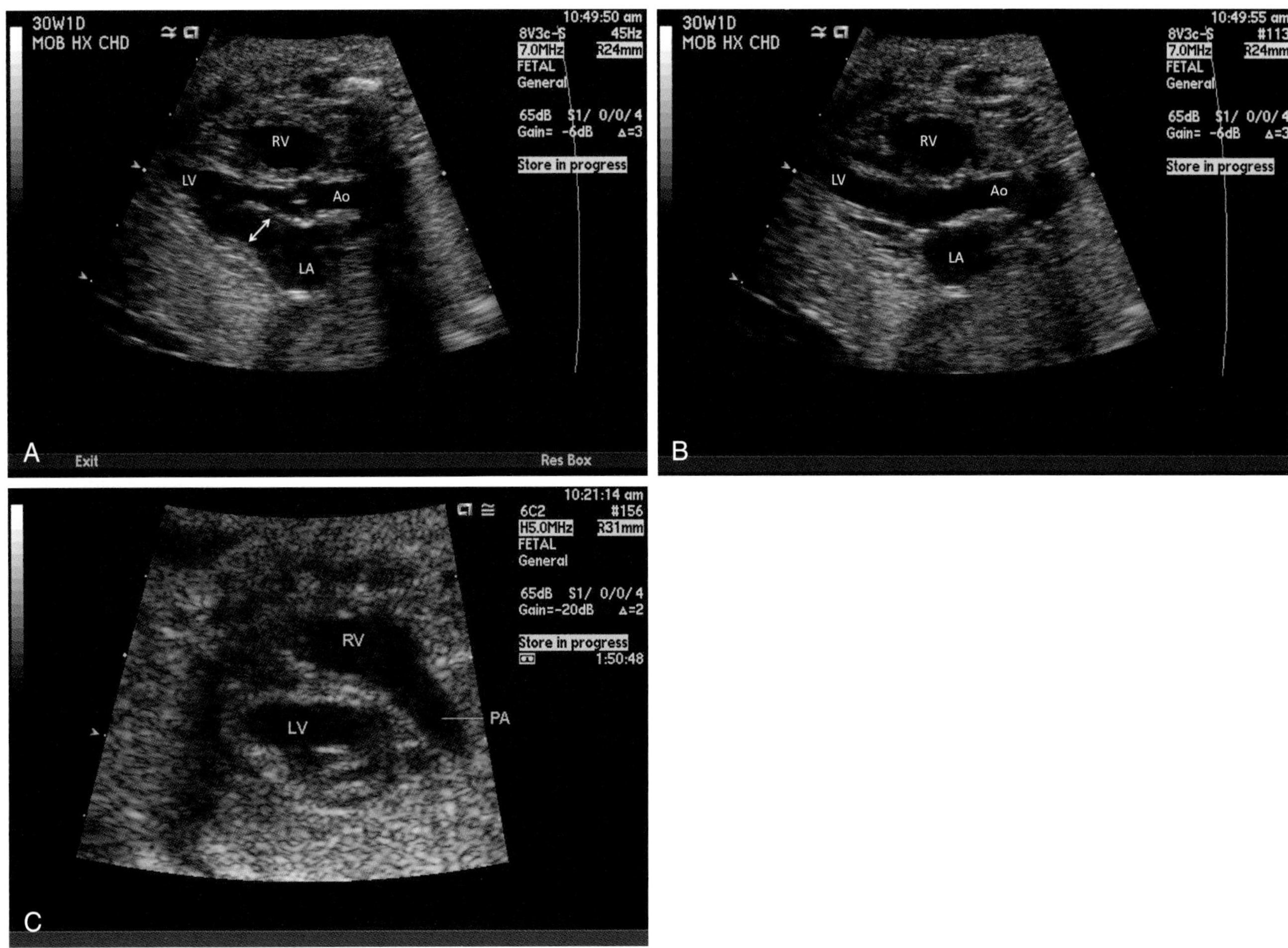

Figure 3-14. **(A)** Long-axis view of the LV in diastole. The *arrow* denotes the mitral valve, which is open. The aortic valve (Ao) is closed. The RV cavity is seen superiorly. **(B)** Long-axis view of the LV in systole. The mitral valve is closed and the aortic valve is open. **(C)** Long-axis view of the RV and right ventricular outflow tract with the PA arising from the RV.

(infundibulum). Conal deviation such as in tetralogy of Fallot is best appreciated in this view. Conoventricular septal defects are seen in this view adjacent to the tricuspid valve (at 3 o'clock). Slight angulation to the left will allow for visualization of the main pulmonary artery, the branch pulmonary arteries, and the origin of the DA. Sweeping caudad and toward the apex of the heart will demonstrate a short axis of the left and right ventricles, the architecture of the mitral valve, and the ventricular septum (Figure 3-16). In the short-axis view, M-mode sampling through the anterior wall of the right ventricle, right ventricular cavity, ventricular septum, and left ventricular cavity provides important information concerning wall thickness, cavity volumes, and systolic function. Measurements of the ventricular septum can be made and compared against standards for gestational age in order to identify abnormal thickness such as in maternal diabetes or fetal cardiomyopathy.[3] Systolic function of the left ventricle can be measured by calculation of the shortening fraction, which is the end-diastolic diameter minus the systolic diameter divided by the end-diastolic diameter, recorded as a % fraction. Normal left ventricular shortening fraction is greater than 25%.

Caval Long-axis View

In the caval long-axis view, the entry sites for the superior and inferior vena cava are aligned in a single plane as they enter into the right atrium (Figure 3-17). The right pulmonary artery is seen in cross-section behind the superior vena cava. Occasionally, the azygous vein can be seen entering the superior vena cava, creating the appearance of an arch. Color flow imaging will demonstrate venous flow toward the heart and should help to avoid confusion between the azygous vein and the aortic arch. The atrial septum can be seen as it normally bows from right to left.

Ductal and Aortic Arch Views

The fetus has two arterial arches. The aortic arch has an acute curvature as it originates from the central position of the aorta (Figure 3-18). Head and upper limb vessels are seen arising from the peak of the aortic arch, which can distinguish it from the ductal arch (Figure 3-19). The

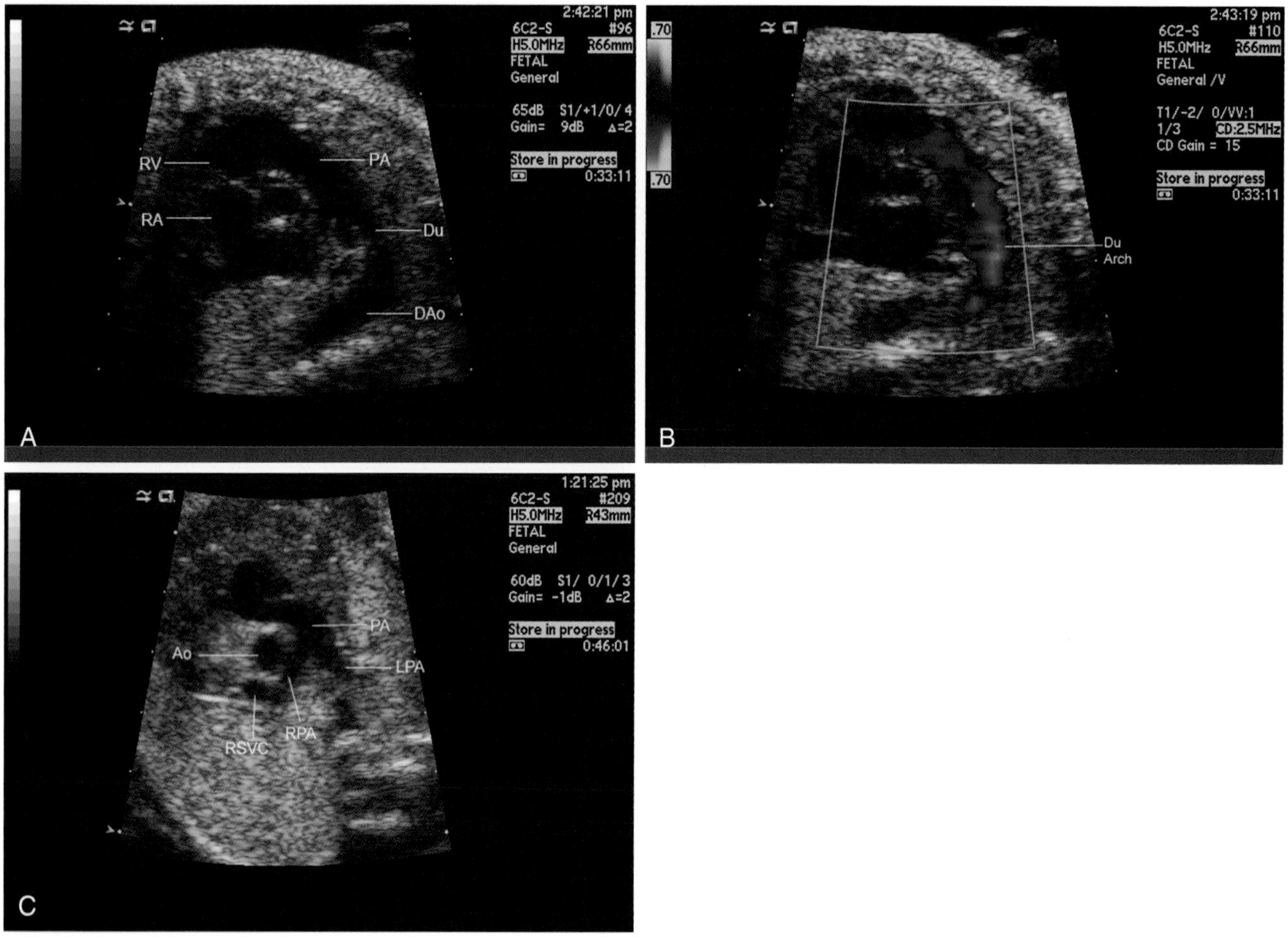

Figure 3-15. **(A)** Short-axis view demonstrates the aorta in the center with structures surrounding, in a clockwise manner: RA, RV, PA, ductus arteriosus (Du), and DAo. The proximal aspects of the branch RPA and LPA are also seen arising from the MPA. **(B)** Color flow imaging across the right ventricular outflow tract, PA, and ductal arch (Du Arch). **(C)** Superior and cephalad sweep demonstrates the relationship between the aorta (Ao), the right superior vena cava (RSVC) positioned anterior to the RPA, and the bifurcation of the branch RPA and LPA from the main pulmonary artery (PA).

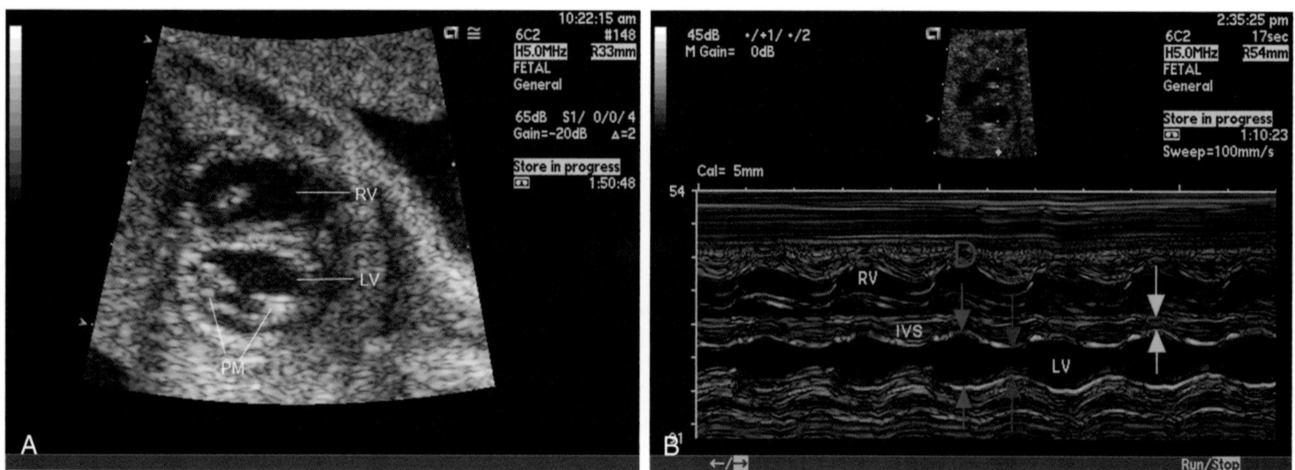

Figure 3-16. **(A)** Short-axis view at the level of the midportion of the ventricles. The superior ventricle has one papillary muscle in its center and is the RV; the inferior ventricle has two papillary muscles (PM) and is the LV. **(B)** M-mode tracing short-axis ventricle view. This image allows for accurate measurement of cardiac walls and cavities. The maximal excursion of the interventricular septum (IVS) from the LV posterior free wall is the cavity dimension in diastole (D; *blue arrows*). The point of greatest proximity between the IVS and the LV posterior free wall is the cavity dimension in systole (S; *red arrows*). % shortening fraction = ([D − S]/D] × 100. The *green arrows* depict the site for measurement of the wall thickness of the IVS in D.

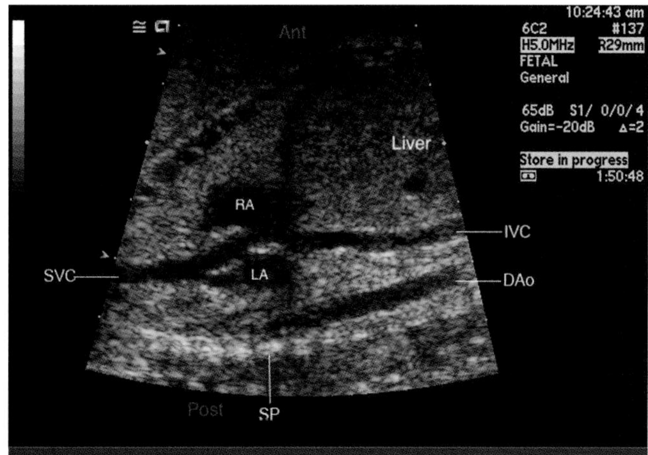

Figure 3-17. Long-axis vena cava view. Both the superior vena cava (SVC) and the inferior vena cava (IVC) are seen entering the RA. The LA is posterior. The DAo is seen adjacent to the spine (SP).

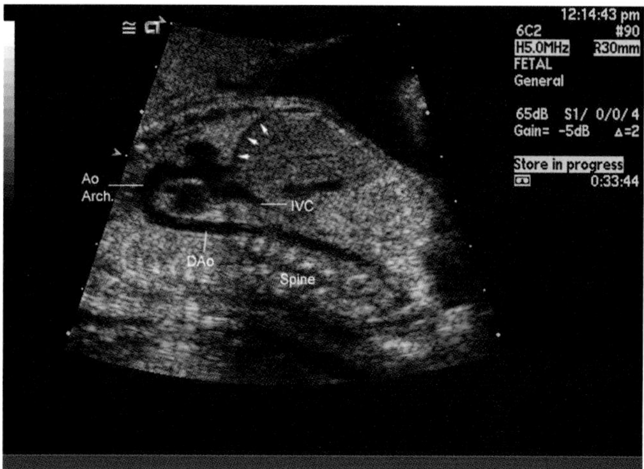

Figure 3-18. Aortic arch view with visualization of the arch from its central origin in the heart down to the level of the lower abdomen. The *arrows* delineate the echolucency of the diaphragm.

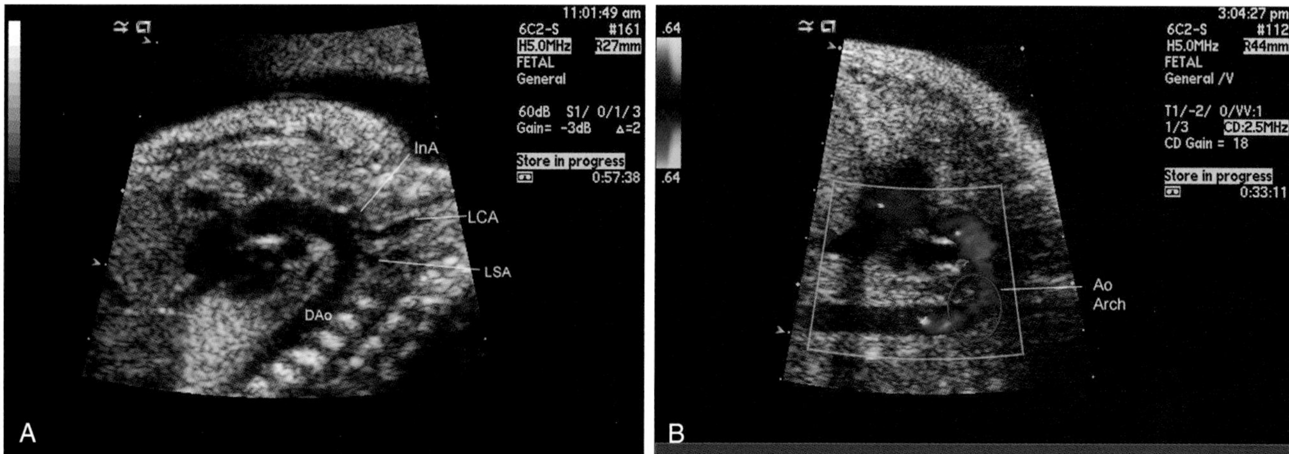

Figure 3-19. (A) View of the aortic arch with the innominate artery (InA), left carotid artery (LCA), and left subclavian artery (LSA) arising. (B) Color flow imaging of the aortic arch (Ao Arch) with visualization of the DAo. The *red circle* denotes the aortic isthmus, which narrows as it joins the DAo. The aortic isthmus is the section of the aortic arch with the smallest diameter.

ductal arch has a wider, less acute curvature as it originates from the bifurcation of the branch pulmonary arteries (Figure 3-20). The ductal arch is normally larger in diameter than the aortic arch, and there is absence of head/upper limb vessels arising from it. The ductal arch joins the *isthmus* or the aortic arch as they both insert into the descending aorta. Doppler interrogation of the ductal arch and the aortic isthmus normally demonstrate pulsatile antegrade flow toward the descending aorta.

Three-vessel View and Cephalad Sweep

From a cardiac short-axis view, a sweep cephalad demonstrates the origin of the great vessels from the heart as well as the superior vena cava to the right. From fetal right to left and in increasing size order, the three vessels seen are the superior vena cava, ascending aorta, and pulmonary artery (Figure 3-21). Recognition of the relationship of these three vessels to one another and their relative size is an important diagnostic tool.[4,5] The aorta and pulmonary artery can be traced further cephalad until the ductal and aortic arches come into view and connect. This provides excellent visualization of the transverse aortic arch and aortic isthmus and allows for assessment of aortic or isthmul hypoplasia. Further sweeping cephalad will allow for visualization of aortic arch sidedness, as a normal left aortic arch coursing over the left mainstem bronchus or a right aortic arch coursing over the right mainstem bronchus. Another indirect method for determining arch sidedness is to identify the course of the first brachiocephalic vessel that arises from the aortic arch. If the first vessel off the arch courses to the right, the arch is left sided; if the first vessel off the arch is to the left, the arch is right sided. A careful cephalad sweep in this plane will also allow for the

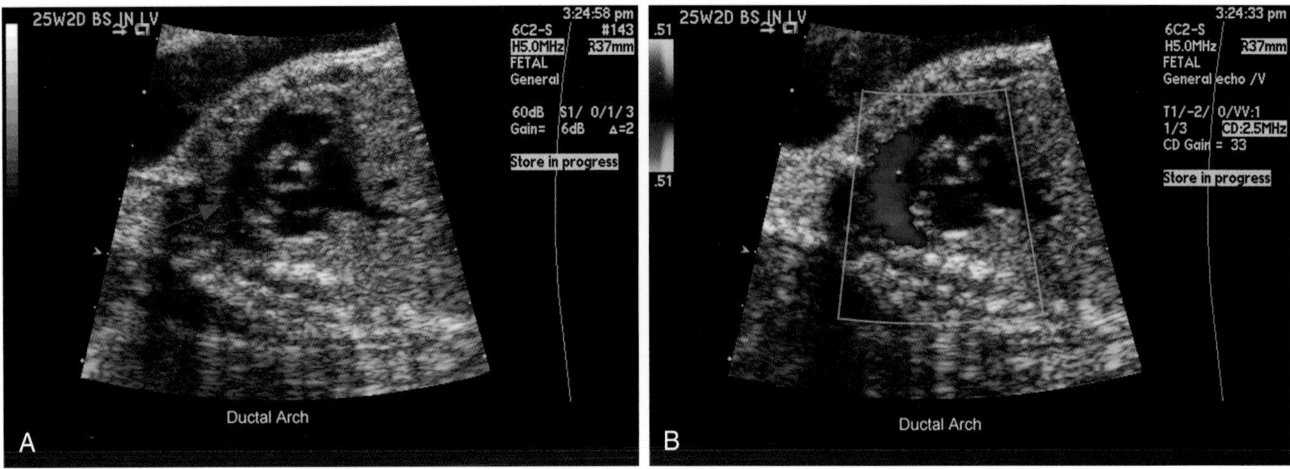

Figure 3-20. **(A)** View of the origin of the ductal arch *(red arrow)*. **(B)** Color flow imaging of the ductal arch. Note the origins of the ductal arch from the margin at the edge of the heart and from the PA, unlike the aortic arch, which originates from the center of the heart.

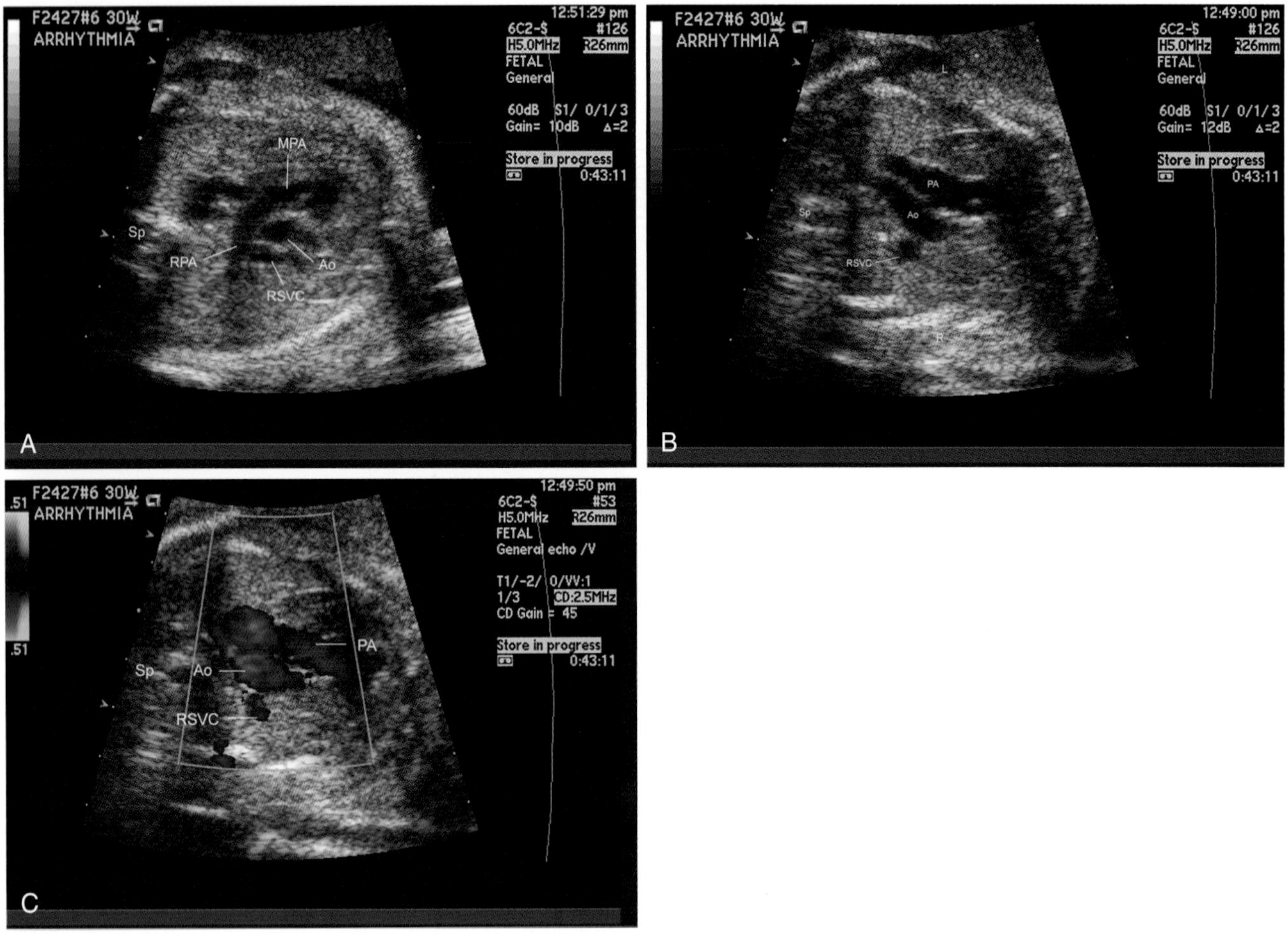

Figure 3-21. **(A)** View of the vessels within the mediastinum as they arise from the heart. The origin of the MPA and the branch take-off of the RPA as it wraps behind the aorta (Ao) and RSVC are shown. **(B)** Sweeping further cephalad within the mediastinum is the three-vessel view with visualization of the PA, aorta (Ao), and RSVC from fetal left to right. Note the size order from largest vessel to smallest vessel is from fetal left to right with the PA larger than the Ao, and the Ao larger than the RSVC. **(C)** Color flow imaging slightly more cephalad demonstrates the junction between the DA and the aorta.

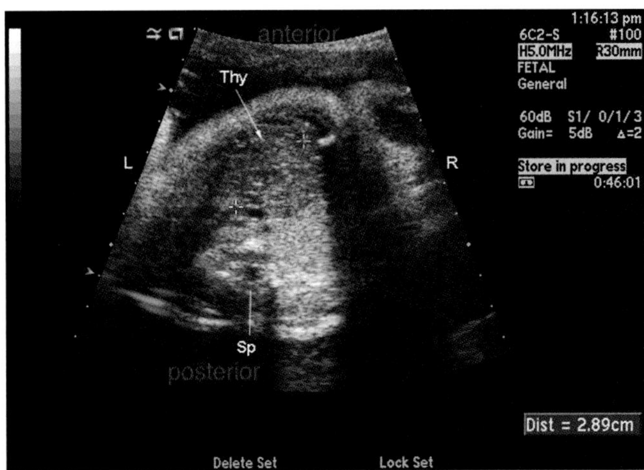

Figure 3-22. Transverse view through the upper chest demonstrates the position of the thymus (Thy).

identification of an *aberrant right subclavian artery (ARSA)*, which will arise from the descending aorta beyond the ductal insertion, after the other head vessels and left subclavian, and will course to the right. The finding of isolated ARSA may suggest the presence of trisomy 21.[6]

Located just anterior to these three vessels is the thymus (Figure 3-22). The relative position of these vessels to the anterior chest wall can be indicative of thymic hypoplasia and, in conjunction with a conotruncal anomaly, may suggest the possibility of chromosome 22q11 deletion.[7]

Table 3-4 reviews the cardiovascular structures best visualized in the various views and sweeps.

Dimensions for the various chambers and valves of fetal heart throughout gestation have been extensively described with multiple references available in the literature.[8-10] In order to compare the dimensions of structures from subjects at different gestational ages and different weights, *Z-score* values (the number of standard deviations from the mean for that age or weight population) for cardiac dimensions are useful.[11,12] A positive Z-score implies a value above the mean, and a negative Z-score implies a value less than the mean. A normal value for a particular measure will lie in the Z-score range between +2 and −2.

Table 3-4 Structures Best Identified in the Various Views and Sweeps

VIEW/SWEEP	STRUCTURE
Transverse abdomen and sweep cephalad into the chest	• Position of the stomach • Position of the liver • Position of the aorta • Position of the inferior vena cava • Size of the azygous vein • Position of the heart and cardiac apex
Four-chamber apical view	• Atria and atrial septum • Ventricular morphology • Ventricular septum • Ventricular function in long axis • Atrioventricular valves (mitral, tricuspid, or common) • Pulmonary veins • Coronary sinus
Ventricular long axis view and sweep anteriorly	• Long axis of the left ventricle • Left ventricular outflow tract • Ventricular septum • Aortic valve • Ascending aorta • Right ventricular outflow tract • Pulmonary valve • Main pulmonary artery • Origin of the ductus arteriosus
Short-axis view and sweep	• Aortic valve • Right ventricular outflow tract • Conal septum • Conoventricular septum • Pulmonary veins • Tricuspid valve • Pulmonary valve • Pulmonary artery bifurcation • Branch pulmonary arteries • Proximal ductus arteriosus • Anterior ventricular septum • Muscular ventricular septum • Mitral valve architecture
Caval long-axis view	• Superior vena cava • Inferior vena cava • Eustachian valve • Right atrial appendage • Atrial septum • Right pulmonary artery • Pulmonary veins • Azygous vein
Ductal and aortic arch views	• Main pulmonary artery • Branch pulmonary arteries • Ductus arteriosus • Aortic arch (ascending, transverse, and isthmus) and head/upper limb vessels
Three-vessel view and cephalad sweep	• Superior vena cava • Innominate vein • Ascending aorta • Arch sidedness and arch branching • Pulmonary artery • Ductus arteriosus • Aortic isthmus • Thymus

Applications of Doppler Echocardiography: Sites Evaluated, Information Learned

Whereas two-dimensional imaging provides for assessment of structure and *form*, Doppler echocardiography elucidates *function* of the fetal cardiovascular system through an evaluation of the motion characteristics of blood flow. Patterns of normal flow and abnormal flow have been extensively described for key structures and vascular sites, with the information gleaned through Doppler echocardiography providing for an understanding of blood flow physiology and the overall state of wellness or unwellness of the fetus.[13]

The following cardiac structures and vascular sites are candidates for interrogation through Doppler techniques and are, in our view, a part of the comprehensive fetal echocardiographic evaluation.

Atrioventricular Valve and Ventricular Inflow

Doppler echocardiography of the AV inflow provides information on diastole and the relaxation properties of the heart. The Doppler sample is placed at the inflow portion of the ventricle beneath the level of the AV valve annulus. Normally, two waveforms are seen (Figure 3-23). The first waveform corresponds to the *early filling* phase of diastole, which occurs after opening of the AV valve and corresponds to the passive, rapid rush of blood from atrium to ventricle (E wave). There is a short period of rest referred to as *diastasis,* and then a second waveform appears that corresponds to atrial contraction and is called *active filling* (A wave). In the fetus, diastasis is very short or nonexistent, due to the relatively rapid heart rates and short time period of diastole. Because the fetal heart is relatively noncompliant and much stiffer than the mature postnatal heart, the dominant waveform is the second peak, related to atrial contraction. Hence, peak velocities and the integrated area under the Doppler waveform, referred to as the *velocity time integral,* is higher for the A wave than for the E wave in fetal life. The opposite is true in the adult mature heart, and through early childhood, there is a transition toward E wave predominance. As the right ventricle becomes more compliant, a greater amount of diastolic filling takes place during passive early filling, with less dependency upon active atrial contraction for ventricular filling.[14,15]

As gestation progresses, peak velocities for both the E wave and the A wave increase (Figure 3-24); however, the E wave increases to a greater degree such that the E/A velocity ratio increases from 15 weeks to term (Figure 3-25).

Under disease conditions in which there is myocardial hypertrophy or ventricular dysfunction, filling characteristics of the ventricle and Doppler inflow patterns will be affected. As ventricular compliance worsens, A wave dominance increases. Fusion of the E and A waves into a single peak inflow pattern can occur in either very rapid heart rates or disorders of marked myocardial hypertrophy and/or ventricular dysfunction (Figure 3-26).

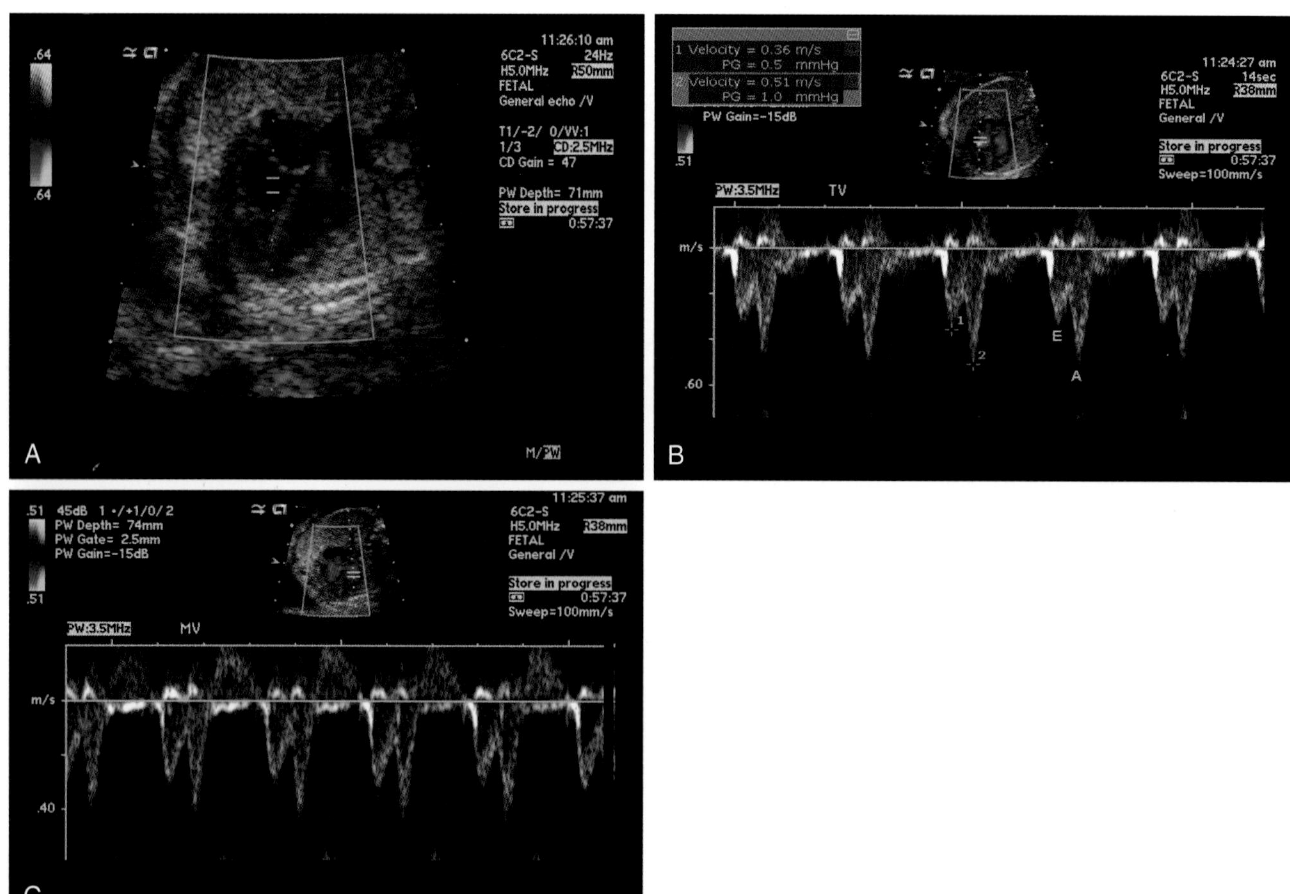

Figure 3-23. (A) Four-chamber apical view. The cursor is placed across the tricuspid valve for Doppler sampling. (B) Doppler tracing of flow across the tricuspid valve (TV). Note the normal double-peak inflow pattern with the early diastolic flow (E wave) peak velocity less than the atrial contraction diastolic flow (A wave) peak velocity. (C) Doppler tracing of flow across the mitral valve (MV) with a normal double-peak inflow pattern.

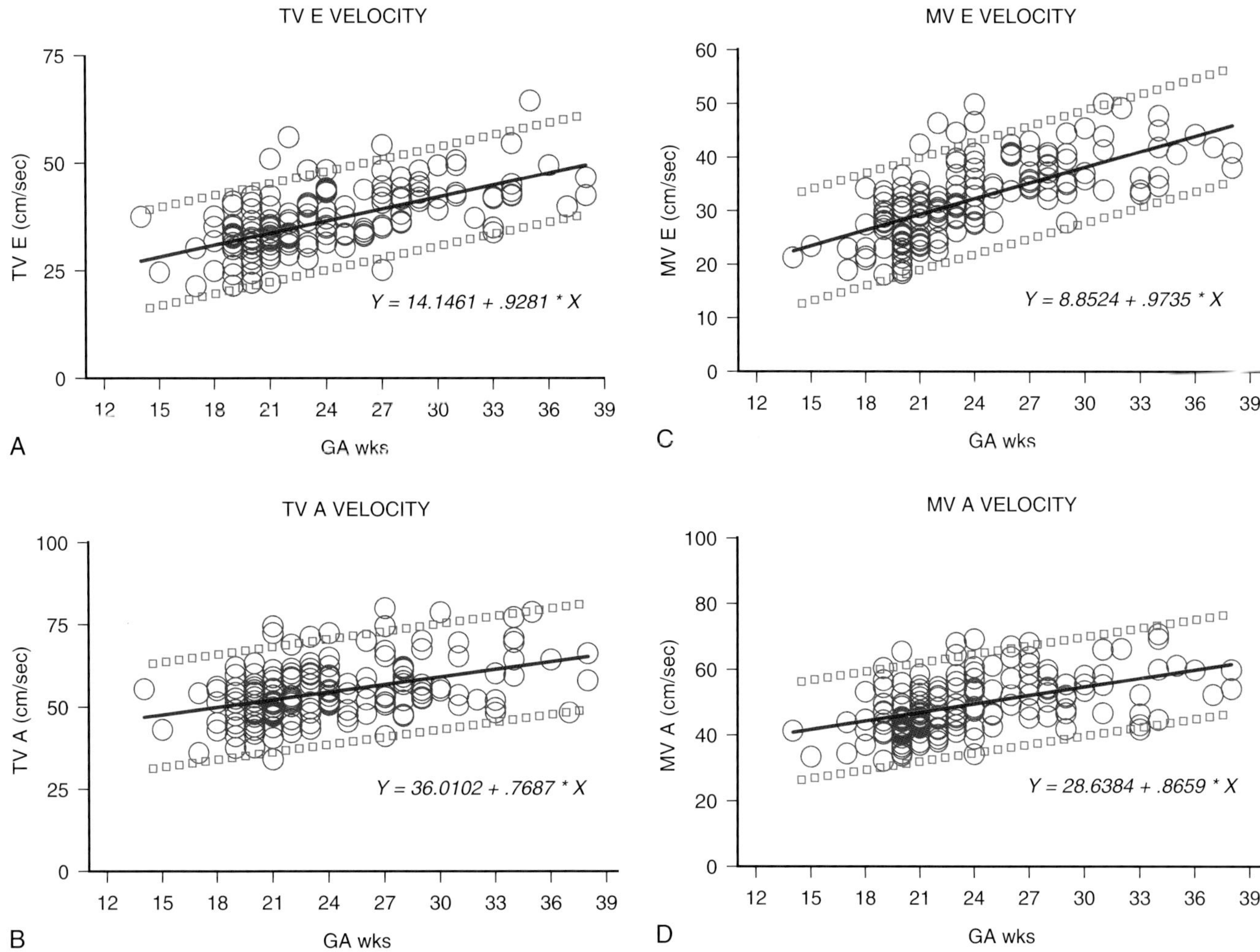

Figure 3-24. Relationship of peak velocities of flow across the TV and MV in relation to gestational age (GA). This data are derived from 150 normal fetuses seen at the Fetal Heart Program at the Children's Hospital of Philadelphia. The *solid red line* is the mean value and the *green dotted lines* represent the upper and lower 95% confidence limits. **(A)** TV peak E wave velocity versus GA. **(B)** TV peak A wave velocity versus GA. **(C)** MV peak E wave velocity versus GA. **(D)** MV peak A wave velocity versus GA.

Hepatic Veins and Inferior Vena Cava Flow

Doppler-derived flow patterns in the hepatic veins and inferior vena cava have a similar appearance to each other. The waveform is triphasic with two waves of forward antegrade flow (Figure 3-27): the first one corresponding to ventricular systole and the second to early diastole. The third wave is typically small and demonstrates reversal of flow (retrograde) and coincides with atrial contraction (Figure 3-28). The ratio of the peak velocity and velocity time integral of the reversal waveform to forward flow can be measured as an indicator of altered ventricular compliance or as a reflection of right atrial pressure (if right atrial pressure is elevated, reversal of flow is increased). A very prominent atrial waveform is seen in lesions such as tricuspid atresia. Blunting of the ventricular systolic wave and decreased systolic velocity is seen in severe tricuspid valve regurgitation.

Ductus Venosus

Doppler evaluation of the ductus venosus yields important information and is of great interest. Assessment of this site has emerged as an important aspect of overall fetal cardiovascular health and should be routinely included as part of the fetal echocardiogram.[16-18]

The ductus venosus is a vascular junction that bridges the umbilical venous circulation to the floor of the right atrium. The structure itself is slightly narrower than the vessel proximal to it, so there is typically aliasing with an increased velocity when assessed using color flow imaging. The method of identifying the ductus venosus is, in fact, to search for this region of color aliasing within the body of the liver (Figure 3-29). As a rule, spectral flow in the ductus venosus should always normally be antegrade.[19] Unlike the umbilical vein (see later), there is a phasic aspect to the waveform in which there is decreased flow velocity with atrial contraction; however, flow should still

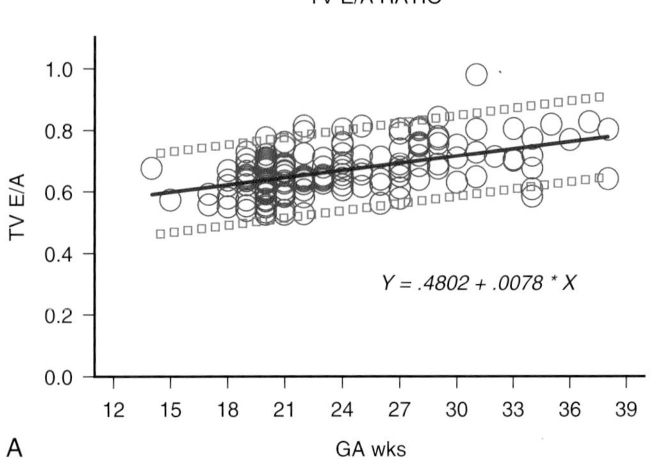

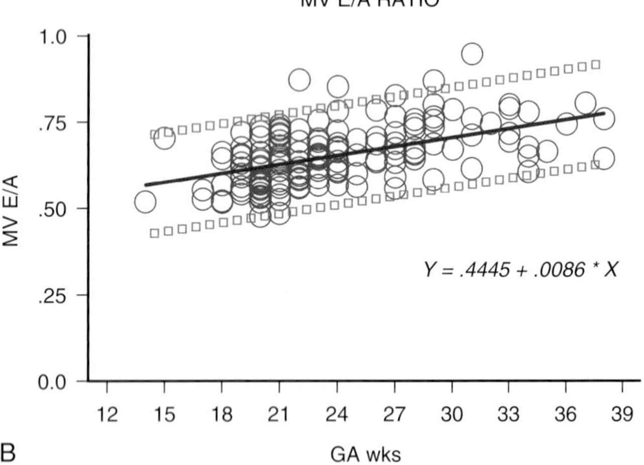

Figure 3-25. **(A)** The ratio of TV peak E wave velocity to peak A wave velocity versus GA for 150 normal fetuses. There is a steady linear increase in TV E/A ratio with increasing GA, suggesting a greater prominence of early diastolic filling as the fetus matures. **(B)** The ratio of MV peak E wave velocity to peak A wave velocity.

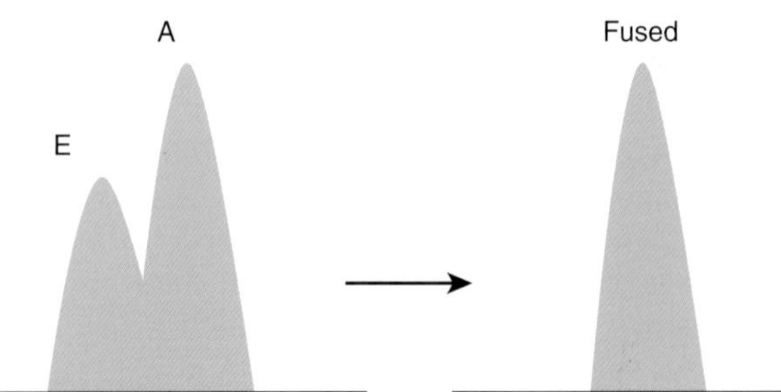

Figure 3-26. Cartoon depicting the early diastolic (E wave) and late diastolic/atrial contraction phase (A wave) pattern seen in the normal fetus. In conditions of altered diastolic compliance and poor diastolic function, these waves can fuse into a single peak, with an overall decrease in diastolic filling time as well.

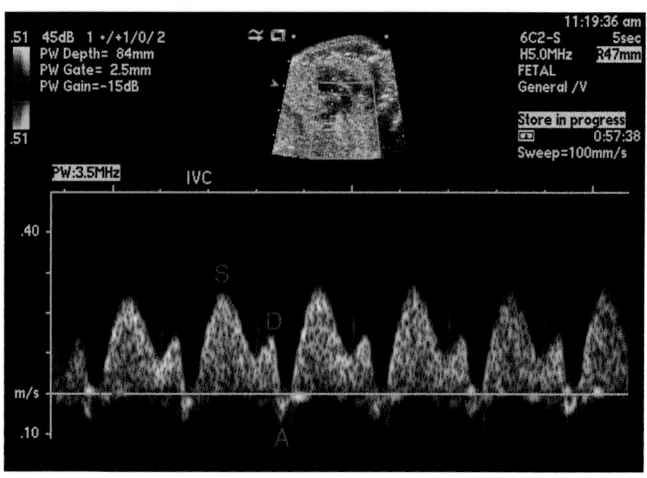

Figure 3-27. Doppler flow pattern obtained from the IVC. There are three components: a systolic wave (S), an early diastolic wave (D), and a retrograde atrial contraction wave (A).

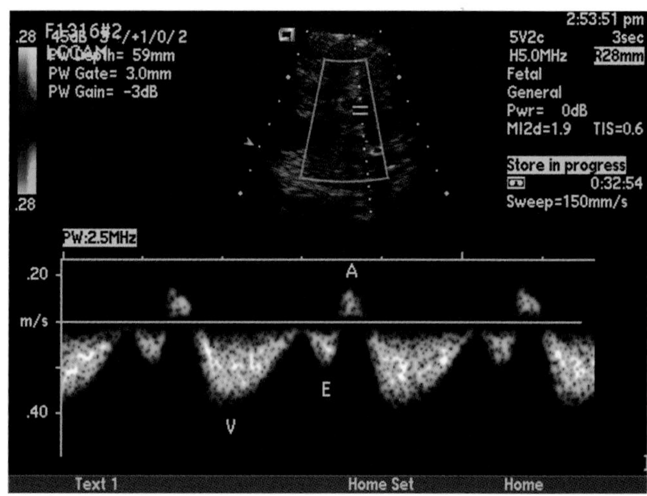

Figure 3-28. Doppler flow pattern obtained from a hepatic vein. The sweep speed is increased to 150 mm/sec in order to highlight the morphology of each of the individual waves. The pattern is similar to that in the IVC in which there is a systolic wave (V), an early diastolic wave (E), and a retrograde wave (A) as seen above the baseline.

all be forward and antegrade (Figure 3-30). Some investigators report that a small amount of reversal of flow in the ductus venous is normally acceptable before 17 weeks gestation, reflecting the normal stiffness and poor compliance of the early gestational fetal heart. Certainly, beyond 17 weeks, such reversal should be considered abnormal.

The amount of flow through the ductus venosus can vary during gestation and during periods of stress.[20,21] Reversal of flow in the ductus venosus with atrial contraction may be an indicator of a poor circulatory state (Figure 3-31), and in some conditions such as intrauterine growth restriction, it can predict poor outcome.[21] However, it is important to understand the fundamental physiology behind why reversal of flow in the ductus venosus is present. For example, in the fetus with tricuspid atresia or pulmonary atresia and a hypoplastic right ventricle, right atrial pressures are normally elevated as a consequence of the underlying anatomical substrate. In such circumstances, reversal of ductus venosus flow, although not "normal," is perfectly acceptable and expected.

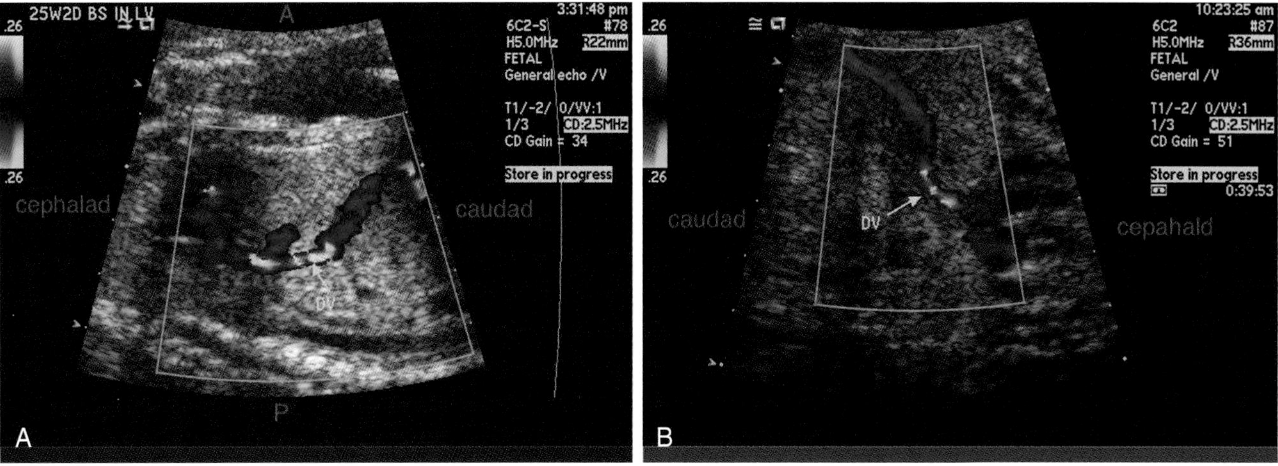

Figure 3-29. (A) Color flow imaging long axis view of the abdomen. This plane highlights the course of the UV connection to the ductus venosus (DV). The DV is the narrowest portion of this pathway and is identified by the presence of color aliasing. (B) Color flow imaging allows for identification of the site of the DV.

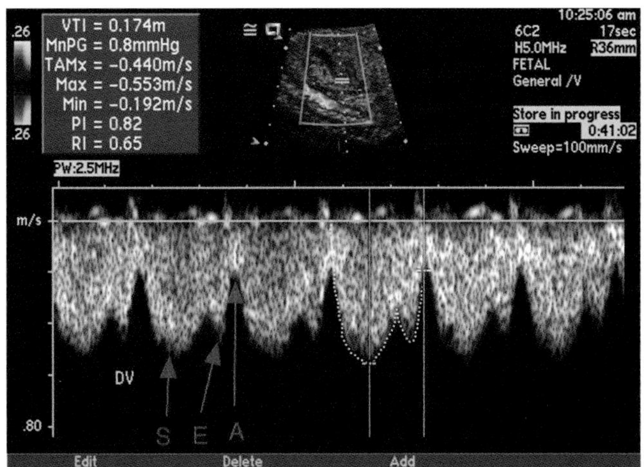

Figure 3-30. Doppler pattern of flow in the normal DV. Note that all of the flow is in the same direction, antegrade (below the baseline). The waveform is triphasic with a component related to ventricular systole (S), early diastole (E), and a decrease in flow with atrial contraction (A). Although not an arterial waveform, a PI can be calculated, which will characterize the velocity of the atrial contraction component to the entire waveform (the greater the diminution in flow with atrial contraction, the higher the calculated PI).

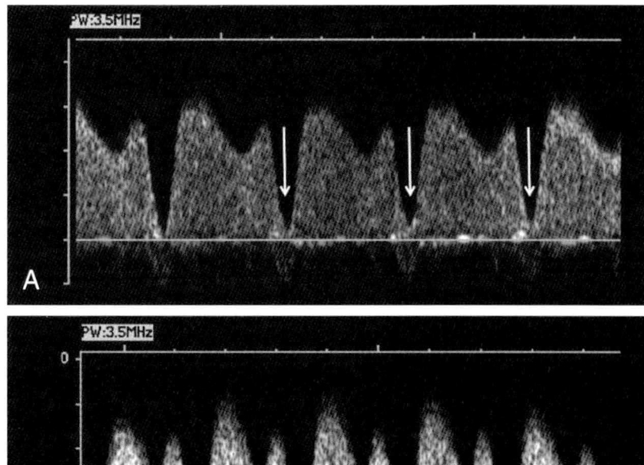

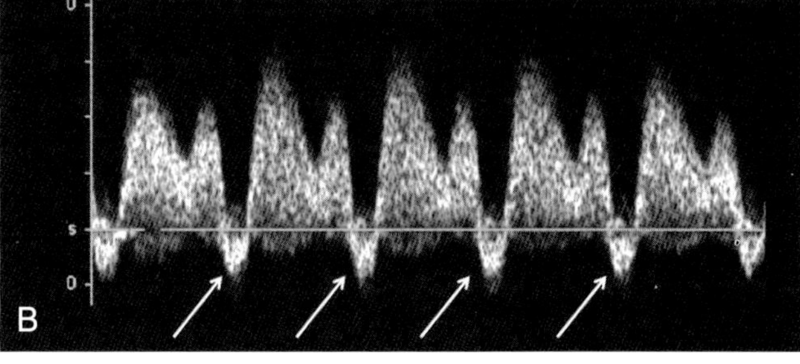

Figure 3-31. (A) DV Doppler flow pattern. There is decreased velocity with atrial contraction reflecting poor distal compliance during atrial contraction. This may be due to a stiff ventricle or congenital heart disease such as tricuspid atresia or pulmonary atresia with RV hypoplasia. (B) DV Doppler flow pattern with reversal of flow during atrial contraction. *Arrows* point to retrograde flow (below the baseline). This suggests a severe downstream abnormality, typically reflecting poor RV compliance.

The degree of diminution or reversal of flow with atrial contraction can be quantified by measuring the peak velocity of A wave contraction and comparing it with the peak systolic velocity.

Umbilical Cord: Umbilical Vein and Umbilical Artery

Color flow imaging of the umbilical cord demonstrates the normal presence of two UAs and one umbilical vein. Spectral tracings of Doppler samples obtained from the umbilical cord can vary based on the site of sampling. Hence, it is recommended that, for consistency, a free loop of umbilical cord is identified for analysis midway between the fetus and the placenta. The Doppler sample cursor is placed over both the artery and the vein and two waveforms are generated, one above and one below the baseline (Figure 3-32).

The umbilical vein carries return from the placenta to the fetus. Umbilical venous flow is normally nonphasic, continuous, low-velocity flow.[22] In late third trimester, mild undulations can normally be seen with fetal attempts at respiration, but these changes will not coincide with any elements of the cardiac cycle. A phasic appearance of flow within the umbilical vein, with a rhythmic cardiac cycle decrease in velocity, or appearance of *pulsation,* is

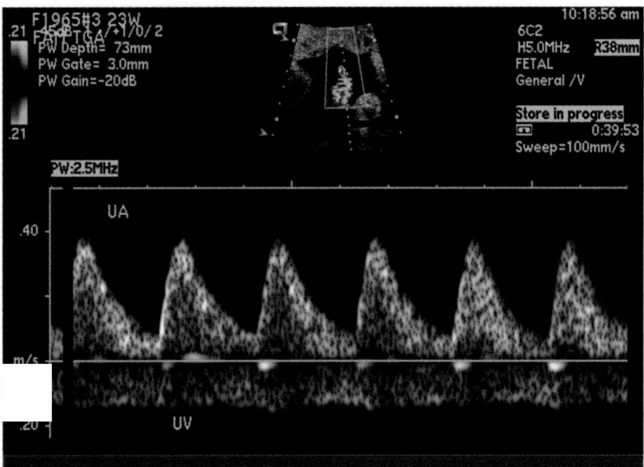

Figure 3-32. Doppler interrogation of the umbilical cord yields a signal of flow for both the UA and the UV.

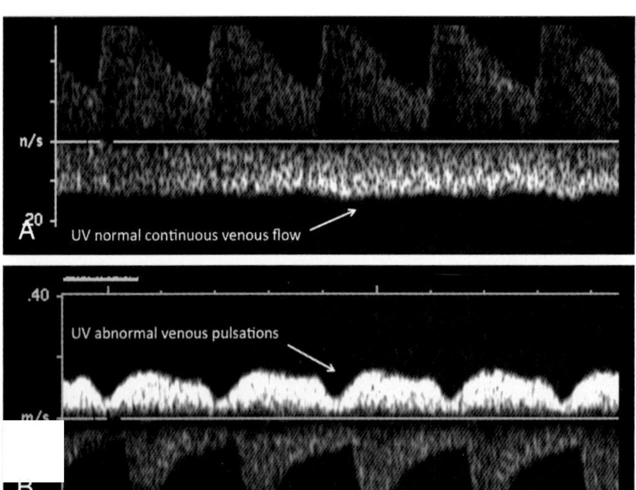

Figure 3-33. (A) Umbilical venous flow (below the baseline) is continuous, low velocity. (B) Umbilical venous flow (above the baseline) exhibits venous pulsations. There is a decrease in umbilical venous velocity during ventricular diastole, at the tail end of the arterial waveform, seen below. This suggests that the venous pulsation is occurring when the atrioventricular valves are open during diastole and is likely related to markedly abnormal diastolic compliance.

abnormal and an ominous sign (Figure 3-33). The corresponding umbilical arterial waveform can act as a guide to the cardiac cycle events, which may explain the cause of an umbilical vein pulsation. If the decrease in umbilical vein velocity occurs during ventricular systole (at the same time as the umbilical arterial systolic waveform), it may be due to severe tricuspid regurgitation. If the decrease in umbilical vein velocity occurs during ventricular diastole, which is commonly the case, it reflects severely altered ventricular compliance and myocardial diastolic dysfunction. Umbilical venous flow pulsations are seen only once the ductus venosus is abnormal as well, because both are influenced by distal downstream forces within the heart, but the ductus venosus is closer to the heart. Abnormalities of increased umbilical venous flow can occur when there is increased umbilical venous return in conditions such as chorioangioma or agenesis of the ductus venosus. The umbilical vein will appear dilated in these cases.

The UAs supply the fetal circulation to the placenta. Placental resistance is normally very low, and hence, there is typically a significant amount of diastolic flow relative to systolic flow seen on the Doppler echocardiographic spectral tracing (Figure 3-34). The pulsatility index (PI) measure provides information concerning the resistance of the distal placental circulatory bed. UA PI decreases during gestation but may increase slightly at the tail end of the third trimester.[23] Abnormally elevated UA PI values are seen in conditions such as intrauterine growth restriction and in the donor in twin-twin transfusion syndrome. Congenital heart defects have not been demonstrated to impact upon umbilical arterial pulsatility indices alone so long as cardiac function remains adequate.[24]

Middle Cerebral Artery

Cerebrovascular flow can be evaluated through Doppler assessment of the middle cerebral artery (MCA).[25,26] MCA sampling can take place just after biometric assessment of the head circumference. The MCA is identified as it emerges from the circle of Willis and courses toward the lateral aspect of the fetal cranium. The color imaging scale is lowered to highlight low-velocity flow and the Doppler sample cursor is placed midway between the origin of vessel from the circle of Willis centrally and the cranial free wall laterally (Figure 3-35). The MCA vascular resistance is normally higher than the UA vascular resistance; hence, the MCA PI value is normally higher than the UA PI value (see later).

Maternal Uterine Artery

Although somewhat out of the realm of the fetal cardiovascular system, we have found assessment of the maternal uterine artery to be of importance and value in the overall evaluation of cardiovascular health of the maternal-fetal unit.[27] The maternal uterine arteries carry blood to the placenta, which provides for fetal oxygenation and nutrition; thus, maternal uterine circulatory disturbances may influence fetal well-being. Assessment of the maternal uterine artery provides context for abnormalities that may be seen in the fetal UA. The right or left maternal uterine artery can be identified as it originates at a right angle from the internal iliac artery. This is best visualized by scanning in the maternal right upper groin region. Doppler sampling reveals a pulsatile waveform with a systolic and diastolic component. In the normal healthy state, there should be an abundance of diastolic flow suggesting a very low resistance (Figure 3-36). The calculated PI should be lower in the maternal uterine artery than in the fetal UA. Hence, a *vascular resistance gradient* exists in the fetus with a healthy circulation, in which MCA resistance and PI are highest, with UA resistance and PI lower, and maternal uterine artery resistance and PI lower still. Increased maternal uterine

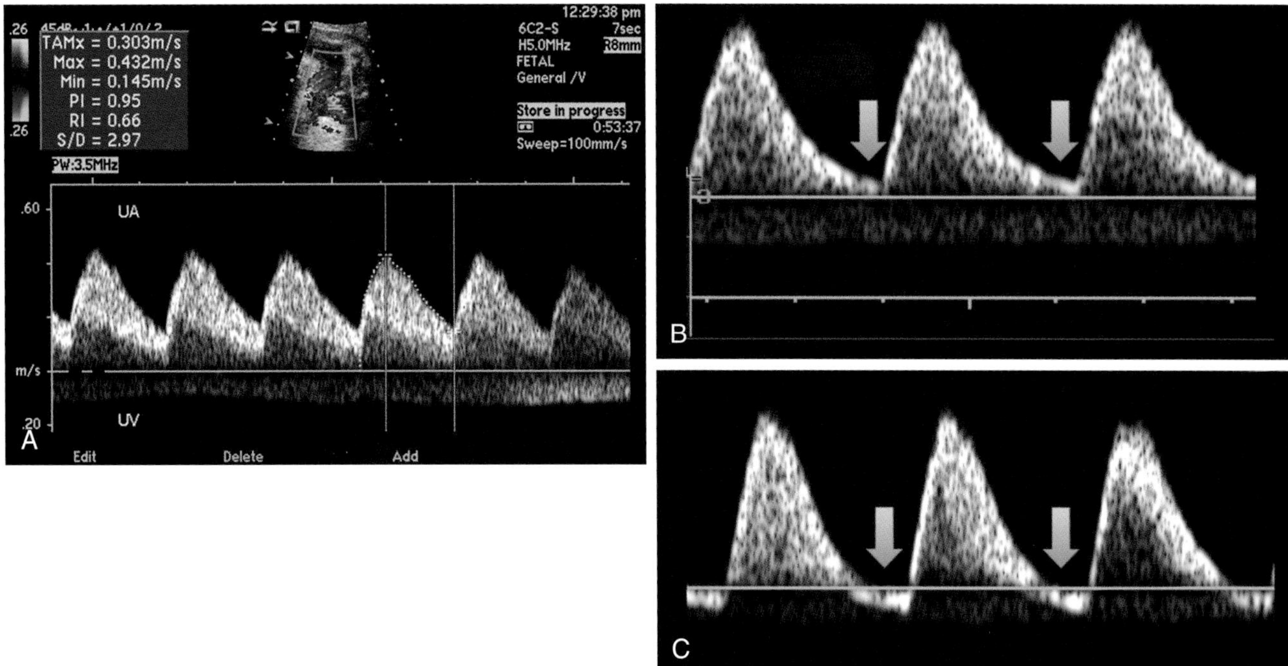

Figure 3-34. (A) Automated calculation of the PI of the UA in a normal fetus. Note the abundance of diastolic flow. (B) UA Doppler tracing with decreased diastolic flow (*arrows*) consistent with elevated placental resistance. (C) UA Doppler tracing with reversal of flow in diastole (*arrows*) suggesting severely elevated placental resistance. Diastolic reversal of UA flow implies a higher impedance to flow into the placenta in diastole than impedance of flow back to the fetus. This is an ominous sign because blood will take the pathway of least resistance away from the placenta, which may herald fetal demise.

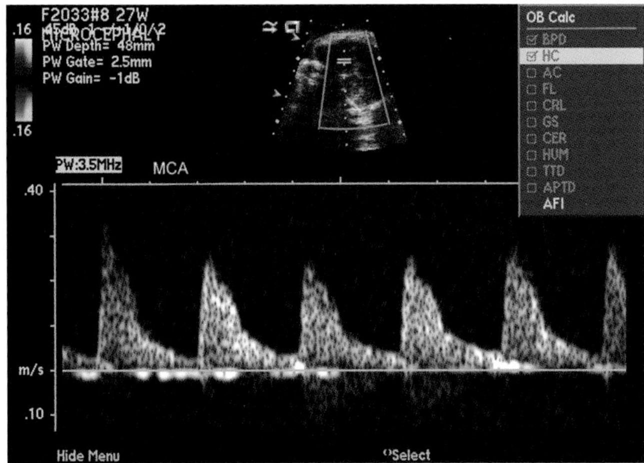

Figure 3-35. MCA Doppler flow tracing.

artery PI and the presence of *notching* is associated with complications such as preeclampsia, stillbirth, and intrauterine growth restriction (Figure 3-37).[28] The role of maternal uterine artery analysis in the evaluation of the fetus with congenital heart disease has not yet been fully explored.

Ductus Arteriosus

The DA connects the main pulmonary artery to the descending aorta and, thus, directs right ventricular ejection toward the descending aorta. In the normal state, the DA is larger than the adjoining aortic isthmus, which is carrying blood ejected by the left ventricle. Flow is always antegrade with a dominant waveform in systole and a persistent smaller waveform of antegrade flow in diastole (Figure 3-38).[29,30] The DA can change in caliber and undergo constriction in utero. This can result in an increase in diastolic flow because not all of the right ventricular systolic ejected blood volume can complete passage through the DA in systole. Flow then persists into diastole with continued elastic recoil into diastole as an impetus driving blood forward. The DA PI will decrease as diastolic flow increases. DA PI can be used as a measure of ductal constriction due to exogenous agents such as nonsteroidal anti-inflammatory agents or salicylates.

In congenital heart disease, the presence of significant left- or right-sided heart disease will influence the size and flow patterns through the DA. For example, in hypoplastic left heart syndrome (HLHS), the DA is quite large and systolic velocities are increased, reflecting the fact that nearly all of the cardiac output must traverse the DA. Alternatively, in cases of severe pulmonary stenosis or pulmonary atresia, the DA is smaller than normal and may have a different shape as it arises from the underside of the aorta to perfuse the pulmonary arteries. Flow is then retrograde in the DA, and the Doppler pattern reflects the high pulmonary vascular resistance of the fetal pulmonary circulation.

Aortic Isthmus

The aortic isthmus is defined as the region of the aorta between the take-off of the left subclavian artery and the insertion of the DA to the descending aorta. Based on its

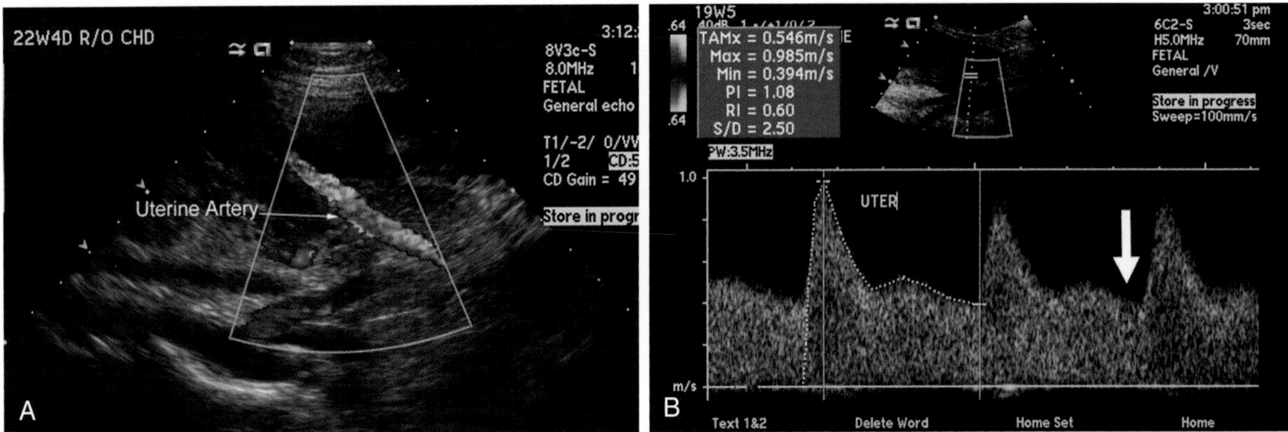

Figure 3-36. (A) Color flow imaging identification of the maternal UA at its origin from the internal iliac. This image is acquired by scanning in the maternal groin region. (B) Doppler tracing for a normal maternal UA at approximately 20 weeks' gestation. Note the abundance of diastolic flow (*arrow*) consistent with very low vascular resistance. The calculated PI is low (1.08).

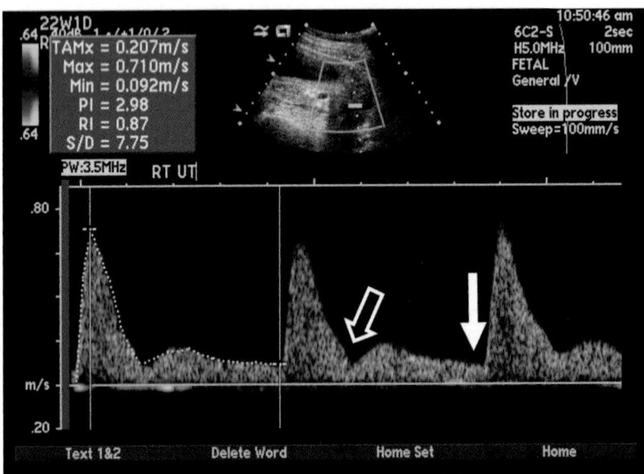

Figure 3-37. Doppler tracing from a maternal UA at 22 weeks' gestation. There is notching of the waveform *(open arrow)* with a dip in velocity immediately after systole, suggesting very high distal resistance. The end-diastolic velocity is low *(white arrow)*. The calculated PI is very high (2.98).

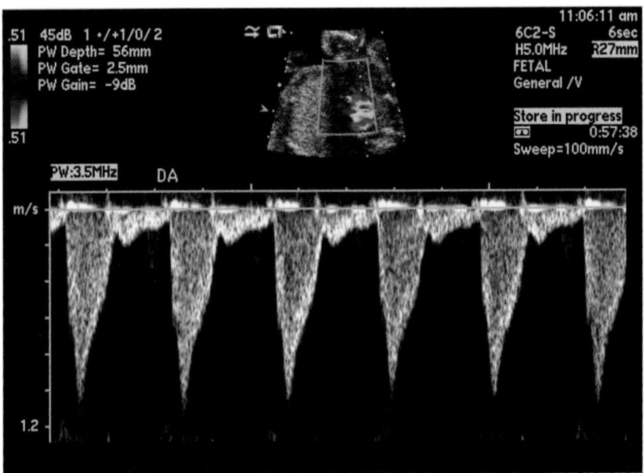

Figure 3-38. Doppler flow tracing derived from the DA.

location, it is described as being of unique importance and value.[31] Investigators consider the aortic isthmus the "bridge" between two regional circulations—that perfused by the left ventricle, namely, the upper circulations of the myocardium, upper limbs, and cerebrovasculature, and that perfused by the right ventricle, namely, the lower body, lower limbs, and placental circulation. In the normal state, flow is antegrade in systole and in diastole as the isthmus joins the DA and descending aorta. Forward flow in diastole reflects the ratio of relative vascular resistances, with *caudad* vascular resistance normally lower than *cephalad* vascular resistance, due to the placenta's connection to the caudad circulation. Retrograde flow in diastole is seen in the aortic isthmus when the ratio of vascular resistances is such that cephalad vascular resistance is abnormally lower than caudad.[32] This may occur in conditions of cerebral hypoxemia or impaired perfusion, with a decrease in cerebrovascular resistance and an attempt to autoregulate and increase cerebral blood flow.[33] Retrograde flow in the aortic isthmus is seen during systole when there is inadequate left ventricular forward ejection such as in anatomical lesions such as aortic atresia, HLHS, or transverse arch hypoplasia and coarctation of the aorta. Retrograde systolic flow in the aortic isthmus is also seen when there is severe left ventricular dysfunction and inadequate forward flow into the ascending aorta.

Pulmonary Veins

The pulmonary veins carry venous return from the right and left lungs to the left atrium. In prenatal life, pulmonary venous return is much less than after birth as blood flow to the lungs is limited. The color flow imaging sector is focused on the hilum and the region behind the left atrium and the color flow imaging scale is lowered to approximately 20 to 40 cm/sec in order to highlight the pulmonary veins (Figure 3-39). Doppler interrogation produces a spectral display in which there are three

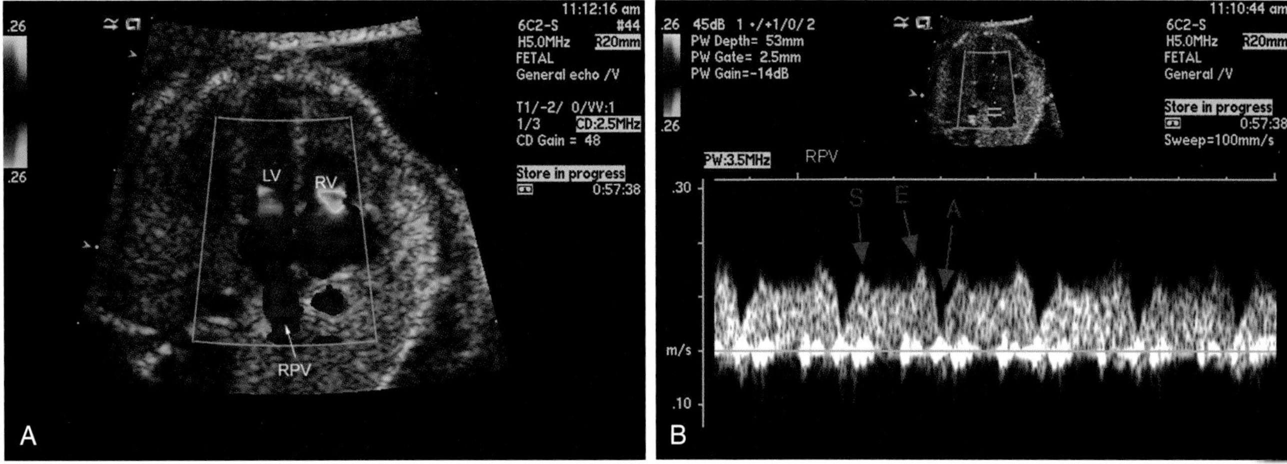

Figure 3-39. (A) Apical four-chamber view with focus on the pulmonary veins. Note the color scale is lowered to 26 cm/sec in order to enhance low-velocity venous flow. (B) Doppler flow tracing of the right pulmonary vein (RPV). The flow pattern is triphasic with a systolic (S), an early diastolic (E), and an atrial contraction (A) component.

phases: a systolic wave (S wave), an early diastolic wave (D wave), and an atrial contraction wave (A wave). In the normal state, the S wave is dominant, with the highest velocity; the D wave is next, and the A wave has the lowest velocity. S wave and D wave flow are always normally antegrade into the left atrium. In early gestation, there may be some A wave reversal of flow, but as pulmonary blood flow increases slightly toward the end of gestation, A wave flow will be antegrade. Abnormalities that result in increased left atrial pressure such as left ventricular dysfunction or poor left ventricular compliance will result in progressive increase in A wave reversal velocity and time velocity integral.[34,35] Mitral stenosis or atresia with restriction at the atrial level will also lead to an increase in A wave reversal and has been studied extensively in the HLHS[36] (see Chapter 22).

Applications of Echocardiography: Understanding Abnormal Hemodynamic States and Myocardial Dysfunction

Doppler Tissue Imaging

Doppler techniques can be applied to the assessment of myocardial tissue in the same way it is used to assess blood flow. By altering the velocity scale to very low velocity movements and adjusting the signal filter, myocardial tissue direction and velocities can be ascertained and displayed in a spectral manner (Figure 3-40). Doppler tissue imaging (DTI) offers another way to assess functional aspects of the heart by looking directly at myocardial dynamics as opposed to blood flow dynamics.[37] Furthermore, analysis of DTI tracings can provide a read on a complete cardiac cycle because the myocardium is constantly moving in both systole and diastole, whereas assessment of blood flow can be performed only during the phase of the cardiac cycle in which blood is moving (i.e., mitral valve flow during diastole, aortic valve flow during systole).

The Doppler sample cursor is placed at the junction of the right ventricular free wall and the tricuspid valve annulus for assessment of right ventricular mechanics and at the level of the junction between the left ventricular free wall and the lateral aspect of the mitral valve for assessment of left ventricular mechanics. Values for normal myocardial tissue velocities throughout gestation for systole (Sa wave), early diastole (Ea wave), and atrial contraction (Aa wave) have been reported (Figure 3-41). Doppler tissue velocities for both the right and the left ventricle increase with gestational age.[38] Similar to flow-related velocities, the ratio of velocity of tissue motion of Ea wave–to–Aa wave increases with gestational age (Figure 3-42). The ratio of early diastolic blood flow velocity across the AV valve (E wave) to the early diastolic myocardial tissue velocity of the ventricular free wall (Ea wave) is described as reflecting the filling pressure of the ventricle and is thought to be an index of diastolic function and relaxation.[39] The higher the E/Ea ratio, the greater the velocity of blood flow in relation to the movement of the myocardium reflecting elevated atrial pressure and poor relaxation, and the lower the E/Ea ratio, the lower the blood flow velocity in relation to velocity of movement of the myocardium, reflecting lower atrial pressure and improved relaxation. The E/Ea ratio for both the right and the left ventricle decreases with gestation as compliance of the ventricle and diastolic relaxation improves with gestation (Figure 3-43).

DTI has been helpful in the analysis of complex fetal arrhythmias by observing for the onset and timing of myocardial movement[40] and in the assessment of myocardial deformation such as strain and strain rate (see later).

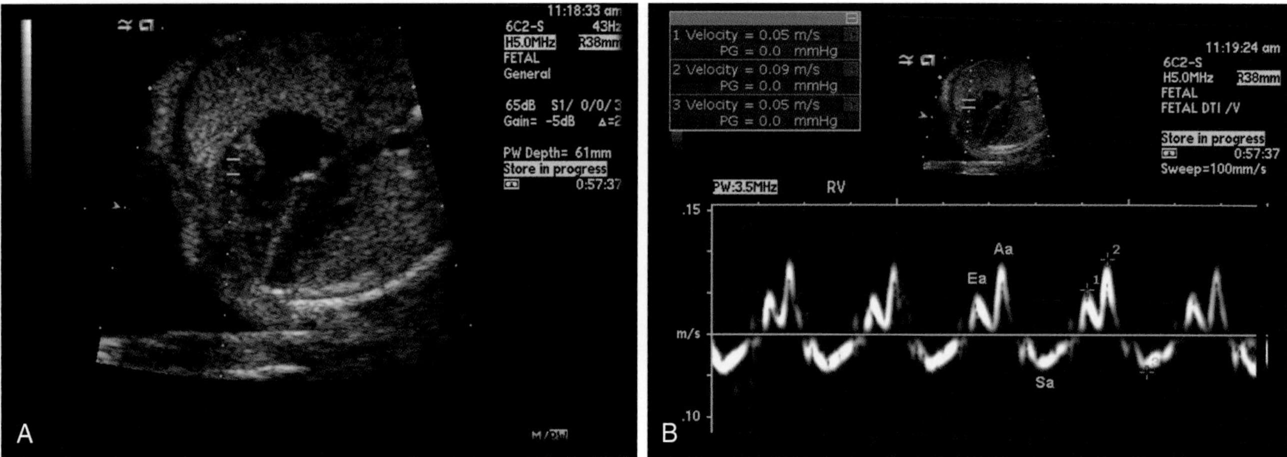

Figure 3-40. **(A)** Four-chamber apical view for Doppler tissue imaging (DTI). The Doppler cursor is placed on the RV free wall just beneath the TV annulus. **(B)** Spectral display of Doppler signal obtained from the RV free wall. Note the peak velocities of myocardial movement are much lower than they are for blood flow. The suffix lowercase "a" is added onto the identifiers for the waveforms of tissue-derived signals. There are myocardial motion waveforms generated for early diastole (Ea), atrial contraction (Aa), and ventricular systole (Sa). DTI signals include both the systolic and the diastolic phases in the same tracing, because the myocardium moves in different opposing directions throughout the cardiac cycle. Diastolic waveforms (Ea and Aa) are above baseline with movement of the RV free wall expanding toward the transducer position; the systolic waveform (Sa) is below the baseline as the heart contracts and moves away from the transducer position.

RV Sa VELOCITY
RV Sa (cm/sec)
Y = 2.0561 + .1267 * X
GA wks
A

RV Aa VELOCITY
RV Aa (cm/sec)
Y = 5.0739 + .1559 * X
GA wks
C

RV Ea VELOCITY
RV Ea (cm/sec)
Y = .9495 + .1793 * X
GA wks
B

LV Sa VELOCITY
LV Sa (cm/sec)
Y = 1.1631 + .1246 * X
GA wks
D

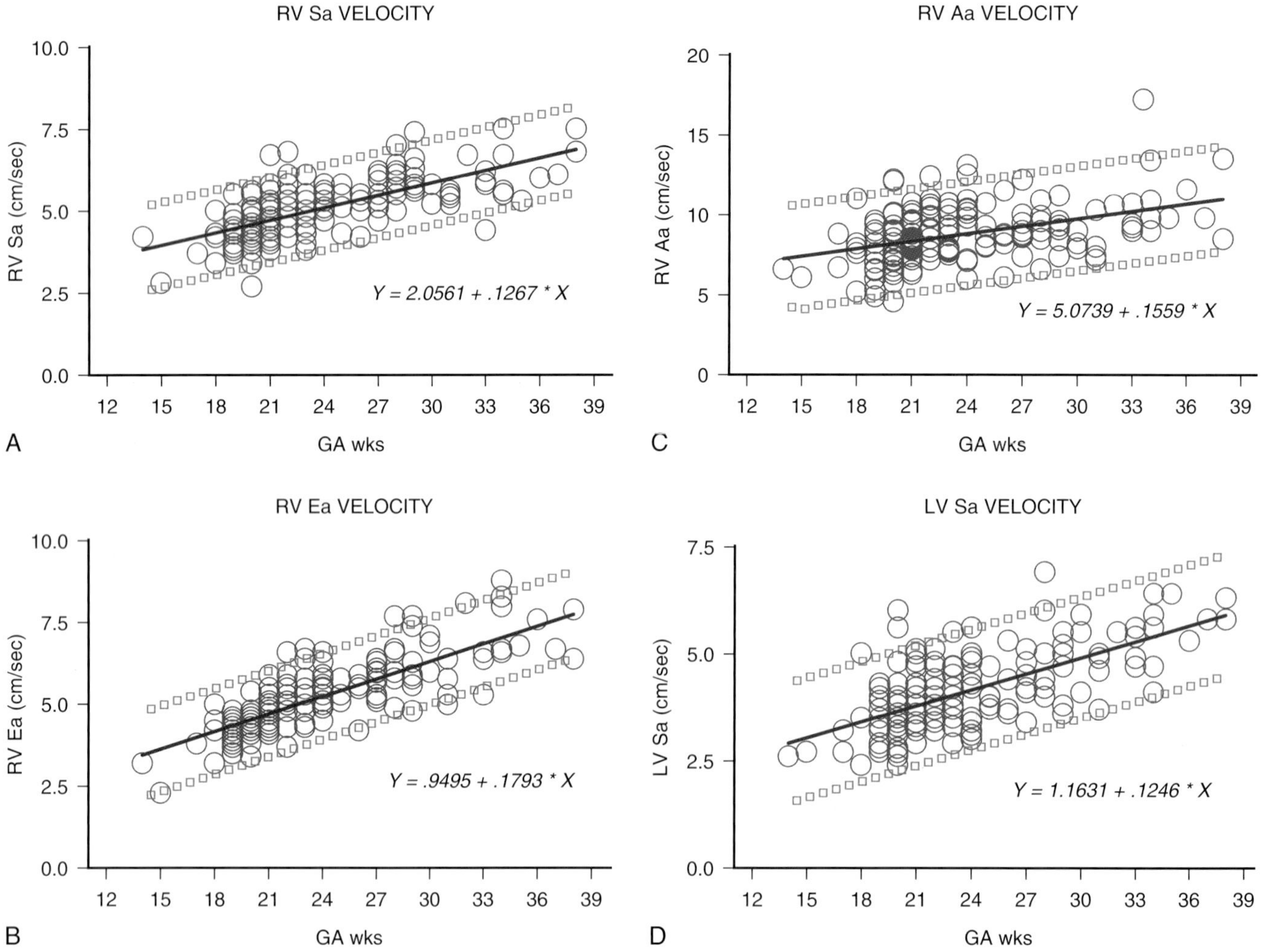

Figure 3-41. DTI velocities were acquired in 150 normal fetuses at the Fetal Heart Program at The Children's Hospital of Philadelphia and plotted against GA. RV signals were obtained from the RV free wall portion of the myocardium beneath the TV annulus. LV signals were obtained from the LV free wall portion of the myocardium just beneath the MV annulus. All velocities increased with GA. The *red line* depicts the average, and the *green dotted lines* are the 95% upper and lower confidence interval limits. **(A)** RV peak systolic (Sa) velocity versus GA. **(B)** RV peak early diastolic velocity versus GA. **(C)** RV peak late diastolic, atrial contraction velocity versus GA. **(D)** LV peak Sa velocity versus GA.

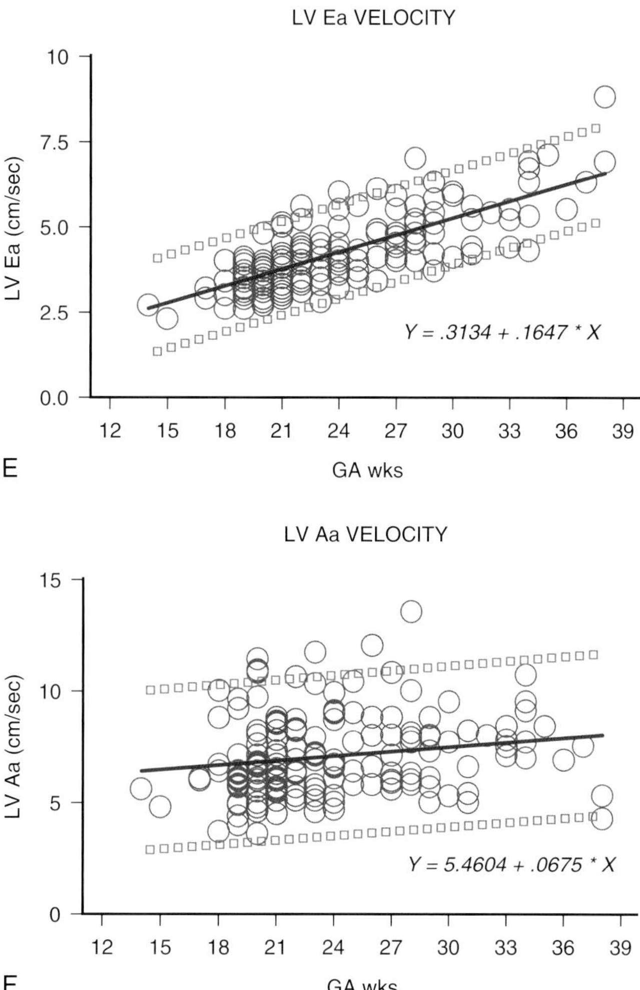

Figure 3-41, cont'd (**E**) LV peak early diastolic velocity versus GA. (**F**) LV peak late diastolic, atrial contraction velocity versus GA.

Ratio of Umbilical Artery—to–Middle Cerebral Artery Pulsatility Index

Distribution of blood flow in the fetus is dictated by relative resistance ratios of vascular circuits. The relative resistance ratio of placental flow (as reflected by the UA) to cerebral flow (as reflected by the MCA), or the UA-PI/MCA-PI ratio, is an important indicator of overall fetal wellness. In the healthy state, placental resistance is much lower than cerebrovascular resistance, UA-PI is lower than MCA-PI; hence, the ratio is normally less than 1.0.[41,42] This relationship and numerical ratio describes the fact that blood flow is preferentially directed toward the placenta in a healthy state. When a diseased state is present, adaptive mechanisms are triggered that increase blood flow to the vital organs such as the brain (Figure 3-44), which can be characterized by a change in the UA-PI/MCA-PI ratio.[42] When cerebrovascular resistance drops to a level that is lower than placental resistance (UA-PI/MCA-PI ratio > 1.0), a *steal* phenomenon may be present with greater impetus for blood to travel toward the head instead of the placenta. This process of change in distribution of blood flow is referred to as *cephalization*. It is important to realize that these indices reflect resistance and not flow, because it is expected that when resistance drops in a vascular bed, flow will increase to a significant degree. Hence, a UA-PI/MCA-PI ratio change suggests an attempt by regulatory systems to adapt to a new state and to improve flow. Such a response may or may not adequately compensate for a disease state with adequate restoration of perfusion. Nevertheless, the UA-PI/MCA-PI ratio change itself suggests an underlying need to adapt to a new condition that may be placing the fetus at risk, and hence, this ratio can be used as a marker for fetal unwellness.

The UA-PI/MCA-PI ratio may abnormally increase in conditions that increase the placental resistance or conditions that lower cerebrovascular resistance (Figure 3-45). Intrauterine growth restriction, abnormalities of placental cord insertion, or the twin-twin transfusion syndrome may increase the UA-PI and, hence, increase the UA-PI/MCA-PI ratio. Low cardiac outputs states due to ventricular dysfunction, cardiomyopathy, or arrhythmia can lower MCA-PI and, hence, increase the UA-PI/MCA-PI

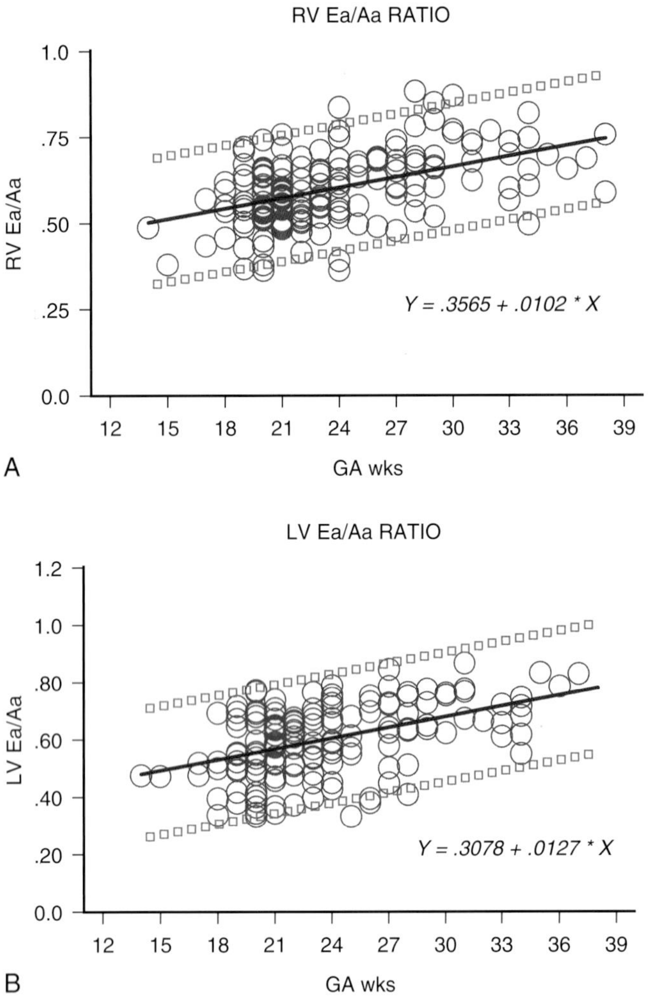

RV Ea/Aa RATIO

RV Ea/Aa

GA wks

Y = .3565 + .0102 * X

A

LV Ea/Aa RATIO

LV Ea/Aa

GA wks

Y = .3078 + .0127 * X

B

Figure 3-42. The ratio of DTI peak early diastolic (Ea wave) velocity to peak atrial contraction (Aa wave) velocity versus GA. Although Aa remains dominant throughout gestation, the ratio of RV Ea/Aa increases as GA increases. **(A)** RV Ea/Aa ratio versus GA. **(B)** LV Ea/Aa ratio versus GA.

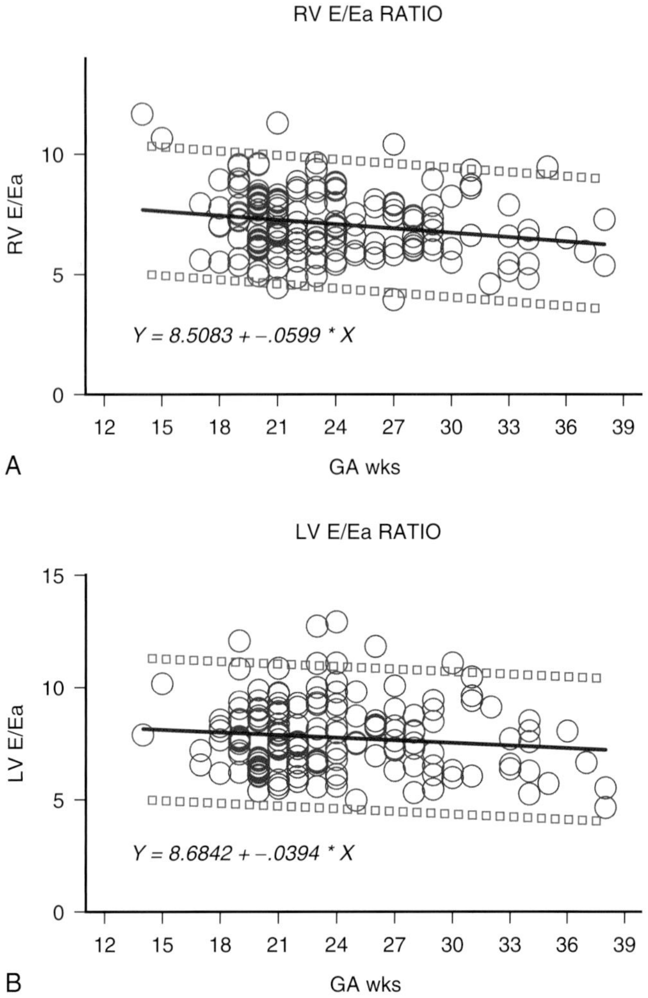

RV E/Ea RATIO

RV E/Ea

GA wks

Y = 8.5083 + -.0599 * X

A

LV E/Ea RATIO

LV E/Ea

GA wks

Y = 8.6842 + -.0394 * X

B

Figure 3-43. The ratio of early diastolic peak blood flow velocity to early diastolic myocardial motion peak velocity (E/Ea). The greater the E/Ea ratio, the higher the atrial filling pressure. The E/Ea decreases slightly throughout gestation. **(A)** RV E/Ea versus GA. **(B)** LV E/Ea versus GA.

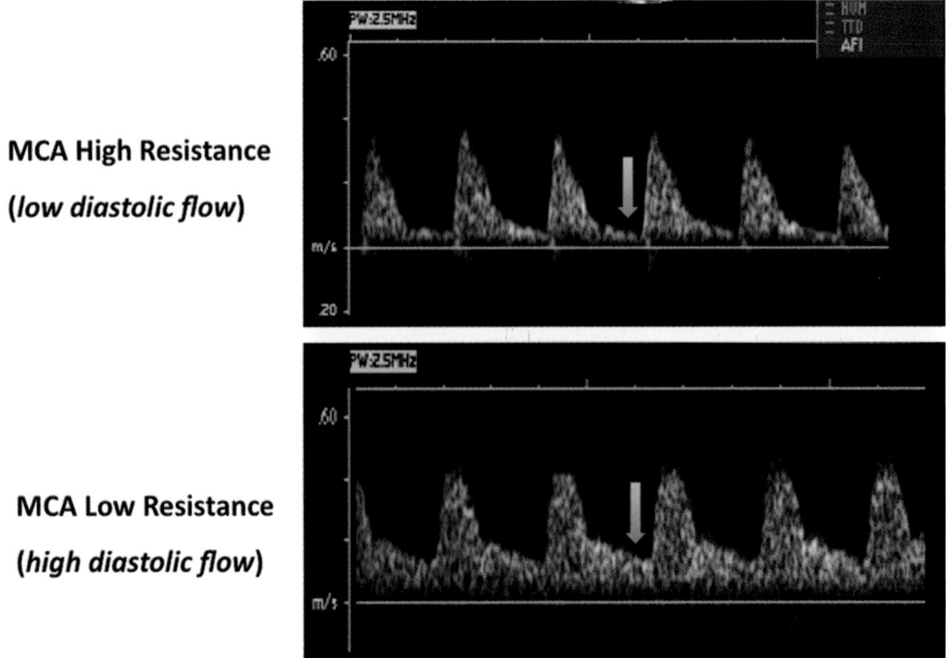

Figure 3-44. Doppler flow tracings of the MCA. **Top,** A normal flow pattern with high resistance in which there is low diastolic flow (*arrow*). **Bottom,** Increased diastolic flow (*arrow*) suggests low resistance and an attempt to increase perfusion.

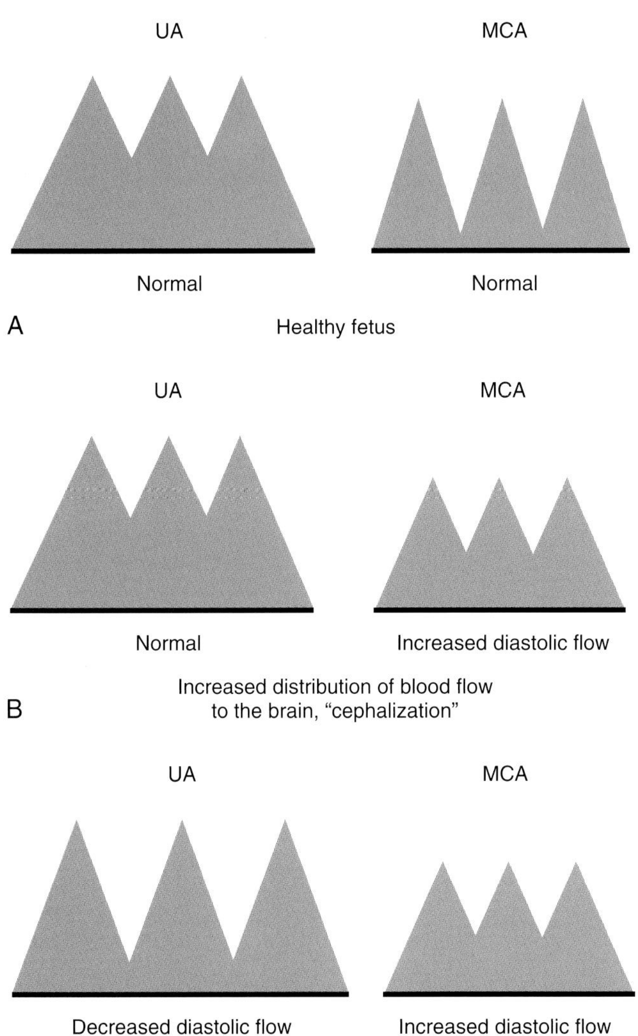

Figure 3-45. Pictorial display of the comparative appearance of Doppler flow patterns for the UA and MCA. A quick visual inspection of the appearance of the Doppler flow patterns from these two vascular beds, the relative size of the peaks of systolic flow and the valleys of diastolic flow, which can provide important information about fetal cardiovascular health. **(A)** In the normal, healthy state, UA diastolic flow is much higher than MCA diastolic flow, or the valleys of the MCA are much deeper than the valleys of the UA. **(B)** Under conditions of impaired cerebral blood flow and cerebral hypoxia such as in the low cardiac output state of cardiomyopathy or structural impediment to cerebral flow such as in aortic arch hypoplasia, the valleys of the UA and MCA appear equal with increased MCA diastolic flow. **(C)** In the fetus with placental insufficiency or intrauterine growth restriction, the UA valley is deeper than the MCA valley, which is consistent with an elevated UA resistance and a compensatory attempt to increase cerebral blood flow by lowering the MCA resistance.

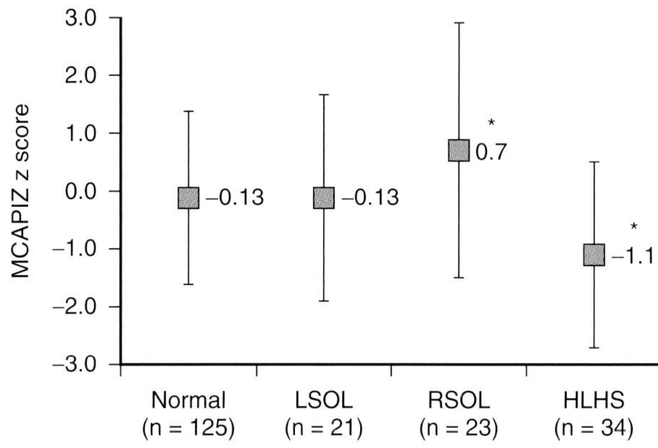

Figure 3-46. Graph of the Z-scores of MCA PI values and standard deviations for fetuses with completely normal anatomy (n = 125), left-sided obstructive lesions (LSOLs) but with two-ventricles (e.g., coarctation of the aorta) (n = 21), right-sided obstructive lesions (RSOLs) but with two ventricles (e.g., tetralogy of Fallot) (n = 23), and hypoplastic left heart syndrome (HLHS) in which flow in the aortic arch is reversed with perfusion retrograde from the ductus arteriosus (n = 34). Note, normal fetuses have a mean Z-score close to 0 (−0.13) as do the LSOLs (−0.13) but with a wider standard deviation. In these fetuses, blood flow patterns to the brain are undisturbed by the anatomy and a normal complement of blood flow is delivered to the carotid arteries. However, in the fetuses with RSOL, the mean MCA PI Z-score is 0.7, which is significantly higher than normal, and in the HLHS group, the mean PI Z-score is −1.1, which is significantly lower than normal. This can be explained in the following manner. In lesions such as tetralogy of Fallot, a greater complement of blood volume is shunted into the aorta, and hence, the carotid arteries carry the potential for a higher quantity of blood flow. The cerebrovasculature clamps down in order to increase resistance, regulate flow, and limit perfusion to a more normal degree of blood flow. Hence, the MCA PI values in such lesions are *higher* than normal. In contrast, in HLHS, because flow is retrograde from the DA through a hypoplastic arch, blood volume is shunted away from the aorta. Blood flow into the carotid arteries is potentially limited due to the structural anatomy. Hence, the cerebrovasculature relaxes in order to decrease resistance and increase perfusion to compensate for the anatomical limitations to flow. As a consequence, MCA PI values are significantly *lower* than normal ($^*P < 0.01$).

ratio. Serial follow-up of UA-PI/MCA-PI ratio can be helpful in monitoring the evolution of a particular disease or in assessing for response to therapy (i.e., if cardiac output improves in response to therapy or naturally over time, UA-PI/MCA-PI ratio can decrease or normalize to <1.0).

Congenital heart malformations alter the pathways in which blood flow reaches the cerebrovasculature influencing the MCA-PI, which may, therefore, form the foundation for an alteration in UA-PI/MCA-PI ratio.[43] In a study from our group, Kaltman and coworkers[43] compared the MCA-PI of fetuses with HLHS to fetuses with right-sided heart disease, fetuses with left-sided heart disease, and normal fetuses (Figure 3-46). The fetuses with HLHS had significantly lower MCA-PI values and the fetuses with right-sided congenital heart disease had significantly higher MCA-PI values in comparison with normal. This makes sense on a structural anatomical basis. Fetuses with HLHS have impaired antegrade flow and complete retrograde perfusion of a small aortic arch via the DA. This anatomical basis for limited cerebral blood flow promotes regulatory mechanisms that lead to attempts to increase flow through cerebral vasodilation, manifested as a decrease in the MCA-PI. Similarly, in fetuses with right-sided heart disease such as tricuspid atresia or pulmonary atresia, the entire cardiac output is diverted to the left side and all of the blood returning the heart is ejected into a large aorta. Hence, in order to protect the cerebral circulation from an inordinate amount of increased flow, regulatory mechanisms lead to an increase in cerebrovascular resistance, manifested as an increase in the MCA-PI (Figure 3-47). This phenomenon suggests that cardiac structural differences in the fetus with congenital heart disease have an important influence on the development of distal, extracardiac structures through alterations in blood flow perfusion patterns to the various organs.[44] The influence of these altered patterns of blood flow delivery on postnatal organ functionality, such as neurocognitive outcome, is yet to be fully investigated.

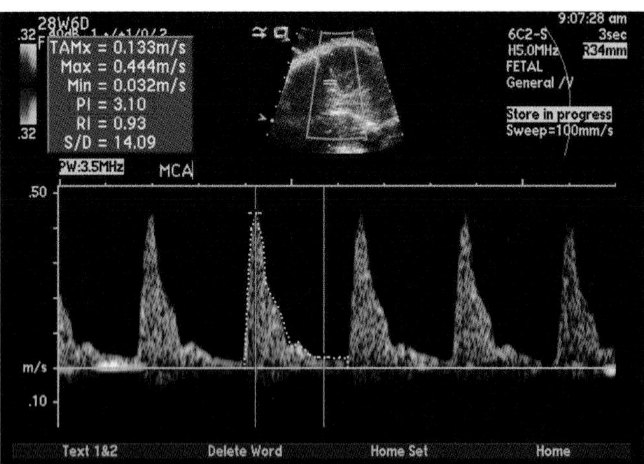

Figure 3-47. Doppler tracing of the MCA in a fetus with tetralogy of Fallot and severe pulmonary stenosis. Because all of the venous return makes its way into the aorta from both the RV and the LV, the amount of blood ejected into the aorta with every stroke is substantially higher than normal. Hence, the brain attempts to autoregulate flow by increasing resistance so as not to flood the brain with blood. This is manifested as an increased peak systolic velocity in relation to diastolic velocity and a very high PI. This phenomenon can be consistently found in the fetus with right-sided congenital heart disease and good cardiac output.

Pulmonary Vasoreactivity in Response to Maternal Hyperoxygenation

Doppler signals obtained form the fetal pulmonary artery are characteristically very "spiky" with a rapid upstroke, a short systolic time interval and no, or only a small degree of, diastolic flow (Figure 3-48). This reflects the normally elevated pulmonary vascular tone in the fetus, before the lungs expand with the first breath at birth. Investigators have found that, at the end of the second trimester and through the third trimester of pregnancy, the normal healthy fetal pulmonary vasculature will vasodilate in response to maternal hyperoxygenation.[45] This vasodilatory response is manifested as a decrease in the PI of the spectral pulmonary arterial flow tracing (Figure 3-49). Absence of vasodilation reflects abnormal pulmonary vasculature. Hence, the presence of pulmonary vasodilation can be assessed in fetuses at risk for abnormally pulmonary vasculature such as those with congenital diaphragmatic hernia[46] or hypoplastic left heart with intact atrial septum.[47]

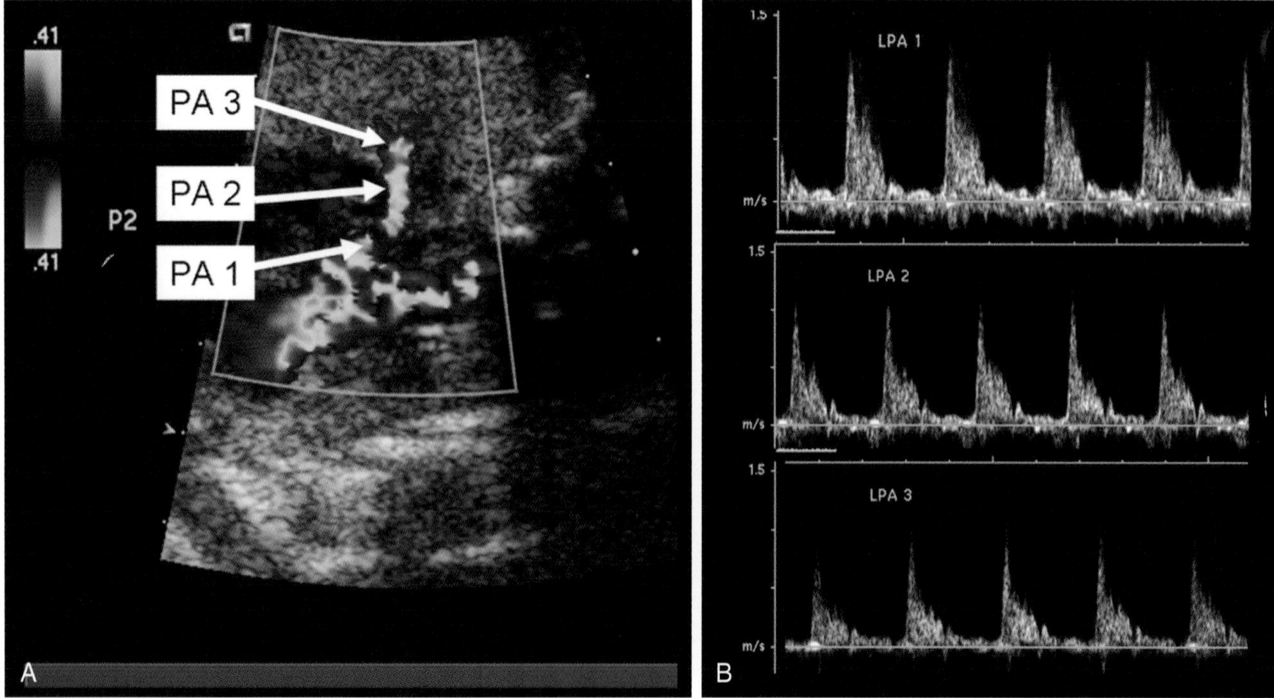

Figure 3-48. Color flow image of the MPA in a fetus with HLHS. **(A)** The branch RPA is isolated and three segments are identified: PA 1, the proximal branch take-off; PA 2, midportion of the pulmonary artery; and PA 3, the intraparenchymal portion of the RPA. Each site will manifest a slightly different Doppler flow pattern. **(B)** Doppler tracings from PA site 1, PA site 2, and PA site 3. Note that there is less diastolic flow and a narrower waveform as the Doppler sample is moved out from the proximal branch take-off (PA site 1) to the intraparenchymal position (PA site 3).

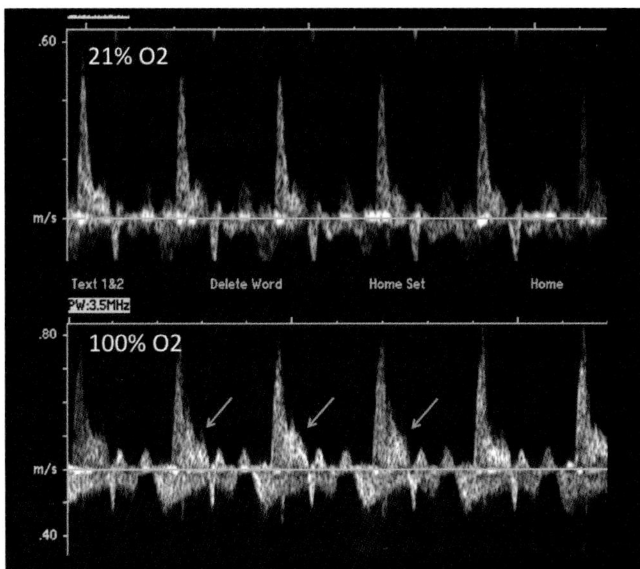

Figure 3-49. Change in the Doppler flow pattern in response to maternal hyperoxygenation, taken at PA site 3. **Top,** The waveform seen in room air (21% O_2), a very narrow rapid upstroke with a rapid downstroke. **Bottom,** The waveform seen after 20 minutes of maternal hyperoxygenation in 100% O_2. Note the broadening of the waveform *(arrows)* indicating a decrease in impedance and an increase in pulmonary artery blood flow.

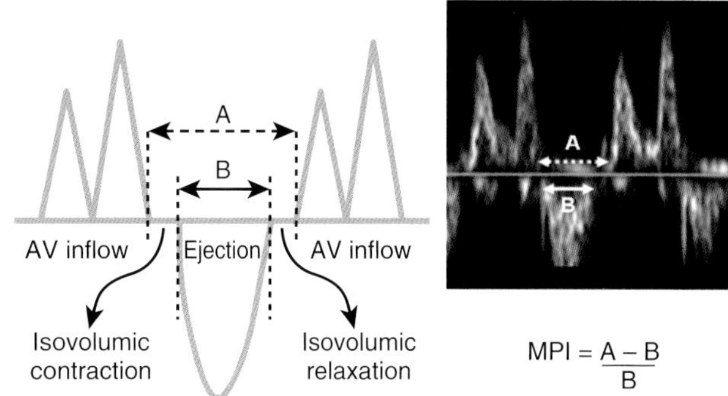

Figure 3-50. Myocardial performance index (MPI) is calculated as the time interval between atrioventricular (AV) valve closure to AV valve opening (time A) minus the ejection time across the semilunar valve (time B) divided by time B. This provides an index of the combined isovolumic contraction and isovolumic relaxation times in relation to the ejection time and can be thought of as a measure of ventricular efficiency and global myocardial performance.

Cardiac Function: Myocardial Performance Index

Analysis of Doppler-derived time intervals during the cardiac cycle can provide information that aids in understanding heart function. Tei and colleagues developed a useful measure called the *myocardial performance index (MPI)*, which is an index measure of global myocardial performance, inclusive of both systole and diastole. One of the benefits of the MPI is its independence from geometric assumptions because it is solely derived from flow parameters and not from changes in ventricular shape during the cardiac cycle. It can be used for the right ventricle, left ventricle, or single ventricle in various types of congenital heart disease.[48-52]

The MPI is obtained by measuring the time interval between AV valve closure and AV valve opening and measuring the ejection time derived from the flow signal across the semilunar valve arising from the ventricle of interest (Figure 3-50). The time interval between AV valve closure and opening includes the ejection time but also the time between AV valve closure and opening of the semilunar valve, or the isovolumic contraction time (ICT) and the time after semilunar valve closure but before AV valve opening, the isovolumic relaxation time (IRT). By subtracting the ejection time (value B) from the time interval between AV valve closure and opening (value A) one obtains the sum of both the ICT and the IRT. Indexing the *global* isovolumic time intervals of ICT and IRT to the ejection time (A – B/B) is the MPI. This simple formula is an intuitive method for measuring global myocardial function, because it is in essence the ratio of time for isovolumic activity in relation to ejection or volumic change. Isovolumic activity can be thought of as the time it takes for the ventricle to gird itself and prepare for ejection, and ejection time reflects cardiac output and perfusion. The shorter the isovolumic time and the greater the ejection time, the lower the MPI value, which reflects good global myocardial performance. Conversely, the longer the isovolumic time and the shorter the ejection time, the higher the MPI, and the worse the global myocardial performance.

When interested in the MPI of the left ventricle, a Doppler signal is obtained by placing the sample cursor at the junction of inflow and outflow in order to optimize a signal than can allow for measurement of AV valve time interval as well as ejection time interval within one tracing. This method is not possible for assessment of right ventricle MPI, because the pulmonary artery is too distant from the tricuspid inflow in order to obtain a simultaneous inflow and outflow signal. A separate signal reading must, therefore, be obtained from AV inflow and then semilunar valve outflow. Such can be achieved in a rapid, serial manner, and the values can be used so long as there are no significant changes in heart rate between the time the AV inflow signal and the outflow ejection signal are recorded. In order to get around this problem, some investigators have advocated the use of Doppler tissue signals in order to obtain the MPI, because this method provides both systolic and diastolic signals in the same tracing.

Normal values for the left and right ventricle MPI have been described. The fetal MPI remains essentially unchanged throughout gestation with perhaps a slight increase as gestation increases. In one series of 125 normal fetuses between 20 and 40 weeks; gestation, left ventricular MPI was 0.36 ± 0.06 and the right ventricular MPI was 0.35 ± 0.05.[48] In another large series of 557 fetuses between 19 and 39 weeks' gestation, left ventricular MPI was seen to increase slightly with MPI = 0.33 + 0.001 × gestational age in weeks.[49] As a general guideline in our laboratory, we have used an upper limit for normal right ventricular MPI of 0.45 and an upper limit of normal left ventricular MPI of 0.4 throughout gestation.

As for most of the various indices of myocardial function that exist, the values are load dependent and do not necessarily reflect inherent myocardial function in an independent manner. The MPI value is load dependent; as volume load increases, MPI increases. Nevertheless, it is a useful tool, which can be used in a serial evaluation of the fetus with impaired cardiovascular function.

Cardiac Function: Cardiac Output

Doppler techniques allow for the calculation of flow across a region of interest. Cardiac output of the left ventricle (LCO), right ventricle (RCO), and the fetal combined cardiac output (CCO) can be measured. CCO provides important information in lesions with high-output states, such as fetal anemia, AV malformations, and sacrococcygeal teratoma, and in low-output states, such as cardiomyopathy, heart block with bradycardia, and congenital cystic adenomatoid malformation in which ventricular volume filling is limited.[14]

Measurement of cross-sectional area (CSA) times the Doppler-derived velocity-time integral (VTI) of flow across the area of interest times the heart rate (HR) will provide the flow in mL/min (CO = CSA × VTI × HR). For assessment of RCO, flow across the tricuspid valve is possible; however, the pulmonary valve is the optimal site for assessment, because assumptions of shape and CSA can be more safely made. The diameter of the pulmonary valve is measured and divided by 2 to obtain the radius. Because the valve annulus can be assumed to be a circle, the CSA is 3.14 × (pulmonary valve radius)^2. The Doppler flow signal across the pulmonary valve is then traced to obtain the VTI. Time intervals between beats provide for the HR. The same can be done for the LCO by calculating the CSA of the aortic annulus and obtaining a Doppler flow signal across the aortic valve (Figure 3-51).

Care must be taken in calculating the Doppler-derived cardiac output because there are a number of potential pitfalls. First, any error in diameter measurement results in a compounded error in the derived flow because this value is squared in the CSA calculation. Second, the

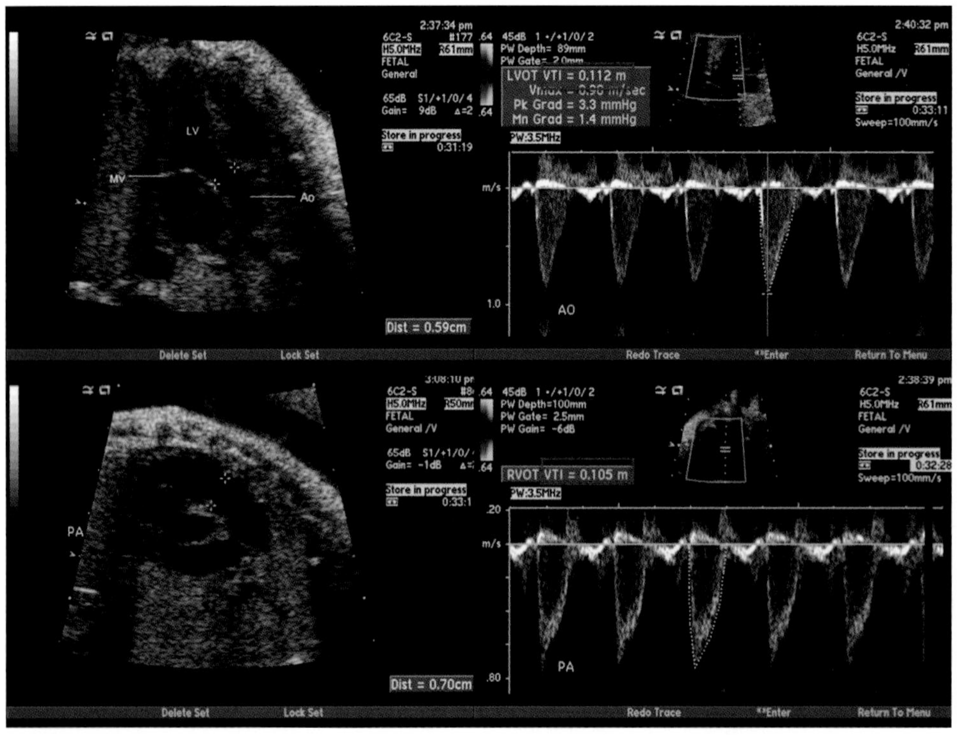

Figure 3-51. Calculation of combined cardiac output in this fetus with a normal cardiovascular system. The fetus is 32 weeks' gestation and the estimated fetal weight is 2.2 kg. **Top left,** The measurement of the aortic valve annulus. The annulus measures 0.59 cm; hence, the radius is 0.295 cm, and the aortic cross-sectional area is 3.14 × 0.295^2 = 0.273 cm^2. **Top right,** The Doppler tracing of flow across the aortic valve. The velocity-time integral (VTI) is 11.2 cm. The heart rate is 140 bpm. The left-sided cardiac output is the aortic cross-sectional area × heart rate × aortic VTI, which is 0.273 cm^2 × 140 bpm × 11.2 cm = 428 mL/min. Indexed to weight, the left-sided cardiac output is 195 mL/kg/min. **Bottom left,** The measurement of the pulmonary artery annulus. The annulus measures 0.70 cm; hence, the radius is 0.35 cm, and the pulmonic valve cross-sectional area is 3.14 × 0.35^2 = 0.385 cm^2. **Bottom right,** The Doppler tracing of flow across the pulmonic valve. The VTI is 10.5 cm. The right-sided cardiac output is the pulmonic cross-sectional area × heart rate × pulmonic VTI, which is 0.385 cm^2 × 140 bpm × 10.5 = 566 mL/min. Indexed to weight, the right-sided cardiac output is 257 mL/kg/min. The combined cardiac output is 452 mL/kg/min (normal), with the right side of the heart contributing 57% of flow and the left side of the heart contributing 43% of flow (normal ratio of flow).

Doppler signal must be obtained as best as possible "head-on" parallel to flow with little angle variation in order accurately reflect flow. Third, care must be taken in using consistent units; CSA should be calculated in centimeters and the VTI tracing result imported as centimeters, thus the cardiac output value will be provided as cubic centimeters, which is equivalent to milliliters, the desired unit. The volume per minute value is then indexed to the estimated fetal weight to provide for the desired value as milliliters per kilogram per minute (mL/kg/min) of flow.

Normal values for cardiac output have been reported.[53,54] RCO is normally higher than LCO, with the right-to-left proportion equal to approximately 60:40.[55] In our laboratory, a series of 76 normal fetuses at a mean gestational age of 26 ± 5 weeks' gestation had CCO of 477 ± 79 mL/kg/min. In a series of 212 normal fetuses between 18 and 41 weeks' gestation, average CCO was 400 mL/kg/min throughout. In general in our laboratory, we use a range of 400 to 500 mL/kg/min as the normal CCO throughout gestation beyond 18 weeks' gestation, with lower CCO of 300 to 400 mL/kg/min at less than 18 weeks' gestation.

Cardiac Function: Speckle Tracking and Myocardial Deformation Analysis

Investigators have started to look at fetal myocardial mechanics using the concept of *speckle tracking*. Each region of myocardial tissue has a unique ultrasound scatter pattern that can be identified and "tagged" as it moves through the cardiac cycle. As such, the relationship of movement of one region of myocardium to another can provide information on the *strain* and *strain rate* of the myocardium, where strain is the percent deformational change, and the strain rate is the rate of deformational change during either systole or diastole.[56,57] Strain [S(%)] is a unitless measure of percent change in deformation and is reported by convention as a negative value, reflecting contraction of the myocardium. Systolic strain rate [SRs(s^{-1})] is the rate of myocardial deformation during systole (contraction) and is similarly reported as a negative value, and diastolic strain rate [SRd(s^{-1})] is the rate of myocardial deformation during diastolic expansion and is, therefore, reported as a positive value.

Myocardial deformational analysis is currently still an investigational tool and is not yet readily used in clinical practice; however, it does provide for interesting new information and offers a number of benefits over conventional Doppler echocardiography. The software can be applied onto any previously acquired high-quality cine loop image, the method is relatively angle independent, and it is applicable regardless of geometry; hence, it is of value in assessing right ventricular function and the single ventricle of irregular geometry. Deformation of the myocardium can be analyzed in either a longitudinal, a radial, or a circumferential plane. Thus far, most of the investigational work in the fetal heart has been in looking at longitudinal strain acquired from cine loops of the four-chamber apical view. Software is available to look at specific regions of the myocardium; however, because

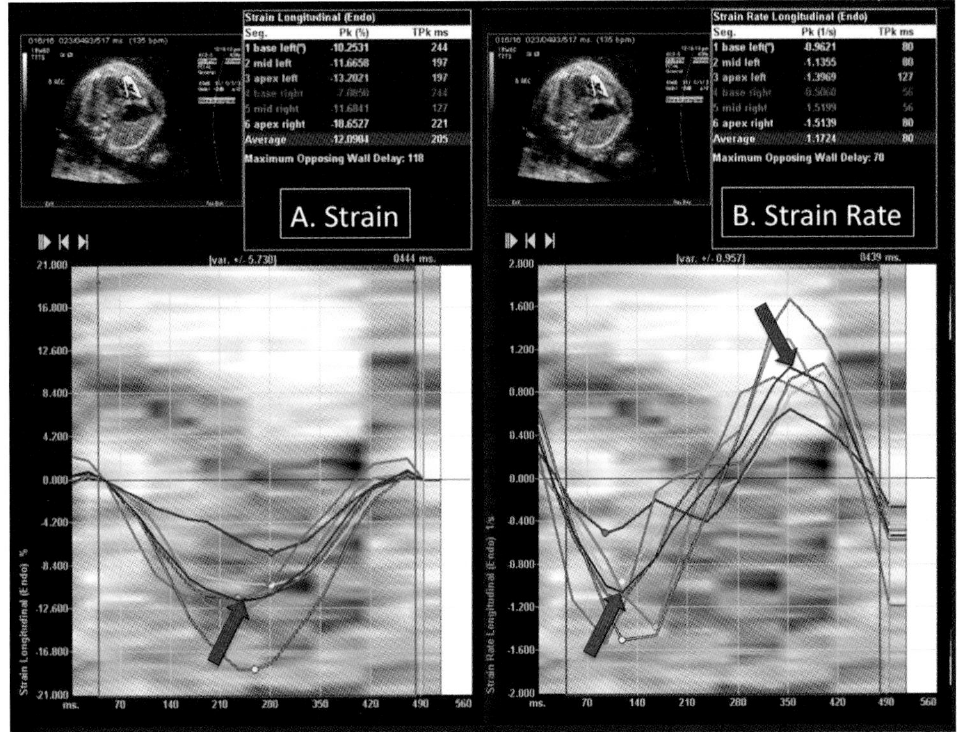

Figure 3-52. Myocardial deformation imaging analysis using vector velocity imaging software (Siemens). The endocardium is traced, and through speckle tracking techniques, longitudinal left and right ventricular myocardial deformation parameters of strain and strain rate can be generated. **Left,** Strain. **Right,** Strain rate. In this particular application, once the myocardial border is traced, the ventricular myocardium, RV or LV, is automatically divided into six segments (base left, mid left, apex left, base right, mid right, and apex right). The myocardial region is tagged and strain or strain rate curves for each segment are generated for the cardiac cycle. A summation, or average curve for all segments of the ventricle, is also generated and is seen as a black curve *(red arrow)*. The peak value for strain, systolic strain, or diastolic strain rate can be obtained and recorded. Myocardial deformation analysis is still currently an investigational tool to help understand complex pathophysiology. Strain is expressed as negative value percent; systolic strain rate as a negative value, and diastolic strain rate as a positive value.

CARDIOVASCULAR PROFILE SCORE (10 POINTS = NORMAL)

	Normal	−1 point	−2 points
Hydrops	None (2 pts)	Ascites *or* pleural effusion *or* pericardial effusion	Skin oedema
Venous Doppler (umbilical vein and ductus venosus)	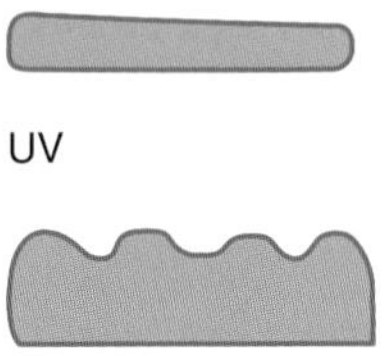 UV DV (2 pts)	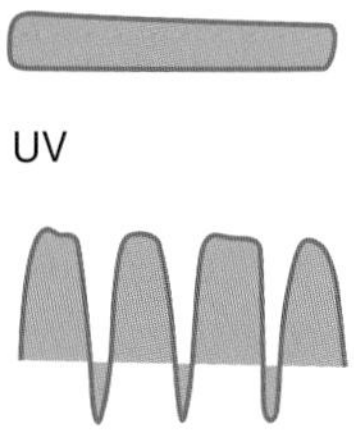 UV DV	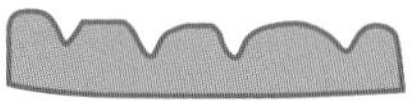 UV pulsations
Heart size (heart area/chest area)	>0.20 and <0.35 (2 pts)	0.35–0.50	>0.50 or <0.20
Cardiac function	Normal TV and MV RV/LV S.F. >0.28 Biphasic diastolic filling (2 pts)	Holosystolic TR *or* RV/LV S.F. <0.28	Holosystolic MR *or* TR dP/dt 400 *or* monophasic filling
Arterial Doppler (umbilical artery)	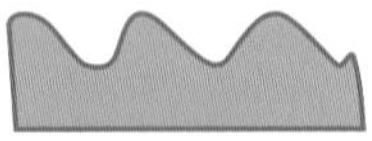 UA (2 pts)	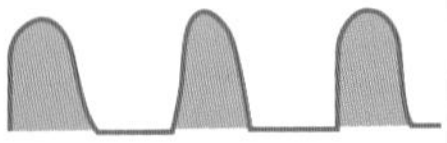 UA (AEDV)	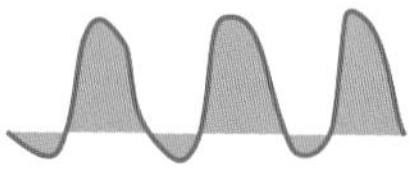 UA (REDV)

Figure 3-53. The cardiovascular profile score. MR, mitral regurgitation; TR, tricuspid regurgitation. (From Huhta JC. Fetal congestive heart failure. *Semin Fetal Neonatal Med.* 2005;10:542-552.)

the fetal heart dimensions are quite small relative to the mature adult heart, average longitudinal deformation analysis for the entire right ventricle or entire left ventricle provides for much greater reproducibility of data (Figure 3-52).[58,59]

Cardiac Function: The Cardiovascular Profile Score

A composite cardiovascular profile score (CPS) has been developed that combines a number of parameters into a comprehensive picture of the fetal cardiovascular status.[60] The five elements of the CPS are (1) presence or absence of hydrops, (2) assessment of venous Doppler of the umbilical vein and ductus venosus, (3) heart size, (4) heart function as determined by the ventricular shortening fraction (systolic function) or single- or double-peak inflow pattern (diastolic function), and (5) Doppler flow pattern within the UA (Figure 3-53). A score of 10 is achieved if each of the parameters are normal, with points deducted for various abnormalities present. The CPS provides a general overall sense of cardiovascular wellness, it has correlated with abnormal myocardial performance index values,[61] and it is a predictor of poor outcome in complex congenital heart disease and growth-restricted fetuses.[62]

Timing of Fetal Cardiovascular Imaging: The Early Scan

Obstetrical ultrasound is performed at a variety of levels of detail and scrutiny at various intervals. Current practice is to commonly perform a rudimentary ultrasound assessment of fetal number and size within the first trimester (<13 wk′ gestation). Evaluation of nuchal translucency is also now commonly performed at the first trimester. More detailed anatomical obstetrical ultrasound scans are undertaken in the mid-second trimester typically at 18 to 22 weeks' gestation. Fetal echocardiography and detailed assessment of the cardiovascular system is largely performed beyond 18 weeks' gestation only after suspicion has been raised by the second-trimester anatomical scan or through the presence of various risk factors. Yet, technological advances currently allow for ultrasound information concerning anatomy and functionality to be obtained as early as 11 to 13 weeks' gestation. A number of reports describe the accuracy of such early fetal cardiovascular imaging and its growing use.[63,64] The role early fetal cardiovascular scanning will play in the future is still evolving as it becomes clear that most of the aforementioned tools for assessment of the fetus can be reliably applied earlier in gestation, pushing back the time with which care and management can be offered.

References

1. Rychik J, Ayres N, Cuneo B, et al. American Society of Echocardiography guidelines and standards for performance of the fetal echocardiogram. *J Am Soc Echocardiogr*. 2004;17:803-10.
2. Lee W, Allan L, Carvalho JS, et al. ISUOG consensus statement: what constitutes a fetal echocardiogram? *Ultrasound Obstet Gynecol*. 2008;32:239-242.
3. Allan LD, Joseph MC, Boyd EG, Campbell S, Tynan M. M-mode echocardiography in the developing human fetus. *Br Heart J*. 1982; 47:573-583.
4. Yagel S, Arbel R, Anteby EY, Raveh D, Achiron R. The three vessels and trachea view (3VT) in fetal cardiac scanning. *Ultrasound Obstet Gynecol*. 2002;20:340-345.
5. Zalel Y, Wiener Y, Gamzu R, Herman A, Schiff E, Achiron R. The three-vessel and tracheal view of the fetal heart: an in utero sonographic evaluation. *Prenat Diagn*. 2004;24:174-178.
6. Borenstein M, Minekawa R, Zidere V, Nicolaides KH, Allan LD. Aberrant right subclavian artery at 16 to 23 + 6 weeks of gestation: a marker for chromosomal abnormality. *Ultrasound Obstet Gynecol*. 2010;36:548-52.
7. Barrea C, Yoo SJ, Chitayat D, et al. Assessment of the thymus at echocardiography in fetuses at risk for 22q11.2 deletion. *Prenat Diagn*. 2003;23:9-15.
8. Tan J, Silverman NH, Hoffman JI, Villegas M, Schmidt KG. Cardiac dimensions determined by cross-sectional echocardiography in the normal human fetus from 18 weeks to term. *Am J Cardiol*. 1992; 70:1459-1467.
9. Firpo C, Hoffman JI, Silverman NH. Evaluation of fetal heart dimensions from 12 weeks to term. *Am J Cardiol*. 2001;87:594-600.
10. Steed RD, Strickland DM, Swanson MS, et al. Normal fetal cardiac dimensions obtained by perpendicular imaging. *Am J Cardiol*. 1998;81:1059-1062.
11. Schneider C, McCrindle BW, Carvalho JS, Hornberger LK, McCarthy KP, Daubeney PE. Development of Z-scores for fetal cardiac dimensions from echocardiography. *Ultrasound Obstet Gynecol*. 2005;26: 599-605.
12. Lee W, Riggs T, Amula V, et al. Fetal echocardiography: Z-score reference ranges for a large patient population. *Ultrasound Obstet Gynecol*. 2010;35:28-34.
13. Hecher K, Campbell S, Doyle P, Harrington K, Nicolaides K. Assessment of fetal compromise by Doppler ultrasound investigation of the fetal circulation. Arterial, intracardiac, and venous blood flow velocity studies. *Circulation*. 1995;91:129-138.
14. Rychik J. Fetal cardiovascular physiology. *Pediatr Cardiol*. 2004; 25:201-209.
15. Szwast A, Rychik J. Current concepts in fetal cardiovascular disease. *Clin Perinatol*. 2005;32:857-875, viii.
16. Kiserud T, Eik-Nes SH, Blaas HG, Hellevik LR. Ultrasonographic velocimetry of the fetal ductus venosus. *Lancet*. 1991;338:1412-1414.
17. Kiserud T. In a different vein: the ductus venosus could yield much valuable information. *Ultrasound Obstet Gynecol*. 1997;9:369-372.
18. Kiserud T. The ductus venosus. *Semin Perinatol*. 2001;25:11-20.
19. Kessler J, Rasmussen S, Hanson M, Kiserud T. Longitudinal reference ranges for ductus venosus flow velocities and waveform indices. *Ultrasound Obstet Gynecol*. 2006;28:890-898.
20. Tchirikov M, Schroder HJ, Hecher K. Ductus venosus shunting in the fetal venous circulation: regulatory mechanisms, diagnostic methods and medical importance. *Ultrasound Obstet Gynecol*. 2006; 27:452-461.
21. Kiserud T, Kessler J, Ebbing C, Rasmussen S. Ductus venosus shunting in growth-restricted fetuses and the effect of umbilical circulatory compromise. *Ultrasound Obstet Gynecol*. 2006;28: 143-149.
22. Baschat AA, Harman CR. Venous Doppler in the assessment of fetal cardiovascular status. *Curr Opin Obstet Gynecol*. 2006;18:156-163.
23. Arduini D, Rizzo G. Normal values of pulsatility index from fetal vessels: a cross-sectional study on 1556 healthy fetuses. *J Perinat Med*. 1990;18:165-172.
24. Meise C, Germer U, Gembruch U. Arterial Doppler ultrasound in 115 second- and third-trimester fetuses with congenital heart disease. *Ultrasound Obstet Gynecol*. 2001;17:398-402.
25. Harman CR, Baschat AA. Comprehensive assessment of fetal well-being: which Doppler tests should be performed? *Curr Opin Obstet Gynecol*. 2003;15:147-157.
26. Mari G, Hanif F. Fetal Doppler: umbilical artery, middle cerebral artery, and venous system. *Semin Perinatol*. 2008;32:253-257.
27. Sciscione AC, Hayes EJ. Uterine artery Doppler flow studies in obstetric practice. *Am J Obstet Gynecol*. 2009;201:121-126.
28. Smith GC, Yu CK, Papageorghiou AT, Cacho AM, Nicolaides KH. Maternal uterine artery Doppler flow velocimetry and the risk of stillbirth. *Obstet Gynecol*. 2007;109:144-151.
29. Dugoff L, Lynch AM, Cioffi-Ragan D, et al. First trimester uterine artery Doppler abnormalities predict subsequent intrauterine growth restriction. *Am J Obstet Gynecol*. 2005;193:1208-1212.
30. Mielke G, Benda N. Blood flow velocity waveforms of the fetal pulmonary artery and the ductus arteriosus: reference ranges from 13 weeks to term. *Ultrasound Obstet Gynecol*. 2000;15:213-218.
31. Fouron JC. The unrecognized physiological and clinical significance of the fetal aortic isthmus. *Ultrasound Obstet Gynecol*. 2003;22: 441-447.
32. Sonesson SE, Fouron JC. Doppler velocimetry of the aortic isthmus in human fetuses with abnormal velocity waveforms in the umbilical artery. *Ultrasound Obstet Gynecol*. 1997;10:107-111.
33. Fouron JC, Gosselin J, Amiel-Tison C, et al. Correlation between prenatal velocity waveforms in the aortic isthmus and neurodevelopmental outcome between the ages of 2 and 4 years. *Am J Obstet Gynecol*. 2001;184:630-636.
34. Lenz F, Chaoui R. Reference ranges for Doppler-assessed pulmonary venous blood flow velocities and pulsatility indices in normal human fetuses. *Prenat Diagn*. 2002;22:786-791.
35. Lenz F, Chaoui R. Changes in pulmonary venous Doppler parameters in fetal cardiac defects. *Ultrasound Obstet Gynecol*. 2006;28: 63-70.
36. Chintala K, Tian Z, Du W, Donaghue D, Rychik J. Fetal pulmonary venous Doppler patterns in hypoplastic left heart syndrome: relationship to atrial septal restriction. *Heart*. 2008;94:1446-1449.
37. Nii M, Roman KS, Kingdom J, Redington AN, Jaeggi ET. Assessment of the evolution of normal fetal diastolic function during mid and late gestation by spectral Doppler tissue echocardiography. *J Am Soc Echocardiogr*. 2006;19:1431-1437.
38. Gardiner HM, Pasquini L, Wolfenden J, et al. Myocardial tissue Doppler and long axis function in the fetal heart. *Int J Cardiol*. 2006;113:39-47.
39. Aoki M, Harada K, Ogawa M, Tanaka T. Quantitative assessment of right ventricular function using Doppler tissue imaging in fetuses with and without heart failure. *J Am Soc Echocardiogr*. 2004;17: 28-35.
40. Rein AJ, O'Donnell C, Geva T, et al. Use of tissue velocity imaging in the diagnosis of fetal cardiac arrhythmias. *Circulation*. 2002; 106:1827-1833.
41. Baschat AA, Gembruch U. The cerebroplacental Doppler ratio revisited. *Ultrasound Obstet Gynecol*. 2003;21:124-127.
42. Ebbing C, Rasmussen S, Kiserud T. Middle cerebral artery blood flow velocities and pulsatility index and the cerebroplacental

pulsatility ratio: longitudinal reference ranges and terms for serial measurements. *Ultrasound Obstet Gynecol*. 2007;30:287-296.
43. Kaltman JR, Di H, Tian Z, Rychik J. Impact of congenital heart disease on cerebrovascular blood flow dynamics in the fetus. *Ultrasound Obstet Gynecol*. 2005;25:32-36.
44. Guorong L, Shaohui L, Peng J, et al. Cerebrovascular blood flow dynamic changes in fetuses with congenital heart disease. *Fetal Diagn Ther*. 2009;25:167-172.
45. Rasanen J, Wood DC, Debbs RH, Cohen J, Weiner S, Huhta JC. Reactivity of the human fetal pulmonary circulation to maternal hyperoxygenation increases during the second half of pregnancy: a randomized study. *Circulation*. 1998;97:257-262.
46. Done E, Allegaert K, Lewi P, et al. Maternal hyperoxygenation test in fetuses undergoing FETO for severe isolated congenital diaphragmatic hernia. *Ultrasound Obstet Gynecol*. 2011;37:264-271.
47. Szwast A, Tian Z, McCann M, Donaghue D, Rychik J. Vasoreactive response to maternal hyperoxygenation in the fetus with hypoplastic left heart syndrome. *Circ Cardiovasc Imaging*. 2010;3:172-178.
48. Eidem BW, Edwards JM, Cetta F. Quantitative assessment of fetal ventricular function: establishing normal values of the myocardial performance index in the fetus. *Echocardiography*. 2001;18:9-13.
49. Hernandez-Andrade E, Figueroa-Diesel H, Kottman C, et al. Gestational-age-adjusted reference values for the modified myocardial performance index for evaluation of fetal left cardiac function. *Ultrasound Obstet Gynecol*. 2007;29:321-325.
50. Friedman D, Buyon J, Kim M, Glickstein JS. Fetal cardiac function assessed by Doppler myocardial performance index (Tei index). *Ultrasound Obstet Gynecol*. 2003;21:33-36.
51. Szwast A, Tian Z, McCann M, et al. Impact of altered loading conditions on ventricular performance in fetuses with congenital cystic adenomatoid malformation and twin-twin transfusion syndrome. *Ultrasound Obstet Gynecol*. 2007;30:40-46.
52. Szwast A, Tian Z, McCann M, Donaghue D, Rychik J. Right ventricular performance in the fetus with hypoplastic left heart syndrome. *Ann Thorac Surg*. 2009;87:1214-1219.
53. Vimpeli T, Huhtala H, Wilsgaard T, Acharya G. Fetal cardiac output and its distribution to the placenta at 11-20 weeks of gestation. *Ultrasound Obstet Gynecol*. 2009;33:265-271.
54. Kiserud T, Ebbing C, Kessler J, Rasmussen S. Fetal cardiac output, distribution to the placenta and impact of placental compromise. *Ultrasound Obstet Gynecol*. 2006;28:126-136.
55. Mielke G, Benda N. Cardiac output and central distribution of blood flow in the human fetus. *Circulation*. 2001;103:1662-1668.
56. Younoszai AK, Saudek DE, Emery SP, Thomas JD. Evaluation of myocardial mechanics in the fetus by velocity vector imaging. *J Am Soc Echocardiogr*. 2008;21:470-474.
57. Di Salvo G, Russo MG, Paladini D, et al. Two-dimensional strain to assess regional left and right ventricular longitudinal function in 100 normal foetuses. *Eur J Echocardiogr*. 2008;9:754-756.
58. Peng QH, Zhou QC, Zeng S, et al. Evaluation of regional left ventricular longitudinal function in 151 normal fetuses using velocity vector imaging. *Prenat Diagn*. 2009;29:1149-1155.
59. Pu DR, Zhou QC, Zhang M, Peng QH, Zeng S, Xu GQ. Assessment of regional right ventricular longitudinal functions in fetus using velocity vector imaging technology. *Prenat Diagn*. 2010;30:1057-1063.
60. Huhta JC. Fetal congestive heart failure. *Semin Fetal Neonatal Med*. 2005;10:542-552.
61. Falkensammer CB, Paul J, Huhta JC. Fetal congestive heart failure: correlation of Tei-index and cardiovascular-score. *J Perinat Med*. 2001;29:390-398.
62. Makikallio K, Rasanen J, Makikallio T, Vuolteenaho O, Huhta JC. Human fetal cardiovascular profile score and neonatal outcome in intrauterine growth restriction. *Ultrasound Obstet Gynecol*. 2008;31:48-54.
63. McAuliffe FM, Trines J, Nield LE, Chitayat D, Jaeggi E, Hornberger LK. Early fetal echocardiography—a reliable prenatal diagnosis tool. *Am J Obstet Gynecol*. 2005;193:1253-1259.
64. Carvalho JS. Fetal heart scanning in the first trimester. *Prenat Diagn*. 2004;24:1060-1067.

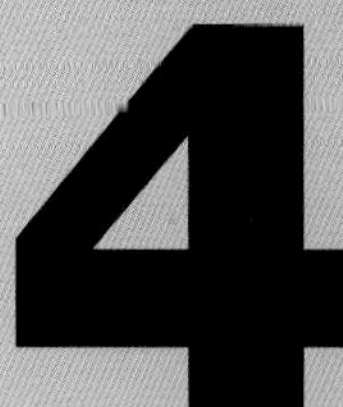

Three- and Four-Dimensional Imaging in Fetal Echocardiography

Simcha Yagel, Sarah M. Cohen, and Ori Shen

Introduction

Recent years have seen an ever-burgeoning literature based on three-dimensional ultrasonography (3DUS) of the fetus. 3DUS of the fetal heart presented particular challenges, related to the difficulties of imaging a moving object in three dimensions. With improvements in technology and data processing came methods of gating and image correlation that meet these challenges and allow near–real-time 3DUS of the fetal heart. Spatiotemporal image correlation (STIC) technology, introduced in 2003, adds the fourth dimension (time). Today, it is customary to refer collectively to 3D/4DUS of the fetal heart, encompassing the many combinations of acquisition and post-processing modalities and techniques available.

In this chapter, we describe these techniques briefly (with minimal technical information: the interested reader will refer to technical materials supplied by the vendor), beginning with the acquisition modalities and continuing with post-processing modalities; then moving on to their practical application, including traps and pitfalls to avoid; and finally, when and where various methods are most useful in the work of fetal echocardiography.

The International Society of Ultrasound in Obstetrics and Gynecology (ISUOG) has published guidelines for the performance of the "basic" and "extended basic" fetal cardiac scan.[1] These guidelines include all the cardiac parameters necessary for complete fetal echocardiography. The sequential segmental approach to fetal cardiology divides the heart into three basic segments, the atria, ventricles, and great arteries.[2] These are interfaced by the atrioventricular valves and the ventriculoarterial junctions. By applying the five planes of fetal echocardiography methodology,[3,4] which is based on a 2DUS sweep from the fetal upper abdomen to the upper mediastinum, five short-axis planes of the fetal heart are visualized that provide the examiner with all the elements of the heart as described by the sequential segmental approach[2] and include all the parameters cited by the ISUOG guidelines.[1]

Volume Acquisition

3D/4DUS scans are based on a volume block of data made up of numerous voxels (volume display units [volume pixels]). Once acquired and saved, this block of data is available for manipulation and analysis. Some displays are available almost immediately and can be viewed with the patient still present, whereas others require considerable time and effort and are usually achieved after the patient is dismissed.

Spatiotemporal Image Correlation

STIC acquisition is the mainstay of 3D/4DUS of the fetal heart. The modality has been extensively described and numerous publications have been based on its use. STIC is an indirect, offline, motion-gated scanning mode. The operator scans the region of interest in a sweep (in the fetal heart, this would be a sweep beginning just caudal to the four-chamber view and then moving cephalad to the upper mediastinum). The array in the transducer makes this automated volume acquisition possible. The array performs a single slow sweep of 7.5 to approximately 30 seconds, for a sweep angle of 20 to 40 degrees (depending on the size of the fetus) and a frame rate of up to 150 frames/sec. An acquisition of 10 seconds and 25 degrees, therefore, would include approximately 1500 sequential B-mode images. Following this acquisition sweep, the STIC program uses mathematical algorithms to process the volume data. It identifies the systolic peaks that will be used to calculate the fetal heart rate. These peaks then act as triggers for correlation of the spatial and temporal position of each B-mode image. STIC acquisition is designed to mimic the traditional abdomen-to-mediastinum sweep of 2DUS, and a well-executed and acquired STIC volume will contain all five short-axis planes of fetal echocardiography[3,4] and all the data necessary for fetal cardiac examination as set out by the ISUOG guidelines[1]. In practice, owing to fetal breathing movements and other sources of interference, two or more acquisitions are usually required for a complete heart scan.

B-Flow

B-Flow is an ultrasound technology that images blood flowing in its vessels, without relying on Doppler shift. B-Flow is made possible by the digital encoding of one ultrasound beam into two sub-beams: one beam provides structural B-mode display and the other contains B-mode flow display of blood flow and part of the lumen. This flow display is enhanced to make up for the weak signal from blood cell reflectors. B-Flow uses faster frame rates than Doppler flow mapping and provides better spatial resolution.[5] Because it is not based on Doppler shift, B-flow is angle-independent and avoids image drop-out at orthogonal scanning angles. The greater sensitivity of B-flow makes it an excellent tool for the measurement of blood vessel dimensions.[6] When B-flow is used in tandem with STIC to image the fetal heart, the threshold is set high to eliminate the surrounding tissue and show the enhanced, high-intensity B-flow signal. The result is a 3D moving impression of blood flowing in the heart and great vessels that we have found remarkably sensitive for imaging the normal heart as well as great vessels anomalies such as transposition of the great arteries and others[7-9] (Figure 4-1).

Doppler Applications

Doppler applications, color Doppler, power Doppler, and high-definition power flow Doppler (HDPD) have been used extensively in combination with 3D/4DUS.[10-15] Static 3DUS acquisition is preferable for use with

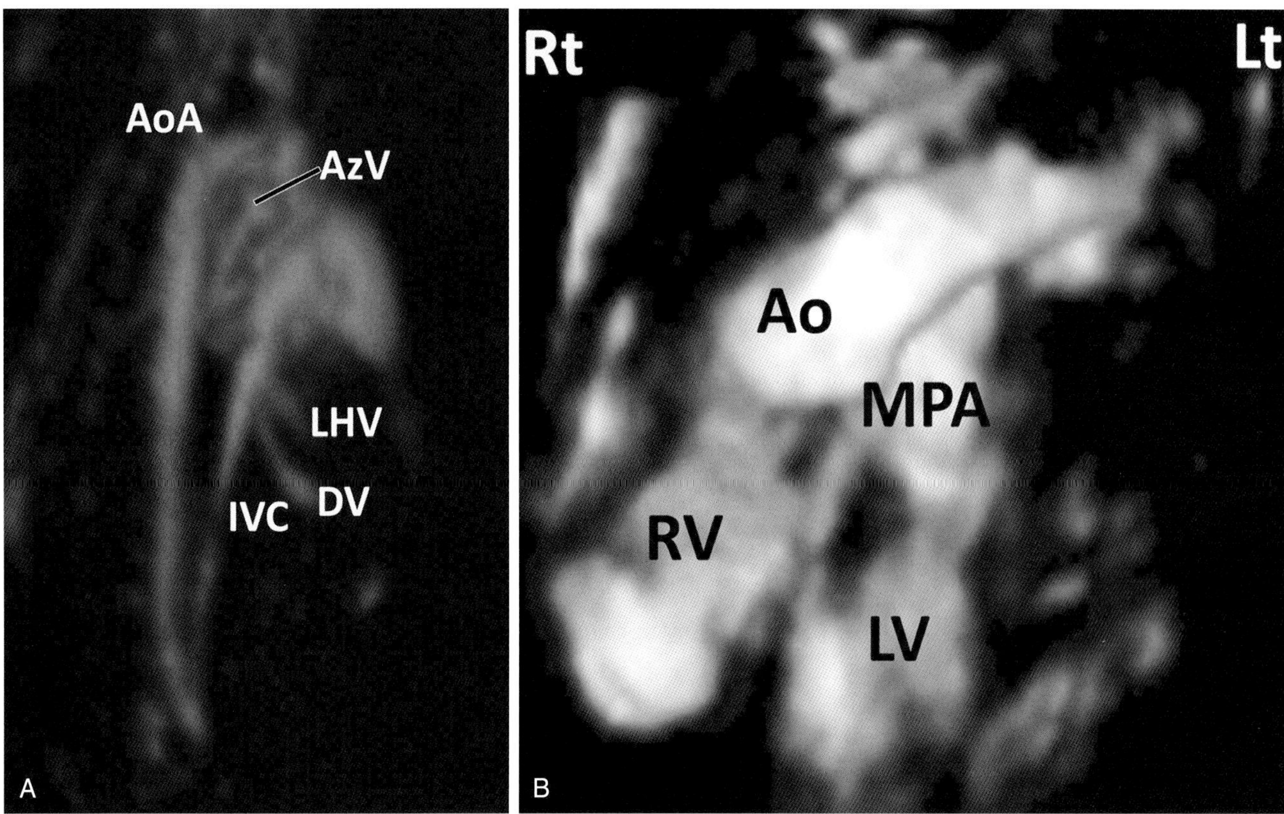

Figure 4-1. **(A)** The normal heart and great vessels imaged in B-flow. This volume was acquired with spatiotemporal image correlation (STIC) with B-flow activated. This view shows heart and aortic arch (AoA), azygos vein (AzV), and the inferior vena cava (IVC) as well as the left hepatic vein (LHV) and ductus venosus (DV). Compare with **B.** **(B)** A case of transposition of the great arteries imaged in B-flow. This volume was also obtained with STIC and B-flow and shows the right (RV) and left (LV) ventricles with the aorta (Ao) and main pulmonary artery (MPA) transposed in a crossover formation.

three-dimensional power Doppler (3DPD),[11,13] and STIC acquisition can be combined with color Doppler or with HDPD.[10,14] HDPD is a bidirectional color Doppler mode that operates at lower velocity than either standard color Doppler or power Doppler. But whereas power Doppler is unidirectional, HDPD has the added advantage of directionality. Its greater sensitivity provides a cleaner image with less blooming of color beyond vessel walls than in regular or power Doppler (Figure 4-2).[14]

Post-processing Applications

Once the volume block has been acquired and stored to the ultrasound machine, it is available for extensive manipulation and analysis in post-processing. Each application allows manipulation of different aspects of the volume data; the applications can also be combined sequentially to a given saved volume to extract biometric and functional parameters.

Multiplanar Reconstruction

In order to analyze the acquired volume block effectively, it is necessary to "slice" it into two-dimensional planes. The multiplanar reconstruction (MPR) application displays three orthogonal planes from the volume and allows the operator to navigate within the volume along three axes. The point of intersection of all three planes is anchored at a navigation dot that assists the operator in orientation within the volume (Figure 4-3A).[16] In the case of stored STIC volumes, which contain temporal information, it is also possible to scroll forward and backward in time and to review the beating heart in a virtual cine loop of the heart cycle.

Three-Dimensional Rendering

3D rendering is familiar from surface-rendered images of the fetal face, body, and limbs. When applied to the fetal heart, 3D rendering is applied to the MPR display in post-processing. Once the desired plane is achieved in MPR display, a bounding box is placed around the region of interest and the rendered image is shown in the fourth frame of the display (see Figure 4-3B).[16] The rendered image has the advantage of including depth, which reflects the thickness of the slice through the volume (i.e., the width of the bounding box). For example, when applied to imaging the interventricular septum, the characteristic trabeculations of the right ventricle are clearly seen.[17,18] If the original acquisition was combined with STIC and/or color Doppler, these parameters are available in the rendered image.

Tomographic Ultrasound Imaging

Whereas MPR displays three orthogonal planes of a volume, and 3D rendering adds depth to one selected plane from the MPR display, tomographic ultrasound imaging (TUI) allows for the display of a matrix of sequential parallel planes. This capability shows the reference plane at the center of the matrix, with its adjacent slices arranged in order around it. The number of slices displayed and the distance between them are set by the operator. This capability has been applied to fetal echocardiography[19] in normal and anomalous hearts and allows the display of some or all of the five planes of fetal echocardiography simultaneously (Figure 4-4).[14] As is the case with MPR and rendering, when STIC acquisition is used, temporal information is available in the TUI display and, if combined with Doppler mapping, color will be available.

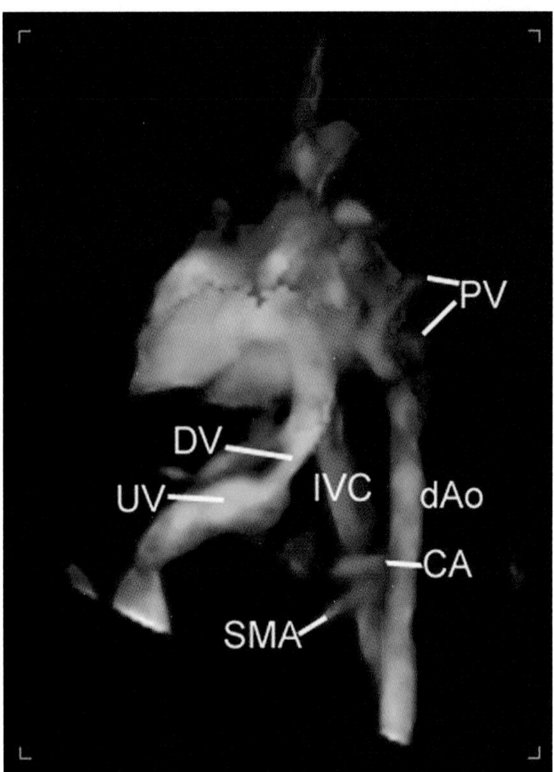

Figure 4-2. The fetal heart and vessels imaged in a volume acquired with STIC and high-definition power flow Doppler (HDPD). The umbilical vein (UV), ductus venosus (DV), superior mesenteric artery (SMA), celiac artery (CA), and pulmonary veins (PVs) are shown in addition to the inferior vena cava (IVC) and descending aorta (dAo). (Reproduced with permission from Yagel S, Cohen SM, Shapiro I, Valsky DV. 3D and 4D ultrasound in fetal cardiac scanning: a new look at the fetal heart. *Ultrasound Obstet Gynecol.* 2007;29:81-95.)

Virtual Organ Computer-Aided Analysis

Virtual organ computer-aided analysis (VOCAL) is used in post-processing to measure the volume of a target organ. The application performs a rotational measurement of volume as the dataset is rotated 180 degrees around a fixed central axis through a preset number of rotation steps based on the angle of rotation (i.e., 6 steps of rotation 30 degrees apart, for example, in the case of a regular-shaped object, or 12 steps 15 degrees apart, where necessary). Thus, the contours are traced manually or automatically at each plane in sequence, and the system reconstructs a contour model and provides a volume measurement.

Inversion Mode

Inversion mode (IM), as its name implies, is a post-processing application that inverts the color of acquired voxels so that echogenic (solid) areas are displayed in black, and fluid-filled areas are displayed in gray. This modality has been applied to the fetal heart to create "digital casts" of the fetal heart ventricles and great vessels[20]; however, B-flow is more effective for this purpose.

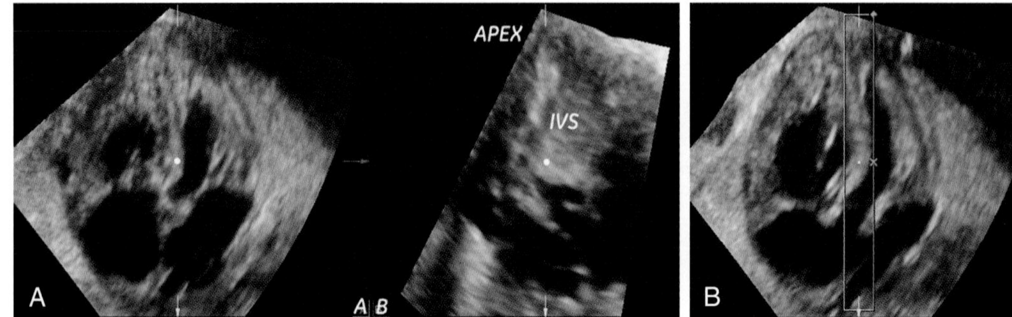

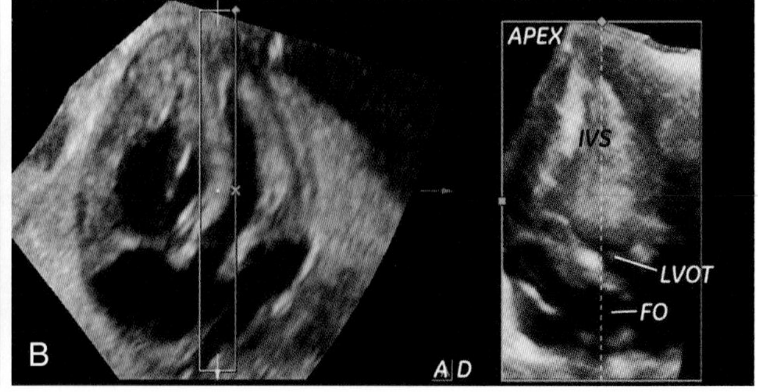

Figure 4-3. **(A left)** The four-chamber view from a STIC acquisition, displayed in the A-plane of the multiplanar reconstruction (MPR) screen, with the navigation dot placed on the ventricular septum. **(Right)** The orthogonal B-plane from the MPR screen shows the interventricular septum (IVS) in en face view. Apex of the heart is indicated. **(B left)** Another four-chamber view from the same volume dataset. The bounding box is placed tightly around the ventricular septum with the active orientation placed in the left ventricle *(green line)*. **(Right)** The rendered image of the IVS from within the left ventricle appearing in the D-plane of the rendering screen, with the left ventricle outflow tract (LVOT) and foramen ovale (FO). Note the smooth quality of the ventricular wall. (**A** and **B**, Reproduced with permission from Yagel S, Cohen SM, Valsky DV, Messing B. 3D and 4D ultrasound in fetal cardiac screening and the evaluation of congenital heart defects. *Expert Rev Obstet Gynecol.* 2009;4:261-271.)

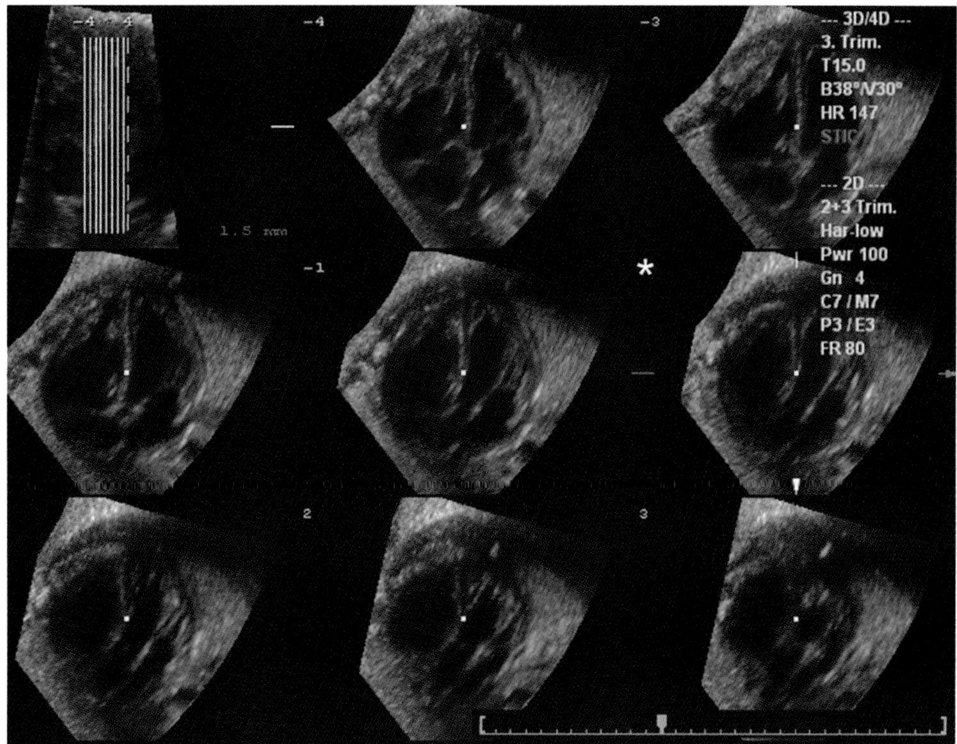

Figure 4-4. Tomographic ultrasound imaging (TUI). **(Top center)** The −4 plane shows the four-chamber view. **(Asterisk, middle right)** The zero plane shows the outflow tracts view. **(Bottom right)** The +3 plane shows the great vessels. (Reproduced with permission from Yagel S, Cohen SM, Shapiro I, Valsky DV. 3D and 4D ultrasound in fetal cardiac scanning: a new look at the fetal heart. *Ultrasound Obstet Gynecol.* 2007;29:81-95.)

The Methodology of 3D/4D Fetal Echocardiography

As stated previously, STIC is the mainstay of 3D/4DUS of the fetal heart. The optimal acquisition technique has been described at length elsewhere.[14,21] Briefly, the fetus should be in a quiet state without breathing movements and in supine lie. The operator identifies the four-chamber view, initiates the STIC application, and sweeps the fetal body from the upper abdomen to the upper mediastinum. Ideally, this acquired volume will contain all the images necessary for complete examination of the fetal heart. In practice, part of the volume may be degraded by maternal or fetal motion or breathing, and another volume acquisition will be necessary. Because the first processing stage performed by the ultrasound machine requires only seconds, the volume can be reviewed briefly with the patient present and repeated, without untoward delay. We find that most normal scans require two volumes, and extracting the acceptable portions of each will provide all the necessary planes. In cases of suspected or known fetal anomalies, of course, the approach will be focused on the affected parts to optimize visualization still further, and multiple volumes may be necessary.

Planes and Virtual Planes in Fetal Echocardiography

2DUS can effectively image the five planes of fetal echocardiography as well as countless others. However, many planes are not readily accessible in 2DUS. One of the strengths of 3D/4DUS is the possibility to image "virtual planes" that are acquired in the volume block and, through post-processing manipulation, made available for assessment. For example, the interventricular septum can be evaluated to confirm or exclude the presence of ventricular septal defect (VSD). At the beginning of the evaluation, the operator scrolls through the volume to obtain the four-chamber view in the A-plane of the MPR display. By placing the navigation dot on the interventricular septum, the orthogonal B-plane will show the septum en face, a plane not generally accessible in 2DUS. By applying 3D rendering and placing the bounding box tightly around the septum, the D-frame on the lower right of the display will show the en face view of the ventricular septum and the foramen ovale with the advantage of the depth the bounding box provides (see Figure 4-3). In either case, temporal information in the STIC volume allows the resulting plane to run through the cardiac cycle: this allows for evaluation of the action of the foramen ovale during the heart cycle or of blood flow across the VSD.

The same algorithm may be applied to visualizing the coronal atrioventricular valve (CAV) plane. Beginning from the four-chamber view, with the navigation dot placed on the crux of the heart, the coronal C-plane will show the CAV plane of the heart. With the bounding box placed tightly around the level of the atrioventricular valves in rendering mode, the D-frame will display the

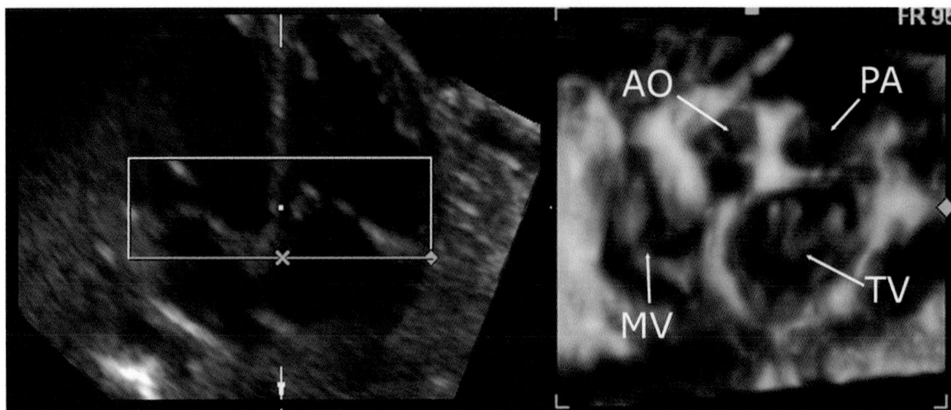

Figure 4-5. Ultrasound image in the normal coronal atrioventricular (AV) plane. **(Left)** The rendering box is placed tightly around the level of the AV valves and fine-tuned with the X-rotation option to image the great vessel valves as they begin to open and close. **(Right)** The rendered image of the coronal atrioventricular valves (CAVs) plane in end-diastole: the tricuspid (TV) and mitral (MV) valves are closed, and the aortic and pulmonary valves are beginning to open. Note the aortic valve cusp just visible in the orifice. AO, aorta; PA, pulmonary artery. (Reproduced with permission from Yagel S, Benachi A, Bonnet D, et al. Rendering in fetal cardiac scanning: the intracardiac septa and the coronal atrioventricular valve planes. *Ultrasound Obstet Gynecol.* 2006;28:266-274.)

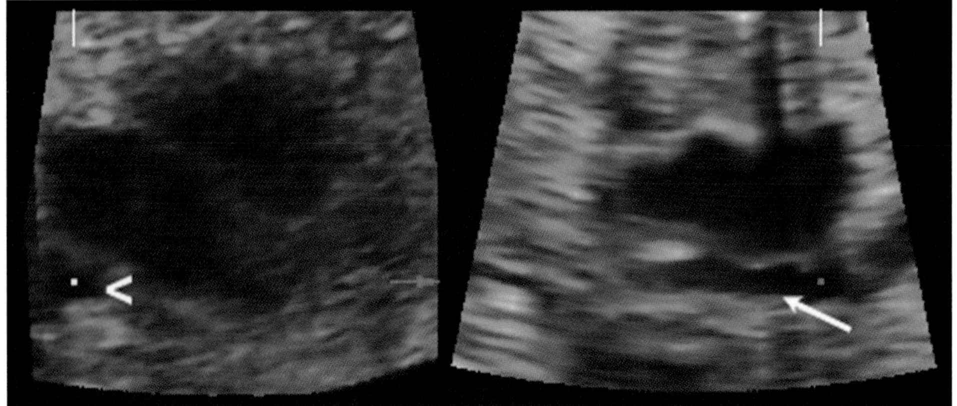

Figure 4-6. The orthogonal planes in MPR. **(Left)** In the A-plane, a suspicious circular finding *(arrowhead)* was seen. **(Right)** The navigation dot was placed on the finding and the B-plane showed this to be a vessel when viewed at an angle of 90 degrees *(arrow)*. This was shown to be the characteristic vertical vein in a case of total anomalous pulmonary venous connection. (Reproduced with permission from Yagel S, Cohen SM, Shapiro I, Valsky DV. 3D and 4D ultrasound in fetal cardiac scanning: a new look at the fetal heart. *Ultrasound Obstet Gynecol.* 2007;29:81-95.)

CAV plane. This plane facilitates evaluation of the patency of the atrioventricular and arterial valves (Figure 4-5).[17]

Applying 3D/4DUS to Fetal Echocardiography

Each 3D/4DUS modality brings different advantages to fetal echocardiography. The following examples illustrate the application of various modalities to the diagnosis of fetal cardiac anomalies.

Multiplanar Reconstruction and Tomographic Ultrasound Imaging

MPR is the first-line approach to analysis of an acquired volume block and allows the operator to view three orthogonal planes simultaneously. With the help of the navigation dot, the operator can compare the same point in space in three planes positioned at right angles to each other. Figure 4-6 shows a case of suspicious finding in the A-plane, which proved to be an anomalous blood vessel when viewed in the orthogonal B-plane. This was identified as the characteristic vertical vein of total anomalous pulmonary venous connection, leading ultimately to the diagnosis.[14]

TUI is an extension of MPR because it displays the selected MPR frame as the center plane in a series of parallel planes. This can be useful to evaluate cardiac structures at several planes simultaneously. The relative positions and orientations of structure can thereby be evaluated. Figure 4-7 shows the aorta, right ventricle, and pulmonary artery in three frames of one screen in this case of transposition of the great arteries with pulmonary atresia.

MPR combined with color Doppler is shown in Figure 4-8. In this case of pulmonary artery–to–pulmonary vein shunt, the 2DUS gray-scale four-chamber view showed an

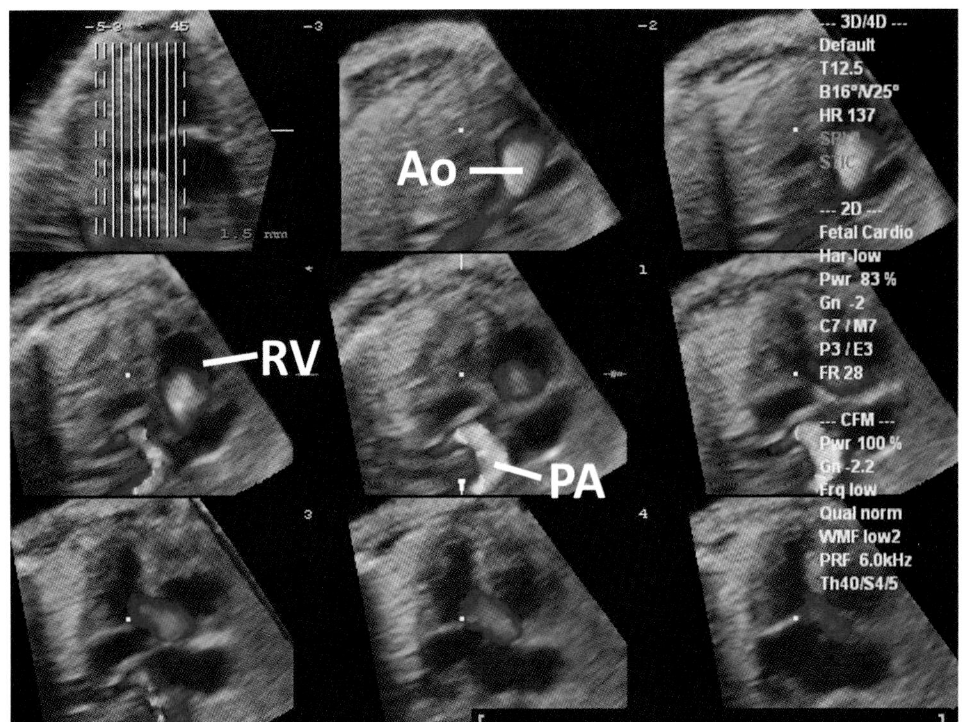

Figure 4-7. TUI display with HDPD. In this case of transposition of the great arteries with pulmonary atresia. TUI shows blood flow in the aorta, right ventricle, and pulmonary artery in one display. **(Upper left)** The planes imaged in each of the other frames and the distance between frames. The center plane and corresponding frame (in this case, the pulmonary artery plane) are marked with asterisks. Ao, aorta; PA, pulmonary artery; RV, right ventricle.

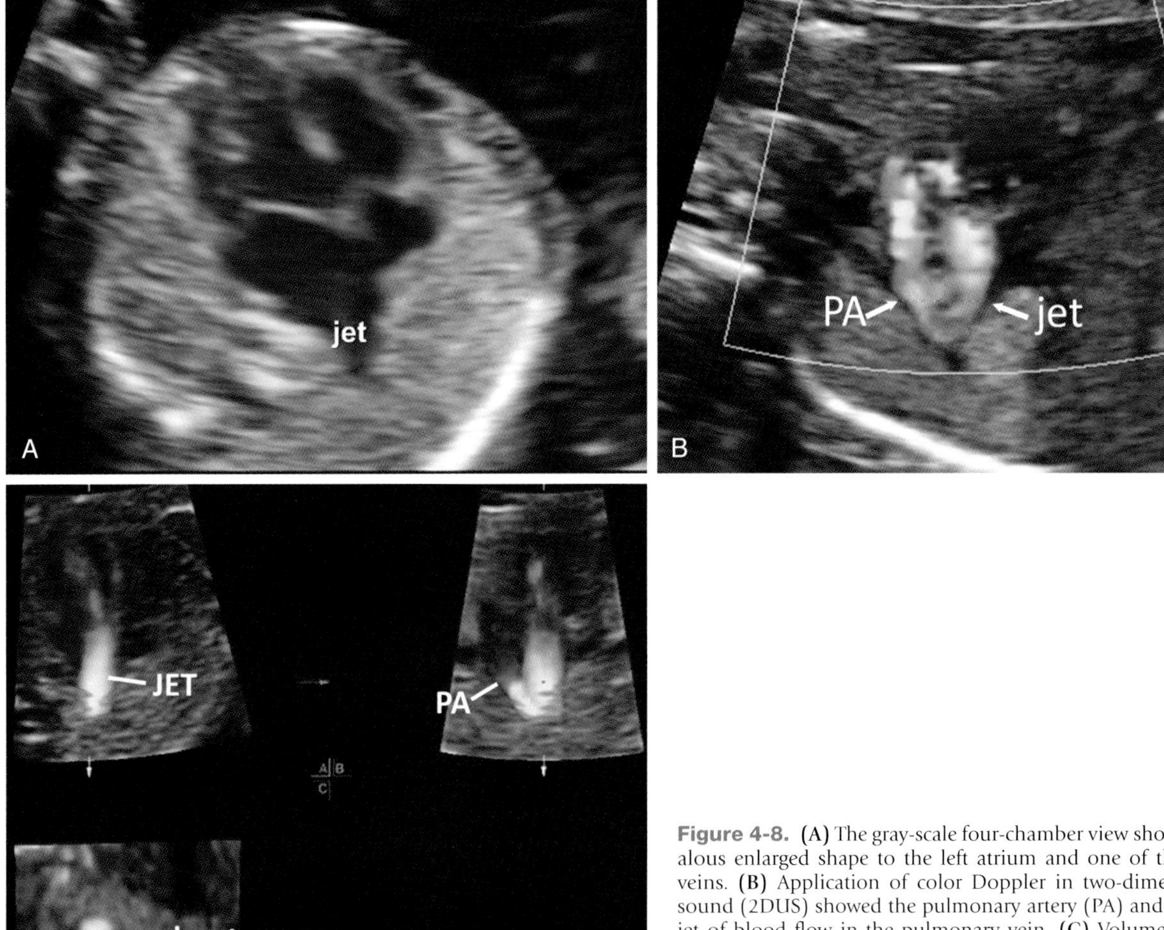

Figure 4-8. **(A)** The gray-scale four-chamber view showed an anomalous enlarged shape to the left atrium and one of the pulmonary veins. **(B)** Application of color Doppler in two-dimensional ultrasound (2DUS) showed the pulmonary artery (PA) and an impressive jet of blood flow in the pulmonary vein. **(C)** Volume was acquired with STIC and HDPD. In the MPR display, the three orthogonal planes show the jet in the pulmonary vein in the A-plane, the jet as well as flow in the pulmonary artery (PA) in the B-plane, and the shunt junction in the coronal C-plane.

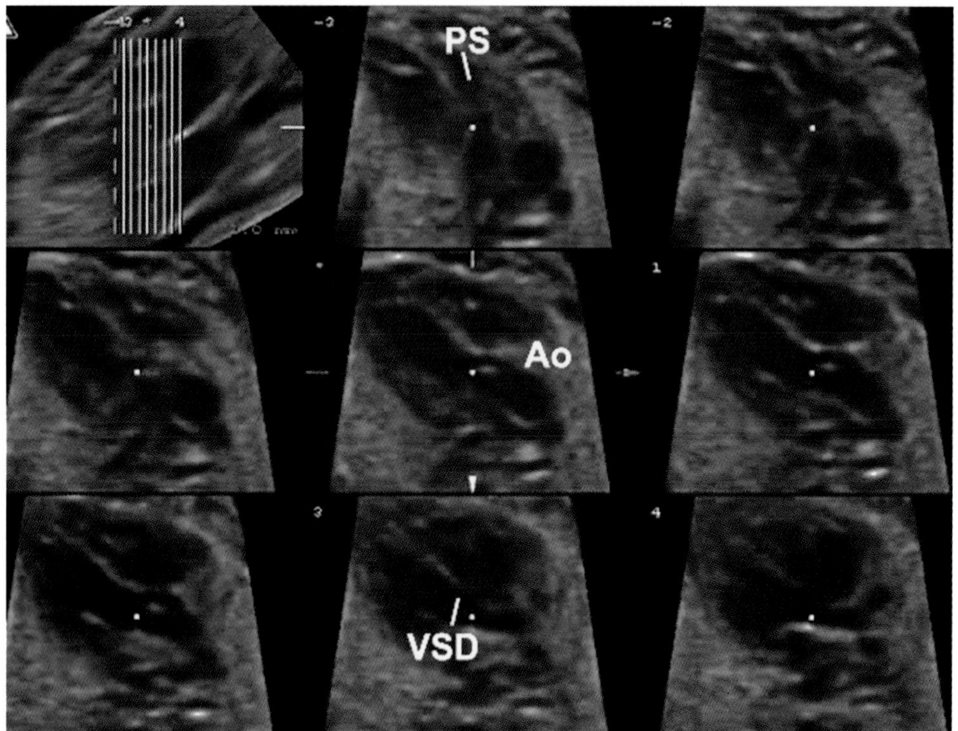

Figure 4-9. TUI in gray scale shows three pathognomonic elements of tetralogy of Fallot in one display: the pulmonary stenosis (PS; **top center)** overriding aorta (Ao; **middle center)**; and ventricular septal defect (VSD; **bottom center).** Note the navigation dot, which is anchored in all the planes, is placed on the aortic valve; in the VSD frame, the dot is seen directly above the defect, confirming the overriding aorta.

enlarged anomalous shape to the left atrium and one of the pulmonary veins. 2DUS with color Doppler showed jetting of blood flow into the pulmonary vein. 4DUS with color Doppler was applied, and post-processing analysis with MPR clearly showed two-directional blood flow, with a jet toward the left atrium and the arteriovenous shunt junction in the coronal C-plane.

Figure 4-9 shows a case of tetralogy of Fallot evaluated with TUI. On a single display, three of the pathognomonic elements are shown together: pulmonary stenosis, overriding aorta, and perimembranous VSD.

3D Rendering

3D rendering adds depth and texture to MPR images. This can have important implications in some situations. For example, in transposition of the great arteries, the degree of restriction of the foramen ovale can affect postnatal care and prognosis. In these cases, evaluation of the foramen ovale can provide useful information for preoperative consultation. As shown in Figure 4-10,[17] 3D rendering with the interatrial septum plane shows the foramen ovale, and because the STIC volume contains temporal information, the operator can evaluate the range of movement of the foramen ovale throughout the course of the heart cycle.

As is well known, the most common cardiac anomaly—and the most commonly missed—is VSD. By applying 3D rendering and the interventricular septum plane, it is possible to view the ventricular septum en face and, by adjusting the width of the bounding box, to tweak the depth of the image. The operator can identify the characteristic trabeculations of the right ventricle wall, for example. In a case of VSD, the lesion or lesions will be shown and made available for measurement. If the volume is acquired with color Doppler, the presence and directionality of blood flow across the defect can also be evaluated (Figure 4-11).[18]

The CAV plane is obtained similarly to the IVS plane, but the bounding box is placed tightly around the area of the atrioventricular valves, at the level of the cardiac crux (see Figure 4-5). The resulting rendered image shows the relative position of the valves, the valve leaflets, and their range of motion. If color Doppler is applied, directionality of blood flow across the valves can also be evaluated. In a case of pulmonary stenosis, the CAV plane clearly shows reversed, meager blood flow in the pulmonary artery (Figure 4-12).[17]

STIC volumes acquired with HDPD are also amenable to post-processing with 3D rendering. HDPD is a bidirectional, very sensitive Doppler modality. Figure 4-13 shows the heart and great vessels in a case of aberrant right subclavian artery. In the three vessels and trachea (3VT) plane, the aberrant artery is seen arising from the ascending aorta. The rendered image is shown here in color rendering mode, which highlights Doppler flow isolated from surrounding tissue. Although HDPD is very sensitive for imaging small vessels (e.g., when applied to the ductus venosus, it shows blood flow in systole and

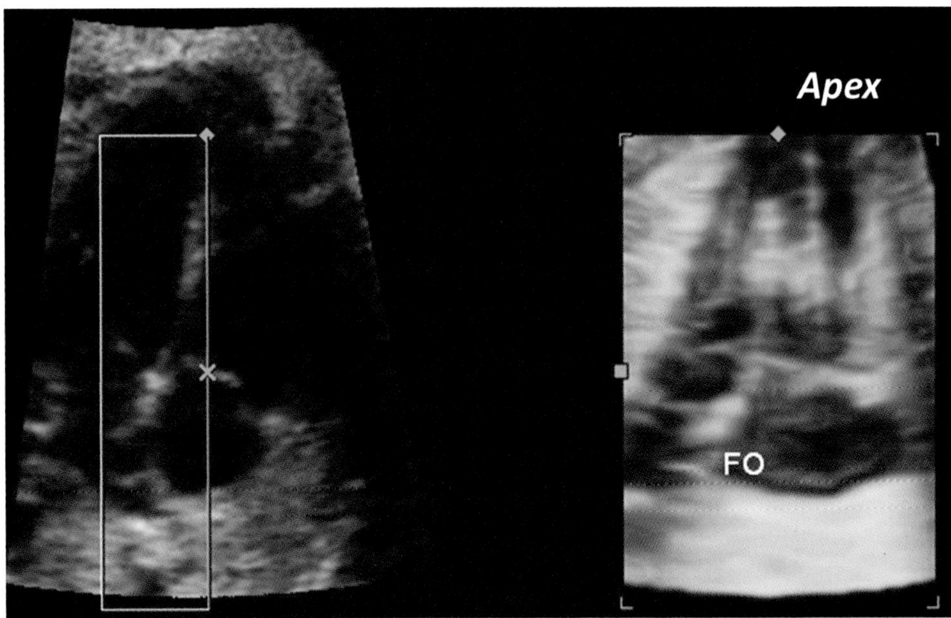

Figure 4-10. Restrictive foramen ovale evaluated with three-dimensional (3D) rendering. **(Left)** The A-plane from the MPR screen with the heart in four-chamber view and the bounding box placed tightly around the interatrial and interventricular septa. **(Right)** The rendered image of the en face view of the interatrial septum and the foramen ovale (FO). When the volume runs in cine loop in this plane, the range of motion of the FO can be evaluated. (Reproduced with permission from Yagel S, Benachi A, Bonnet D, et al. Rendering in fetal cardiac scanning: the intracardiac septa and the coronal atrioventricular valve planes. *Ultrasound Obstet Gynecol.* 2006;28:266-274.)

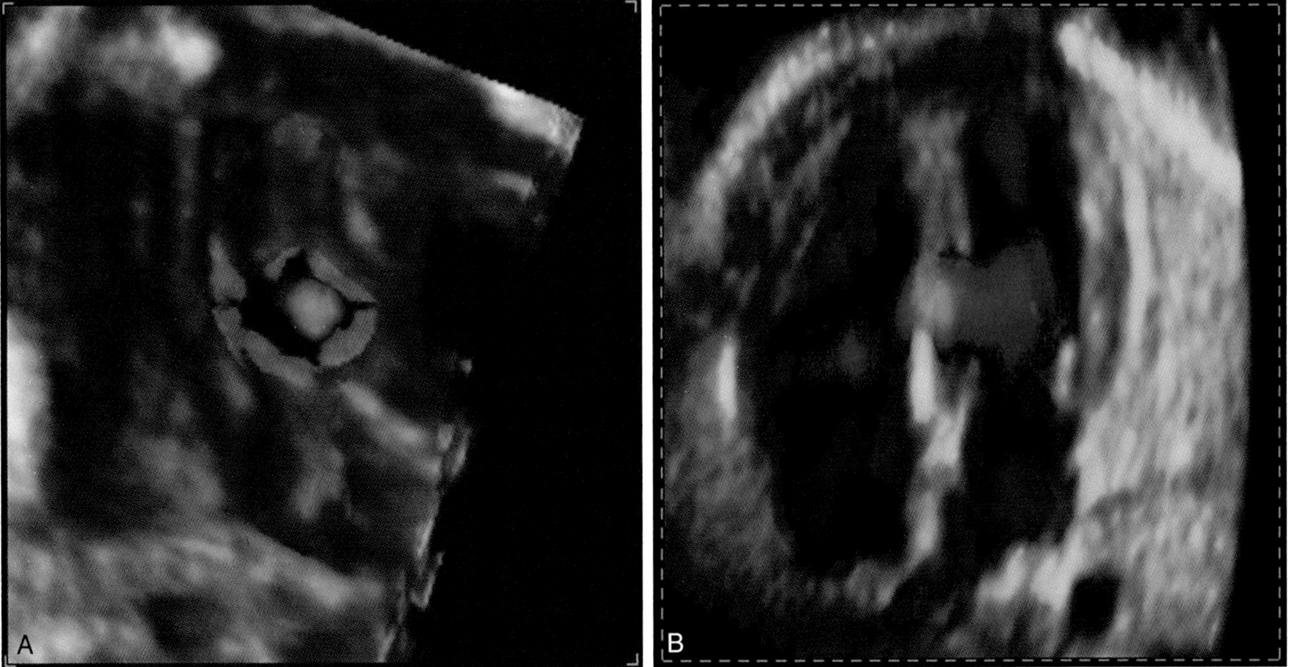

Figure 4-11. VSD evaluated with the aid of virtual planes. With the four-chamber view in the A-plane, the bounding box is placed tightly around the interventricular septum. **(A)** The corresponding rendered image shows the en face view of the septum, clearly displaying the large VSD. **(B)** With the addition of color Doppler, the degree of blood flow shunting across the defect can be evaluated. (**A** and **B**, Reproduced with permission from Yagel S, Valsky DV, Messing B. Detailed assessment of fetal ventricular septal defect with 4D color Doppler ultrasound using spatio-temporal image correlation technology. *Ultrasound Obstet Gynecol.* 2005;25:97-98.)

diastole) and produces images with less "bleeding" of color than conventional Doppler, it is not ideal for vessel diameter measurements.

By applying the VOCAL volume measurement tool in post-processing, the volume of anomalous findings can be determined. This is illustrated in this case of right ventricle aneurysm (Figure 4-14). MPR revealed a well-defined addendum protruding from the right ventricle, and B-flow imaging displayed blood flowing into and draining from this area. With the help of VOCAL, the volume of the aneurysm was determined.

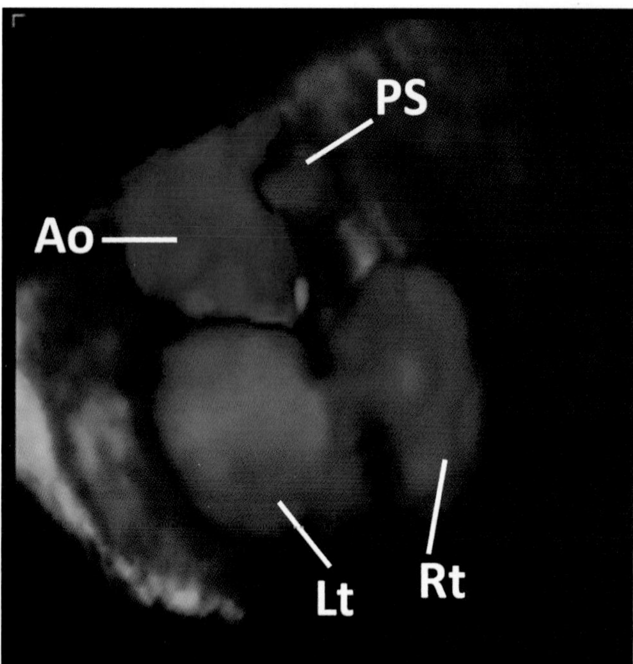

Figure 4-12. Pulmonary valve stenosis (PS) displayed with the virtual CAV plane. Beginning from the four-chamber view in the A-plane, the bounding box is placed tightly around the level of the AV valves. The corresponding rendered image shows the CAV plane. With the addition of color Doppler, the reversed, meager blood flow across the stenotic valve is displayed. Lt, left ventricle; Rt, right ventricle. (Reproduced with permission from Yagel S, Benachi A, Bonnet D, et al. Rendering in fetal cardiac scanning: the intracardiac septa and the coronal atrioventricular valve planes. *Ultrasound Obstet Gynecol.* 2006;28:266-274.)

B-Flow

B-Flow is an underutilized modality in 3D/4DUS scanning. However, it is a highly sensitive tool for imaging blood flowing in the heart and vessels and, as such, is invaluable in fetal echocardiography. B-flow images produce a digital "cast" of the scanned target. B-flow can also aid in the diagnosis of anomalies of the great vessels and smaller vessels such as the ductus venosus. Right aortic arch is a not uncommon embryonic variant. Kommerell's diverticulum may be present as a small protrusion from the arch at the point of confluence of the ligamentum arteriosum (rudimentary left aortic arch) into the left subclavian artery. B-Flow imaging of the heart and great vessels in this case of right aortic arch shows the characteristic four vessels originating from the arch and the subtle finding of Kommerell's diverticulum (Figure 4-15).

Another subtle embryonic variant is the interrupted inferior vena cava (IVC). The IVC is made up of four segments during the embryonic period, and failure of the hepatic segment to form results in an interrupted IVC. In this case, blood from the lower body returns to the right atrium via the azygos and hemiazygos veins (Figure 4-16).[22] B-Flow clearly showed the interrupted IVC with azygos vein continuation to the superior vena cava (SVC).

The preceding anomalies may oftentimes be clinically silent, and doubtless, many cases go undiagnosed in the general population. Agenesis of the ductus venosus (ADV), however, may have significant impact on fetal and neonatal development. Many studies have described the wide variability in outcome of these fetuses, apparently owing to differences in the site of umbilical vein drainage,

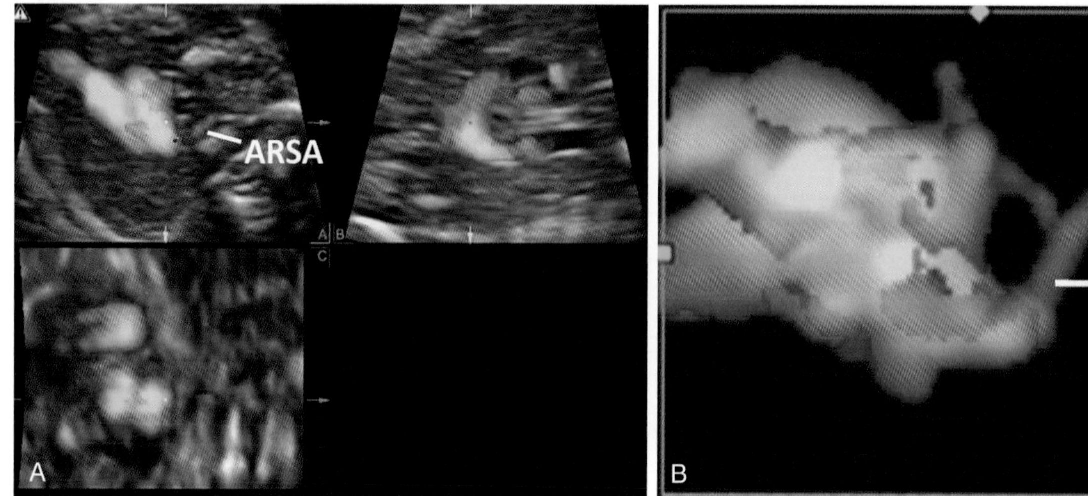

Figure 4-13. STIC acquired with HDPD shows the aberrant right subclavian artery (ARSA) anomaly. **(A)** MPR display of the three vessels and trachea (3VT) plane shows the ARSA arising from the ascending aorta. **(B)** The heart and great vessels displayed in glass body transparency mode, which highlights Doppler flow isolated from surrounding tissue.

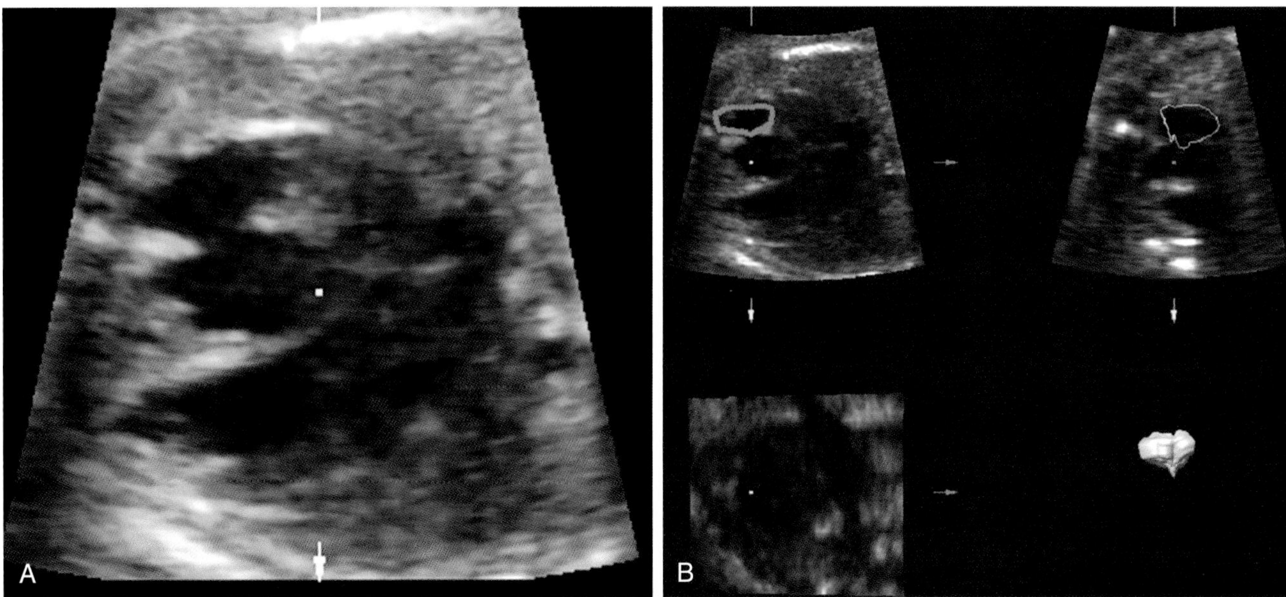

Figure 4-14. RV aneurysm. **(A)** MPR display of the four-chamber view in the A-plane shows an anomalous shape to the RV. **(B)** Virtual organ computer-aided analysis (VOCAL) mode was applied to measure the volume of the aneurysm. The A-plane shows the manual trace of the area of interest, and the rendered D-plane displays a 3D model of the measured volume.

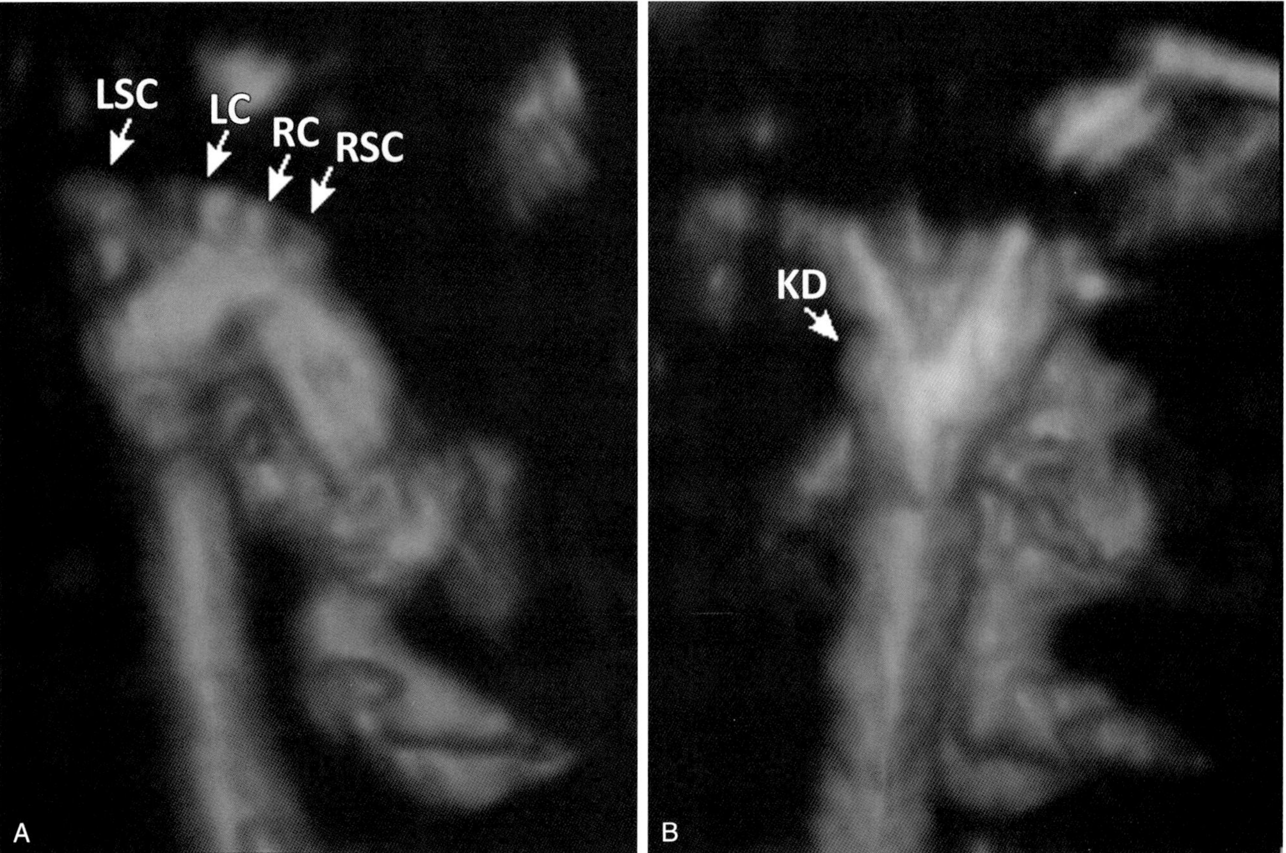

Figure 4-15. Right aortic arch with Kommerrell's diverticulum (KD). B-Flow sensitively images the heart and great vessels. **(A)** In the right aortic arch anomaly, four vessels originate from the aortic arch: the right subclavian (RSC), right carotid (RC), left carotid (LC), and left subclavian (LSC) arteries. **(B)** The posterior view shows the subtle finding of KD.

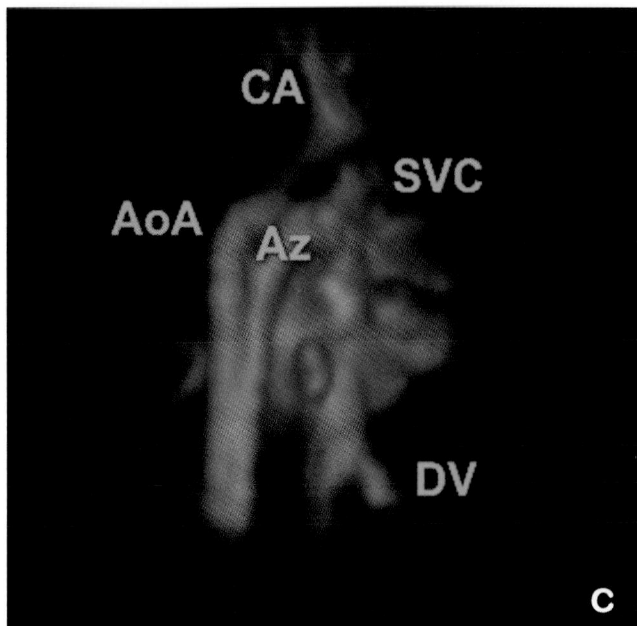

Figure 4-16. Interrupted IVC. B-Flow shows the continuation of the azygos (Az) vein draining into the superior vena cava (SVC). AoA, aortic arch; CA, carotid artery; DV, ductus venosus. (Reproduced with permission from Yagel S, Kivilevitch Z, Valsky DV, Achiron R. The fetal venous system: normal embryology, anatomy, and physiology and the development and appearance of anomalies. In Yagel S, Silverman N, Gembruch U, eds. *Fetal Cardiology.* 2nd ed. New York: Informa; 2009.)

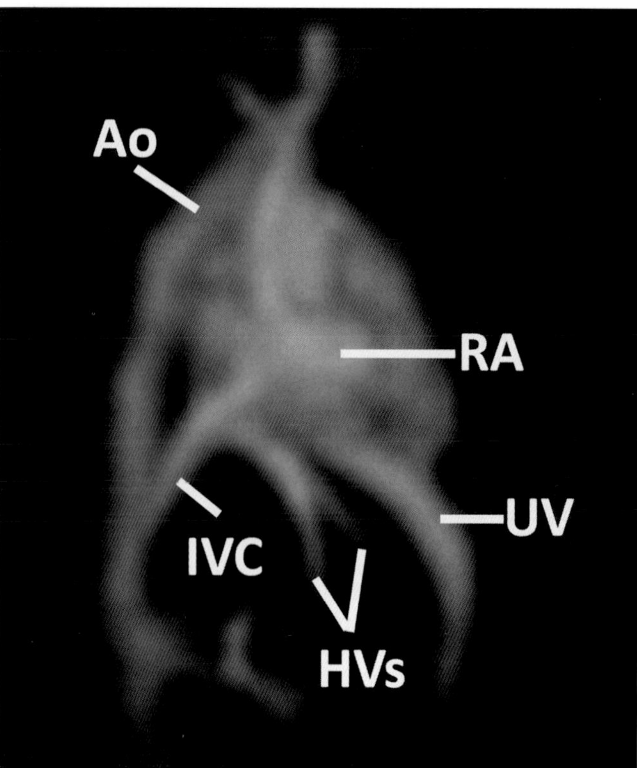

Figure 4-17. B-Flow scan in a case of agenesis of the ductus venosus with drainage of the umbilical vein (UV) to the right atrium (RA). The heart and great vessels, including the hepatic veins (HVs) draining into the IVC, and the aorta (Ao), are shown.

whether intra- or extrahepatic, and perhaps, in the case of the latter variant, depending on the dimensions of the extrahepatic shunt.[23,24] Whenever ADV is suspected, thorough investigation of the fetal cardiovascular system, particularly the fetal portal venous system, is warranted. Figure 4-17 shows a case of ADV with drainage to the right atrium, diagnosed with B-flow.

3D/4DUS for Fetal Cardiac Functional Assessment

In addition to anatomic evaluation of the fetus, ultrasound is an indispensable tool in functional assessment of fetal well-being in general and cardiac function in particular. 3D/4DUS has provided new tools in fetal cardiac functional assessment. Description of the range of applications for the evaluation of the fetus with intrauterine growth restriction (IUGR), cardiac compromise, or congenital heart disease is beyond the scope of this chapter.

3D/4DUS can be applied to quantification of the cardiac ventricle volume and ventricular myometrial mass. By applying VOCAL and IM modalities, we[25] and others[26,27] have shown that it is feasible to quantify the volume of the fetal cardiac ventricles as well as the mass of the ventricular myocardium.[28] These applications may be useful in the evaluation of heart function cardiac anomalies and in evolving cardiac compromise. The methods for ventricle volumetry and mass quantification using VOCAL and IM have been described in detail elsewhere[25,28]; briefly, after STIC acquisition, the operator initializes the IM application to isolate the fluid-filled area of the ventricle then, using VOCAL application, traces the contour of each ventricle in turn. The system compiles the sequential traces to produce an image of the interior of the ventricle and calculates the volume. To obtain the mass measurement, the trace is drawn around the entire ventricle, including the septum, and the intraventricular volume (determined with IM) is subtracted from the total. The result is then multiplied by 1.050 g/cm^3 (myocardial density). Fetal cardiac ventricular volume and mass measurements are shown in Figure 4-18.

Minimal Projection Mode

The rendering algorithm minimal projection mode, or minimal rendering mode, uses a very high transparency; thereby anechoic structures such as the heart or stomach are highlighted as compared with the surrounding more echogenic structures. This was found to be very useful in imaging situs abnormalities or diaphragmatic hernia.[29]

Cautions and Pitfalls

3D/4DUS is prone to the same problems as 2DUS including acoustic shadowing, Doppler signal drop-out, and loss of resolution at greater scanning depth. In addition, 3D/4DUS introduces issues not encountered in 2DUS scanning. A 3DUS volume dataset is only as good as the 2DUS image that preceded it. It is essential to optimize

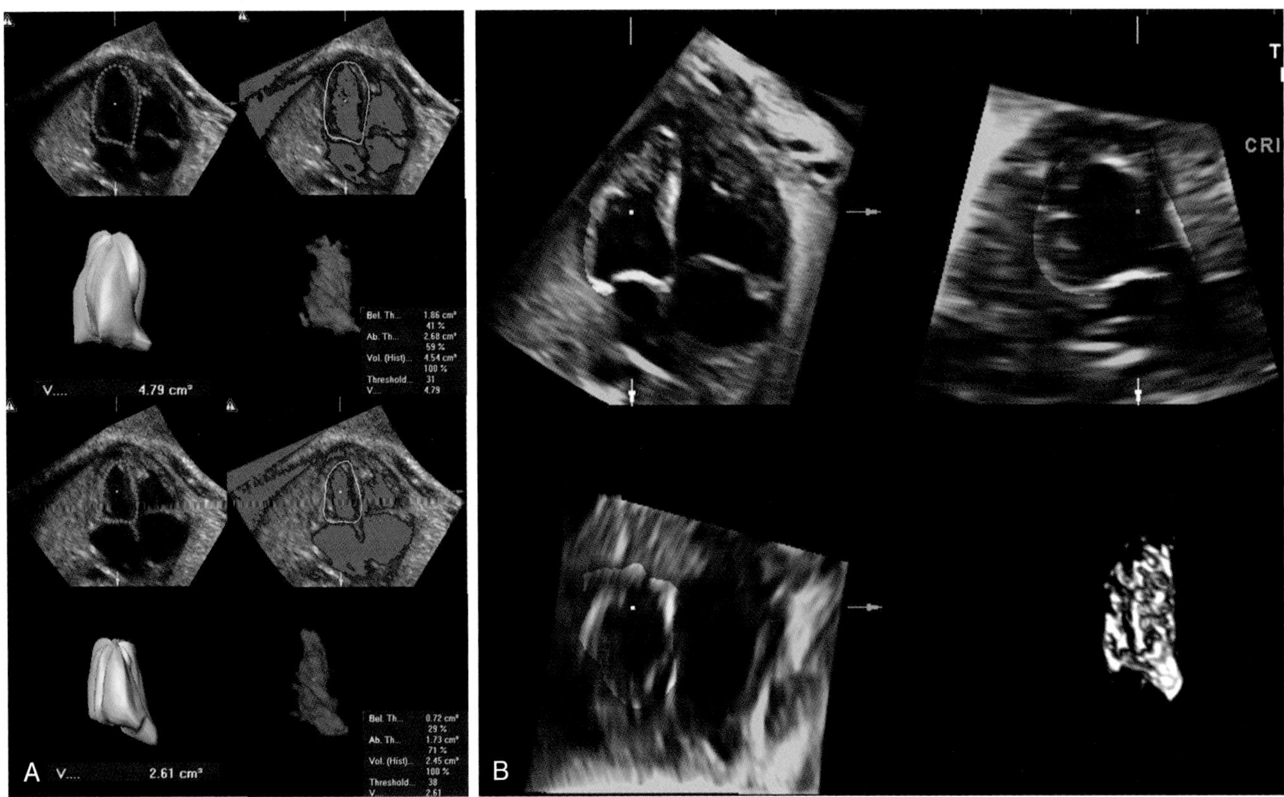

Figure 4-18. (**A**) Cardiac ventricular volume measurement. Post-processing quantification of left ventricle volumetry in end-diastole (**upper panel**) and end-systole (**lower panel**). For each panel, diastole and systole, the top left shows the trace in the A-frame at the level of the four chamber view; the top right shows the same frame with the inversion mode activated; the bottom left shows the 3D models created by the VOCAL tool, that includes the entire traced volume; and the bottom right shows the final intraventricular volume models. (**B**) Ventricular myocardial mass measurement. The mass of the ventricular myocardium can be quantified by applying the same methodology. The VOCAL trace is performed to include the entire ventricle. The intraventricular volume, isolated by application of inversion mode, is subtracted from the total, and the result is multiplied by 1.050 to obtain the mass. (**A**, Reproduced with permission from Messing B, Cohen SM, Valsky DV, et al. Fetal cardiac ventricle volumetry in the second half of gestation assessed by 4D ultrasound using STIC combined with inversion mode. *Ultrasound Obstet Gynecol.* 2007;30:142-151.)

those aspects that can be improved before acquisition is begun. 3D rendering produces virtual images. The algorithms applied to smooth the image can potentially disguise defects.

STIC acquisition is susceptible to motion artifacts introduced by maternal breathing or fetal body or breathing movements. The fetus should ideally be in a quiet state, and the mother can be asked to hold her breath for the few seconds of acquisition. The resulting volume can be quickly reviewed and additional volumes acquired, if motion artifacts are seen. In broad terms, if the upper right B-plane appears sound in the MPR screen, the volume is most likely acceptable.

Acoustic shadowing is evident on 2D scanning. When 3D volumes are acquired, the volume block may contain acoustic shadows that were not apparent in the 2D image. These may subsequently appear as a defect during post-processing manipulation of the volume. Whenever a defect is suspected, therefore, it should be confirmed by repeated scanning to exclude acoustic shadow artifact.

Directional Doppler studies are an essential part of fetal echocardiography, and STIC volumes acquired with Doppler are available for post-processing manipulation. This manipulation often includes rotation of the volume around its axes: color Doppler flow directions can be misinterpreted. As with acoustic shadowing, suspected pathologies should be confirmed or excluded by verification of whether blood flow was toward or away from the transducer in the initial acquisition, and scanning repeated if necessary.

Accuracy of 3D/4DUS in Fetal Echocardiography

Since its introduction, 3D/4DUS has been found to make an important contribution to fetal echocardiography. However, no studies have shown that addition of 3D/4DUS to screening echocardiography improves diagnostic accuracy. In our experience of over 11,000 examinations in a mixed low-risk and referral population in a tertiary referral center, we found that of 155 cases of CHD, in only 11 did 3D/4DUS have added value in reaching a diagnosis.[30] In all these cases, other anomalies or findings observed in the 2DUS scan prompted detailed cardiovascular evaluation.[30] Additional well-powered prospective studies are required to establish the added value of 3D/4DUS modalities to the screening accuracy of fetal echocardiography.

Imaging Essentials and Important Points

- A 3D/4DUS volume is only as good as the 2DUS scan that preceded it.
- A well-performed STIC volume will contain all the standard planes for complete fetal echocardiography.
- MPR with the navigation dot is indispensable in navigating within the volume and comparing orthogonal planes.
- "Virtual planes" of the fetal heart will be available within the saved volume, which would not normally be accessible in 2DUS.
- TUI extends the ability of MPR and displays sequential parallel planes: from a well-executed STIC acquisition, TUI can simultaneously display all five classic planes of fetal echocardiography.
- B-Flow is more sensitive for imaging blood vessels when measurement is desired because it is not prone to the "bleeding" seen in HDPD.
- Rendering algorithms can mask defects by smoothing the image.
- Directionality in color Doppler that was acquired in a 4DUS volume must be reconfirmed with repeated 2DUS scanning to avoid confusion of flow direction resulting from rotation of the volume in post-processing.

References

1. International Society for Ultrasound in Obstetrics and Gynecology. Cardiac screening examination of the fetus: guidelines for performing the "basic" and "extended basic" cardiac scan. *Ultrasound Obstet Gynecol.* 2006;27:107-113.
2. Carvalho JS, Ho SY, Shinebourne EA. Sequential segmental analysis in complex fetal cardiac abnormalities: a logical approach to diagnosis. *Ultrasound Obstet Gynecol.* 2005;26:105-111.
3. Yagel S, Arbel R, Anteby EY, Raveh D, Achiron R. The three vessels and trachea view (3VT) in fetal cardiac scanning. *Ultrasound Obstet Gynecol.* 2002;20:340-345.
4. Yagel S, Cohen SM, Achiron R. Examination of the fetal heart by five short-axis views: a proposed screening method for comprehensive cardiac evaluation. *Ultrasound Obstet Gynecol.* 2001;17:367-369.
5. Deng J, Rodeck CH. Current applications of fetal cardiac imaging technology. *Curr Opin Obstet Gynecol.* 2006;18:177-184.
6. Volpe P, Campobasso G, Stanziano A, et al. Novel application of 4D sonography with B-flow imaging and spatio-temporal image correlation (STIC) in the assessment of the anatomy of pulmonary arteries in fetuses with pulmonary atresia and ventricular septal defect. *Ultrasound Obstet Gynecol.* 2006;28:40-46.
7. Bord A, Valsky DV, Messing B, Rosenak D, Cohen SM, Yagel S. B-Flow modality combined with STIC in the normal fetal echocardiography examination. *Ultrasound Obstet Gynecol.* 2006;28:447.
8. Bord A, Valsky DV, Rosenak D, Cohen SM, Yagel S. B-Flow modality combined with STIC in the evaluation of malalignment of the great vessels. *Ultrasound Obstet Gynecol.* 2006;28:447.
9. Bord A, Rosenak D, Valsky DV, Cohen SM, Yagel S. B-Flow modality combined with STIC in the evaluation of fetal venous anomalies. *Ultrasound Obstet Gynecol.* 2006;28:556-557.
10. Chaoui R, Hoffmann J, Heling KS. Three-dimensional (3D) and 4D color Doppler fetal echocardiography using spatio-temporal image correlation (STIC). *Ultrasound Obstet Gynecol.* 2004;23:535-545.
11. Chaoui R, Kalache KD. Three-dimensional power Doppler ultrasound of the fetal great vessels. *Ultrasound Obstet Gynecol.* 2001; 17:455-456.
12. Chaoui R, Kalache KD, Hartung J. Application of three-dimensional power Doppler ultrasound in prenatal diagnosis. *Ultrasound Obstet Gynecol.* 2001;17:22-29.
13. Sciaky-Tamir Y, Cohen SM, Hochner-Celnikier D, Valsky DV, Messing B, Yagel S. Three-dimensional power Doppler (3DPD) ultrasound in the diagnosis and follow-up of fetal vascular anomalies. *Am J Obstet Gynecol.* 2006;194:274-281.
14. Yagel S, Cohen SM, Shapiro I, Valsky DV. 3D and 4D ultrasound in fetal cardiac scanning: a new look at the fetal heart. *Ultrasound Obstet Gynecol.* 2007;29:81-95.
15. Goncalves LF, Romero R, Espinoza J, et al. Four-dimensional ultrasonography of the fetal heart using color Doppler spatiotemporal image correlation. *J Ultrasound Med.* 2004;23:473-481.
16. Yagel S, Cohen SM, Valsky DV, Messing B. 3D and 4D ultrasound in fetal cardiac screening and the evaluation of congenital heart defects. *Expert Rev Obstet Gynecol.* 2009;4:261-271.
17. Yagel S, Benachi A, Bonnet D, et al. Rendering in fetal cardiac scanning: the intracardiac septa and the coronal atrioventricular valve planes. *Ultrasound Obstet Gynecol.* 2006;28:266-274.
18. Yagel S, Valsky DV, Messing B. Detailed assessment of fetal ventricular septal defect with 4D color Doppler ultrasound using spatio-temporal image correlation technology. *Ultrasound Obstet Gynecol.* 2005;25:97-98.
19. Espinoza J, Kusanovic JP, Goncalves LF, et al. A novel algorithm for comprehensive fetal echocardiography using 4-dimensional ultrasonography and tomographic imaging. *J Ultrasound Med.* 2006; 25:947-956.
20. Goncalves LF, Espinoza J, Lee W, et al. A new approach to fetal echocardiography: digital casts of the fetal cardiac chambers and great vessels for detection of congenital heart disease. *J Ultrasound Med.* 2005;24:415-424.
21. Goncalves LF, Lee W, Espinoza J, Romero R. Examination of the fetal heart by four-dimensional (4D) ultrasound with spatio-temporal image correlation (STIC). *Ultrasound Obstet Gynecol.* 2006; 27:336-348.
22. Yagel S, Kivilevitch Z, Valsky DV, Achiron R. The fetal venous system: normal embryology, anatomy, and physiology and the development and appearance of anomalies. In Yagel S, Silverman N, Gembruch U, eds. *Fetal Cardiology.* 2nd ed. New York: Informa; 2009.
23. Berg C, Kamil D, Geipel A, et al. Absence of ductus venosus-importance of umbilical venous drainage site. *Ultrasound Obstet Gynecol.* 2006;28:275-281.
24. Sothinathan U, Pollina E, Huggon I, Patel S, Greenough A. Absence of the ductus venosus. *Acta Paediatr.* 2006;95:620-621.
25. Messing B, Cohen SM, Valsky DV, et al. Fetal cardiac ventricle volumetry in the second half of gestation assessed by 4D ultrasound using STIC combined with inversion mode. *Ultrasound Obstet Gynecol.* 2007;30:142-151.
26. Bhat AH, Corbett VN, Liu R, et al. Validation of volume and mass assessments for human fetal heart imaging by 4-dimensional spatiotemporal image correlation echocardiography: in vitro balloon model experiments. *J Ultrasound Med.* 2004;23:1151-1159.
27. Bhat AH, Corbett V, Carpenter N, et al. Fetal ventricular mass determination on three-dimensional echocardiography: studies in normal fetuses and validation experiments. *Circulation.* 2004;110: 1054-1060.
28. Messing B, Valsky DV, Rosenak D, Cohen SM, Yagel S. 3D/4D ultrasound for fetal cardiac ventricle mass measurement in the second half of gestation in normal and anomalous cases. *Ultrasound Obstet Gynecol.* 2008;32:335.
29. Achiron R, Gindes L, Zalel Y, Lipitz S, Weisz B. Three- and four-dimensional ultrasound: new methods for evaluating fetal thoracic anomalies. *Ultrasound Obstet Gynecol.* 2008;32:36-43.
30. Yagel S, Cohen SM, Rosenak D, Messing B, Lipschuetz M, Valsky DV. Does 3D/4DUS improve diagnostic accuracy in congenital heart malformations? *Ultrasound Obstet Gynecol.* 2009;34:170.

5

Prenatal Practice Care Model and Delivery of the Fetus with Cardiovascular Disease

Jack Rychik

Practice care models for the fetus with cardiovascular disease are varied, evolving, and continuously improving. Diagnostic capacities are increasing through the use of targeted ultrasound and fetal echocardiography. Fetal cardiovascular health is the focus of multiple disciplines including primary maternal caretakers (obstetricians, perinatologists, maternal-fetal medicine specialists), primary infant caretakers (pediatric cardiologists, neonatologists), and medical imagers (sonographers, radiologists). Whether through the auspices of pediatric cardiology or perinatology/maternal-fetal medicine, the goals are the same and include:

1. Accurate diagnosis.
2. Compassionate and knowledge-based counseling and family education.
3. Facilitation of a safe transition from fetus to newborn with creation of a delivery plan that is maternally safe and optimizes outcome for the newborn.

Practitioners will approach these goals in a variety of fashions. Importantly, it should be stated that there is no one correct way to approach caring for these patients. In this chapter, we discuss some of the operational systems and strategies we have developed to care for fetal cardiovascular disease—for the fetus, mother, and family—as well as methods of transition to postnatal care, all within the framework of an academic pediatric cardiology center.

The Fetal Heart Program Practice Care Model

In 2001, we realized the importance of establishing a separate, dedicated section within our clinical group to focus attention on fetal heart disease and, therefore, started our "Fetal Heart Program." Fetal echocardiography can be performed within a general pediatric echocardiography laboratory; however, the time commitment necessary for imaging performance and counseling, and the logistics necessary to provide truly comprehensive optimal care, suggested to us the need to create a separate "clinical unit" focused on fetal heart matters. Creation of a focused fetal heart section allows for program specific endeavors such as creation of a separate adult-focused outpatient waiting area, the purchase of ideal fetus-specific imaging equipment, and identification of staff and personnel specifically trained to deal with the pregnant patient.

Since inception, our "Fetal Heart Program" has grown in size and currently consists of a unit/section physician director and a core staff of attending physicians experienced and trained in fetal cardiovascular imaging and prenatal management. Dedicated nurse coordinators help facilitate care and are individually assigned to patients, which aids tremendously with continuity of care. The nurse plays a key role in the initial counseling sessions and continues the educational process throughout gestation, shepherding families through to the point of delivery. A social worker is assigned to join in counseling sessions and to assist families with whatever logistical support is necessary. The social worker performs a psychological assessment for each patient and provides support and counseling during what is an extremely stressful time. Charts for record keeping are created for each patient, which includes a general maternal and family history "intake questionnaire" (Box 5-1), referring physician records (obstetrical or pediatric cardiology), as well as fetal echo reports, testing data results (blood or amniocentesis), and letters summarizing visits. Notations from nursing and social worker evaluations are generated throughout the pregnancy encounter and are also included. These charts establish a running record of information concerning prenatal care, which accompanies the fetus to postnatal management in the intensive care unit.

Measuring the Impact of a Prenatal Heart Defect: The Fetal Cardiovascular Disease Severity Grading Scale

An essential part of counseling for congenital heart disease before birth involves the designation and conveyance of the severity of the anomaly. Counseling typically involves detailed explanations of what is found, what interventions or surgeries might be necessary, and what the overall prognosis and quality of life will be for the fetus, infant, child, and beyond. Scales for complexity of congenital heart disease have been developed for the

Box 5-1 Examples of Elements to Include in an Intake Questionnaire Form for Families Possibly Carrying a Fetus with Congenital Heart Disease

- Maternal demographic information
- Partner demographic information
- Referring physician information
- Maternal allergies
- Chronic medical problems
- Prescription medications
- Over-the-counter medications
- Natural remedies
- Family history for medical or genetic problems
- Obstetrical health history
- Previous pregnancy history
- Present pregnancy: Spontaneous conception? Assisted reproductive technology? If so, what type?
- Psychosocial history
- Exposure history (e.g., tobacco, alcohol, radiation, toxic substances, febrile/viral illness)

cardiothoracic surgeon and primarily relate to complexity of the surgery and operative outcome. A prenatal severity scale would be of value in a number of ways. It would create uniformity in gauging severity of caseload across centers, aid in counseling, and may be a useful tool for research studies. Such a "fetal cardiovascular severity scale" needs to incorporate surgical complexity as it relates to survival, but also many other factors that can influence severity of a disorder such as (1) likelihood of fetal demise, (2) potential hemodynamic instability after birth but before intervention, (3) number of total lifetime anticipated interventions/surgeries, and (4) functional status and quality of life after intervention/surgery.

In order to attempt to establish a standardized consensus, we are developing a tool we call the "Fetal Cardiovascular Severity Grading Scale." This is a seven-point scale ranging from grade = 1, very mild disorders with excellent outcome, to grade = 7, the most severe form of disease in which perinatal survival is of question. The system is being validated through consensus opinion of pediatric cardiologists across the United States, and continues to evolve through modification. Table 5-1 lists the grading system in its current iteration (2011) and the criteria for each grade. Table 5-2 lists examples of common diagnoses of congenital heart defects and their proposed severity grades, using the current grading system. It is important to note that these grades are based purely on isolated forms of heart disease and do not take into consideration the presence of other variables such as prematurity, additional extracardiac malformations, genetic abnormalities, and chromosomal abnormalities or syndromes, all of which certainly add to the severity of the cardiovascular condition.

Table 5-1 Fetal Cardiovascular Disease Severity Grading Scale

STATUS	DEFINITION	TREATMENT	PROGNOSIS/ANTICIPATED OUTCOME	BRIEF SUMMARY DESCRIPTION	2 V	1 V
Level 1	Cardiovascular finding with minimal, if any, negative impact on well-being.	None	Excellent/normal quality of life.	No significant disease	✓	✗
Level 2	Cardiovascular abnormality where treatment *may* be necessary. Postnatal follow up is necessary.	Medical management may be required in utero or after birth. Surgery or catheter therapy is *possible* but will need to await postnatal assessment to be certain.	Excellent/normal quality of life.	Mild disease, need for intervention (surg/cath) possible.	✓	✗
Level 3	Cardiovascular abnormality/*simple* form of congenital heart disease (two-ventricle).	Surgery or catheter therapy will, with *certainty*, be required.	Excellent/normal quality of life.	One intervention (surg/cath) necessary with excellent outcome.	✓	✗
Level 4	Cardiovascular abnormality/*complex* form of congenital heart disease (two-ventricle).	Surgery will, with *certainty*, be required. Further additional interventions or surgery *may* be necessary at some point in life.	Good/close to normal quality of life.	One intervention necessary, multiple interventions (surg/cath) are possible over lifetime; good outcome.	✓	✗
Level 5	Cardiovascular abnormality/*complex* form of congenital heart disease, single-ventricle or two-ventricle type.	Fontan surgical palliation strategy required for single-ventricle patients; or surgery for two-ventricle repair will, with *certainty*, be required and further intervention or surgery will, with *certainty*, be necessary in the future.	Prognosis is fair-to-good; infant is likely to survive surgery. Quality of life *may* be impaired or duration of life *may* be limited.	Single-ventricle strategy, low risk; two-ventricle strategy, with definite need for additional procedures over lifetime; fair-to-good overall outcome.	✓	✓
Level 6	Cardiovascular abnormality/*complex* form of congenital heart disease, single-ventricle or two-ventricle type.	Fontan surgical palliation strategy required, but is at high risk; or two-ventricle repair but at high risk.	Prognosis is poor-to-fair. Risk of death is possible; long-term complications are highly likely. Survival beyond childhood is poor.	Single-ventricle strategy, high risk; two-ventricle strategy with variable outcome and limited life expectancy.	✓	✓
Level 7	Cardiovascular abnormality/*complex* form of congenital heart disease with very poor prognosis.	Intervention may be offered, but expected outcome is poor.	Fetal or perinatal demise likely, despite intervention.	Poor outcome. Survival beyond early period of life not expected.	✓	✓

cath, catheterization; surg, surgery; 1 V, single-ventricle; 2 V, two-ventricle.

Table 5-2 Examples of Common Forms of Fetal Cardiovascular Disease and Their Proposed Severity Grade

FETAL CARDIOVASCULAR DISORDER	SEVERITY GRADE
Echo bright spot in the left ventricle	1
Small muscular ventricular septal defect	1
Premature atrial contractions	1
Aortic stenosis or pulmonic stenosis, moderate	2
Large ventricular septal defect	3
Pulmonic stenosis, severe	3
Transposition of the great arteries, simple	3 or 4
Tetralogy of Fallot	3 or 4
Truncus arteriosus	5
Tricuspid atresia, mild pulmonic stenosis	5
Hypoplastic left heart syndrome, open atrial septum	5
Tetralogy of Fallot, pulmonary atresia with aortopulmonary collaterals	5 or 6
Hypoplastic left heart syndrome, intact atrial septum	6 or 7
Heterotaxy syndrome, single ventricle, total anomalous pulmonary venous connection	6 or 7
Ebstein's anomaly with hydrops	7

The Transition from Fetus to Neonate: A Delivery Classification System

Identification of congenital heart disease before birth obligates the fetal caretaker team to develop an appropriate strategy for delivery with a plan of action for postnatal care. Mode of delivery for the vast majority of congenital heart disease is completely dependent upon maternal concerns and desires. A vaginal delivery is safe and perhaps even desirable in most cases. In a review of fetuses delivered at our institution with prenatal diagnosis of hypoplastic left heart syndrome, we found no advantage of a cesarean section delivery over a vaginal delivery when looking at surrogate markers of hemodynamic stability and well-being (e.g., blood gas measures, serum lactate, serum creatinine) (Table 5-3).[1] Cord blood gas was in fact slightly lower for those with elective C-section in comparison with vaginal delivery and those delivered via urgent C-section. Follow-through of newborns into the first delivery room blood gas and the first intensive care unit blood gas continued to show no advantage for a C-section delivery. Factors such as distance of family from the site of care and maternal variables and desires should come into play in deciding the mode of delivery. Our data support the notion that for a single-ventricle anomaly with ductal dependence for systemic blood flow, a vaginal delivery is safe and fetuses tolerate such extremely well.

Oftentimes, the delivery room care necessary for the birth of a fetus with congenital heart disease is quite minimal because, for many defects, the condition is anticipated to be stable at birth. Frequently, vascular access is indicated in order to be able to infuse prostaglandin or administer fluids or inotropic agents. At other times, arterial blood gas assessment and real-time blood pressure measures are of value, so an umbilical arterial line may be placed. Less commonly, it is clear from fetal evaluation that the newborn will be unstable at birth and will require urgent resuscitation as soon as it is separated from placental maternal support. Such neonates require a different level of preparation and urgent postnatal care.

We have devised a tool to help identify the immediate neonatal needs of infants with prenatally diagnosed cardiovascular disease through a class designation (Table 5-4). Our "Delivery Classification Scale" is a means of labeling a particular delivery for a fetus with heart disease, communicating to all parties the degree of anticipated instability and the needs of the neonate in the delivery room.

The scale consists of four classes:

1. Class 1: A fetus for which no special care is anticipated at delivery. Examples include a simple large ventricular septal defect, balanced complete atrioventricular canal defect, or truncus arteriosus with normal truncal valve function.
2. Class 2: A fetus anticipated to be stable at birth, however, is dependent upon patency of the ductus arteriosus for either systemic or pulmonic blood flow and requires initiation of prostaglandin infusion. Placement of venous access is indicated, typically an umbilical venous catheter. Umbilical arterial line placement is elective, is commonly not placed, and is left to the discretion of the neonatal resuscitation team. Examples include stable neonates with pulmonary atresia or hypoplastic left heart syndrome with open atrial septum.
3. Class 3: A fetus with a form of heart disease in which instability is possible or likely. Hypoxemia, hypotension, or acidosis is possible and in addition to prostaglandin infusion, other agents such as fluid or inotropes may be indicated. Venous access through an umbilical vein, as well as arterial access, is of value. Such fetuses may require joint delivery room care from both neonatology and cardiology at birth in order to achieve stability. Examples include transposition of the great arteries, in which the atrial septum may be restrictive and an urgent balloon septostomy required, or total anomalous pulmonary venous return with obstruction in which rapid stabilization and transport to the operating room for urgent repair may be necessary.
4. Class 4, IMPACT (**im**mediate **p**ostpartum **a**ccess to **c**ardiac **t**herapy) Procedure: A fetus in whom marked instability is anticipated as soon as it is separated from placental circulation. These are uncommon disorders

Table 5-3 Blood Gas Measurements in 79 Fetuses with Hypoplastic Left Heart Syndrome*†

	ALL SUBJECTS	VAGINAL DELIVERY	ELECTIVE CD	UCD/OVD	*P* VALUE
N	79	49 (62.0%)	18 (22.8%)	12 (15.2%)	
Gestational age (wk)	38.6 ± 1.2	38.8 ± 1.0	37.9 ± 1.3	39.1 ± 1.3	0.01
Birth weight (g)	3148 ± 567	3168 ± 539	2993 ± 734	3320 ± 280	0.3
Umbilical Cord Arterial Blood Gas					
pH	7.28 ± 0.08	7.29 ± 0.08	7.23 ± 0.07	7.24 ± 0.07	0.03
PO_2 (mmHg)	25.3 ± 9.6	26.5 ± 10.5	23.6 ± 9.3	23.5 ± 6.8	0.61
PCO_2 (mmHg)	54.2 ± 15.1	49.9 ± 12.7	63.6 ± 19.1	56.2 ± 11.1	0.007
Base deficit (mmol/L)	2.8 ± 3.5	2.8 ± 3.7	2.0 ± 3.2	4.0 ± 3.0	0.38
Infants with pH ≤7.1 (*N*)	0 (0%)	0 (0%)	0 (0%)	0 (0%)	1
First Delivery Room Arterial Blood Gas					
pH	7.20 ± 1.0	7.30 ± 0.1	7.20 ± 0.1	7.20 ± 0.0	0.016
PO_2 (mmHg)	45.2 ± 14.2	46.4 ± 16.9	43.1 ± 7.2	43.7 ± 9.5	0.922
PCO_2 (mmHg)	43.1 ± 9.6	40.9 ± 7.9	50.0 ± 10.2	34.3 ± 6.7	0.006
Base deficit (mmol/L)	8.5 ± 3.9	7.6 ± 3.9	9.3 ± 3.5	12.7 ± 2.9	0.066
Infants with pH ≤7.1 (*N*)	4 (5.7%)	1 (2.4%)	3 (17.6%)	0 (0%)	0.06
First ICU Arterial Blood Gas					
pH	7.33 ± 0.05	7.34 ± 0.05	7.28 ± 0.05	7.34 ± 0.04	0.0002
PO_2 (mmHg)	42.48 ± 9.86	43.3 ± 10.3	40.8 ± 10.4	41.8 ± 7.1	0.81
PCO_2 (mmHg)	41.8 ± 7.3	40.7 ± 5.6	46.4 ± 10.1	39.3 ± 6.0	0.01
Base deficit (mmol/L)	3.87 ± 2.53	3.4 ± 2.4	4.9 ± 2.8	4.3 ± 2.5	0.09
Infants with pH ≤7.1 (*N*)	0 (0%)	0 (0%)	0 (0%)	0 (0%)	1
First 24 Hours					
Peak serum lactate level (mmol/L)	4.2 ± 2.7	4.0 ± 2.8	3.5 ± 1.5	5.5 ± 3.5	0.14
Peak serum creatinine level (mg/dL)	0.9 ± 0.2	0.9 ± 0.1	0.8 ± 0.1	0.9 ± 0.2	0.06

*Samples were obtained as an umbilical cord gas, in the delivery room, and at initial arrival in the ICU.

†All data are presented as *N* (%) or mean ± standard deviation.

CD, cesarean delivery; ICU, intensive care unit; PCO_2, partial pressure of carbon dioxide; PO_2, partial pressure of oxygen; UCD/OVD, urgent cesarean delivery or operative vaginal delivery (planned vaginal, but circumstances dictated otherwise).

Table 5-4 Delivery Classification Scale for Fetal Cardiovascular Disease

	DEFINITION	EXAMPLES	ACTION	PERSONNEL
Class I	No hemodynamic instability.	VSD, AV canal, truncus arteriosus	Evaluation and monitoring.	Neonatology
Class II	Ductal-dependent lesions, stable hemodynamics anticipated.	Pulmonary atresia, critical coarctation or AS, HLHS	Vascular access, PGE infusion, ± arterial line.	Neonatology
Class III	Possibility or likelihood of hemodynamic instability.	TGA, TAPVR	Vascular access, PGE infusion, arterial line.	Neonatology + cardiology
IMPACT	Hemodynamic instability is anticipated at separation from placental circulation.	HLHS + IAS, Ebstein's, CHB, hydropic fetus	Cesarean section in cardiac facility (operating room or cath laboratory) with neonatal resuscitation in adjacent cardiac room.	Cardiac intensive care, cath laboratory, cardiac anesthesia, cardiac surgery, as necessary.

AS, aortic stenosis; AV, atrioventricular; CHB, complete heart block; cath, catheterization; HLHS, hypoplastic left heart syndrome; IAS, intact atrial septum; IMPACT, immediate postpartum access to cardiac therapy; PGE, prostaglandin E infusion, TAPVR, total anomalous pulmonary venous return; TGA, transposition of the great arteries; VSD, ventricular septal defect.

in which the respiratory or circulatory systems may rapidly fail without urgent, immediate action at birth. Examples may include hypoplastic left heart syndrome with an intact atrial septum or complete heart block with marked bradycardia. For each of these, an immediate intervention can be life-saving: urgent opening of the atrial septum or pacing of the heart, respectively. The IMPACT delivery is a carefully planned strategy tailored to the needs of the anomaly. The infant is delivered via a C-section at term in a cardiac procedure facility (operating room or catheterization laboratory) and the newborn is taken to an adjacent room for rapid evaluation, resuscitation, and performance of whatever procedure is necessary. The IMPACT procedure may involve cardiac surgery, cardiac catheterization interventionalists, anesthesia, and cardiac imaging staff. In order to create efficiency, coordination of duties and assignment of roles is discussed and mapped out before delivery at a pre-IMPACT meeting of participating staff.

The Delivery Classification Scale designates complexity and care needs at delivery and the immediate neonatal period and is to be distinguished from the Fetal Cardiovascular Disease Severity Grading Scale, which describes overall disease severity and prognosis. For example, there may be anomalies in which delivery is perhaps expected to be precarious but long-term outcome is quite good. Transposition of the great arteries is one such example, in which marked hypoxemia may occur at delivery, requiring close neonatal attention and significant effort (e.g., possible urgent balloon atrial septostomy), but long-term prognosis after surgery is quite good.

At regular multidisciplinary meetings, which include fetal cardiology, maternal-fetal medicine, obstetrics, cardiac surgery, and neonatology, all fetal patients with heart disease are discussed and a delivery classification is designated. This improves communication between multiple services and is an efficient and clear way to manage the delivery of a fetus with cardiovascular disease.

We have developed a number of systems that aid in managing the fetus with heart disease. These systems may or may not be of value to other centers, because variable facilities, varying styles of practice, and interdisciplinary relationships at different institutions may influence the management of delivery. Operational tools, clinical care models, and management strategies continue to be developed and tailored to optimize care for these unique patients.

Reference

1. Peterson AL, Quartermain MD, Ades A, Khalek N, Johnson MP, Rychik J. Impact of mode of delivery on markers of perinatal hemodynamics in infants with hypoplastic left heart syndrome. *J Pediatr*. 2011;159:64-69.

6

Counseling and Support for the Family Carrying a Fetus with Cardiovascular Disease

Jack Rychik and Denise Donaghue

The process of counseling families carrying a fetus with congenital heart disease (CHD) is perhaps one of the most difficult and challenging tasks professionals in the field of fetal medicine are asked to perform. The synthesis of complex bits of information into a logical diagnosis that medical caretakers can understand and act upon is one thing. Conveying that information in a cogent, comprehensible manner and explaining the options for a plan of action to a patient and family is quite another.

Whereas resources are available for the professional to learn how to interpret ultrasound images and understand the science and pathophysiology of fetal cardiovascular disease, there is very little guidance on how to effectively speak to families, convey findings, and "counsel." The term "counseling" itself has an interesting connotation in that the presumption is that simple, straightforward conveyance of factual information is insufficient, which is true. Rather, an interpretation of the facts must be made and the essence of the meaning of the data then transmitted, with *advice* as to how to proceed. This, of course, makes sense because families cannot be expected to understand, on their own, the meaning of the medical information discovered at evaluation. Very few families will understand the implications of a particular structural anomaly or an abnormal Doppler flow pattern without a careful and thoughtful explanation with overall context provided by a healthcare professional.

This all becomes very challenging when one adds to the mix the extremely high level of stress and anxiety created by the situation at hand. Pregnancy and gestation is all about anticipation and hope. From the moment the news of pregnancy arrives, families begin their process of imagining what the future will bring. From delivery, to baby care, to child rearing and beyond, thoughts and actions are focused on preparation for a new life. Months of mental preparation pass before the actual arrival of the infant. This allows for the development of a cognitive model of expectations that becomes fixed in the minds of parents to be. The disruptive impact following the diagnosis of a fetal anomaly can be psychologically shattering with a myriad of overpowering thoughts rushing forward. One common immediate reaction is grief at the loss of the envisioned future. Emotions flood forward, blocking cognitive faculties at a time when complex material is being presented. Questions—such as *How* can this happen to me? *Why* did this happen to me? *What* did I do to bring this about?—can intrude, clouding the mind of anyone trying to listen and understand what is being transmitted. The combination of emotional charge on the part of the patient with the need to convey complex information on the part of the professional makes for a challenging encounter, with implications toward effective decision making.

The ideal goals of fetal counseling are to have the patient and family leave the encounter with (1) a complete understanding of the ultrasound findings, (2) a full comprehension of the implications for perinatal and postnatal care, (3) a sound sense of the prognosis, both short and long term, (4) an understanding of all management strategies and options that are available, and (5) a balanced, healthy mental state on the part of the patient, with appropriate expectations for care and outcome. Admittedly, it is rare that all of these goals are achieved at the initial visit or, at times, at all.

How can the medical professional achieve at least some, if not all, of these goals? In the next few paragraphs, the authors would like to describe what they believe to be the principles and essentials of prenatal counseling. We must admit, that we do so with an element of trepidation, because we have found this to be one of the most personal experiences to be shared between a medical professional and her or his patient. Each of us has our own subjective method and technique, and we suspect that there are a number of different correct ways to do this. Some readers may take issue with the suggestions and recommendations we are about to make. Perhaps there are other notions as to how to best achieve the goals or one may completely disagree with our views on the goals to be achieved. Nevertheless, there is a surprising paucity of literature on this subject and very few suggested guidelines as to how to go about performing this incredibly important, but daunting, task. After providing prenatal counseling to hundreds of families carrying a fetus with complex cardiovascular disease, we venture an attempt at tackling this issue. Here is what we have learned.

Principles of Prenatal Counseling for Fetal Cardiovascular Disease

The Setting

For pediatric cardiologists, most fetal echocardiography takes place within the confines of a pediatric echocardiography laboratory. This, unfortunately, can be a suboptimal environment for prenatal care and counseling. For the family about to receive important news concerning their unborn child, an evaluation within the setting of other infants and children awaiting an echocardiogram can be awkward and uncomfortable. Because the prenatal counseling session about to occur may focus on alteration of expectations, watching other children playing in a waiting room may further reinforce false expectations and hopes. It may also cause unnecessary stress to families to see other children when their own pregnancy may not result in such an outcome. Perinatologists and maternal-fetal specialists are better equipped from this perspective; however, some pediatric cardiologists and specialized "fetal centers" have remedied this problem by creating a separate location and setting for prenatal assessment and counseling.

A dedicated, separate area for fetal echocardiography and prenatal counseling is optimal. The waiting room design and environs should be adult oriented with appropriate reading materials and literature concerning pregnancy available. Counseling should take place right after the imaging evaluation but, in our view, should not take place in the same room as the ultrasound examination. The scenario of the physician entering the ultrasound room with the patient lying on the examination table still covered in ultrasound gel and proceeding to immediately discuss the findings is one to be avoided. Such action can create a sense of "physician dominance" over the patient, is unnecessary, and can be the setup for an inappropriate social dynamic that may impede the free flow of questions. Ideally, one should allow the study to be completed and have the patient clean up and use the lavatory if necessary. A separate, quiet room should be assigned for prenatal counseling. The patient may have additional family members in the waiting area who may wish to join her at the counseling session. Ideally, all parties should be seated at a round table, with all members at equal eye level. This provides an open and inviting environment for discussion and verbal exchange. Although this may all seem somewhat mundane, we believe that the subtleties of such psychodynamics play a key role in achieving the prenatal counseling goals listed previously.

The Personnel

Medical staff entering a counseling session may include the echocardiogram-interpreting attending physician and supportive staff such as a nurse or social worker. At our center, we have established as our standard protocol that a physician and a dedicated fetal heart nurse coordinator are at attendance at *every* patient counseling session. In this manner, the patient creates a bond with two members of the prenatal counseling team—a physician and a nurse. This truly broadens the scope of care and advice that can be provided. We have discovered that there are certain inquiries that are made to a nurse that would otherwise not typically be raised with the physician, regardless of the gender of either. There should also be sensitivity to the fact that the overall number of staff members entering a counseling session may need to be limited. Because many of these activities take place within the setting of a teaching hospital, trainees will oftentimes be included in prenatal counseling sessions. Each member of the counseling team should identify themselves; patient wishes should be respected if there is a desire not to include trainees in the counseling session. In our experience, it is the rare family that will complain about the presence of trainees but, if so, this request should be respected. Also, one should be aware of the "us versus them" psychodynamic that can be created if there are too many staff in attendance relative to the patient and her family. Hence, the number of staff assigned to participate should be judged and decided upon before entry into the counseling session.

The sonography staff are part of the team offering overall services to the patient. At times, an anxious patient will directly question the sonographer during the fetal echocardiogram as to the findings and their implications. Our sonographers are specifically trained to provide a supportive encounter with words of encouragement, but to limit the reporting of specific findings directly to the patient. The sonographers will reassure families that all of the information will be provided at the counseling session and all questions answered at that time, with the counseling team placing the echocardiogram findings within the context of the history and other medical information. Most families, although perhaps still anxious, will be satisfied with this approach.

The Discussion

The person leading the discussion, let us call him or her the "counselor," must convey both confidence and honesty throughout the session. The discussion must not be rushed, with ample time allowed for questions and answers. We typically expect that prenatal counseling for newly diagnosed heart disease will take approximately 1 hour. Follow-up visits are variable in the time spent. Factors that contribute to the quantity of time expenditure in counseling relate to the complexity of the heart disease as well as patient-/family-related variables such as maternal temperament, level of stress, psychological state, and cognitive capacity. Here are some tips and pointers:

- Start the conversation through introductions. Describe the role of the various staff (e.g., nurse, social worker). We will frequently begin by asking the patient how she learned about the possibility of the presence of a "birth defect of the heart." This allows for a review of the current knowledge to date about the pregnancy, a review of the referring physician's findings, and what impressions have been conveyed, that is, What is the patient's understanding of the problem?
- Following this introduction, state and confirm that there is a problem with the fetal heart. Outline to the patient/family what you are about to do. Typically, we tell them that we will discuss what the normal fetal heart looks like, describe how the fetal heart differs from normal, and what the implications are for the pregnancy, delivery, neonatal care, and beyond (Box 6-1).
- During the discussion, be honest and do not "sugar coat" the data. It is hard to convey bad news, but it is our job as professionals to do so in as clear and sensitive a manner as possible. As in all things, experience and practice will help. Prenatal counseling is a skill that improves with time.
- If the diagnosis is certain, be firm and say so. If it is not and there are still unknowns, admit this as well and describe to what degree the unknowns may affect overall management and prognosis.
- Describe the ultrasound findings and how they contribute to the diagnosis. Write down the actual name of the diagnosis, because this may help families as they seek additional information through other resources such as the internet/web or a library.

Box 6-1 A Step-by-Step Listing of Important Elements to Include in the Family Counseling Session after a Prenatal Diagnosis of Heart Disease

1. Introduction of team members.
2. Dialogue with the patient as to how she learned of the suspicion of an anomaly, with review of history of present pregnancy, family history of CHD, risk factors, and other issues.
3. State to the family that the fetal echocardiography confirms the presence of an anomaly.
4. Outline what will come next in the counseling, so as to provide a sense of structure (e.g., say "I will discuss the normal heart, how your fetus's heart differs, and what the implications are for the pregnancy and beyond in the next few minutes—please stop me if there is something I have said that you do not understand, in addition I will stop for questions along the way").
5. Describe and demonstrate the normal heart.
6. Describe and demonstrate how the patient's fetal heart differs from the normal heart from an anatomical and physiological perspective.
7. Discuss the implications of the fetal diagnosis for the remainder of the pregnancy (e.g., frequency of visitations, additional testing necessary such as amniocentesis or further obstetrical imaging).
8. Discuss the impact upon the delivery (e.g., mode of delivery, additional monitoring that may be necessary).
9. Discuss the implications for neonatal care (what type of care will be necessary and where that care should offered, e.g., specialized facility, neonatal intensive care unit, cardiac intensive care unit).
10. Discuss therapeutic options including medical treatment, surgery, and the time course and complexity of treatment.
11. Discuss anticipated prognosis, short and long term.
12. Discuss the option of termination of pregnancy with clear articulation of time limits (as appropriate, based on legal regulatory limits and gestational age).

- Describe the implications of the diagnosis for the remainder of the pregnancy and any potential impact toward mother's health, if appropriate.
- Describe the management options for prenatal and postnatal care.
- Describe the prognosis and outcome, based on knowledge of the most recent contemporary outcomes for medical or surgical care for the anomaly or disease at hand. This, therefore, requires an up-to-date knowledge of current strategies and outcomes for CHD (hopefully something this book and other resources will help you to achieve!).
- Some families exhibit immediate sudden outbursts of emotion such as fear or extreme sadness. Crying is common and to be expected. Other families exhibit frustration through anger or rage. It is critically important to create an air of respect and dignity for the patient and their predicament, regardless of who they are or their reaction to the information you are conveying. Families will commonly apologize after such outbursts.
- Use ample print materials—figures, illustrations, and diagrams—to help explain, first, the normal anatomy, and then, the abnormal findings. Allow time for the family to digest and comprehend the differences in the structure between the normal and the abnormal. A side-by-side comparison of anatomy can help. The use of figures portrayed on a computer screen or drawn on a board can also be helpful and illustrative at the time of counseling; however, these are limited by the inability of the family to take these educational aids home for further study and review.
- Explain, explain, and explain—but stop intermittently to allow for questions and ask the family if they understand. One technique is to ask the family to repeat what they have just learned and to explain back to you in their own words what they have heard, if there is suspicion of a poor understanding of the material.
- Judge when enough is enough . . . it can become a huge challenge for some families to absorb dense blocks of data once given the initial shock of the diagnosis. The counselor must develop skills in reading facial cues and body language. Sometimes a quick summary and essential aspects of diagnosis and prognosis are all that the patient and family will allow. For example, discussing the physiological benefits of volume unloading at the second stage of surgical palliation for hypoplastic left heart syndrome when it is evident that the patient is about to erupt into an emotional outburst or fit of crying does not serve any purpose. It is unlikely that such a patient is truly going to absorb what has been explained, and as counselors, we need to be able to read patient/family responses to the counseling content conveyed.
- Occasionally, a break is needed for a "time out." Such a break can benefit both patient and counselor and should be used as a moment to regroup and gather thoughts on all ends. At times, bits and pieces of information need to be doled out in packages, with full details reserved for subsequent counseling sessions.
- Provide the option for additional future counseling sessions, either with other family members to be invited or simply to hear things through for a second time. Such a session may need to be scheduled relatively soon after the initial encounter.

- Provide contact information for the family to call, or email if the practice will allow, following the initial session. In our fetal heart program, the assigned nurse coordinator functions as an easily accessible liaison to the patient and can answer most questions or direct them to the attending physician as needed.
- Make it clear that follow-up evaluations and counseling sessions are anticipated. These serve the purpose of monitoring for anatomical or physiological changes that can occur in the fetus and allow opportunities for continued family education and counseling. Families will frequently come back at follow-up visits with good questions based on a prior counseling session. Gaps in knowledge can be easily ascertained with more focused and attentive counseling offered at these follow-up sessions. We typically see patients with fetal cardiovascular disease at 4-week intervals from time of initial evaluation until point of delivery, with the intent of providing further counseling and education at each and every encounter.

The Hardest of Talks: The Option of Pregnancy Termination

Each and every patient should be made aware of her option to choose termination of pregnancy, based on legal limits as determined by state and local authorities. In most regions of the United States today, termination of pregnancy is possible up to, but no later than, 24 weeks of gestation. Being made aware of the option of termination and its legal limits is the right of every patient and the obligation of the counselor to convey to the patient. Actively advising and suggesting to patients to choose termination is an action we do not believe is within the purview of the prenatal counselor, regardless of the severity of the disease. For example, in cases of severe fetal disease for which no reasonable successful treatment options are available (e.g., trisomy 18 with complex heart disease, conjoined twins with a single heart amalgam, or single-ventricle type CHD with large diaphragmatic hernia), the task of the counselor is to convey as effectively as possible the potential futility of pursuing treatment. If the family declines the option of pregnancy termination after careful time spent in describing the situation and after acquiring an honest sense that the family understands the prognosis, non-intervention at birth is another possible option to be pursued.

We believe it is our task to provide as much information as possible to the family in order to help them come to their own conclusions and to make the right decision for themselves. Criticizing families for expressing interest in termination or intentionally not discussing this option in pregnancies under 24 weeks' gestation is inappropriate. As caretakers and practitioners, we all bring our own opinions, experiences, and life views to the counseling table; however, one should resist the urge to project our own personal beliefs or values, be they cultural, political, or religious, onto our patients. Once a decision toward termination or continuation of pregnancy is made, we convey support for that decision because it is the right one for the family.

Doctor, what would you do? This is a commonly asked question and can be handled in a number of different ways. One should respond honestly and state clearly that one patient's choice may not be appropriate for another patient, because so many variables enter into the decision of whether to continue a pregnancy or to terminate. As a physician or nurse, our conditions may be vastly different than that of the family being counseled, and this factor should be explained to the patient and family. Hence, the physician's or nurse's personal decision in relation to a particular case as to "what we would do" may not be applicable to other families in whom conditions will almost always vary to some degree. In general, caretakers need to avoid the hubris of thinking that they "know best" and avoid a paternalistic or maternalistic approach. Although it can be a huge challenge, careful explanation of the facts and conveyance of the latest data on prognosis, or in rare and unusual cases, a description of the outcome of similar patients or experiences, can all contribute to families making their own judgments and decisions.

Another common request that arises is a desire on the part of the family to speak with other families who have had similar diagnoses and have gone through the same process of prenatal management and postnatal care. On the surface, this may seem like a good idea; however, it is not something that we strongly encourage for fear of inadvertently creating a bias. Those families willing to share their decisions and their story saga are, by nature, the ones with a successful course and a good outcome. Families for which aggressive care is chosen but outcome is unfortunately poor are naturally less willing to participate in such an encounter. This creates a select group of willing families that may not convey a balanced view. Nevertheless, if families ask, we do facilitate such encounters with the added caveat of explaining the possibility of a biased opinion.

One point we have found to be of value in conveying to families during prenatal counseling is the notion of a "fluid prognosis." When describing the prognosis for a congenital anomaly or fetal disorder, in particular for long-term outcome, one can discuss how patients are doing at the current point in time, as far out as data can provide. However, families should understand that care and management of cardiovascular disease is improving steadily. Problems that long-term survivors currently face at the time of fetal counseling may have ready solutions 10 to 20 years henceforth. In the same way that 20 years ago, it would be considered "science fiction" to be able to sit with a family and accurately diagnose complex CHD in a fetus at 20 weeks' gestation, 20 years henceforth, whatever difficulties currently exist for survivors may similarly be more effectively managed and perhaps even resolved. Hope and optimism are integral parts of human nature; when fact based and potentially realistic, these should not be held in reserve when offering prenatal counseling.

Prenatal Counseling: The Nurse's and Social Worker's Perspective

Considering that a majority of prenatal diagnosis of CHD occurs between 18 and 28 weeks' gestation, expectant families will then have anywhere from 12 to 22 weeks to learn as much as possible about their child's diagnosis, to research options for surgical management and expected outcomes, and to make decisions. In the late 1990s, prenatal identification of CHD was occurring with increased frequency, which prompted us to examine how we introduce families into our Cardiac Center at the Children's Hospital of Philadelphia (CHOP). Specifically, we needed to change the timing of when families were brought into this complex continuum of care. In response to this challenge, we designed the Fetal Heart Program, with the primary aim to provide resources at an earlier point in gestation and utilize that time, from prenatal diagnosis to delivery, and help families better prepare for a child with CHD. Our Fetal Heart Program (FHP) was introduced in 2001 and has matured as a multidisciplinary program with dedicated fetal cardiologists, sonographers, nurses, social workers, and administrative assistants. What follows are the operational aspects of the encounter with our patients in which fetal cardiovascular disease is suspected and discovered. Although in our program the physician professional is a fetal cardiologist, the role described later can be played by a maternal-fetal medicine or skilled experienced perinatologist as well.

The Initial Visit

Upon arrival for the initial FHP evaluation, patients are asked to complete an intake questionnaire that provides us with basic background information about the pregnancy, maternal and paternal health history, family histories, cultural/language differences, and other issues. A fetal echocardiogram (echo) is performed by a skilled sonographer with interpretation by a fetal cardiologist. Immediately after the fetal echo, families with a diagnosis of CHD meet with a multidisciplinary team for counseling. The team consists of a fetal cardiologist, a nurse coordinator, and a social worker. The cardiologist is the person leading the counseling and she or he reviews the interpretation of the fetal echo and provides a diagnosis for the patient/family (see earlier). The cardiologist reviews diagrams of the normal heart and one that reflects how their baby's heart is different, which depicts the specific form of CHD that has been identified. They discuss the diagnosis, options for surgical management, outcomes, hospital stay, expectations for quality of life, and need for lifelong follow-up with a cardiologist. If the patient is diagnosed before 24 weeks, the options discussed include termination of pregnancy. Because this is a sensitive subject, we recognize it is an important aspect to include as part of counseling in a nonbiased manner. It has been our experience that approximately 10% to 15% of families we initially counsel for prenatal diagnosis of CHD elect to terminate the pregnancy.

Learning that your unborn baby has a congenital heart defect is a stressful, often devastating, experience for families. A multidisciplinary team approach to delivering bad news affords the nonphysician members of the team the opportunity to strike a balance, ensuring adequate support for the patient/family, while the cardiologist focuses on imparting important clinical information about the details and implications of the diagnosis. We have learned a great deal from our patients and families over the years and have come to have a deeper appreciation that prenatal diagnosis really is just the beginning of a long journey. Once a diagnosis of CHD is confirmed, and counseling has been provided, patients and families are left with many questions. Some of these questions are clinical in nature, some are more pragmatic about logistics, follow-up appointments, finances, lodging, and so on. This certainly makes sense when you think about it. Families report, that "their heads are swimming with new worries and questions." Concerns will range from length of hospitalization, to breastfeeding, to what to tell their other children. Patients specifically have many questions about delivery, asking "Will I need a C-section? Where will I deliver? Will I be able to hold the baby? Can I still breastfeed"? It is not surprising then to discover that families are receptive to working with a team of people from multiple disciplines, each knowledgeable in their own areas. This provides the patient and family access to comprehensive care to meet many needs, from clinical information to coordination of clinical activities and consultations, access to on-going education, support for emotional and psychosocial needs, and resources to help manage logistical issues.

How Do Families Get to Us?

Most patients/families rely on their primary physicians (perinatologists, obstetricians, or pediatric cardiologist) to refer them for further fetal cardiac evaluation. Once a diagnosis of CHD has been confirmed, many families go into what is called "consumer mode." Many people will spend hours online searching the Web for information about their child's diagnosis, seeking physicians/institutions that have expertise in pediatric cardiac care. Typically, they are focused on obtaining data about case volume, surgical outcomes, and any other information they can gather to help them better understand what they are facing and prepare for their baby with CHD. One patient intimated that when she learned her unborn baby had a heart defect, "she felt like she was being inducted into an exclusive club, that she never knew existed, and had no desire to be a member of." She was amazed that so many people she met in person and online knew someone who had a child with CHD. Conversely, we have patients who report feeling incredibly isolated and alone. When families are feeling so isolated and desperate, the Web has sometimes been the only place to find information or connect with other parents who have children with CHD. We worry about the reliability and accuracy of some of the information online. This is one point that families and professionals tend to agree upon—the Web and the current world of social media can be a blessing and a curse. Once a patient has been evaluated in the FHP, we encourage them to utilize the FHP team as informational resources moving forward. Interestingly, a vast majority of patients will reach out by phone or email within 7 to 10 days after their last appointment, most often to the nurse coordinator or social worker, to discuss additional questions/concerns as they arise. These intermittent contacts helps establish a rapport and reinforces for the patient that this is a complicated situation, and that is why we are here to partner with them. The overarching theme is preparation. We have found that providing patients/families accessible, ongoing education and support on the front end (during the prenatal period) has tremendous pay-off when they are in the intensive care unit with their baby. Parents and our colleagues in intensive care have acknowledged that this preparation in FHP facilitates a smoother transition from prenatal to postnatal care.

The Precounseling Huddle

Our practice has come to include an informal precounseling informal conference or "huddle" with the cardiologist, sonographer, nurse, and social worker to discuss any pertinent information revealed on the intake questionnaire, diagnosis made by the cardiologist, and any observations about the family's understanding of why they are here, their demeanor, and other issues. Did they come in to this appointment suspecting or knowing a diagnosis of CHD exists? Or is this going to be new information? If the nurse or social worker had contact with the patient before their appointment by phone, it is important to share that assessment. It has been helpful to hear the sonographer's impression of the patient/family's demeanor during the scan. Were they tearful? Asking questions? Anxious? Laughing? All of this information helps us to approach the counseling session more prepared and gives us a sense of where the family is emotionally, psychologically, and functionally.

Counseling

Patients referred for evaluation for possible suspected CHD seem to fall into a variety of categories. The first category of patient arrives for the appointment organized and in control. They have researched the suspected/working diagnosis given to them by the referring perinatologist or pediatric cardiologist and often have binders full of information they have gathered and pages of questions prepared for the meeting. If they have been counseled elsewhere before their FHP evaluation, they are typically stable and composed throughout. Often such patients may express emotions subsequent to the physician counseling, while meeting separately with the nurse and social worker. Some physicians have likened this phenomenon to the "good cop–bad cop" phenomenon. The physician describes the findings and delivers the prognosis whereas the nurse/social worker can help interpret and provide further context. The absence of emotions and absence of "letting down of guard" with the physician may reflect the patient/family's desire to have some modicum of control whenever possible. The second wave of counseling, or wrap-up, is performed by the nurse/social worker, which continues once the physician leaves. This is a period of relief, where emotions can flood to the surface. When a patient/family does get through the counseling with the cardiologist without crying, it is almost certain that the nurse and social worker can anticipate a swell of emotions at this closure portion of the counseling session. In our experience, this phenomenon occurs in approximately 60% of counseling.

The second category of patient we commonly see in our program seems to be more fragile, appearing overwhelmed and more emotional from the outset. Whereas they are not prepared for a diagnosis of CHD, neither are they particularly surprised to learn that there is in fact something very wrong. This group tends to be very emotional at the counseling with the physician and their anxiety is almost palpable right from the outset. Another category of patient referred for fetal echo and consultation come with no worry or suspicion of a problem whatsoever. Often they have come to the appointment alone, with plans to return to work as soon as they are done with the visit. They are shocked when they hear about a diagnosis of CHD. Their reactions are understandably more extreme, almost raw. They range from crying hysterically to intense anger and denial; some have even walked out from counseling before completion.

This is an extremely vulnerable time for all of these families. Regardless of how they arrive, we have a standard approach to counseling that ensures that the patient/family receives a comprehensive review of the fetal echo findings and its implications. This standard approach provides a foundation and creates structure so that we can objectively and logically introduce pertinent clinical information. Many families are distraught and even desperate for encouragement and hope. We will frequently have patients ask the same question two or three different ways during counseling in an attempt to get a more hopeful response. Uncertainty about what exactly they can expect after birth (e.g., will the infant require a single-ventricle or a two-ventricle surgical pathway) can be even more stressful for patients and families, as opposed to knowing with certainty that the baby has a definitive single-ventricle physiology and will require three surgeries in the first few years of life. We are cautious in our approach, because it is human nature to want to comfort families and tell them "everything is going to be fine." We may want to soften the blow when delivering bad news, which can be done, as long as the message is clear. We refrain from a paternalistic, protective approach because this is their life, and they need to know all of the details of what they are facing.

Our methodical manner of counseling has become fairly routine and, in our experience, naturally seems to facilitate further discussion and prompt questions from the patient and family. Once we move onto the discussion/question phase of counseling, we are dealing more with human dynamics and we take our cues from the patient's/family's responses and reactions. During this discussion, families are typically very open about what they are thinking. Families often ask: "Are there any other questions we *should* be asking?" What they really are telling us is that they want to trust us and that they need to be able to trust us. They are vulnerable and in unchartered territory. It is our responsibility to help them navigate their way by filling in any information gaps that we identify so that we can ensure that they have not missed anything.

Benefits of Multidisciplinary Counseling

One of the primary benefits of multidisciplinary counseling is that each discipline brings a different skill set to the table. As a team, we are able to assess each family member's reaction and understanding of the diagnosis and plan. Although it may seem foreboding or overwhelming to have three or four people involved in the counseling, we have found that it creates a more fluid dynamic and naturally promotes opportunity for discussion about everything the family needs and wants to discuss. We are better able to partner with families when we introduce "the team" right from the start. At the end of the counseling with the entire team, the nurse and social worker remain with the family. The nurse asks the patient and family if they understood everything that Dr. X was discussing. It is a great opportunity to acknowledge how overwhelming this experience is, how difficult it can be to process all of the information being provided in one meeting. We reinforce that they are not alone and that we are here to provide information and will have additional opportunities to speak further in person and/or by phone. Frequently, patients and families wish to review the diagrams to clarify the anatomy and review their understanding of the plan moving forward. Patients often want to discuss things that they feel are less important, and they state that they "don't want to bother the doctor with this but ...." It may be a clinical question about the postoperative hospital course or medications or something like lactation, hospital visitation, or something as simple as availability of parking. Sometimes patients and families actually seem embarrassed or pressured when asked if they have any questions, and they do not. We do not typically find that this means that they do not understand what has been discussed, but rather, they "got it." Oftentimes they simply have had enough discussion for the time being and are exhausted. Finally, at the end of the session, our social worker remains with the family to conduct a more formal psychosocial assessment. This provides an entirely different set of data from which to craft plans for the family.

Debriefing

Routinely after each counseling, we informally review how the counseling seemed to go from each person's perspective. It is a debriefing of sorts with colleagues after counseling, because these are often emotionally charged meetings that warrant at least a brief analysis. It is interesting to note that this is a time that highlights the difference in how physicians, nurses, and social workers assess families. Each discipline has its own perspective/vantage point, making this a valuable experience for all. We continue to learn "best practices for counseling" from our colleagues and families. To be honest, these counseling sessions can be incredibly draining for professionals as well as the patients/families. This reconvening of the group helps us recharge as we prepare to counsel the next patient/family.

Patient Scenarios Illustrating the Value of Multidisciplinary Counseling

Scenario A: G1/P0, 28 Weeks' Gestation, Dx: Tetralogy of Fallot, Normal Amniocentesis: 46XY

After a 1-hour counseling session with cardiologist, nurse, and social worker, the patient and her husband seemed to understand the anatomy of the heart well, could verbalize an understanding of tetralogy of Fallot (TOF) and plans moving forward toward delivery and postnatal surgery. They asked insightful questions about prognosis and expected outcome, both short and long term. When there were no further questions for the physician, the couple was left to continue the discussion with the nurse and social worker. The husband of the patient became notably quiet when the physician left the room and almost immediately broke down crying. Given the positive tone of the counseling and the thorough discussion that ensued, the team was caught off guard. We acknowledged how stressful the experience can be for families, particularly because we had reviewed a tremendous amount of information in a relatively short time. The social worker was equally surprised by his reaction and asked "What just happened? ... What are you thinking about right now?" He was still tearful and said "so I can bring my basketball trophies up from the basement?" Not understanding where he was heading, we waited. After a minute he took a deep breath, smiled, and simply stated, "So my son *will* be able to shoot hoops with me after all!" When he had learned 48 hours earlier from their obstetrician that there was suspicion of a heart defect, one that would likely require open-heart surgery, he assumed that his son would not be able to participate in any physical activity. As soon as they got home from that appointment, he put all of his trophies in a box and took them down to the basement so that his son would never have to know what he was missing.

We think of this as "tiers of counseling," a process that entails three levels of support and education at each visit—from physician, nurse, and social worker. The percentage of time spent by each professional varies based on the family's needs at that time of visit. First, there is the initial in-depth clinical counseling that involves all three disciplines, with the physician leading. It is beneficial to have the entire team present for this portion so that nurse and social worker will have heard what the family was told and, at the same time, assess how the family is processing information. We are assessing what components of the counseling should be reiterated for the family once they have had a little time to digest what they have been told. Time and time again, patients and families have reported that "once you hear something is wrong with the baby's heart, the rest is a blur. You try to listen to what the doctor is saying but it's hard, it's overwhelming." This is our rationale for providing this second tier of counseling, as an opportunity for families to continue with questions after the initial portion of counseling has been completed by the physician. When the patient and family have exhausted questions for the nurse, they are left to meet with our social worker one-on-one. This is the third and final tier of counseling. Typically, the initial comprehensive counseling can take approximately 90 minutes. We employ this three-tiered approach at each subsequent visit, with each of these subsequent sessions requiring slightly less time, but typically close to 60 minutes. How that hour is allocated among the team members varies depending on the patient's/family's questions and needs at that visit. Some matters are best addressed by the physician, some by the nurse, and others by the social worker. But it is often the nonclinical questions that lead to deeper discussions and better understanding of where the patient/family is situated emotionally and psychologically. This in turn helps the greater team at large to provide support in a more personalized, meaningful, and effective manner.

Scenario B: G3/P1, 24 Weeks' Gestation, Dx: Hypoplastic Left Heart Syndrome, with Intact Atrial Septum, Declined Amniocentesis. Indication for Fetal Echo Was "Unable to Visualize Fetal Heart Adequately, Please Rule Out CHD"

The couple seemed relaxed, not anticipating anything to be wrong with their fetus's heart. Complex CHD (hypoplastic left heart syndrome [HLHS] with intact atrial septum) was diagnosed by the physician. The sonographer communicated her impression that the patient was completely unaware of why she was sent for imaging to look at the fetal heart. The patient in fact stated to the sonographer that she "thought it was crazy that her husband insisted on coming to this appointment, because she planned to be in and out, and immediately head back to work." After the fetal echo was completed, the family was escorted to the consultation room. The nurse stopped in to greet the family and let them know that the team would be in to meet with them in just a few minutes. The patient was visibly agitated and said "something serious is wrong, isn't it?" The nurse confirmed that there was in fact something wrong and that the team would be in shortly to provide the family with a complete picture. This was a situation in which it was important for members of the counseling team to be aware of the family's state of agitation and stress before commencing the counseling session. It was agreed at the precounseling huddle that we needed to go into the consultation room and get right to the point. While the patient had arrived not anticipating a problem, she was becoming increasingly frantic not knowing what exactly was wrong.

Immediately upon hearing this sad news, it was clear that the patient was visibly grieving the loss of the perfect, healthy baby she had envisioned. She was understandably overwhelmed, frightened and very angry. She demanded to know, "How could this happen?" and "Why didn't someone tell me this a month ago?" After counseling with the team, the couple continued to be in shock, reeling from the devastating diagnosis and grave prognosis that it carried. We offered to leave for a few minutes to give the couple some private time and returned 15 minutes later. The couple, although devastated, was able to focus sufficiently to ask about options available to them. They listened intensely to the limited clinical scenarios that included immediate intervention at birth, non-intervention/palliative care, or experimental fetal intervention to open the atrial septum. When they were ready to leave, the patient was distraught, exhausted, and just so angry that she stormed down the hall.

The nurse placed a call to the patient 10 days later but got the answering machine. The patient did in fact call back a few weeks later. She spent a good deal of time talking about what a "dark day" her visit had been for her. She was teary and apologetic for the anger she expressed and stated that she was embarrassed by her behavior, particularly because everyone had been so patient and compassionate. The patient was reassured that her reaction was genuine, honest, and certainly understandable. Sadly, there was not much hope to share in this situation and the family chose non-intervention and palliative care at birth. Before the conversation ended, the patient stated "For what it's worth, I could tell this was a dark day for all of you as well as for me, which in some odd way made you more human, and that was a comfort to me." One year later the family returned for early first-trimester fetal cardiovascular imaging, which revealed a normal, healthy pregnancy with a structurally normal heart. The family expressed tremendous gratitude for the services previously provided and were pleased to share the joy of this new pregnancy with our staff.

Conclusions

Comprehensive counseling with a multidisciplinary team is an essential part of our practice. Feedback from patients and families has greatly influenced the evolution of our care. We continue to strive to improve our approach to counseling and are continuously seeking to better understand what this experience is like for patients and families. Analyzing the counseling process and its impact on families can and should be studied in a rigorous way, similar to the methods employed for reviewing the medical aspects of fetal cardiovascular disease. By doing so, we hope to glean insight to better understand parental stress during this vulnerable time and identify new strategies and resources that we can employ to potentially decrease levels of stress and improve overall outcomes.

Suggested Readings

Allan LD, Huggon IC. Counselling following a diagnosis of congenital heart disease. *Prenat Diagn*. 2004;24:1136-1142.

Bijma HH, van der Heide A, Wildschut HI. Decision-making after ultrasound diagnosis of fetal abnormality. *Reprod Health Matters*. 2008;16:82-89.

Menahem S, Grimwade J. Counselling strategies in the prenatal diagnosis of major heart abnormality. *Heart Lung Circ*. 2004;13:261-265.

Menahem S, Grimwade J. Effective counselling of pre-natal diagnosis of serious heart disease—an aid to maternal bonding? *Fetal Diagn Ther*. 2004;19:470-474.

Menahem S, Grimwade J. Pregnancy termination following prenatal diagnosis of serious heart disease in the fetus. *Early Hum Dev*. 2003;73:71-78.

Congenital Heart Anomalies: Septal Defects

7 Ventricular Septal Defects

Deepika Thacker and David J. Goldberg

Key Echocardiographic Features

- Location of defect on the ventricular septum.
- Size of defect in relation to aortic annulus.
- Direction of shunting across the defect.
- Presence or absence of valve tissue (i.e., tricuspid valve) through the defect.
- Any associated findings such as outflow tract obstruction, semilunar valve narrowing, or coarctation of the aorta.

Anatomy and Anatomical Associations

The ventricular septum is a helical structure that separates the right and left ventricles. More than simply a wall of separation, it is a complex structure made up of many different components. It is predominantly made up of a small thin membranous septum and a larger muscular septum. The membranous septum is bounded superiorly by the aortic valve at the junction of the right and noncoronary cusps and inferiorly by the muscular septum. The muscular septum is further divided into a posterosuperior inlet septum contributing to the separation between the mitral and the tricuspid valves, a trabecular septum in the middle and extending to the apex, and an anterosuperior smooth-walled outlet or conal septum. Endocardial cushion tissue further contributes to the ventricular septum between the two atrioventricular (AV) valves, the "atrioventricular (AV) canal" septum. Looking at it geographically, the "inlet" portion of the septum adjacent to the AV valves is composed of the AV canal septum and the posterior muscular septum. The "outlet" portion of the septum is composed of the muscular conal septum. A ventricular septal defect (VSD) is a communication between the right and the left ventricles due to a defect in the ventricular septum.

Postnatally, the most common type of VSD involves the membranous septum and typically extends into the surrounding structures. This is referred to as a *conoventricular* or *perimembranous* VSD (Figure 7-1) and accounts for up to 80% of cases.[1-3] This defect lies below the aortic valve when viewed from the left ventricle and underneath the septal leaflet of the tricuspid valve when viewed from the right ventricle. It can be covered by tricuspid valve tissue leading to partial or complete closure of the defect. Conoventricular VSDs can be associated with other forms of congenital heart disease. Additionally, subaortic membrane, prolapse of the aortic cusp with development of aortic insufficiency, and right ventricular muscle bundles are some of the associations that can develop postnatally but are rarely, if ever, seen before birth.

Defects in the muscular trabecular septum account for 5% to 20% of all VSDs. They are further classified depending on location: apical, central, posterior, and anterior muscular defects, with apical defects being the most common subtype of muscular defects. Multiple defects in the trabecular septum can give it a "Swiss cheese" appearance and can be particularly challenging to manage after birth. The incidence of muscular defects is significantly higher in the prenatal period and declines after birth owing to a high rate of spontaneous closure of small muscular VSDs in utero.[4] In fact, some consider the presence of a muscular defect in the fetus to be so common as to be considered a variant of normal because, on subsequent scanning, many are no longer seen and are thought to spontaneously close. This, however, raises the question of whether there is simply a high rate of "false-positive" identification. Small jets noted along the septum on color Doppler imaging may be spuriously suspected of being a tiny muscular defect.

The inlet septum is located between the two AV valves, inferior to the membranous septum and posterosuperior to the trabecular septum. A VSD in the inlet septum is often referred to as an *inlet* or *AV canal type* VSD and is found in approximately 5% to 8% of patients with VSDs.

The outlet or the conal septum is located anterosuperior in relation to the trabecular septum and inferior to the aorta and the pulmonary artery. The conus is the region beneath the pulmonary valve that lifts the pulmonary valve above the level of the other three heart valves. The conal septum separates the outlet portion of the right ventricle on the right side from the region beneath the aortic valve on the left side. Defects in this region can be of either the conal septum malalignment type or an actual deficiency in conal tissue referred to as *conoseptal hypoplasia type*. Conal defects constitute 5% to 7% of all VSDs. The conal malalignment type involves varying degrees of displacement or malalignment of the conal septum with respect to the remainder of the ventricular septum. In a patient with normally related great arteries, anterior malalignment of the conal septum can cause subpulmonary obstruction. This type of VSD is typically seen in association with tetralogy of Fallot and is associated with aortic override. Posterior malalignment of the conal septum can cause subaortic stenosis and may be associated with coarctation of the aorta or interruption of the aortic arch.

Frequency, Genetics, and Development

Aside from a bicuspid aortic valve, VSDs are the most common of all congenital heart defects. The incidence has been reported to be 1% to 2% among live-born infants.[1,5,6] Prenatally, however, VSDs are only the fifth most common congenital heart defect to be identified echocardiographically.[7] Over the years, possibly due to improved diagnostics, the incidence of children diagnosed with a VSD is rising.[6,8]

In utero, partitioning of the primitive heart tube starts at the beginning of the fourth week of gestation and is completed by the eighth week.[9] The right and left ventricles are formed with the septation of the primordial ventricle and the bulbus cordis (see Chapter 2). Initially, development of the muscular septum starts as a ridge in the floor of the primordial ventricle. The free wall of the ridge is concave and is separated from the endocardial cushions posterosuperiorly and the bulbus cordis anterosuperiorly by a crescent-shaped interventricular foramen. Meanwhile, there is active proliferation of mesenchymal cells in the endocardial cushions as well as in the right and left bulbar ridges within the walls of the bulbus cordis. The membranous part of the interventricular septum is derived from an extension of tissue from the endocardial cushions. Closure of the interventricular foramen and completion of the membranous septum results from fusion of tissue derived from the endocardial cushions,

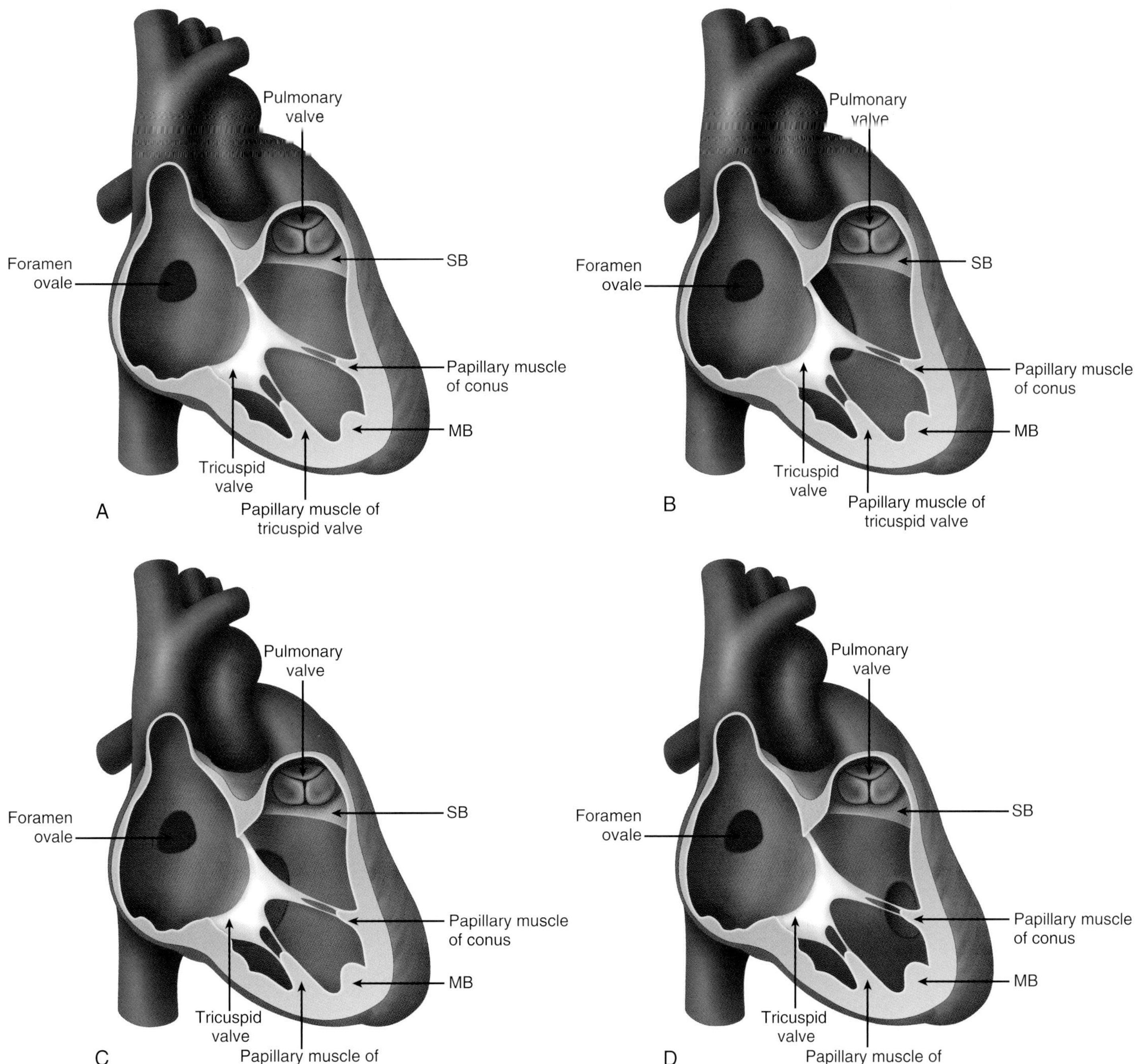

Figure 7-1. (A) View of the ventricular septum from the right ventricle identifies the various anatomical landmarks used to help localize and label various types of ventricular septal defects (VSDs). The moderator band (MB) is a bundle of muscle that runs along the apical anterior aspect of the right ventricle and is in continuity with the large papillary muscle of the right ventricle. The septal band (SB) separates the conus (infundibulum) from the sinus or inlet portion of the right ventricle. (B) Conoventricular or large perimembranous VSD. The defect is located under the septal leaflet of the tricuspid valve and extends up to underneath the aortic valve on the left ventricle side. (C) Atrioventricular cabal type or "inlet" type of VSD located alongside the tricuspid valve incorporating the inlet rim of the septum. Note that the outlet portion under the SB is intact. (D) Anterior muscular VSD located anterior to the MB.

Continued

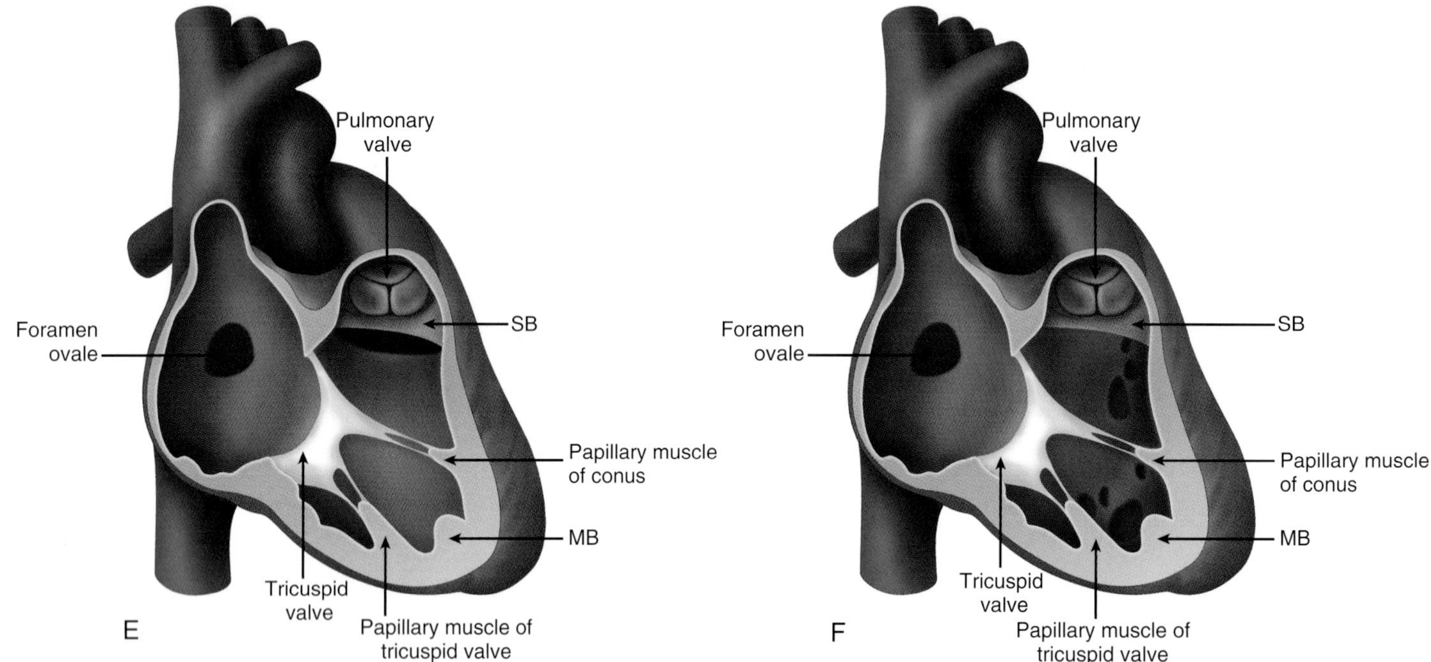

Figure 7-1, cont'd (E) Malalignment type of VSD located completely beneath the SB of the conus. The infundibular (conal) septum is commonly either malaligned and positioned anteriorly encroaching upon the pulmonary outflow or malaligned posteriorly encroaching upon the aortic outflow. Displacement of the infundibular (conal) septum from the rest of the ventricular septum is what defines the limits of the septal defect. These defects are always large and are often referred to as "outflow" septal defects. (F) Multiple muscular defects located anteriorly and in the right ventricle apex. This is often referred to as a "Swiss cheese" septum.

the bulbar ridges, and the muscular septum. A VSD can result either from maldevelopment or failure of fusion of one of the components or from excess resorption of myocardial tissue in the formation of the trabeculae in the muscular septum.

Although a majority of VSDs are isolated lesions, they are associated with other cardiac anomalies in 18% of fetuses and extracardiac and chromosomal anomalies (e.g., trisomy 21, 13, and 18) in as many as 47% of cases.[4,7,10,11] VSDs are also one of the most common teratogen-associated cardiac defects[12,13] and are known to occur with prenatal exposure to alcohol and marijuana.[13] The exact etiology of VSDs, however, does not follow a fixed genetic pattern and is believed to be multifactorial. When one parent has a VSD, the risk in the fetus is increased to 3% to 4%.[14,15] The risk in the fetus is increased to 2% to 5% when a previous sibling has a VSD and to 10% to 15% with two affected siblings.[3,16]

Prenatal Physiology

In the fetus, the right ventricle pumps against a high resistance in the pulmonary vascular bed and into the systemic circulation through a patent ductus arteriosus. The right ventricular pressure is, thus, equal to the left ventricular pressure throughout fetal life. An isolated VSD usually does not cause any significant hemodynamic effects prenatally. Application of color Doppler imaging onto a VSD may not demonstrate much shunting of flow on fetal echocardiography. Nevertheless, because the left ventricle normally contracts a few milliseconds before the right ventricle, one may see left-to-right shunting across a VSD during systole.

Prenatal Management

An isolated VSD does not require any alteration in normal obstetrical management. Cardiological evaluation after birth is recommended.

The identification of a VSD on prenatal echocardiography should, however, prompt closer scrutiny for associated cardiac and noncardiac defects including chromosomal anomalies. Studies have reported termination of pregnancy in as many as 15% to 41% of patients with VSDs when associated with extracardiac and chromosomal anomalies.[4,11]

Postnatal Physiology

An isolated VSD is unlikely to cause significant problems in the first few days of life as the pulmonary vascular resistance (PVR) remains high. With a drop in the PVR in the first few weeks of life, there is progressively increased left-to-right shunting of blood across the VSD. Patients with a moderate or large VSD may develop signs of congestive cardiac failure such as tachypnea, tachycardia, hepatomegaly, poor feeding, and poor weight gain as early as 2 weeks of life but, more commonly, between 1 and 6 months of age. If the VSD left untreated, patients with large defects may develop pulmonary vascular disease as early as 2 years of age. Patients with a small VSD are usually asymptomatic with the only sign being the presence of a harsh pansystolic murmur upon auscultation.

Postnatal Management

Isolated VSDs diagnosed on fetal echocardiography merit reevaluation at birth. This should include a thorough cardiac examination and search for noncardiac and chromosomal anomalies. Infants with small defects are unlikely to require any medical or surgical intervention. Infants with moderate or large defects should be followed closely for signs of congestive cardiac failure as the PVR drops. Medical anticongestive measures with digoxin or diuretics or even surgical closure of the defect may be warranted in some of these babies. Newer techniques have been developed that allow for transcatheter closure of some trabecular defects, alleviating the need for surgery in some cases.

Outcomes

In the past, studies have described an intrauterine spontaneous closure rate of isolated VSDs of as high as 74%.[3,6] More recent studies, however, show that approximately 32% of all VSDs undergo spontaneous closure in utero.[4,11] When classified by subtype, approximately 30% of muscular VSDs and 50% of conoventricular VSDs close spontaneously in utero. Postnatally, there is a higher rate of spontaneous closure of muscular defects so that at the end of the first year of life, the rate of closure of conoventricular and muscular VSDs is almost comparable. Smaller defects close more often than larger ones. Malalignment defects are almost always large and are unlikely to undergo spontaneous closure.

Patients with isolated small VSDs have an excellent prognosis. Postnatally, more than 40% of these undergo spontaneous closure,[4,11] with a majority closing in the first 2 years of life.[1] However, even if still open thereafter, these defects do not cause significant hemodynamic disturbances. Patients with muscular VSDs close by overgrowth of surrounding muscle. Perimembranous VSDs may close by filling in of accessory tricuspid valve tissue, which may result in formation of a ventricular septal aneurysm. Rarely, a perimembranous VSD may close by prolapse of an aortic cusp, which may lead to aortic insufficiency and require surgical intervention.

Patients with moderate-sized defects can usually be managed medically without surgical intervention. A large number of these defects will become smaller or close in the first few years of life. Patients with persistent small or moderate defects have only a 6% to 10% chance of closure after adolescence.[17,18] They have a small but increased risk of infective endocarditis, aortic valve prolapse, or late cardiac arrhythmia and, therefore, should continue to be monitored.

Patients with large VSDs can benefit from a trial of medical therapy. If signs of congestive cardiac failure persist, surgical or catheter closure (when amenable) should be performed to prevent the development of progressive pulmonary vascular disease. Large VSDs should be addressed and closed before 1 year of age in order to prevent the development of pulmonary vascular disease.

The vast majority of patients with appropriately managed isolated VSDs, whether large or small, will have a normal lifespan and normal level of activity. VSDs associated with other structural cardiac defects have a less favorable prognosis.

Imaging Essentials and Important Points

- Careful attention should be paid to the ventricular septum with two-dimensional and color Doppler imaging in order to identify the presence of a VSD.
- Focusing on the septum in a regional serial manner can be helpful, starting with the four-chamber view and the inlet septum, moving to the apical septum, and then angling toward the outflow tracts.
- Small VSDs are difficult to diagnose—they can be missed or falsely suspected. False drop-out on two-dimensional imaging in particular in the thinned region of the membranous septum may give the impression of a defect that may not truly be present.
- In order to reduce a false-positive reading, a VSD should be seen in at least two orthogonal planes before confirming the diagnosis.
- On color Doppler imaging, the color jet must be seen originating from the left ventricular septal surface in order to be called a true VSD. Color jets seen just on the right ventricular side not originating from the left ventricular septal surface may be nothing more than blood flow within the right ventricular trabeculations and should not be confused with a true VSD.
- Associated cardiac anomalies, such as coarctation of the aorta, should be searched for when there is a VSD.
- Measuring the size of a VSD, in particular in the muscular region, can be a challenge. A quick visual way to estimate VSD size is to compare it with the size of the aorta. A defect that is equal to or close to being equal to the size of the aortic valve is a large defect. Defects seen only on color Doppler imaging or measuring 1 to 2 mm in diameter at any point in gestation are considered small. However, small defects seen early in gestation, before 20 weeks' gestation, should prompt a serial follow-up fetal echocardiographic reevaluation closer to term to make sure these defects are, in fact, small.

References

1. McDaniel N, Gutgesell HP. Ventricular septal defects. In Allen HD, Driscoll DJ, Shaddy RE, Feltes TF, eds. *Moss and Adams' Heart Disease in Infants, Children, and Adolescents including the Fetus and Young Adult*. Philadelphia: Lippincott Williams & Wilkins; 2008: 667-682.
2. Pieroni DR, Nishimura RA, Bierman FZ, et al. Second natural history study of congenital heart defects. Ventricular septal defect: echocardiography. *Circulation*. 1993;87(2 suppl):I80-I88.
3. Persutte W. Ventricular septal defects. In Drose JA, ed. *Fetal Echocardiography*. Philadelphia: Saunders; 1998:91-104.
4. Axt-Fliedner R, Schwarze A, Smrcek J, Germer U, Krapp M, Gembruch U. Isolated ventricular septal defects detected by color Doppler imaging: evolution during fetal and first year of postnatal life. *Ultrasound Obstet Gynecol*. 2006;27:266-273.
5. Hiraishi S, Agata Y, Nowatari M, et al. Incidence and natural course of trabecular ventricular septal defect: two-dimensional echocardiography and color Doppler flow imaging study. *J Pediatr*. 1992; 120:409-415.
6. Meberg A, Otterstad JE, Froland G, Sorland S, Nitter-Hauge S. Increasing incidence of ventricular septal defects caused by improved detection rate. *Acta Paediatr*. 1994;83:653-657.
7. Allan LD, Sharland GK, Milburn A, et al. Prospective diagnosis of 1,006 consecutive cases of congenital heart disease in the fetus. *J Am Coll Cardiol*. 1994;23:1452-1458.
8. Martin GR, Perry LW, Ferencz C. Increased prevalence of ventricular septal defect: epidemic or improved diagnosis. *Pediatrics*. 1989; 83:200-203.
9. Moore KL, Persaud TVN. The cardiovascular system. In Moore KL, Persaud TVN, eds. *The Developing Human: Clinically Oriented Embryology*. Philadelphia: Elsevier Saunders; 2008:285-337.
10. Meberg A, Hals J, Thaulow E. Congenital heart defects—chromosomal anomalies, syndromes and extracardiac malformations. *Acta Paediatr*. 2007;96:1142-1145.
11. Paladini D, Palmieri S, Lamberti A, Teodoro A, Martinelli P, Nappi C. Characterization and natural history of ventricular septal defects in the fetus. *Ultrasound Obstet Gynecol*. 2000;16:118-122.
12. Jenkins KJ, Correa A, Feinstein JA, et al. Noninherited risk factors and congenital cardiovascular defects: current knowledge: a scientific statement from the American Heart Association Council on Cardiovascular Disease in the Young: endorsed by the American Academy of Pediatrics. *Circulation*. 2007;115:2995-3014.
13. Williams LJ, Correa A, Rasmussen S. Maternal lifestyle factors and risk for ventricular septal defects. *Birth Defects Res A Clin Mol Teratol*. 2004;70:59-64.
14. Driscoll DJ, Michels VV, Gersony WM, et al. Occurrence risk for congenital heart defects in relatives of patients with aortic stenosis, pulmonary stenosis, or ventricular septal defect. *Circulation*. 1993;87(2 suppl):I114-I120.
15. Nora JJ, Nora AH. Recurrence risks in children having one parent with a congenital heart disease. *Circulation*. 1976;53:701-702.
16. Rice MJ, McDonald RW, Pilu G, Chaoui R. Cardiac malformations. In Nyberg DA, McGahan JP, Pretorius DH, Pilu G, eds. *Diagnostic Imaging of Fetal Anomalies*. Philadelphia: Lippincott Williams & Wilkins; 2002:451-506.
17. Gabriel HM, Heger M, Innerhofer P, et al. Long-term outcome of patients with ventricular septal defect considered not to require surgical closure during childhood. *J Am Coll Cardiol*. 2002;39: 1066-1071.
18. Neumayer U, Stone S, Somerville J. Small ventricular septal defects in adults. *Eur Heart J*. 1998;19:1573-1582.

CASES

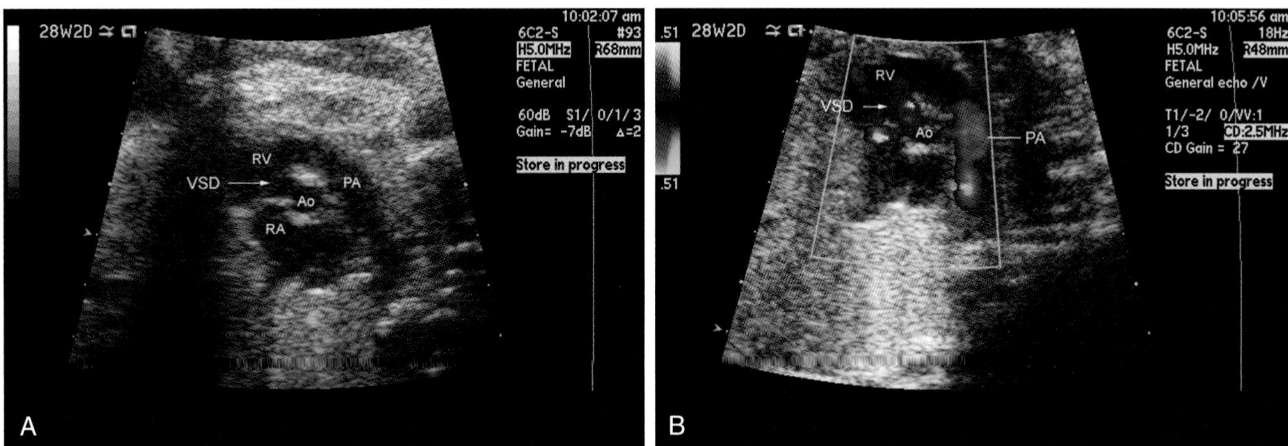

Case 7-1. **(A)** Short-axis view at the level of the aorta (Ao) and the pulmonary artery (PA). The *arrow* points to a large conoventricular ventricular septal defect (VSD). The right ventricle (RV) is seen wrapping around the heart anteriorly. The VSD is deemed to be large because it is centrally equal in size to the aortic annulus. RA, right atrium. **(B)** Color Doppler imaging demonstrates the left-to-right shunting across the large conoventricular VSD.

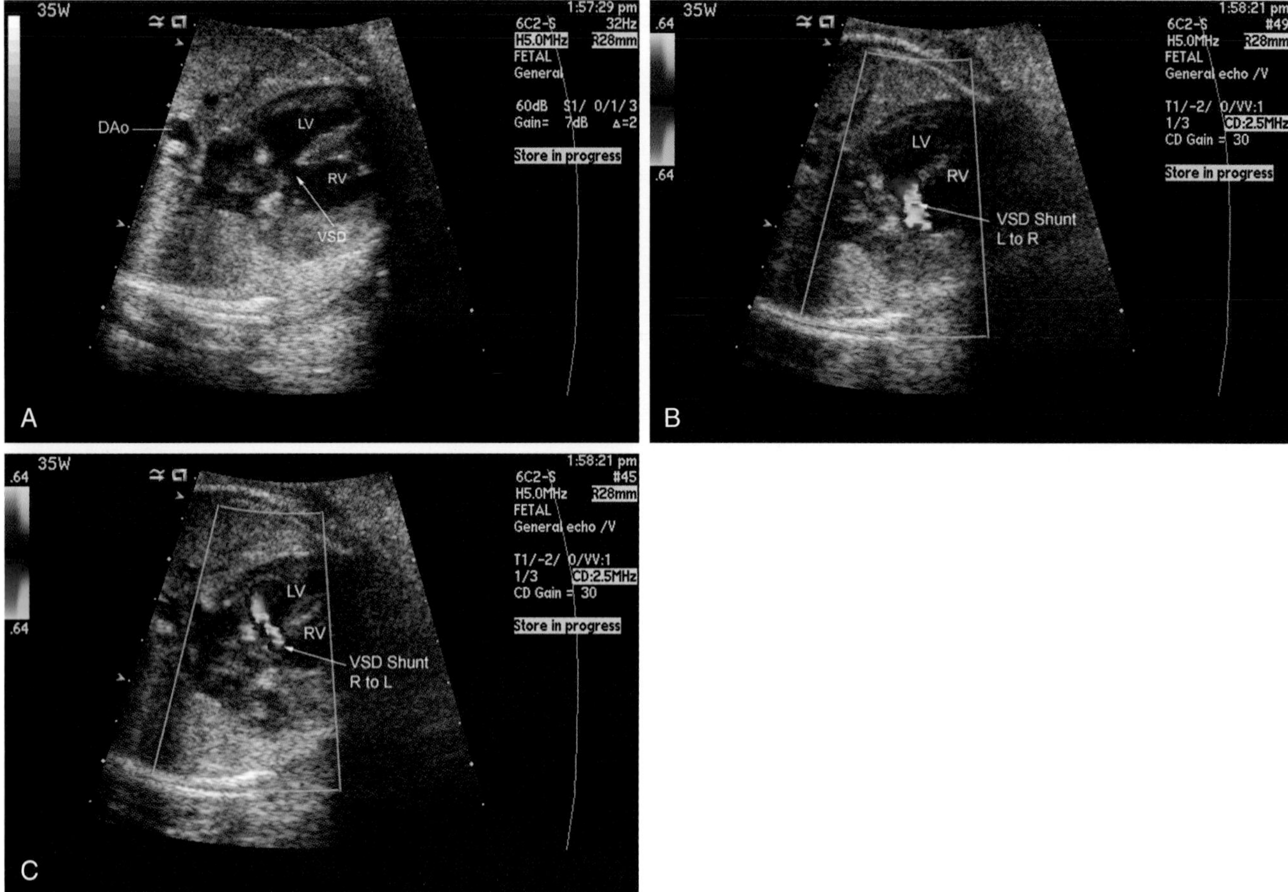

Case 7-2. **(A)** Long-axis view of a large VSD. Notice the left ventricle (LV), which, on its septal surface, is smooth walled without any trabeculations. The RV has a moderator band seen along the surface of the muscular ventricular septum. The *arrow* points to the large VSD. DAo, descending aorta. **(B)** Color Doppler imaging reveals shunting from the LV to the RV. **(C)** At another point in the cardiac cycle, shunting is from the RV to the LV.

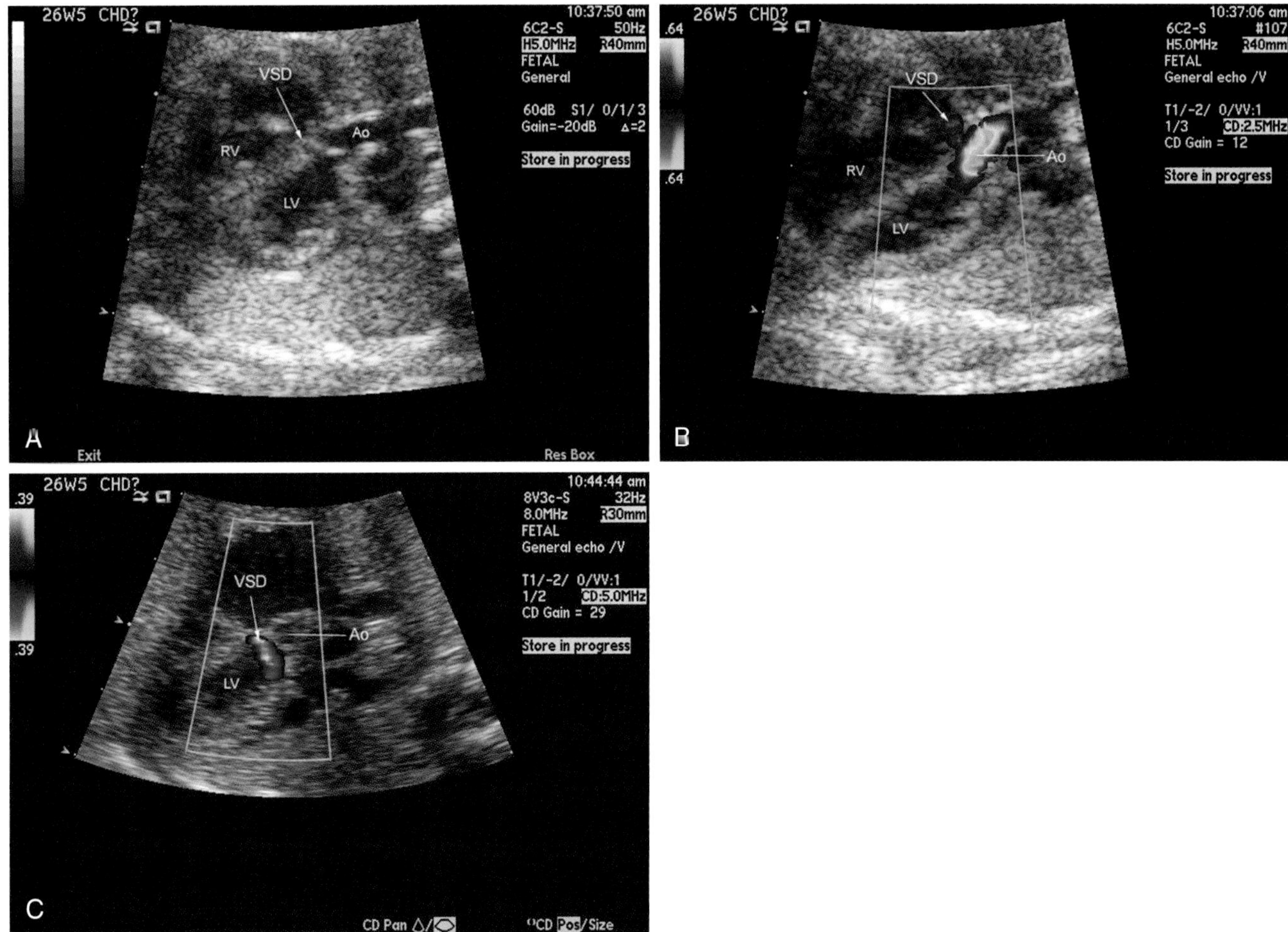

Case 7-3. **(A)** A view of the LV and left ventricular outflow tract. The *arrow* points to a "knuckle" of aneurysm tissue that, on two-dimensional imaging, provides a hint of a possible VSD. At this point in time, it is difficult to tell whether there is any shunting across or whether the defect is of any significance. **(B)** With color Doppler imaging during systole, shunting is seen from the LV to the RV. There is antegrade flow across the aortic valve, which suggests that this image is taken during the systolic phase of the cardiac cycle. Hence, one can deduce that there is LV-to-RV shunting at this portion of the cardiac cycle across this small somewhat restrictive perimembranous VSD. **(C)** Now at a different phase of the cardiac cycle one, a small jet of flow is see angled into the LV *(blue)*. This jet reflects RV-to-LV shunting at a time in which there is no color flow seen in the ascending aorta; hence, we deduce that this is occurring during diastole.

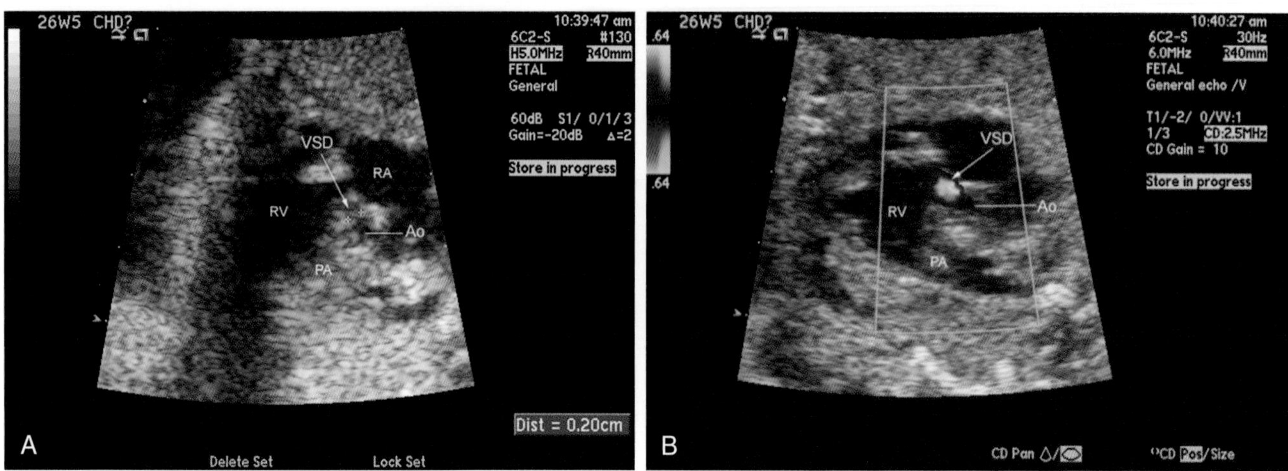

Case 7-4. **(A)** Short-axis view at the level of the left ventricular outflow tract just below the aorta. The *arrow* points to a small perimembranous VSD. Aneurysm tissue is seen as well, partially covering the defect. **(B)** Color Doppler imaging reveals LV-to-RV shunting across the small VSD. The defect on two-dimensional imaging measures approximately 2 mm in diameter; however, this does not truly reflect the effective defect because it is partially covered by aneurysm tissue.

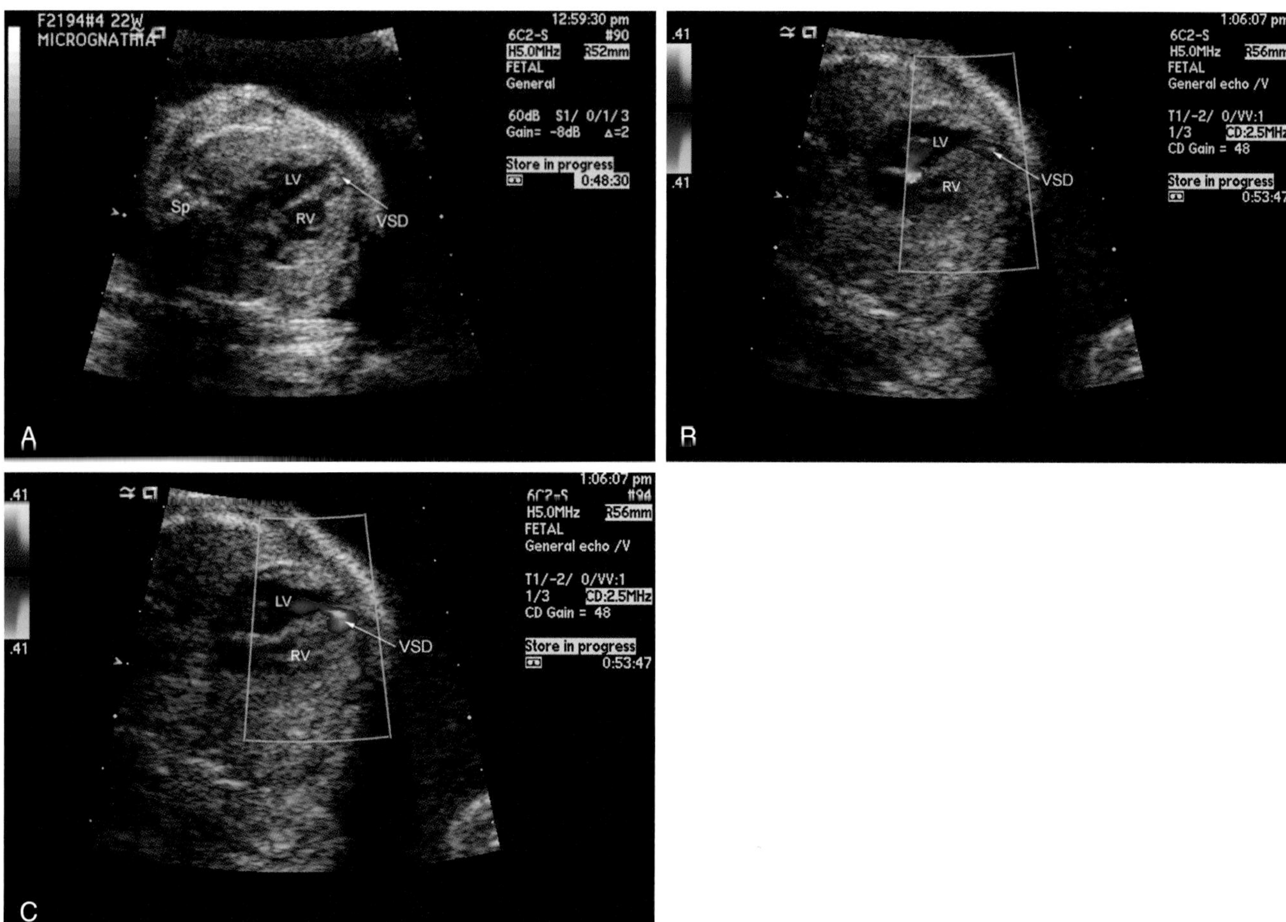

Case 7-5. (A) Long-axis view of the heart demonstrates both the LV and the RV. At the very apex of the heart, two-dimensional imaging reveals a gap that suggests the presence of a VSD of the apical muscular type, small in size. (B) Only with color Doppler imaging do we have confirmation of a defect in the apical muscular region. There is a red jet suggesting RV-to-LV flow across this small apical muscular VSD. (C) At a different phase in the cardiac cycle, there is a blue jet across this small defect, suggesting LV-to-RV shunting.

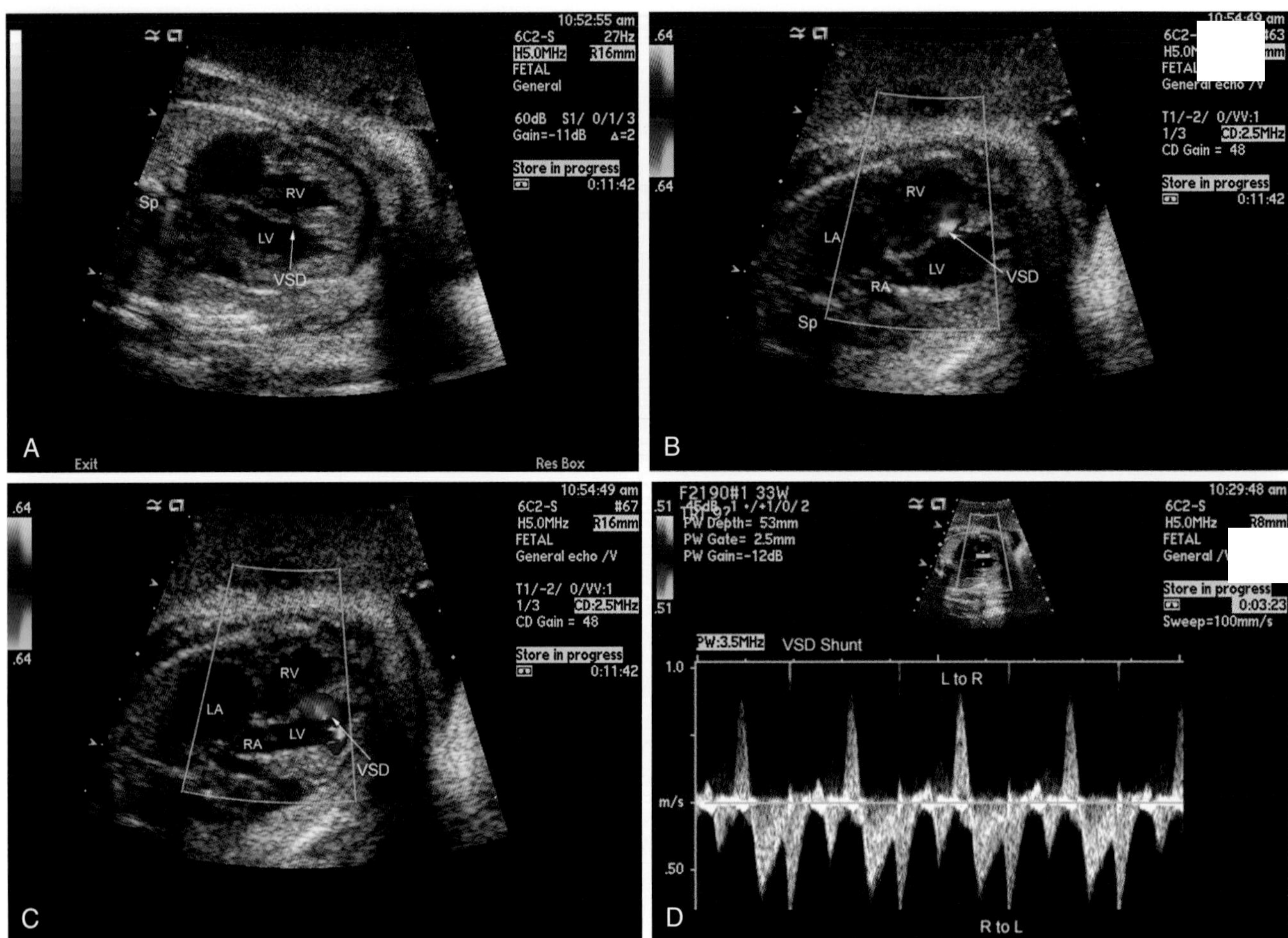

Case 7-6. **(A)** Long-axis view of both the LV and the RV with the ventricular septum aligned in a horizontal manner. There is a gap in the mid-portion of the septum, in the muscular region. This is a muscular VSD. **(B)** Color imaging reveals LV-to-RV shunting across this midmuscular VSD. RA, right atrium. **(C)** At a different point in the cardiac cycle, a blue jet is noted across this midmuscular VSD reflecting shunting from RV to LV. LA, left atrium. **(D)** Pulse Doppler assessment of flow across this defect demonstrates flow above the baseline, which is toward the transducer and hence left-to-right shunting, and then flow below the baseline, suggesting right-to-left shunting. The flow pattern of right-to-left shunting is quite similar to what is seen across the flow of an atrioventricular valve with a double-peak pattern. This suggests that perhaps the right-to-left shunting is occurring in diastole and the flow is subject to the forces that create both an early diastolic filling and a late filling in relation to atrial contraction. The right-to-left shunting is likely a reflection of differences in compliance between the RV and the LV, whereas the left-to-right shunt is likely a reflection of systolic forces driving blood from the LV to the RV.

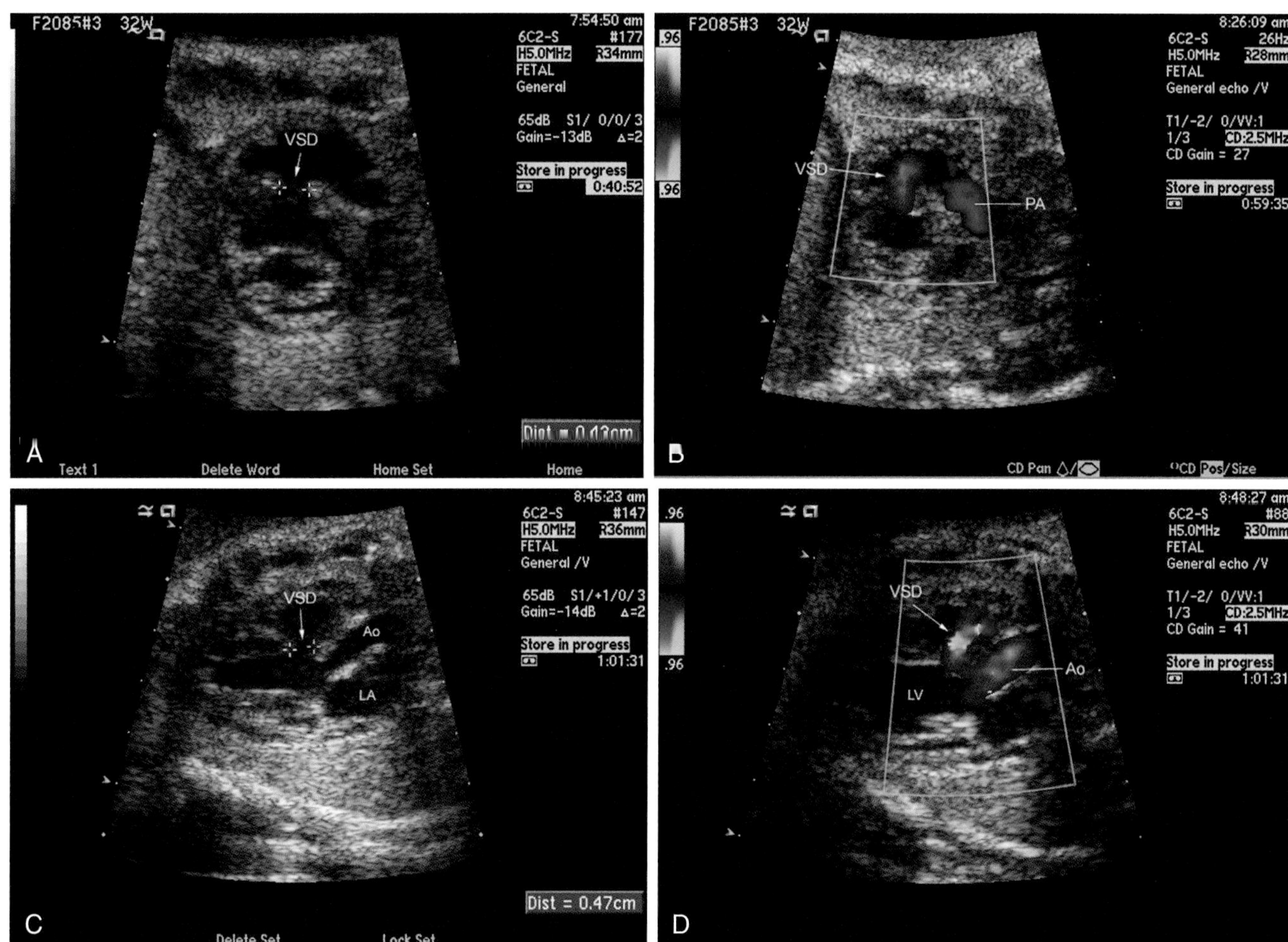

Case 7-7. **(A)** Short-axis view of the heart demonstrates the anterior and posterior leaflets of the mitral valve; just anterior to it is the ventricular septum with a fairly large gap centrally. This is a large anterior muscular VSD. The measurement is approximately 4 to 5 mm in diameter on two-dimensional imaging. **(B)** Color Doppler imaging reveals LV-to-RV shunting as demonstrated by the red jet. This is occurring in systole because there is also a demonstration of antegrade flow across the PA. **(C)** Long-axis view of the LV and the left ventricular outflow tract. This demonstrates the muscular defect in relation to the aorta. **(D)** Color Doppler imaging demonstrates LV-to-RV shunting across the VSD simultaneous with red color flow in the aorta, suggesting that this is occurring during systole.

8

Atrial Septal Defects

David J. Goldberg

Key Echocardiographic Features

- Location of defect on the atrial septum
- Relationship of the defect to the superior and inferior vena cava (sinus venosus type of atrial septal defect)
- Relationship of the defect to the atrioventricular valves (primum atrial septal defect)
- Direction of shunting across the defect

Anatomy and Anatomical Associations

The atrial septum, the part of the heart that separates the left from the right atrium, is not formed as a single structure. It is made up of embryological components that fuse in fetal and early postnatal life to fully separate the left from the right atrium. With the exception of a patent foramen ovale (PFO), any residual communication across the atrial septum after birth is considered an atrial septal defect (ASD).

There are four subtypes of ASD, each named according to its embryological origin and the anatomical location on the atrial septum. A secundum ASD is a residual communication in the area of the fossa ovalis (Figure 8-1). A primum ASD (see Chapter 9) is seen as part of the spectrum of disease associated with endocardial cushion defects or atrioventricular canal defects. Sinus venosus ASDs may be of the superior vena cava (SVC) or the inferior vena cava (IVC) type and are related to incomplete inclusion of the sinus venosus portion of the atrial septum. A coronary sinus ASD is located at the entrance of the coronary sinus into the right atrium and is synonymous with the finding of an unroofed coronary sinus.

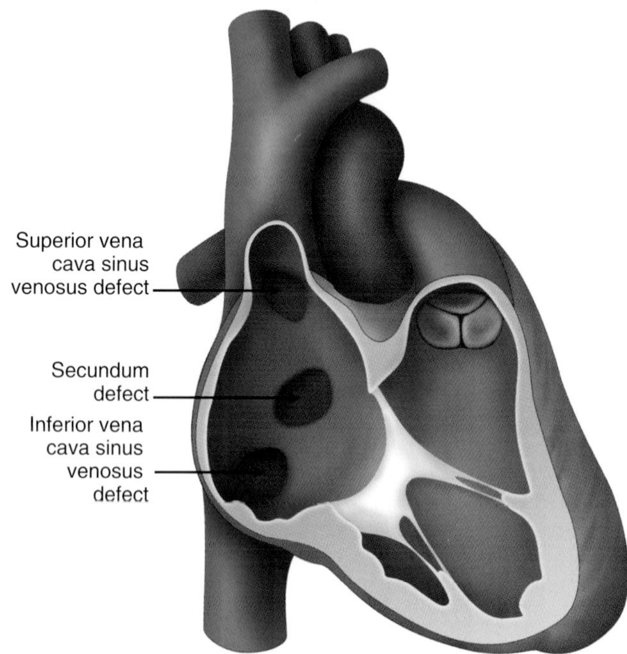

Figure 8-1. Types of atrial septal defect.

The subtypes of ASD may be seen in isolation or as part of more complex congenital heart disease. A coronary sinus ASD may be associated with the presence of a left SVC.

Frequency, Genetics, and Development

ASDs are among the most common congenital heart defects, occurring at a rate of 1 in 1500 live births.[1] Isolated secundum defects make up 6% to 10% of all congenital heart disease in the pediatric population. For an isolated ASD, the female-to-male ratio is approximately 2 : 1.[2]

The development of the atrial septum occurs from the fourth to the eighth week of gestation. The septum primum, a thin membrane, grows from the roof of the primordial atrium toward the endocardial cushions. The ostium primum, the communication that exists between the encroaching septum primum and the endocardial cushions, closes as the septum primum fuses with the endocardial cushions. At the same time, programmed cell death occurs in the more posterior portion of the septum primum, creating the ostium secundum, which allows continued communication between the right and the left atrium. The septum secundum, an infolding of muscular tissue from the ventral wall of the primordial atrium, forms just to the right of the septum primum. By the eighth week of development, fusion of the septum primum and the septum secundum generally has occurred such that the only remaining communication through the septated atria is the foramen ovale, a flap valve formed by the attachment of the septum primum onto the septum secundum. The fossa ovalis is the region of the flap of the foramen ovale as seen from the right atrial side. As the septum primum and septum secundum form, a separate portion of the primordial atrium, the sinus venosus, splits into a right and a left horn. The right horn is the larger of the two and eventually forms the inflow of the IVC and SVC into the right atrium. The left horn fuses with the septum primum and forms the opening of the coronary sinus.

A secundum ASD is thought to arise from abnormal or excessive resorption of the septum primum during the period of programmed cell death. They can occur anywhere along the septum primum but typically occur in the region of the foramen ovale and fossa ovalis.

A sinus venosus ASD forms as a result of incomplete inclusion of the right horn of the sinus venosus into the right atrium and abnormal formation of the septum secundum. These defects are often associated with anomalous pulmonary venous connections and can have significant left-to-right shunting after birth. An ASD involving the coronary sinus results from incomplete fusion of the left horn of the sinus venosus with the septum primum.

An isolated ASD is not generally associated with syndromes or inheritable genetic anomalies, although there are some exceptions and some families with a inheritable form of ASD have been reported. One particular syndrome, Holt-Oram syndrome, is characterized by abnormalities of the upper extremities and cardiac septal defects, predominantly ventricular septal defects or secundum ASD.[3] This syndrome is due to a mutation in the transcription factor TBX5.[4] Other genetic associations include mutations in the genes *NKX2-5* and *GATA4*.[5] In addition, a missense mutation on chromosome 14q12 coding for myosin heavy chain has been shown to be responsible for a subset of inherited ASDs.[6]

Fetal Physiology

The normal fetal circulation includes flow through the foramen ovale from the right atrium into the left atrium. Oxygen-rich blood returning from the placenta by way of the umbilical vein is preferentially directed by the eustachian valve across the atrial septum and into the left atrium. This blood then traverses the mitral valve and is ejected by the left ventricle, allowing the most highly oxygenated blood in the fetus to reach the most vital organs such as the developing fetal brain. The presence of an ASD does not influence this normal shunting in any way and is, therefore, of no hemodynamic consequence. In the absence of associated cardiac defects, an isolated ASD will not have a significant impact on fetal physiology.

Prenatal Management

Owing to the normal fetal flow of blood across the atrial septum, isolated ASDs are very difficult to diagnose in the fetus. However, the fetal circulation is such that an isolated ASD does not have an impact on fetal physiology and, thus, prenatal diagnosis is not essential.

Postnatal Physiology

During the transition from fetal to newborn life, the ductus arteriosus closes and the pulmonary and systemic circulations separate. The left atrium fills completely through the increased pulmonary venous return and, in most cases, the flap valve of the foramen ovale is closed within the first few days of life. Beyond the neonatal period, blood flow across the atrial septum represents an ASD.

In the newborn period and beyond, flow across an ASD is determined by relative compliance of the left and right atria, which are a reflection of the compliances of the left and right ventricles. In the immediate newborn period, the compliance of the left and right ventricle is similar and shunting across an ASD is minimal. However, through childhood and into adulthood, the right ventricle becomes more compliant as fetal ventricular hypertrophy regresses because the chamber now pumps at a lower pressure to the lungs whereas the left ventricle becomes less compliant over time. This then leads to left-to-right shunting across an ASD if present. Children with ASDs are usually asymptomatic but, if the volume of left-to-right flow is great, they may manifest failure to thrive as early as in infancy. Most commonly, ASDs are diagnosed as an incidental finding on routine pediatric examination by auscultation of a pulmonary stenosis type murmur. This murmur is not caused by a true pulmonary valvular abnormality but is instead due to an increased volume of blood going across a normal pulmonary valve as a consequence of left-to-right shunting at the atrial level, creating a flow-to-structure mismatch and "relative" pulmonic stenosis.

Postnatal Management

ASDs do not usually cause hemodynamic impairment in the first few years of life. Nevertheless, the treatment strategy is generally to close these defects before children reach school-age years. Traditionally in the past, this was done surgically using either a primary suture repair or a patch repair. However, since the 1990s, most secundum ASDs are closed using a device deployed by a transcatheter approach. This approach, first described in 1976, continues to be modified as new generations of ASD devices have become available.[7-10] Results are excellent, without the need for open-heart surgery.

Outcomes

ASDs rarely cause significant hemodynamic or rhythm issues in the first two to three decades of life. Indeed, some small secundum ASDs may occasionally close spontaneously.[11,12] However, children with large ASDs can present with failure to thrive that is related to the large left-to-right shunt, right ventricular volume overload and dilation, and increased pulmonary blood flow.[13] Beyond the first two decades, complications related to a persistent unrepaired ASD are more frequent. Individuals with ASDs that have significant shunting are at risk for the development of congestive heart failure,[14] atrial arrythmias,[15] and pulmonary hypertension.[16] Paradoxical emboli leading to stroke are another potential concern and a reason to close an interatrial communication. Indeed, in the natural state, individuals with unrepaired, open ASDs have a significantly diminished life expectancy as compared with the general population.[17] When looking at the excellent current outcomes after intervention, the risk benefit-ratio is such that all ASDs should be closed early in life.

Imaging Points

- Because an interatrial communication is a normal part of the fetal circulation, the diagnosis of an isolated ASD can be quite a challenge. In essence, it comes down to being able to distinguish between a normal versus a larger than normal size communication.
- One method is to observe for the normal flap of the atrial septum bowing into the left atrium. The absence of a bowing flap into the left atrium in the presence of a large deficiency in the septum should raise suspicion of a secundum ASD.
- Prenatal identification of sinus venosus type ASD is very difficult. Deficiency in the atrial septum at the most superior aspect of the atrial septum on a four-chamber view may raise suspicion of a sinus venosus defect. Visualization of the SVC appearing to "override" the atrial septum, with its entry orifice straddling both the left and the right atria, suggests a sinus venosus defect of the superior type.
- Prenatal identification of an isolated coronary sinus type of ASD is extremely rare. A deficiency in the region of the atrial septum just above the level of the atrioventricular valves, but in a posterior aspect of the heart, suggests the presence of coronary sinus type ASD.
- Shunting at the level of the atrial septum is always right to left in the normal fetus. This direction of shunting will be seen in the presence of an ASD in the fetus as well. The presence of left-to-right shunting, however, should prompt inquiry as to the possibility of left-sided heart disease such as mitral valve disease or hypoplastic left heart syndrome. Left-to-right shunting at the atrial level can also be seen when there is an abnormal compliance of the left ventricle due to cardiomyopathy or when there is a torrential return of pulmonary venous flow as seen in the presence of a large pulmonary arteriovenous malformation.
- Small ASDs cannot be reliably detected before birth. We have included a statement to this effect in our report for the normal fetal echocardiogram. If there is a high index of suspicion due to strong family history or some other reason, then a postnatal echocardiogram at a few weeks of life, once the flap of the foramen ovale is potentially closed, is indicated.

References

1. Samanek M. Children with congenital heart disease: probability of natural survival. *Pediatr Cardiol.* 1992;13:152-158.
2. Porter BJ, Edwards WD. *Moss and Adams' Heart Disease in Infants, Children, and Adolescents: Including the Fetus and Young Adult.* 7th ed. Philadelphia: Wolters Kluwer Health/Lippincott Williams & Wilkins; 2008:632-645.
3. Holt M, Oram S. Familial heart disease with skeletal malformations. *Br Heart J.* 1960;22:236-242.
4. Li QY, Newbury-Ecob RA, Terrett JA, et al. Holt-Oram syndrome is caused by mutations in TBX5, a member of the Brachyury (T) gene family. *Nat Genet.* 1997;15:21-29.
5. Srivastava D, Olson EN. A genetic blueprint for cardiac development. *Nature.* 2000;407:221-226.
6. Ching YH, Ghosh TK, Cross SJ, et al. Mutation in myosin heavy chain 6 causes atrial septal defect. *Nat Genet.* 2005;37:423-428.
7. Sideris EB, Sideris SE, Thanopoulos BD, Ehly RL, Fowlkes JP. Transvenous atrial septal defect occlusion by the buttoned device. *Am J Cardiol.* 1990;66:1524-1526.
8. Hausdorf G, Schneider M, Franzbach B, Kampmann C, Kargus K, Goeldner B. Transcatheter closure of secundum atrial septal defects with the atrial septal defect occlusion system (ASDOS): initial experience in children. *Heart.* 1996;75:83-88.
9. Chan KC, Godman MJ, Walsh K, Wilson N, Redington A, Gibbs JL. Transcatheter closure of atrial septal defect and interatrial communications with a new self expanding nitinol double disc device (Amplatzer septal occluder): multicentre UK experience. *Heart.* 1999;82:300-306.
10. King TD, Thompson SL, Steiner C, Mills NL. Secundum atrial septal defect. Nonoperative closure during cardiac catheterization. *JAMA.* 1976;235:2506-2509.
11. Radzik D, Davignon A, van Doesburg N, Fournier A, Marchand T, Ducharme G. Predictive factors for spontaneous closure of atrial septal defects diagnosed in the first 3 months of life. *J Am Coll Cardiol.* 1993;22:851-853.
12. Helgason H, Jonsdottir G. Spontaneous closure of atrial septal defects. *Pediatr Cardiol.* 1999;20:195-199.
13. Lammers A, Hager A, Eicken A, Lange R, Hauser M, Hess J. Need for closure of secundum atrial septal defect in infancy. *J Thorac Cardiovasc Surg.* 2005;129:1353-1357.
14. Murphy JG, Gersh BJ, McGoon MD, et al. Long-term outcome after surgical repair of isolated atrial septal defect. Follow-up at 27 to 32 years. *N Engl J Med.* 1990;323:1645-1650.
15. Shah D, Azhar M, Oakley CM, Cleland JG, Nihoyannopoulos P. Natural history of secundum atrial septal defect in adults after medical or surgical treatment: a historical prospective study. *Br Heart J.* 1994;71:224-227; discussion 228.
16. Steele PM, Fuster V, Cohen M, Ritter DG, McGoon DC. Isolated atrial septal defect with pulmonary vascular obstructive disease—long-term follow-up and prediction of outcome after surgical correction. *Circulation.* 1987;76:1037-1042.
17. Campbell M. Natural history of atrial septal defect. *Br Heart J.* 1970;32:820-826.

CASE

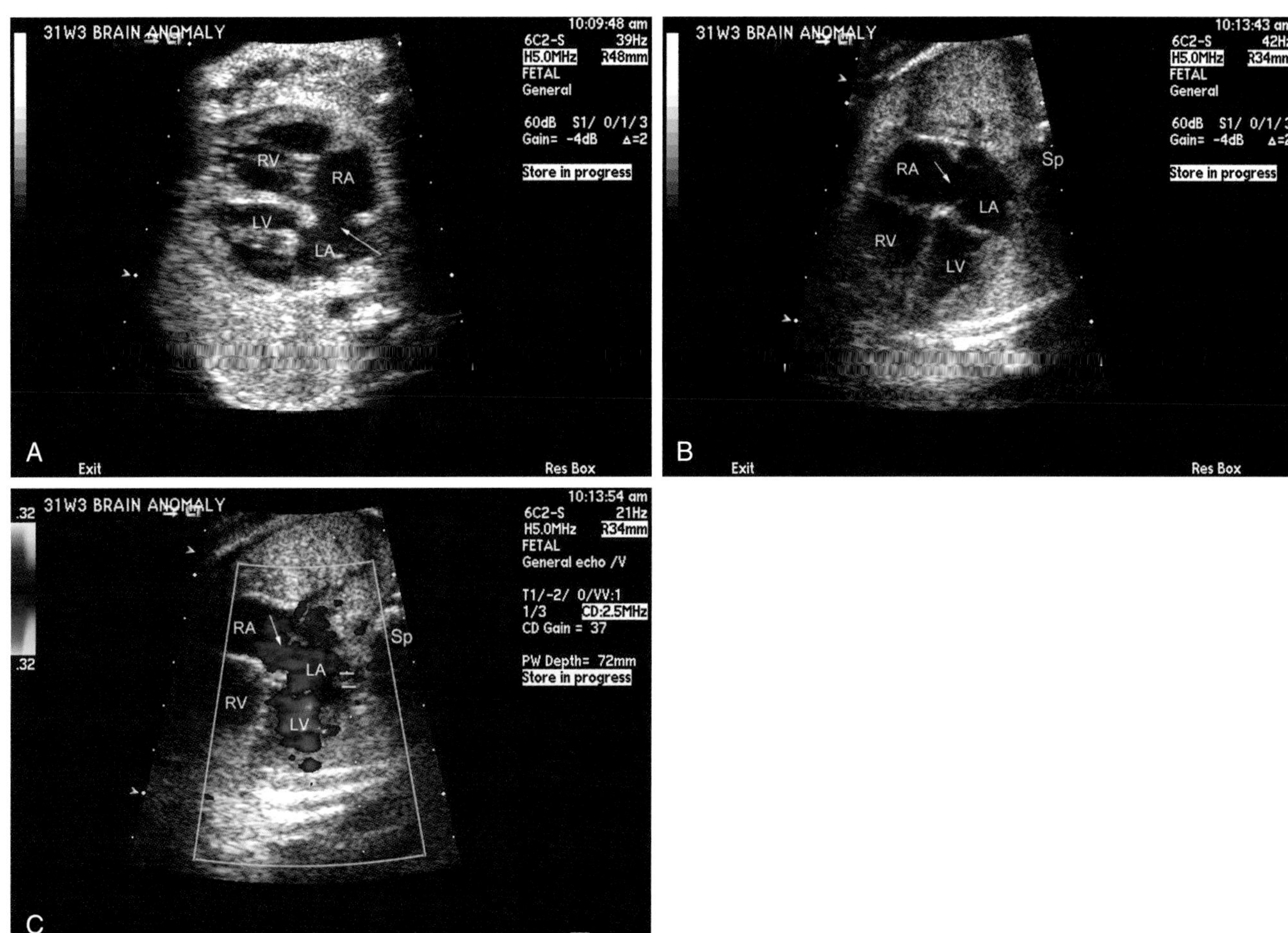

Case 8-1. **(A)** Identification of a secundum atrial septal defect (ASD) in utero is quite challenging because all normal fetuses will have an opening between the atrial chambers, the foramen ovale. However, a dilated fossa ovalis with deficiency in septal tissue can hint at the possible manifestation of an ASD after birth. This is an example of a fetus that presented with a very large fossa ovalis *(arrow)* but with a very thin aneurysmal septum primum. Postnatal evaluation revealed a large secundum ASD. LA, left atrium; LV, left ventricle; RA, right atrium; RV, right ventricle. **(B)** Four-chamber apical view demonstrates a large interatrial communication *(arrow)* as a very large fossa ovalis with a thin membrane bowing into the LA. **(C)** Color flow imaging demonstrates a wide swath of color across the atrial septum consistent with a large interatrial communication *(arrow)* at 31 weeks' gestation. Postnatal imaging revealed a large secundum ASD.

9

Atrioventricular Canal Defects

Meryl S. Cohen

Key Echocardiographic Features

- Size of the atrial septal defect
- Size of the ventricular septal defect (large = complete, small = transitional, none = incomplete)
- Valve attachments to the crest of the septum
- Presence or absence and degree of atrioventricular valve regurgitation
- Degree of balance or unbalance of the atrioventricular valve over the two ventricles
- Relative size of the ventricular cavities
- Presence or absence of left ventricular outflow tract obstruction (valve tissue obstructing or narrowed pathway due to small left ventricular outflow tract)

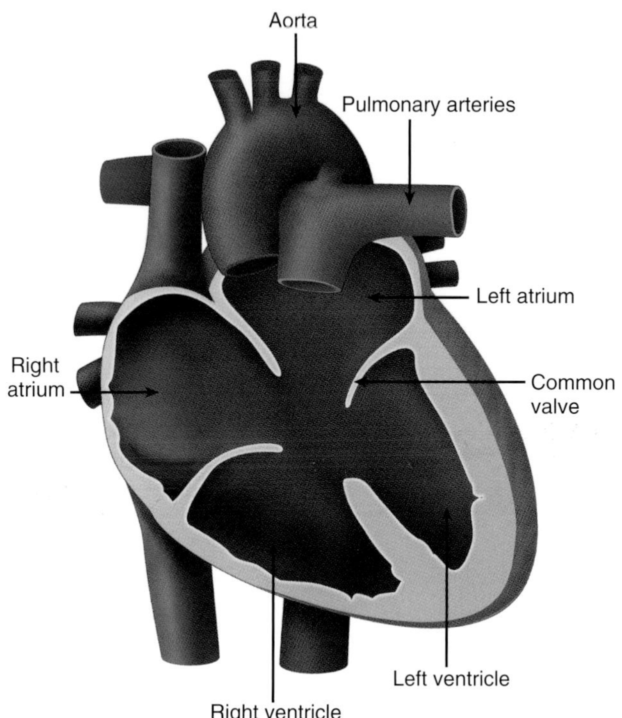

Figure 9-1. Atrioventricular canal (AVC).

Anatomy and Anatomical Associations

The term *common atrioventricular canal* defines a group of cardiac defects characterized by abnormal development of structures derived from the endocardial cushions during embryological development of the heart. Nomenclature varies depending on the school of thought and includes atrioventricular septal defect, endocardial cushion defect, and atrioventricularis communis; atrioventricular canal (AVC), our preference, is used for the purposes of this chapter. In AVC, there is absence of the atrioventricular (AV) portion of the septum as well as maldevelopment of the AV valves resulting in a common inlet to both the right and the left ventricles. The common AV valve is, by definition, abnormal and incompetence (regurgitation) frequently occurs. The defect in the AV septum can result in an exclusive atrial communication, a combined atrial septal defect (ASD) and ventricular septal defect (VSD), or an exclusive ventricular communication. The size and location of these defects dictates the clinical course. Fetal diagnosis of AVC is quite feasible and recognition in utero allows for prenatal counseling and possible identification of other noncardiac defects including chromosomal abnormalities (e.g., trisomy 21).

AVC is typically categorized based on level of septal shunting (Figure 9-1). In all forms of the defect, the absent portion of the AV septum is the same; the septal communication is, therefore, determined by the position of the AV valve within the defect. The *complete* form of the defect is characterized by a large ASD and VSD with the common atrioventricular valve (CAVV) positioned between both defects. The atrial communication, known as an *ostium primum defect,* is located anteroinferior to the margin of the fossa ovalis and adjacent to the AV valves. Importantly, the septum primum portion of the atrial septum is intact. The VSD, known as a canal or inlet type defect, is situated in the posterior ventricular septum along the septal leaflet of the AV valve extending into the membranous septum. This location results in a "scooped out" appearance of the crest of the ventricular septum.

The CAVV anatomy includes a mural leaflet exclusively over the left ventricle and, typically, two leaflets exclusively over the right ventricle. The unique feature of AVC is that in all cases, two leaflets bridge the ventricular septum, one superiorly and one inferiorly.[1] The superior bridging leaflet compromises the AV junction such that the aorta (wedged between the tricuspid and the mitral valve in the normal heart) sits more anterior than normal, resulting in the so-called gooseneck deformity. This abnormality results in foreshortening of the length of the left ventricle from the AV valve annulus to the apex and elongation of the length from the apex to the aortic valve annulus (these measures are equal in length in the normal heart).[2] Patients with AVC are, therefore, at risk for the development of left ventricular outflow obstruction. The inferior leaflet always has chordal attachments to the ventricular septum. With regard to the superior bridging leaflet, these chordal attachments are more variable and are categorized by the Rastelli classification.[3] In Rastelli type A, the superior bridging leaflet is divided at the level of the ventricular septum. Rastelli type A is associated with left ventricular outflow obstruction primarily because the attachments result in increased elongation of the left ventricular outflow tract.[4] Rastelli B is quite rare; the superior leaflet is divided with attachments to a right ventricular papillary muscle that sits more superiorly on the ventricular septum. Type C is commonly associated with

Down syndrome and is considered the most rudimentary of the classifications, with the superior leaflet being "free floating" with no attachments to the septum.

In addition to these classifications, the papillary muscle anatomy of the AV valve may be abnormal. They may be positioned closely or shifted counterclockwise in comparison with the normal heart. The presence of a solitary papillary muscle should be highlighted as a risk factor for repair and may reflect the potential for left ventricular inflow obstruction.[5] In unusual cases of complete AVC, the CAVV is positioned superiorly attaching to the septum primum such that there is a large ventricular communication with no atrial level shunt.

The *incomplete* (also known as partial) form of AVC occurs when the chordae of the CAVV are densely adherent to the ventricular septum such that there is an ostium primum ASD but no VSD component (Figure 9-2). Though there is a common, single AV valve annulus, there are two orifices. The superior and inferior bridging leaflets (as previously described) are attached to the ventricular septum by means of a connecting tongue of chordal tissue, which gives the valve the appearance of a "cleft." Regurgitation through this cleft is quite common.

There is a *transitional* form of AVC as well, quite similar to the incomplete type. In transitional AVC, the chordal attachments are not quite as adherent to the ventricular septum resulting in a restrictive VSD or multiple small VSDs through the chordae.

The CAVV in AVC may be "balanced" over both ventricles or "unbalanced" such that the valve sits disproportionately over one ventricle more than the other. Typically, the contralateral ventricle is hypoplastic. Unbalance occurs in 10% of AVC cases.[6,7] The more common right dominant type of unbalanced AVC is challenging to treat and often associated with other levels of left-sided obstruction such as subaortic stenosis and/or aortic arch obstruction.[6] Right dominant unbalanced AVC can be quite marked, resulting in a variant of hypoplastic left heart syndrome. Left dominant type is less common and right ventricular outflow obstruction may occur.[7]

Associated lesions seen with AVC include patent ductus arteriosus, ostium secundum ASD, coarctation of the aorta, and additional VSDs. Tetralogy of Fallot can also occur with AVC and is seen almost exclusively in patients with Down syndrome. The complete form of AVC with Rastelli C is most commonly associated with tetralogy of Fallot.[8] AVC is often a component of heterotaxy syndrome and seen with other complex congenital heart lesions.

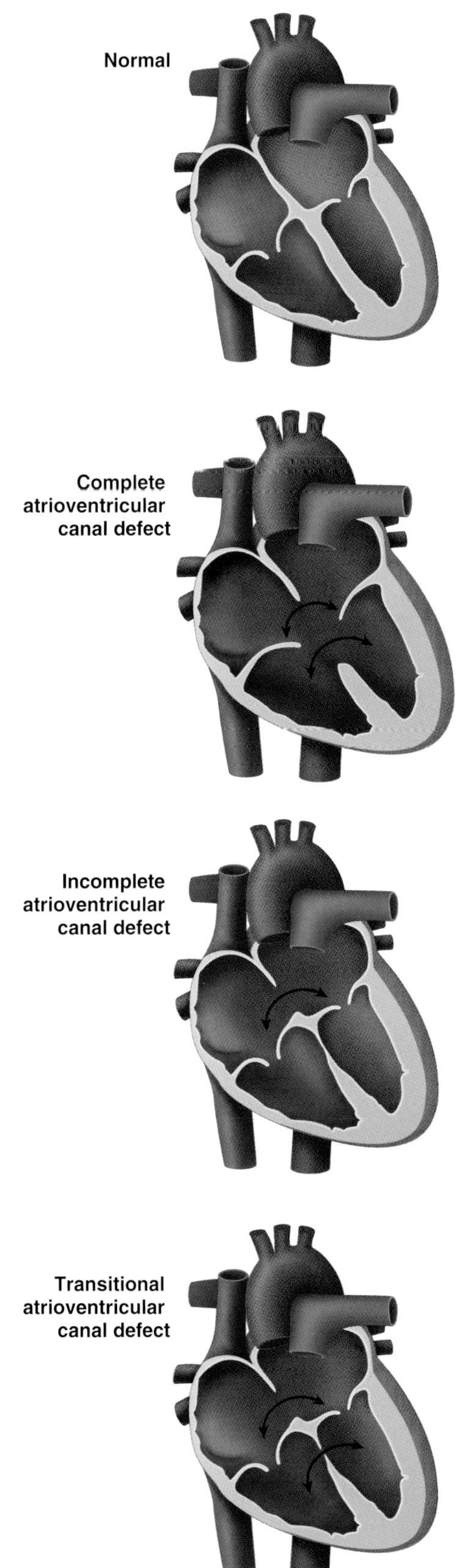

Figure 9-2. Spectrum of AVC defect (complete, incomplete, transitional).

Frequency, Genetics, and Development

AVC occurs in approximately 34.8 per 100,000 live births but is more frequently present in fetal life.[9] It is the ninth most common congenital heart lesion. Termination of pregnancy as well as fetal demise account for the higher prenatal incidence, although the actual number is not known.

There is a very strong association between AVC and Down syndrome. A child with Down syndrome is 1000 times more likely to have AVC than a child with normal chromosomes. The complete form of AVC is the most common seen in Down syndrome, although the other types can also be seen. In Down syndrome, other noncardiac anomalies can be seen including diffuse hypotonia, duodenal atresia, anal atresia, and Hirschsprung's disease. After birth, many children with Down syndrome develop thyroid disease and/or a form of acute lymphocytic leukemia. Alzheimer's disease can also occur in the fourth or fifth decade of life.

Recently, DSCAM (Down syndrome cell adhesion molecule) has been proposed as a possible candidate gene for the development of AVC.[10] Familial clusters with different modes of inheritance have also been reported. AVC is also seen frequently in association with the heterotaxy syndrome, particularly the asplenia type.

Epithelial-to-mesenchymal transformation results in formation of the endocardial cushions (the primordia of the valves and septa).[11] Mouse embryos that fail to develop these cushions experience demise late in gestation. The endocardial cushions are divided into superior, inferior, right, and left cushions. The AV canal septum and the AV valves are formed, at least in part, by the superior and inferior endocardial cushions. When the endocardial cushions fail to fuse, likely as a result of abnormal migration of mesenchymal cells, the canal portion of the atrial and ventricular septum do not develop and the tricuspid and mitral valves become a CAVV.[11]

Fetal Physiology

The physiology of AVC has little impact on the fetal circulation unless there is significant CAVV regurgitation. The ostium primum ASD and the VSD are usually well tolerated in utero. Because the pulmonary vascular resistance is elevated in the fetus, there is little if any left-to-right shunting and, thus, no significant volume burden on the heart.

In contrast to many conotruncal abnormalities, the four-chamber view readily identifies the diagnosis; the AV communication can be seen with the single AV valve over the right and left ventricles. This is in contrast to the normal heart in which the triscupid valve annulus sits inferior to the mitral valve annulus. In balanced AVC, there is usually no discrepancy in size between the ventricles and ventricular shortening is typically normal.

In the short-axis view, the CAVV can often be seen en face with the superior and inferior bridging leaflets crossing into both ventricles. In the incomplete form, the ASD is sometimes difficult to see because a patent foramen ovale is also present. However, the short-axis view identifies the so-called cleft in the left component of the AV valve, which helps confirm the diagnosis. The distinction between incomplete and transitional AVC may be difficult in prenatal diagnosis because there may be minimal if any ventricular level shunting and the VSD may be too small to visualize by two-dimensional (2D) echocardiography.

Color Doppler imaging of balanced AVC typically demonstrates right-to-left shunting at the atrial level and bidirectional shunting at the ventricular level. Color Doppler imaging also readily identifies fetal AV valve regurgitation and its severity. The CAVV is, by definition, an abnormal valve. The mural leaflets may be hypoplastic and/or redundant; in the incomplete form, some element of regurgitation through the cleft is expected after birth. Because loading conditions are different in utero, AV valve regurgitation may not be present in the fetus. In fact, the presence of significant AV regurgitation before birth heralds a significantly abnormal valve, which may have a negative impact on outcome. If the AV valve regurgitation is severe, volume overload develops. Persistence of severe regurgitation often results in fetal compromise with heart failure and the development of hydrops fetalis.

Unbalanced AVC can also be identified prenatally. It should be suspected when AVC is diagnosed in association with ventricular size discrepancy. The severity of ventricular hypoplasia may progress during the pregnancy if there is only minimal inflow into one of the ventricles. When unbalanced AVC is recognized, distal obstruction from the hypoplastic ventricle should be suspected and searched for. In the right dominant type, the aorta is often significantly smaller (based on gestational age Z-scores) than the pulmonary artery. Aortic arch hypoplasia and/or coarctation of the aorta may be seen. Although a pressure gradient across the left ventricular outflow tract may not be observed because of the fetal physiology, direction of flow at the atrial septum can be helpful in determining the severity of disease. Left-to-right shunting at the atrial level signifies severe left-sided obstruction.[12] After birth, these neonates generally require palliation with the Norwood procedure rather than a biventricular repair.

With left dominant type of unbalanced AVC, right ventricular outflow tract obstruction may be identified. In milder forms, the only evidence of pulmonary outflow obstruction may be that the pulmonary artery is smaller than the aorta (in the normal heart, it is larger). In more severe forms, there may be reversal of flow at the level of the ductus arteriosus with flow from the aorta to the pulmonary artery.[12]

Complete heart block is sometimes seen in association with AVC in the fetus. It can occur with isolated AVC or in association with heterotaxy syndrome. The prognosis for this combination of defects with heart block is quite poor even with aggressive postnatal management.[13]

Prenatal Management

Identification of AVC in utero may occur as early as the late part of the first trimester. Increased nuchal translucency, a screening tool for chromosomal and other anomalies of the fetus, can occur as early as 10 to 12 weeks' gestation and can lead to early detection of congenital heart disease.[14] If nuchal thickness is greater than the 95th percentile for fetal size, the risk of congenital heart disease increases from 8 to almost 50 per 1000 fetuses.[15] Fetuses with Down syndrome will often have increased nuchal thickening as well. Early fetal echocardiography can be performed when there is suspicion based on nuchal translucency using transvaginal probes, particularly if the fetal position and/or acoustic window is inadequate for good visualization using the transabdominal approach.

The typical timing of prenatal diagnosis is at 18 to 20 weeks' gestation. If the diagnosis of isolated AVC is made, amniocentesis should be strongly urged during counseling to rule out Down syndrome, because there is such a strong correlation. Families may consider termination of the pregnancy based on these findings. If the pregnancy is continued, monthly follow-up echocardiographic studies are suggested to follow progression of disease. In cases of balanced AVC with minimal or no AV valve regurgitation, the disease generally remains quiescent during gestation with no significant physiological impact on the fetus or the mother. For those with significant AV valve regurgitation, closer follow-up is warranted to assess for development of hydrops fetalis. When the AV valve regurgitation is severe, no good in utero treatment exists because this level of regurgitation generally signifies that the valve is structurally abnormal. Fetal demise from hydrops fetalis may occur and families should be counseled appropriately.

In unbalanced AVC, serial fetal echocardiography determines whether ventricular hypoplasia progresses. Direction of flow at the atrial septum and ductus arteriosus should be performed at each monthly assessment to help establish severity of disease. Serial studies allow for continued consultation with the family and discussion about changes that may have taken place.

The identification of an AVC on fetal imaging is an indication for a detailed obstetrical ultrasound evaluation as well as karyotype testing. From a cardiac standpoint, cesarean section is not necessary if a mother is carrying a fetus with AVC even if Down syndrome is present. Normal labor and delivery is well tolerated and is optimal for fetal transition. In general, fetuses with a diagnosis of AVC have a full-term gestation.

Postnatal Physiology

Because the pulmonary vascular resistance remains elevated after birth, most full-term neonates with AVC are completely asymptomatic in the first few days of life. In fact, there is minimal left-to-right shunting and the physical examination can be essentially normal. Some newborns, in particular those with Down syndrome in whom pulmonary vascular resistance remains high, may exhibit mild central cyanosis as a result of bidirectional shunting at the VSD level. Some children, particularly those *without* Down syndrome, may be discharged home without recognition of cardiac disease unless prenatal diagnosis is made.

Features of Down syndrome include generalized hypotonia, hyperflexibility of joints, brachycephaly with flat occiput, epicanthal folds, Brushfield's spots of the iris, protruding tongue, short neck with loose posterior folds, simian crease of the palm, short fifth finger with clinadactyly, and wide space between the first and the second toes. Although none are seen with 100% frequency, any combination of these phenotypic findings should prompt genetic evaluation to confirm trisomy 21 as well as cardiology consultation, because half of such infants will have cardiac disease.[16] Many of these findings such as brachycephaly, loose neck folds, and wide space between the first and the second toes can be diagnosed on obstetrical ultrasound as well.

Infants with complete forms of AVC will likely begin to exhibit symptoms starting at 4 to 8 weeks of age. The amount of left-to-right shunting at the ventricular level is determined almost exclusively by the pulmonary vascular resistance. The defect is large and unrestrictive with systemic pulmonary artery pressure. As the pulmonary vascular resistance decreases over the first 2 months of life, flow across the VSD increases with a concomitant increase in pulmonary blood flow and volume overload to the left atrium and left ventricle. This eventually evolves into high-output congestive heart failure. If hemodynamically important CAVV regurgitation is present, symptoms may develop sooner than 4 to 8 weeks and can be more severe. The presence of coarctation of the aorta in association with AVC will also result in earlier symptoms. The increased systemic vascular resistance from aortic narrowing causes increased left-to-right shunting at the ventricular level.

The infant with complete AVC will begin to have diaphoresis with feeding, tachypnea, and tachycardia. Weight gain will be poor despite adequate caloric intake because the metabolic demands of the heart are so high. In severe cases, the pulmonary blood flow may be so high that the systemic blood flow becomes compromised. These infants may become lethargic with poor peripheral perfusion and metabolic acidosis.

Infants with incomplete AVC usually remain asymptomatic in the neonatal period. In fact, this form of AVC may go unrecognized through early childhood and sometimes into adulthood. The physiological consequence of this defect is that of an ASD. Atrial level shunting is dependent on the relative compliances of the left and right ventricles. Right ventricular compliance improves after birth with relaxation resulting in increased left-to-right atrial level shunting and subsequent dilation of the right-sided structures. Most infants tolerate this physiology well and are asymptomatic, but dyspnea and/or growth failure can occur in some cases.[17] Similar to the complete form, significant AV regurgitation can result in earlier symptoms and presentation.

The clinical presentation of the transitional form of AVC varies depending on the size of the VSD. This form of AVC is often recognized relatively early because a restrictive VSD causes a loud murmur that alerts the general practitioner to refer the patient to a pediatric cardiologist. The larger the VSD component, the more likely the infant will develop symptoms of high-output congestive heart failure. Those with very small VSDs behave similarly to patients with the incomplete form of AVC.

Unbalanced forms of AVC generally present soon after birth. The right dominant type is usually associated with left-sided obstruction including subaortic stenosis and/or arch obstruction. If unbalance is severe with significant left ventricular hypoplasia, the infant is dependent on the ductus arteriosus to provide adequate systemic perfusion. In these cases, ductal narrowing or closure results in critically diminished cardiac output. Such infants appear gray and mottled with diminished distal pulses. Marked tachypnea develops to compensate for the low cardiac output. If prostaglandin therapy is not initiated urgently, death ensues. Left dominant type of unbalanced AVC usually has a less severe presentation. A heart murmur can be heard in the newborn period if pulmonary outflow obstruction is present.

Postnatal Management

The primary treatment for any form of AVC is surgical repair. These defects do not close on their own and catheter-directed intervention is at present not possible. Type of repair and timing of the operation depend on the type of AVC and whether the defect is balanced or unbalanced.

Any patient with ductal dependent circulation will require a neonatal operation. This occurs almost exclusively in those with right dominant unbalanced AVC with critical arch obstruction. Prostaglandin E_1 infusion must be initiated soon after birth to maintain ductal patency. It is often challenging to judge whether the atrial and ventricular communications can be closed with the arch repair (a biventricular repair) or whether a single-ventricle surgical strategy is required. Morphometric measures of the size and anatomy of the left-sided structures are often helpful and have been developed.[6,18] If a single-ventricle strategy is chosen, the Norwood procedure is typically performed, followed by the bidirectional Glenn (superior cavopulmonary anastomoses) at 4 to 6 months, culminating in the Fontan operation performed at 2 to 4 years of age.

In most cases of balanced AVC, repair can be performed electively. Children with complete AVC may require anticongestive medical therapy before surgery. Medications commonly used during this period include furosemide or a similar loop diuretic, digoxin (Na-K-ATPase pump inhibitor), and/or angiotensin-converting enzyme (ACE) inhibitors. The diuretics are effective in decreasing the pulmonary congestion and fluid retention. The effects of digoxin are poorly understood in the face of high-output cardiac failure (e.g., congestive heart failure despite good ventricular performance), but yet experience has shown this agent to be effective. ACE inhibitors decrease systemic vascular resistance. This is thought to improve forward flow into the aorta in patients with a large VSD or significant AV valve regurgitation.

Poor weight gain is common in those with complete AVC and it typically begins when the pulmonary vascular resistance decreases (4-8 wk of age). In some cases, high-calorie formulas or even nasogastric tube feeding may be required to maintain adequate nutrition. These maneuvers are mainly to optimize the patient's nutritional status before surgery. If weight gain remains poor, early surgical intervention is usually indicated.

Surgical intervention for the complete form of AVC is typically performed electively in the range of 2 to 6 months of age, after the pulmonary vascular resistance has naturally dropped. In children with Down syndrome, this resistance may not completely normalize; often, these infants also have upper airway obstruction, which may play a role in sustaining elevated pulmonary resistance. Surgery should not be delayed beyond 6 to 9 months of age because pulmonary vascular disease can develop; overall outcome is worse for this subset of patients.

Surgical repair consists of closure of the septal defects. Patch closure of the atrial communication is almost invariably performed. A variety of techniques are used to close the ventricular communication including patch (i.e., one or two patches) or direct suture closure (Nunn repair). In addition to closure of the septal defects, most AVC repairs include division of the CAVV into right and left components with at least partial suture approximation of the superior and inferior bridging leaflets (i.e., cleft closure) of the left AV valve.

Patients with incomplete AVC may undergo repair electively in the first several years of life. Earlier repair is indicated if AV valve regurgitation is a concern. Surgical intervention is similar to the complete form of AVC except no VSD closure is required and the CAVV is already divided. Left AV valve cleft closure is still commonly performed. In transitional AVC, VSD closure may be more challenging because the defect is difficult for the surgeon to visualize (it is often covered by AV valve chordal tissue). Suture closure rather than patch closure of the VSD is usually adequate.

Outcomes

If AVC is not repaired in early life, only 4% of patients survive beyond 5 years of age.[19] In general, children who undergo AVC repair have an excellent rate of survival and long-term morbidity is low. Surveillance after repair includes assessment for residual atrial and ventricular communications and/or residual AV valve regurgitation. Residual ASDs are rare but can occur as a result of patch leaks or dehiscence. Small residual VSDs are quite common.[20] Defects less than 2 mm in diameter will usually close spontaneously or never be of hemodynamic importance. Rarely, patch dehiscence can occur and reoperation may be required.

By far, the most common reason for reoperation after AVC repair is residual or new postoperative left-sided AV valve regurgitation. Distortion of the valve can occur when it is being suspended to the VSD patch. Significant AV valve regurgitation seen on the preoperative echocardiogram increases the risk for severe regurgitation after surgery.[21] Postoperative left AV valve regurgitation typically occurs at the interface of the superior and inferior bridging leaflets but can occur at the other commissures as well. Long-term evaluation of patients with AVC is required to ensure that valve regurgitation does not progress. In cases of severe regurgitation, valvuloplasty or even valve replacement may be required.

Most children who undergo successful AVC repair can participate in normal physical activities and have a normal life expectancy. Follow-up with a cardiologist is required over the patient's lifetime. In contrast to the previous surgical era (before the 1980s), surgical intervention is almost always offered to infants with trisomy 21 and AVC. Many adult AVC patients with Down syndrome are still alive who are unrepaired and are inoperable, suffering from pulmonary vascular disease and Eisenmenger's syndrome, which significantly shortens their life expectancy.[22] Those patients with Down syndrome who have a successful AVC repair have the same life expectancy as adults with Down syndrome who have no structural heart disease.

Imaging Essentials and Important Points

- Remember to distinguish between a complete, a transitional, and an incomplete type of AVC because each requires different management strategies and carries a different prognosis (complete = large VSD; transitional = small, restrictive VSD; incomplete = no VSD).
- Short-axis view imaging at the level of the CAVV can demonstrate the position of the valve leaflets in relation to the ventricular septum.
- Long-axis view imaging of the left ventricle and aorta will demonstrate the elongated, "scooped out" or "gooseneck" appearance of the left ventricular outflow tract classically seen in AVC defect.
- Evaluate the degree of "balance" of the CAVV over each ventricle. The CAVV normally sits more so over the right than the left ventricle, approximately 60% over the right ventricle. Anything greater than 60% over the right ventricle suggests right ventricular dominant unbalanced AVC.
- In right dominant unbalanced AVC, left-sided obstructive lesions such as left AV valve inflow obstruction, left ventricular cavity hypoplasia, subaortic stenosis, valvar aortic stenosis, ascending aorta hypoplasia, transverse arch hypoplasia, and coarctation of the aorta are possible and should be looked for.
- Equal sitting of the CAVV over both ventricles or anything greater than 50% over the left ventricle suggests left ventricular dominant unbalanced AVC.
- In left dominant unbalanced AVC, right-sided lesions such as right ventricular hypoplasia, pulmonary stenosis, and branch pulmonary artery narrowing should be looked for.
- AVC can be seen in conjunction with tetralogy of Fallot and is commonly associated with Down syndrome.
- Unbalanced AVC and conotruncal anomaly such as tetralogy of Fallot or double-outlet right ventricle is associated with heterotaxy syndrome of the asplenia type.
- CAVV regurgitation can be seen in utero in AVC defect. If present in more than the mild form, this may reflect a structural abnormality of the valve in addition to the AVC defect. CAVV regurgitation may worsen after birth because loading conditions change with increased preload from increased pulmonary venous return and increased afterload noted after placental separation.

References

1. Barrea C, Levasseur S, Roman K et al. Three-dimensional echocardiography improves the understanding of left atrioventricular valve morphology and function in atrioventricular septal defects undergoing patch augmentation. *J Thorac Cardiovasc Surg.* 2005;129:746-753.
2. Anderson RH, Ho SY, Falcao S, Daliento L, Rigby ML. The diagnostic features of atrioventricular septal defect with common atrioventricular junction. *Cardiol Young.* 1998;8:33-49.
3. Rastelli GC, Ongley PA, Kirklin JW, McGoon DC. Surgical repair of complete form of persistent common atrioventricular canal. *J Thorac Cardiovasc Surg.* 1968;55:299-308.
4. Mahle WT, Shirali GS, Anderson RH. Echo-morphological correlates in patients with atrioventricular septal defect and common atrioventricular junction. *Cardiol Young.* 2006;16(suppl 3):43-51.
5. Chin AJ, Bierman FZ, Sanders SP, Williams RG, Norwood WI, Castaneda AR. Subxyphoid 2-dimensional echocardiographic identification of left ventricular papillary muscle anomalies in complete common atrioventricular canal. *Am J Cardiol.* 1983;51:1695-1699.

6. Cohen MS, Jacobs ML, Weinberg PM, Rychik J. Morphometric analysis of unbalanced common atrioventricular canal using two-dimensional echocardiography. *J Am Coll Cardiol.* 1996;28:1017-1023.
7. Bharati S, Lev M. The spectrum of common atrioventricular orifice (canal). *Am Heart J.* 1973;86:553-561.
8. Gatzoulis MA, Shore D, Yacoub M, Shinebourne EA. Complete atrioventricular septal defect with tetralogy of Fallot: diagnosis and management. *Heart.* 1994;71:579-583.
9. Hoffman JI, Kaplan S. The incidence of congenital heart disease. *J Am Coll Cardiol.* 2002;39:1890-1900.
10. Barlow GM, Chen XN, Shi ZY, et al. Down syndrome and congenital heart disease: a narrowed region and a candidate gene. *Genet Med.* 2001;3:91-101.
11. Loewy KM. *Endocardium, Cardiac Cushions, and Valve Development in Cardiac Development.* New York: Oxford University Press; 2007:119-131.
12. Berning RA, Silverman NH, Villegas M, Sahn DJ, Martin GR, Rice MJ. Reversed shunting across the ductus arteriosus or atrial septum in utero heralds severe congenital heart disease. *J Am Coll Cardiol.* 1996;27:481-486.
13. Cohen MS. Clarifying anatomical complexity: diagnosing heterotaxy syndrome in the fetus. *Progr Pediatr Cardiol.* (Rychik J, ed). 2006;22:61-70.
14. Makrydimas G, Sotiriadis A, Huggon IC, et al. Nuchal translucency and fetal cardiac defects: a pooled analysis of major fetal echocardiography centers. *Am J Obstet Gynecol.* 2005;192:89-95.
15. McAuliffe FM, Hansberger LK, Winsor S, Chitayat D, Chong K, Johnson JA. Fetal cardiac defects and increased nuchal translucency thickness: a prospective study. *Am J Obstet Gynecol.* 2004;191:1486-1490.
16. Jones KL. Down syndrome. In: *Smith's Recognizable Patterns of Human Malformation.* 4th ed. Philadelphia: WB Saunders; 1988:10-15.
17. Weinberg M Jr, Miller RA, Hastreiter AR, Raffensperger JG, Fell EH, Bucheleres HG. Congestive heart failure in children with atrial septal defect. *J Thorac Cardiovasc Surg.* 1966;51:81-87.
18. Cohen MS, Spray TL. Surgical management of unbalanced atrioventricular canal. *Semin Thorac Cardiovasc Surg Pediatr Card Surg Annu* 2005;8:135-144.
19. Berger TJ, Blackstone EH, Kirklin JW, et al. Survival and probability of cure without and with operation in complete atrioventricular canal. *Ann Thorac Surg.* 1979;27:104-111.
20. Yang SG, Novello R, Nicolson SC, et al. Evaluation of ventricular septal defect repair using intraoperative transesophageal echocardiography: frequency and significance of residual defects in infants and children. *Echocardiography.* 2000;17:681-684.
21. Ten Harkel AD, Cromme-Dijkhuis AH, Heinerman BC, Hop WC, Bogers AJ. Development of left atrioventricular valve regurgitation after correction of atrioventricular septal defect. *Ann Thorac Surg.* 2005;79:607-612.
22. Daliento L, Somerville J, Presbitero P, et al. Eisenmenger syndrome. Factors relating to deterioration and death. *Eur Heart J.* 1998;19:1845-1855.

CASES

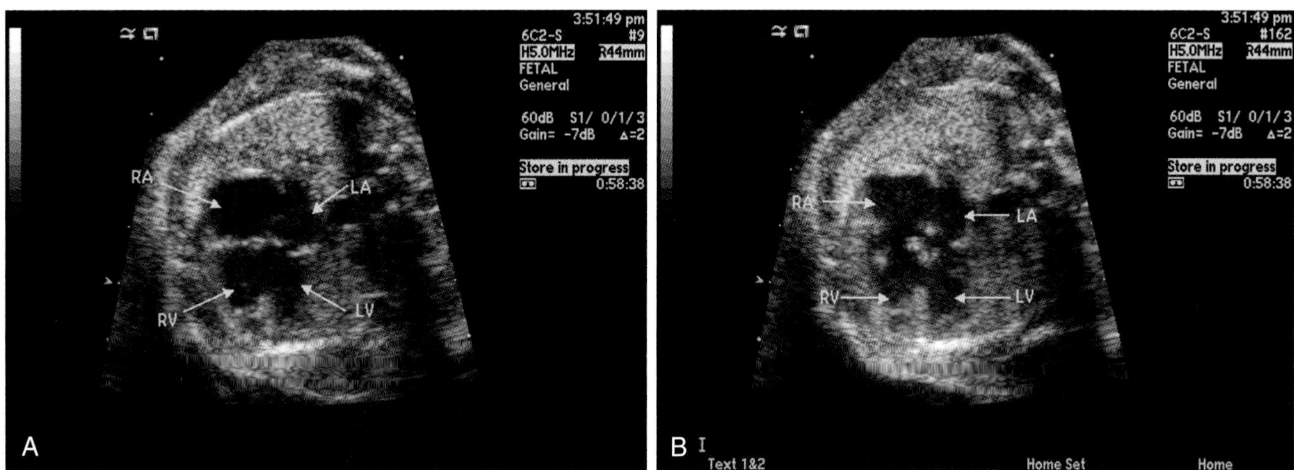

Case 9-1. **(A)** Apical four-chamber view. *Arrows* point to the four chambers of the heart including the right atrium (RA), left atrium (LA), right ventricle (RV), and left ventricle (LV). Note the presence of a gap between the atria as well as between the ventricles, reflecting both an atrial septal defect (ASD) and a large ventricular septal defect (VSD), respectively. In addition, there is a single line of atrioventricular (AV) valve continuity traversing across the middle of the heart separating both the atria and the ventricles. This is the plane of the common AV valve. The current portion of the cardiac cycle is in systole because the common AV valve is closed. **(B)** In the diastole phase of the cardiac cycle, the common AV valve is open because leaflets are open into both the RV and the LV.

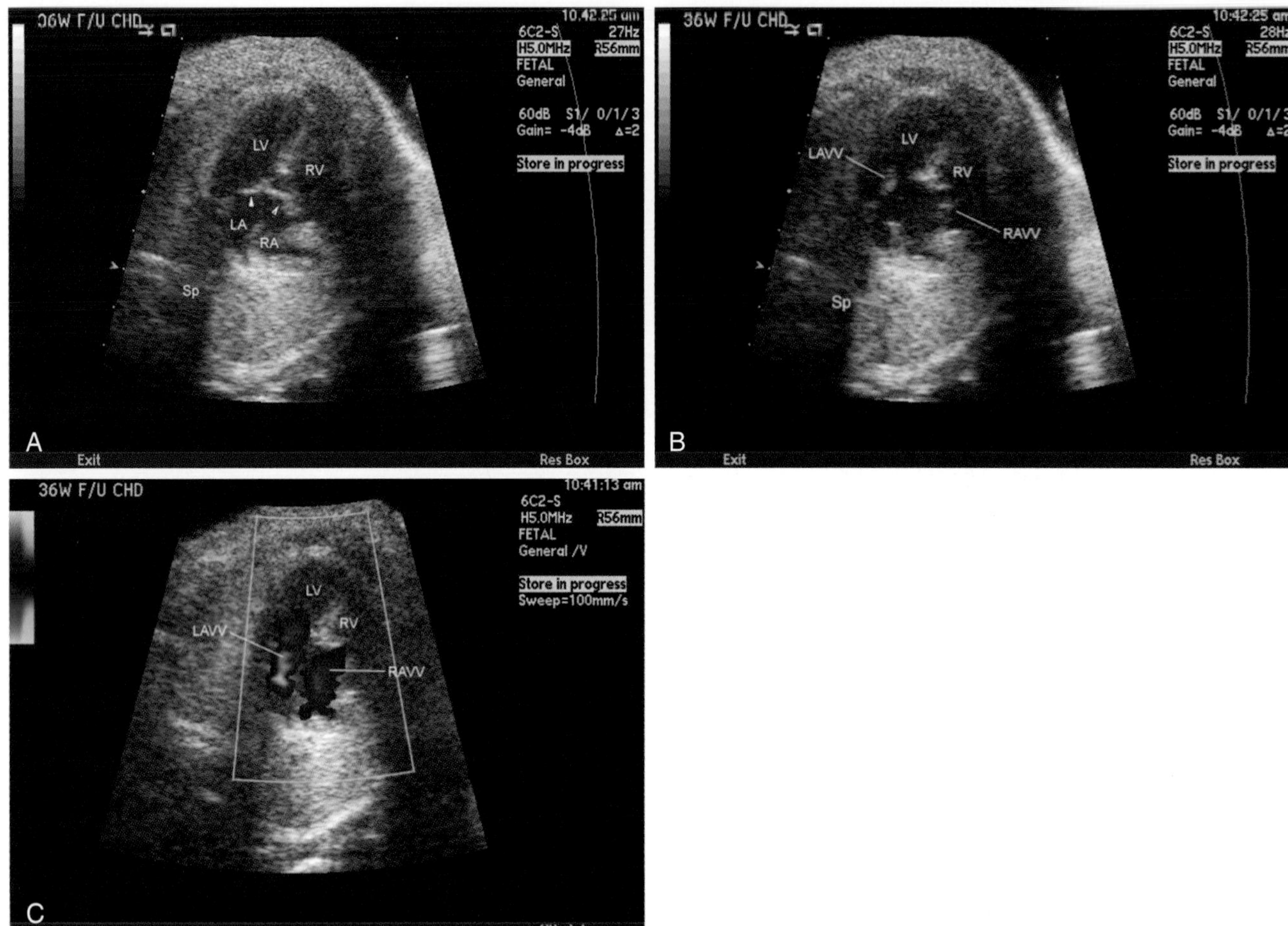

Case 9-2. **(A)** Four-chamber view of the heart with the apex pointing upward. *Arrows* point to the common AV valve. In this fetus, the defect appears to be a transitional AV canal in that the VSD component is somewhat restrictive. The phase of the cardiac cycle is in ventricular systole because the AV valve is currently closed. LA, left atrium; LV, left ventricle; RA, right atrium; RV, right ventricle; Sp, spine. **(B)** In this phase of diastole, the common AV valve is open. A large gap is seen in the atrial septum reflecting the primum ASD. Note again, there is hardly any VSD present, although there does appear to be some thinning of the ventricular septum reflecting suspicion of a transitional AV canal. LAVV, left atrioventricular valve; RAVV, right atrioventricular valve. **(C)** Color Doppler imaging during the phase of ventricular diastole shows inflow across both the LAVV and the RAVV component of the common AV valve. No significant shunting is seen across the ventricular septum.

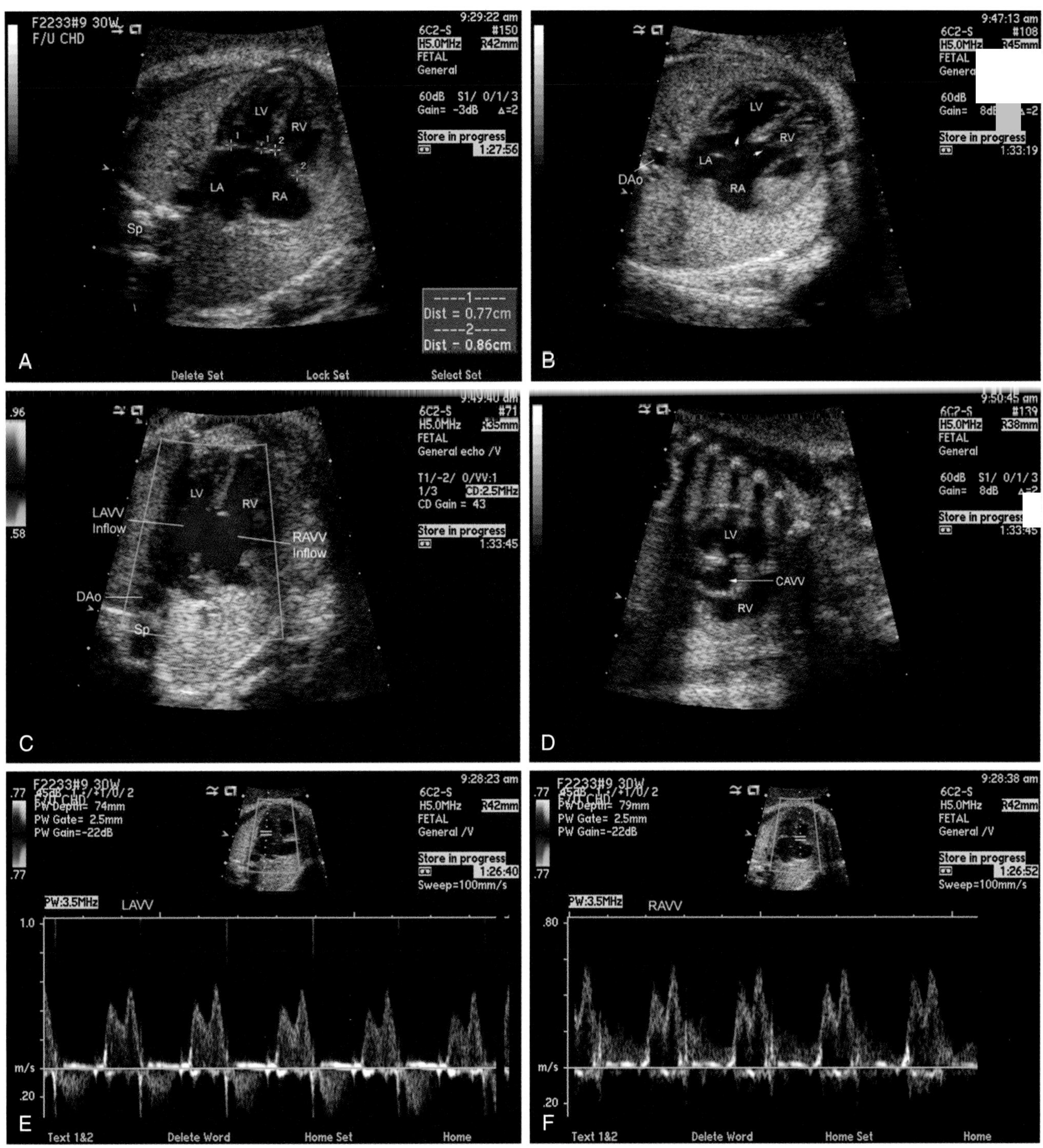

Case 9-3. **(A)** Apical four-chamber view of a primum ASD. This is one form of the spectrum of a common AV canal type defect in which there is an ASD and no VSD component. The crosshairs numbered 1 and 2 reflect the diameter measurements of the left component of the common AV valve and the right component of the common AV valve, respectively. Each of these reflects the potential "mitral" and "tricuspid" valve components, if the common AV valve had developed and differentiated into a normal two-valved heart. Note that the diameter measurement of AV valve 2, which corresponds to the tricuspid valve, is larger than the AV valve component number 1, which corresponds to the mitral valve. In a common AV canal defect, the right valve component inlet into the right ventricle (RV), the tricuspid valve correlate, should be larger than the mitral left AV valve component, as seen here. This is similar to what exists in the normal heart, in which the tricuspid valve annulus is larger than the mitral valve annulus. LA, left atrium; LV, left ventricle; RA, right atrium. **(B)** In ventricular diastole, the common AV valve is open demonstrating inflow into the LV and the RV. The descending aorta (DAo) is seen to the left of the heart just behind the LA in its normal position. **(C)** In diastole with color Doppler imaging, there is inflow into both the RV and the LV. There is no VSD component in this heart. LAVV, left atrioventricular valve; RAVV, right atrioventricular valve. **(D)** Short-axis view of the heart at the level of the RV and LV. The *arrow* points to the common atrioventricular valve (CAVV), which is seen en face and is straddling both cavities of the LV and RV. This image demonstrates the concept of a single valve as a CAVV in fetuses with an endocardial cushion defect. **(E)** Pulse wave Doppler demonstration of inflow across the LAVV component shows a normal E and A wave pattern. **(F)** Pulse Doppler flow assessment of inflow across the RAVV component demonstrates a normal E and A wave pattern.

Continued

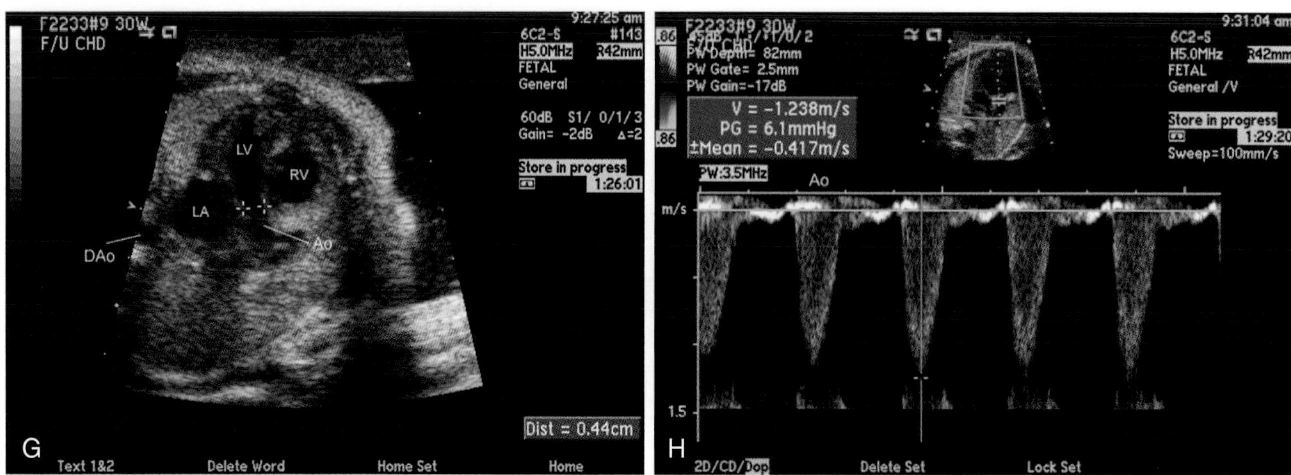

Case 9-3, cont'd (G) Slight anterior angulation provides assessment of the left ventricular outflow tract, which demonstrates no significant narrowing in this fetus with a partial or incomplete AV canal defect. Ao, aorta. (H) Pulse wave Doppler assessment of the left ventricular outflow tract demonstrates a slight increase in velocity; however, the flow is laminar. Because obstruction is possible in patients with an AV canal defect, all fetuses with endocardial cushion type defect should have both two-dimensional and Doppler assessment of the left ventricular outflow tract.

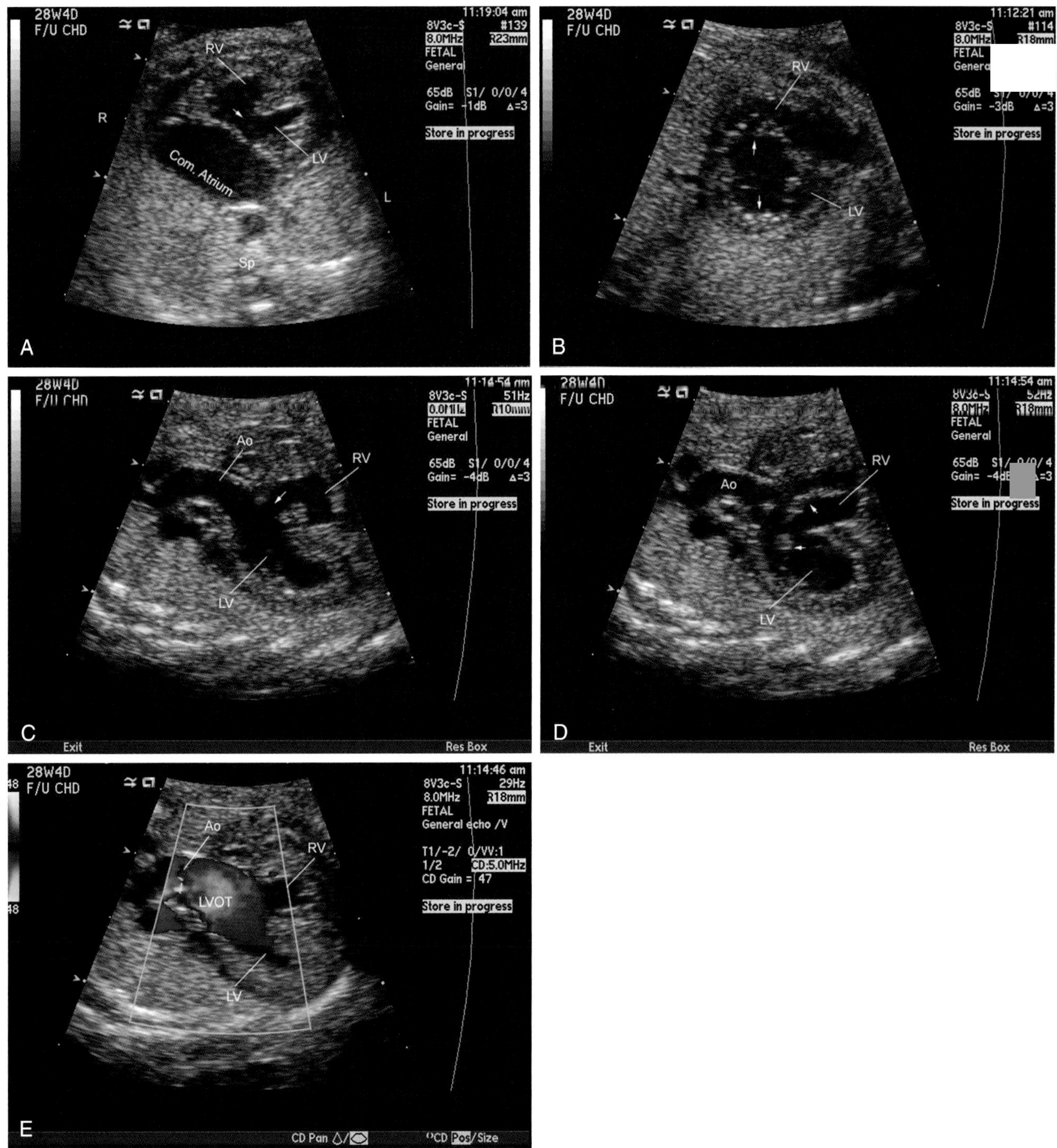

Case 9-4. (**A**) Four-chamber view image of a fetus with a complete AV canal defect. There is a very large VSD component *(arrow)*, as well as a large ASD component, nearly a common (Com.) atrium. (**B**) Short-axis view of the fetal heart with the common AV valve straddling both the RV and the LV. The CAVV is well balanced over both ventricles. The *arrows* point to the RAVV component superiorly and the LAVV component inferiorly. The cardiac cycle is in ventricular diastole because the CAVV is open and seen en face. (**C**) Long-axis view of a fetus with a complete AV canal defect. Notice the geometry of the aorta as it arises from the LV. This is referred to as the "gooseneck" deformity in which the aorta comes off the ventricle in an S-shaped and curved manner. This particular appearance is created by the "scooped out" left ventricular outflow tract caused by the presence of a large CAVC. The *arrow* points to the VSD between the RV and the LV. (**D**) In diastole, one can see in this long-axis view of the LV that the valve appears to be in the way of the left ventricular outflow tract. However, this being diastole, it is the phase for filling of both the LV and the RV. During ventricular systole, the CAVV moves out of the way of the "gooseneck" deformity of the left ventricular outflow tract and there is no obstruction. (**E**) Color Doppler imaging in systole reveals a wide jet of red color in the left ventricular outflow tract (LVOT), demonstrating no LVOT obstruction in this fetus.

Congenital Heart Anomalies: Conotruncal Defects

10 Tetralogy of Fallot

Amanda Shillingford

Key Echocardiographic Features

- Identification of malalignment of the conal septum anteriorly into the right ventricular outflow tract
- Pulmonary annulus size either equal to or smaller than the aortic annulus
- Large ventricular septal defect, beneath the aorta
- Large aorta overriding ventricular septal defect and over both ventricles
- Obstruction of the right ventricular outflow tract (subpulmonic, pulmonary valve, or supravalvar pulmonary stenosis)
- Continuity and confluence of the branch pulmonary arteries
- Size of the branch pulmonary arteries
- Identification of the ductus arteriosus, its location, origin, and connection to the branch pulmonary arteries
- Determine the direction of shunting across the ductus arteriosus
- Search for any additional muscular ventricular septal defects besides the large malalignment type of ventricular septal defect
- Aortic arch sidedness (left or right)

Anatomy and Anatomical Associations

Tetralogy of Fallot (TOF) is an abnormality of conotruncal formation. The *conotruncus* consists of the muscularized conus or conal septum—muscular septal tissue separating the region just beneath the great vessels—and the superiorly adjacent *truncus arteriosus,* which eventually differentiates into the great vessels arising from the heart, the pulmonary artery and aorta. Early in cardiac development, the conotruncus originates from the primitive right ventricle but then shifts leftward over a forming ventricular septum. To complete normal development, septation and rotation of the conotruncus occurs, resulting in a right ventricle–to–pulmonary artery relationship and a left ventricle–to–aorta relationship. In TOF, there is anterior and rightward deviation of the conal septum as well as incomplete rotation of the great arteries and the aorta is much more anteriorly positioned than normal. The ensuing anatomical configuration consists of a large anterior malalignment type ventricular septal defect (VSD), an aorta that "overrides" the VSD, varying degrees of right ventricular outflow tract (RVOT) obstruction at both the pulmonary valve and the subvalvar levels, and right ventricular hypertrophy (Figure 10-1). The pathological associations of TOF were first described by Neils Stenson in 1672, but it was Dr. Etienne Fallot who is credited for correlating the clinical presentation with the anatomy in 1888 referring to the condition as *"la maladie bleue."* In actuality, the term *tetralogy of Fallot* was not popularized until the early 1900s.[1]

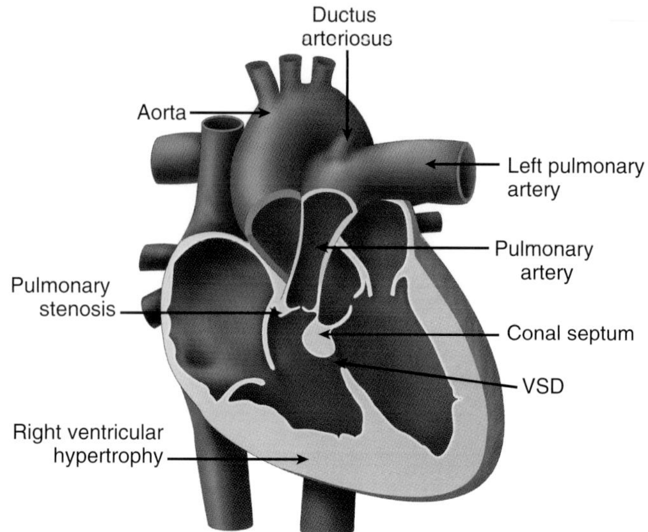

Figure 10-1. Tetralogy of Fallot. VSD, ventricular septal defect.

A number of anatomical variations exist in TOF. The pulmonary valve and subpulmonic region may be only modestly hypoplastic and represent mild degrees of pulmonary stenosis. In contrast, there may be severe valvar hypoplasia or even complete atresia of the pulmonary valve and main pulmonary artery segment. In pulmonary atresia, there is no antegrade flow across the pulmonary valve. The branch pulmonary arteries may originate as a confluence from the ductus arteriosus (DA) or blood flow to the lungs may be supplied by collateral vessels arising from the aorta known as *major aortopulmonary collateral arteries.* Moreover, the branch pulmonary arteries may have varying degrees of hypoplasia, which can affect long-term lung function. Another variant, TOF with absent pulmonary valve syndrome, occurs when the pulmonary valve leaflets are severely underdeveloped or rudimentary, resulting in severe pulmonary insufficiency and dilation of the pulmonary arteries. Associated anatomical considerations include a right aortic arch, which is present in up to 25% of patients with TOF. The DA may be tortuous or absent. Variations of coronary artery anatomy can be seen. An aberrant left anterior descending artery originating from the right coronary artery and crossing the RVOT is noted in approximately 1% to 2% of cases and has important surgical implications. Developmentally, the coronary arteries arise from the region of the ventricle and migrate toward the aorta. In TOF, the aorta is rotated and located more anterior than normal; hence, the left coronary system is prone to link up with the right, which is positioned much more leftward than normal, leading to this finding. A persistent left superior vena cava has been reported in 11% of cases. Additional muscular VSDs can occur, and the combination of TOF and atrioventricular canal defect is strongly associated with trisomy 21.[2]

Frequency, Genetics, and Development

TOF accounts for 7% of all congenital heart disease and is one of the most common forms of cyanotic congenital heart disease, occurring in 0.3 to 0.4 per 1000 live births.[3] Nearly one third of cases of TOF have an associated extracardiac anomaly or chromosomal derangement. Microdeletion of chromosome 22q11 (22q11 del) is present in approximately 90% of patients with DiGeorge syndrome, a genetic disorder associated with multiple extracardiac abnormalities such as palatal abnormalities, feeding and speech difficulties, thymic hypoplasia leading to immunodeficiency and hypocalcemia, varying degrees of developmental, cognitive, and psychological deficits, facial dysmorphism, as well as renal and skeletal abnormalities. Congenital heart disease is estimated to occur in 75% to 80% of patients with 22q11 del, and the most common cardiac defects noted are abnormalities of conotruncal formation, including TOF, interrupted aortic arch, and truncus arteriosus.[4] Conversely, 22q11 has been identified in 16% to 18% of all cases of TOF, and in one half of those patients with TOF and an associated right aortic arch.[4,5] Other important genetic associations with TOF include Alagille syndrome, VACTERL (vertebral abnormalities, anal atresia, cardiac abnormalities, tracheoesophageal fistula and/or esophageal atresia, renal agenesis and dysplasia, and limb defects) association, CHARGE (coloboma, heart disease, atresia choanae, retarded growth and retarded development and/or central nervous system anomalies, genital hypoplasia, and ear anomalies and/or deafness) association, and cat eye syndrome, as well as trisomy 13, 18, and 21 (especially in TOF with common atrioventricular canal defect).

Our understanding of the genetic and molecular basis of this congenital anomaly has increased considerably, although it is still far from complete. Several studies have focused on the role of transcription factors as specific regulators of steps in cardiac development. Gene mutations have been linked to the development of TOF, including *NKX2-5*, *Tbx1* (linked in DiGeorge syndrome), as well as *NOTCH 1 and 2*, and *JAG1* (linked to Alagille syndrome).[6]

Fetal Physiology

The fetus with TOF is typically quite stable from the cardiovascular standpoint. The structural anomalies of (1) an obstruction across the right ventricular outflow to the pulmonary artery and (2) a large communication (VSD) between the two ventricles lead to an alteration in fetal blood flow patterns. There is no alteration in venous return to the right atrium in TOF. As blood enters the right ventricle, there is impetus for shunting across the pathway of least resistance, which in the presence of RVOT obstruction will be right to left across the VSD. Hence, in TOF, there is a greater quantity of blood—a greater stroke volume—ejected into the aorta than normal and less blood ejected into the main pulmonary artery with every beat. This may partly explain the larger than normal size of the aorta in TOF.

In the normal fetal circulation, only 15% to 20% of the right ventricular cardiac output flows into the pulmonary circulation. The majority of blood ejected from the right ventricle bypasses the lungs by crossing the DA and entering the descending aorta.[7] Thus, the presence of RVOT obstruction in utero as seen in TOF can substantially affect the amount of blood that crosses the DA. In the presence of mild RVOT obstruction, a lesser volume of blood flow will cross the DA antegrade (from pulmonary artery to aorta). In general, in TOF, the DA is smaller than normal. In severe pulmonary stenosis or pulmonary atresia, retrograde flow in the DA (aorta to pulmonary artery) can be readily visualized prenatally. The DA often originates from a more vertical orientation adjacent to the underside of the aortic arch or takes a tortuous course, most likely as a consequence of the altered blood flow patterns. Rarely, the DA may be absent altogether.

The degree of RVOT obstruction will influence to what extent the fraction of blood reaching the pulmonary circulation is reduced. Pulmonary perfusion in severe cases of narrowing may receive blood from two sources—antegrade from the right ventricle and retrograde from the DA. In TOF, pulmonary vascular development can be abnormal. Proximal branch pulmonary arteries are smaller than normal and stenosis or narrowing is common. In some cases, small pulmonary vessels may be abnormal and, overall, the pulmonary vascular cross-sectional area can be reduced. Whether this is acquired in utero, secondary to alterations in fetal blood flow patterns and diversion of blood away from the developing lungs, or a primary finding present early at formation simply as an anatomical continuation of RVOT obstruction is unclear.

Cerebral blood flow patterns have been demonstrated to be abnormal in fetuses with TOF, which may in part be related to the alterations in blood flow patterns in the aorta.[8] Newborns with TOF also have smaller anthropometric measurements, including head circumference.[9] In the absence of extracardiac or genetic/chromosomal abnormality, placental function in TOF is believed to be normal.

Prenatal Management

If extracardiac abnormalities are not present, the fetus with TOF is typically stable from a hemodynamic standpoint. Postnatally, the degree of hypoxemia correlates to the degree of severity of RVOT obstruction. Because the pulmonary blood flow demands are limited prenatally, it can be a challenge to accurately predict the magnitude of postnatal hypoxemia based on fetal echocardiography. Moreover, even a mild degree of pulmonary stenosis identified at 20 weeks' gestation can progress to more severe stenosis or atresia by late gestation, which underscores the importance of serial fetal echocardiograms.[10,11] In general, a fetus with a pulmonary valve annulus that is smaller than half the size of the aortic valve annulus will likely have significant hypoxemia at birth. In addition, retrograde flow in the DA is a marker of insufficient flow across the RVOT.[11]

Given the high frequency of associated extracardiac abnormalities, a comprehensive obstetrical ultrasound scan should be performed. The presence of a thymus or a right aortic arch increases the risk of having 22q del. Increased nuchal translucency has been found in nearly half of fetuses with TOF.[12] An amniocentesis should be recommended to every mother carrying a fetus with TOF, because the overall prognosis and tone of counseling to families is strongly linked to the coexistence of extracardiac and chromosomal abnormalities.

Postnatal Physiology

In TOF, there is impediment to forward blood flow from the right ventricle into the pulmonary circulation. Once a baby is detached from fetal circulation, pulmonary vascular resistance decreases and pulmonary blood flow increases dramatically. However, if there is proximal blockage of blood flow as in TOF, blood will take the pathway of least resistance, which may be across the VSD to the left ventricle. Whereas, in utero, such shunting has no impact upon oxygenation, now that the fetus is on its own and separated from placenta, any blood diverted away from the lungs is deoxygenated blood and will be ejected into the aorta, leading to cyanosis.

In patients with a modest degree of obstruction, only a mild degree of hypoxemia may be present with arterial oxygen saturations measured by pulse oximetry of greater than 90%. Alternatively, patients with more significant obstruction will have a deficiency of pulmonary blood flow and develop more significant hypoxemia. The presence of a DA allows for left-to-right shunting (aorta to pulmonary artery), which will augment pulmonary blood flow. Hence, some newborns with even severe RVOT obstruction, but a patent DA, may have adequate oxygenation and saturation levels greater than 90%.

The physical examination of a newborn with TOF reveals a harsh crescendo-decrescendo systolic murmur along the left sternal border, and the intensity of the murmur correlates inversely with the degree of RVOT obstruction (the harsher the murmur, the more blood going across the obstructed region; the softer the murmur, the less blood flow across the obstruction). Varying degrees of hypoxemia will be present depending upon the amount of pulmonary blood flow. Digital clubbing is not appreciated in the newborn period but may be present in older, unrepaired infants and children.

Infants with TOF may also be at risk for intermittent episodes of severe hypoxemia, known as "hypercyanotic spells" or "tet spells." The abrupt change in physiology is related to an increase in right-to-left shunting through the VSD, believed to be related to an acute change in the ratio of pulmonary to systemic vascular resistance. Although short-term therapies to increase systemic vascular resistance may temporarily increase pulmonary blood flow, the occurrence of hypercyanotic spells is an indication to proceed with surgical repair.

Postnatal Management

The postnatal management of TOF is dependent upon the degree of hypoxemia present in the neonatal period. The first decision point is timing for intervention. In a newborn with mild to moderate hypoxemia (arterial oxygen saturations > 80-85%), surgery can be delayed until the infant matures. All fetuses with a diagnosis of TOF should have a cardiology evaluation in the immediate postnatal period. The arterial oxygen saturation is a more reliable indicator of absolute pulmonary blood flow than the pressure gradient across the RVOT. It is also crucial to confirm that supplemental DA flow is absent before establishing the adequacy of antegrade pulmonary blood flow. Assuming oxygen saturations are in an acceptable range and parental education has occurred, the infant can be discharged home with close outpatient follow-up by a pediatric cardiologist and plan for later elective surgery. The timing and surgical approach to repair of TOF is quite variable, with many good, rationale strategies available. At our center, complete primary surgical repair is the procedure of choice in patients with TOF with mild pulmonary stenosis. Ideally, this operation is scheduled electively between 2 and 6 months of age, or earlier if hypoxemia worsens. In neonates with more significant hypoxemia, a prostaglandin infusion is initiated at birth in order to maintain patency of the DA and augment pulmonary blood flow, which allows for stabilization of the infant before a neonatal intervention. Neonatal surgical repair can involve palliation with a shunt or primary complete "repair". Stenting of the right ventricular outflow tract in the cardiac catheterization lab has also been shown to be an effective palliative strategy to augment pulmonary blood flow.[13]

Surgical intervention for TOF was first performed in 1945 stemming from the pioneering work of Blalock, Taussig, and Thomas. The original Blalock-Taussig shunt was created as an anastomosis between the right subclavian artery and the right pulmonary artery. In the current era, a "modified" Blalock-Taussig shunt can be created without sacrifice of the subclavian artery by connecting a 3.5- to 4-mm Gore-Tex graft between the subclavian artery or base of the innominate artery and the pulmonary artery. The first total "repair" was performed in 1954 by Lillehei and numerous modifications to the surgical technique have evolved since then.[14] A complete "repair" involves patch closure of the VSD and augmentation of the RVOT in order to create unobstructed flow into the branch pulmonary arteries. The latter is achieved using a variety of techniques depending on the underlying anatomy, nature, and severity of obstruction. If an adequate-size pulmonary valve annulus is present, a patch can be placed in the RVOT, sparing the pulmonary annulus, and the pulmonary valve leaflets can be opened if necessary to relieve valvar stenosis. If the annulus is small, then this patch may extend across the pulmonary valve annulus (a transannular patch) at the expense of creating a noncompetent pulmonary valve. In cases of severe pulmonary valve hypoplasia or a left anterior descending coronary artery crossing the outflow tract prohibiting an incision in the outflow tract, a conduit can be placed from the right ventricle to the pulmonary arteries. Historically, palliation with a Blalock-Taussig shunt was performed as a primary procedure with a complete repair planned at an older age. However in the current era, complete surgical repair in infancy can be achieved with excellent results.[15,16] An initial palliative shunt or right ventricular outflow tract stent placement is preferable over a complete repair when a complete primary repair is considered high risk. Factors that may add risk to a complete repair include prematurity, low birth weight, coronary artery abnormalities, and the presence of severe extracardiac abnormalities.

Outcomes

Overall surgical outcomes for TOF are excellent. Hospital mortality after neonatal complete surgical repair for all types of TOF is reported as low as 1% to 2% with excellent long-term survival in nonsyndromic infants.[15,17] Pulmonary insufficiency secondary to initial relief of outflow tract obstruction is quite common. Such pulmonary insufficiency is well tolerated in children; however, chronic pulmonary insufficiency in older patients can lead to right ventricular dilation and dysfunction, exercise intolerance, and arrhythmias.[18,19] Many adolescents and young adults are now returning for further surgery to insert a pulmonary valve. There are still unanswered questions concerning the timing of pulmonary valve replacement in repaired TOF, with the possibility that early valve insertion may best preserve right ventricular function long-term. Currently in development are novel techniques for catheter insertion of a pulmonary valve, which will prove very helpful to patients who need it.

Cardiac catheterizations and reoperative procedures, often to address the competency of the pulmonary valve or to replace an outgrown conduit, are common. Re-intervention rates are higher after neonatal repair versus repair in later infancy, prompting some centers to advocate for a staged approach to management of TOF; however, there continues to be a great deal of controversy regarding the optimal surgical management of this population.[20] In essence, different styles have resulted in similarly excellent outcomes, and no single approach can be dictated as styles vary from center to center around the world.

Several studies have demonstrated that some older children may have neurodevelopmental deficits and impaired academic performance after TOF repair, although these patterns have not been specifically linked to any specific surgical strategy.[21] Finally, it is important to emphasize that TOF is a lifelong medical condition, and although most complete surgical repairs are performed in the first year of life, it is anticipated that additional cardiac interventions may be necessary. As a testimony to the tremendous strides made in the successful treatment of TOF, we are now seeing many healthy and well-functioning women with repaired TOF successfully carrying pregnancy to term presenting for evaluation of their fetus. Fetal echocardiographic evaluation is indicated, but as well, such mothers should be considered as having a high-risk pregnancy and require close observation for development of heart failure. Overall, the longevity and quality of life for these patients is expected to be quite good.

Imaging Points

- The aorta is always larger than the pulmonary artery in TOF. In fact, this is one of the telltale, pathognomonic signs of TOF, because in the fetus with normal anatomy, the pulmonary artery is always larger than the aorta.
- Assess for the relative size of the pulmonary artery to the aorta. If it is less than 50% that of the aorta, such fetuses are more likely to have significant obstruction, require postnatal prostaglandin infusion to maintain patency of the DA, and more likely to need a neonatal repair.
- Identify the presence of a large VSD and the aorta overriding the ventricular septum.
- Assess the nature, extent, and severity of the RVOT obstruction starting with the subpulmonary region, the region of conal deviation, the pulmonary annulus, the pulmonary valve, the main pulmonary artery, and the proximal branch pulmonary arteries.
- Identify the presence or absence of antegrade flow across the pulmonary valve upon color Doppler imaging

Continued

Imaging Points—cont'd

- Identify the DA and determine the direction of flow. Normal antegrade flow (pulmonary artery to aorta) across the DA suggests minimal outflow tract obstruction. The combination of antegrade flow in the DA and a pulmonary artery annulus that is greater than 50% of the aortic annulus allows one to confidently counsel families that the newborn will likely be relatively pink and not require an early neonatal surgery.
- Additional muscular VSDs may be present in addition to the large malalignment type VSD and should be searched for. A careful investigation along the length of the muscular septum is warranted.
- Coronary abnormality with origin of left coronary from right may occur; however, this cannot be diagnosed in the fetus with any degree of reliability and should be deferred until postnatal evaluation.
- Aortic arch sidedness should be identified, as well as the presence of any arch anomalies, which are common in TOF.
- Identification of the thymus is important, as absence may suggest the 22q11 deletion (DiGeorge's Syndrome). The proximity of the great vessels in the mediastinum to the anterior chest wall indirectly reflects presence or absence of thymus. If the great vessels are up close against the anterior chest wall, this suggests absent or deficient thymic tissue.
- Serial evaluation in TOF is of utmost importance, because progression of outflow tract obstruction can occur as gestation progresses. Direction of flow across the DA and the overall ratio of pulmonary artery to aorta can change with gestation, influencing postnatal management.

References

1. Evans WN. "Tetralogy of Fallot" and Etienne-Louis Arthur Fallot. *Pediatr Cardiol.* 2008;29:637-640.
2. Siwik ES, Patel CR, Zahka KC, Goldmuntz E. Tetralogy of Fallot. In: *Moss and Adams' Heart Disease in Infants, Children, and Adolescents.* 6th ed. Philadelphia: Lippincott Williams & Williams; 2001.
3. Ferencz C, Rubin JD, McCarter RJ, et al. Congenital heart disease: prevalence at livebirth. The Baltimore-Washington Infant Study. *Am J Epidemiol.* 1985;121:31-36.
4. Goldmuntz E. DiGeorge syndrome: new insights. *Clin Perinatol.* 2005;32:963-978.
5. Kaguelidou F, Fermont L, Boudjemline Y, Le BJ, Batisse A, Bonnet D. Foetal echocardiographic assessment of tetralogy of Fallot and post-natal outcome. *Eur Heart J.* 2008;29:1432-1438.
6. Bruneau BG. The developmental genetics of congenital heart disease. *Nature.* 2008;451:943-948.
7. Artman M, Mahoney L, Teitel DF. *Neonatal Cardiology.* New York: McGraw-Hill Medical Publishing Division; 2002:39-51.
8. Kaltman JR, Di H, Tian Z, Rychik J. Impact of congenital heart disease on cerebrovascular blood flow dynamics in the fetus. *Ultrasound Obstet Gynecol.* 2005;25:32-36.
9. Rosenthal GL. Patterns of prenatal growth among infants with cardiovascular malformations: possible fetal hemodynamic effects. *Am J Epidemiol.* 1996;143:505-513.
10. Pepas LP, Savis A, Jones A, Sharland GK, Tulloh RM, Simpson JM. An echocardiographic study of tetralogy of Fallot in the fetus and infant. *Cardiol Young.* 2003;13:240-247.
11. Hornberger LK, Sanders SP, Sahn DJ, et al. In utero pulmonary artery and aortic growth and potential for progression of pulmonary outflow tract obstruction in tetralogy of Fallot. *J Am Coll Cardiol.* 1995;25:739-745.
12. Poon LC, Huggon IC, Zidere V, Allan LD. Tetralogy of Fallot in the fetus in the current era. *Ultrasound Obstet Gynecol.* 2007;29:625-627.
13. Dohler G, Chaturvedi RR, Benson LN, et al. Stenting of the right ventricular outflow tract in the symptomatic infant with tetralogy of Fallot. *Heart.* 2009;95:142-147.
14. Sarris GE. Questions remaining about the surgical correction of tetralogy of Fallot. *Hellenic J Cardiol.* 2005;46:263-267.
15. Hirsch JC, Mosca RS, Bove EL. Complete repair of tetralogy of Fallot in the neonate: results in the modern era. *Ann Surg.* 2000;232:508-514.
16. Transberger MI, Lechner E, Mair R, et al. Early primary repair of tetralogy of Fallot in neonates and infants less than four months of age. *Ann Thorac Surg.* 2008;86:1928-1935.
17. Michielon G, Marino B, Formigari R, et al. Genetic syndromes and outcome after surgical correction of tetralogy of Fallot. *Ann Thorac Surg.* 2006;81:968-975.
18. Samman A, Schwerzmann M, Balint OH, et al. Exercise capacity and biventricular function in adult patients with repaired tetralogy of Fallot. *Am Heart J.* 2008;156:100-105.
19. Gatzoulis MA, Balaji S, Webber SA, et al. Risk factors for arrhythmia and sudden cardiac death late after repair of tetralogy of Fallot: a multicentre study. *Lancet.* 2000;356:975-981.
20. Fraser CD Jr, McKenzie ED, Cooley DA. Tetralogy of Fallot: surgical management individualized to the patient. *Ann Thorac Surg.* 2001;71:1556-1561.
21. Hovels-Gurich HH, Konrad K, Skorzenski D, et al. Long-term neurodevelopmental outcome and exercise capacity after corrective surgery for tetralogy of Fallot or ventricular septal defect in infancy. *Ann Thorac Surg.* 2006;81:958-966.

CASES

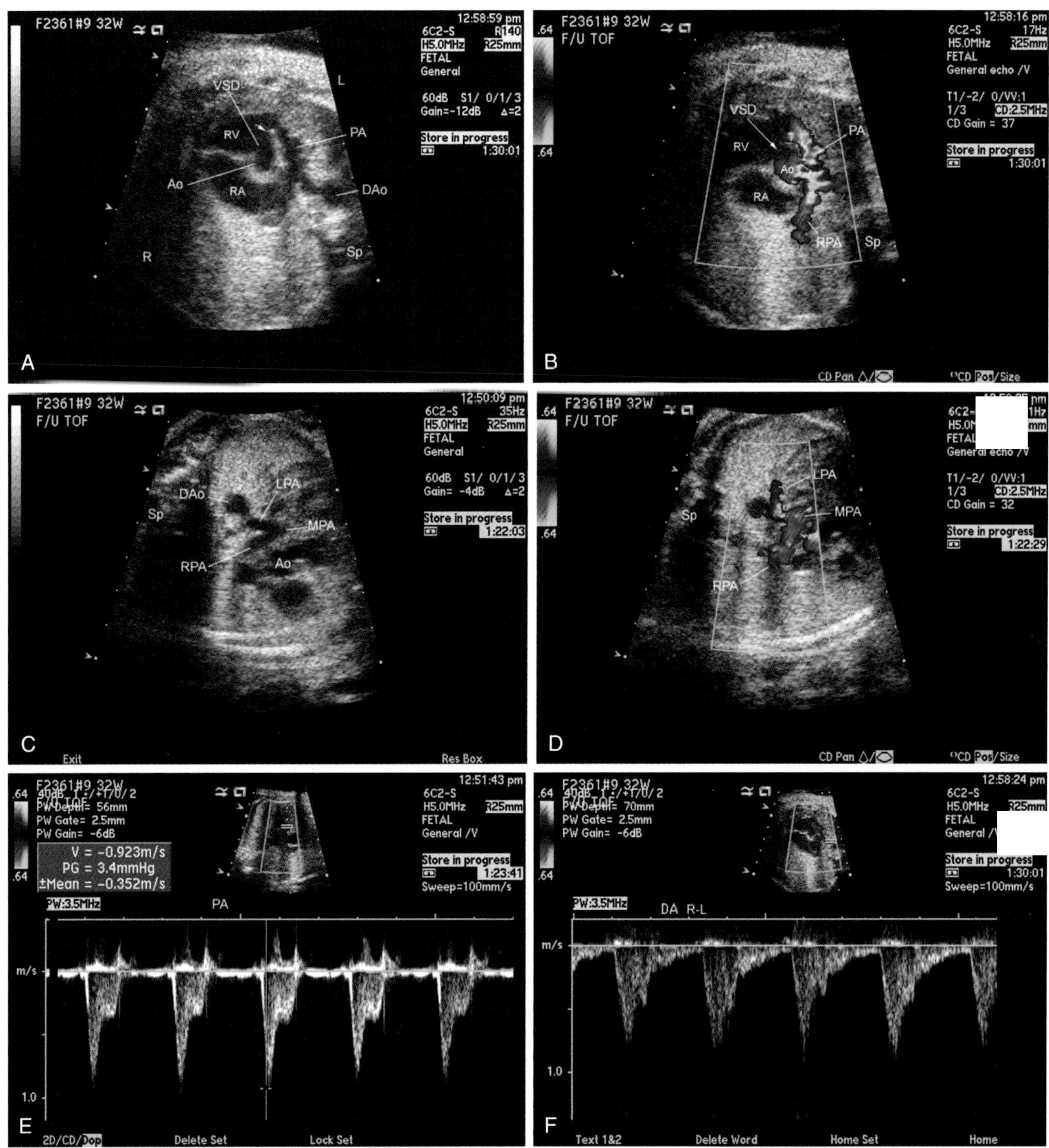

Case 10-1. (**A**) Short-axis view at the level of the outflow tracts of a fetus with tetralogy of Fallot (TOF). *Arrow* points to the infundibular septum, which is anteriorly malaligned toward the right ventricular outflow tract. There is narrowing of the right ventricular outflow tract, the pathway from the right ventricle (RV) to the pulmonary artery (PA). The anterior malalignment of the conal septum away from the remainder of the ventricular septum leads to creation of a ventricular septal defect (VSD). Ao, aorta; DAo, descending aorta; PA, pulmonary artery; RA, right atrium; Sp, spine. (**B**) Color flow imaging across the narrowed right ventricular outflow tract. There is turbulence in the right ventricular outflow due to anterior malalignment of the conal septum. Branch pulmonary arteries are seen; in particular, the right pulmonary artery (RPA) is well displayed. (**C**) This image is acquired by angling superiorly toward the great vessels with focus on the mediastinum. We see a small main pulmonary artery (MPA) and the branching of the MPA into the RPA and left pulmonary artery (LPA). Ao, aorta. (**D**) Color Doppler imaging reveals the LPA to be smaller than the RPA, which is often the case in the fetus with TOF. (**E**) Doppler spectral display of flow in the MPA, note the upstroke and then rapid downstroke with a secondary peak occurring in systole. This "double-peak" pattern is typically seen when there is dynamic right ventricular outflow tract obstruction. The first peak relates to the initial rush of blood into the pulmonary artery (PA). During systole, the right ventricular outflow tract further clamps down and dynamically narrows due to the muscular infundibulum, creating a second peak of flow. (**F**) Doppler sampling in the ductus arteriosus. This information is very important in identifying whether or not there is a need for patency of the ductus arteriosus after birth in the fetus with TOF. Here we see evidence of right-to-left shunting—that is, shunting from the PA to the descending aorta (DA) in a normal manner suggesting an adequate amount of antegrade flow into the MPA and forward into the ductus arteriosus. Reversal of flow with left-to-right shunting from aorta to PA suggests severe narrowing of the MPA and right ventricular outflow tract and will likely indicate the need for prostaglandin infusion after birth to maintain ductal patency and adequate pulmonary blood flow.

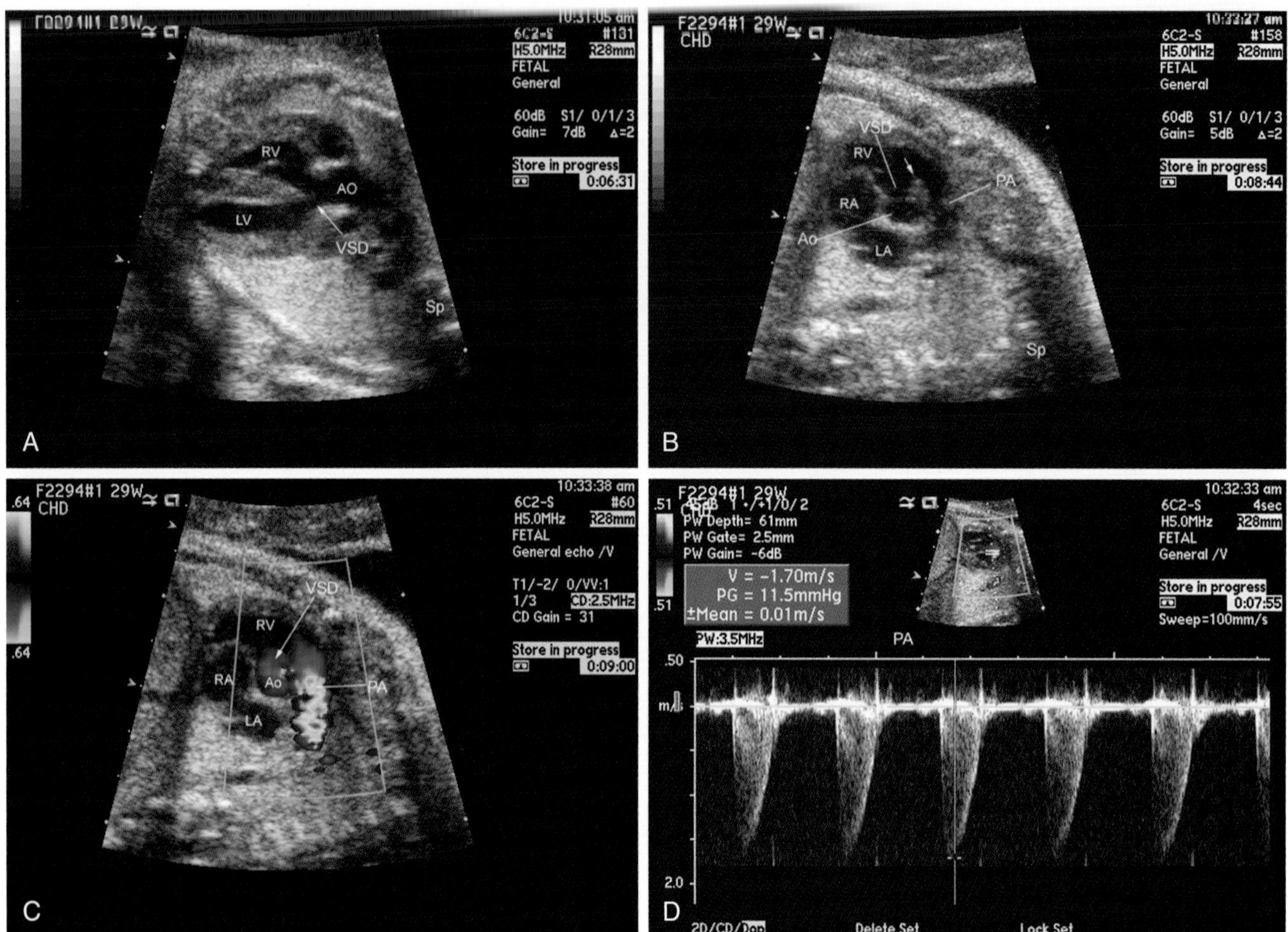

Case 10-2. **(A)** Long-axis view demonstrates the right (RV) and left (LV) ventricles and the overriding aorta (AO) with a ventricular septal defect (VSD). **(B)** Short-axis view demonstrates a thickened and hypertrophied "thumblike" infundibular or conal septum. The septum is malaligned anteriorly encroaching upon the right ventricular outflow tract. VSD is seen. LA, left atrium; PA, pulmonary artery; RA, right atrium; Sp, spine. **(C)** Color flow reveals a blue jet across the VSD, suggesting shunting from the RV into the left ventricular outflow tract and aorta, this occurring during systole. We know this is systole because there is antegrade flow into the PA as well as turbulence in the MPA, suggesting this to be the systolic phase of the cardiac cycle. Only a moderate degree of pulmonary narrowing is seen because the MPA color jet appears to be of relatively good size as blood moves antegrade. **(D)** Doppler interrogation of the main pulmonary artery reveals some turbulence and an increase in velocity to 1.7 m/sec. Typical normal flow of velocity in the MPA should be no greater than approximately 1 m/sec. It is rare to see significant gradients and velocities above 2 m/sec in fetuses with TOF because there is pressure equalization between both of the ventricles and the great vessels due to patency of the ductus arteriosus and presence of a large VSD. Also the lungs are at high resistance downstream; hence, there is no impetus or physiological reason for large pressure gradients across the PA in the fetus.

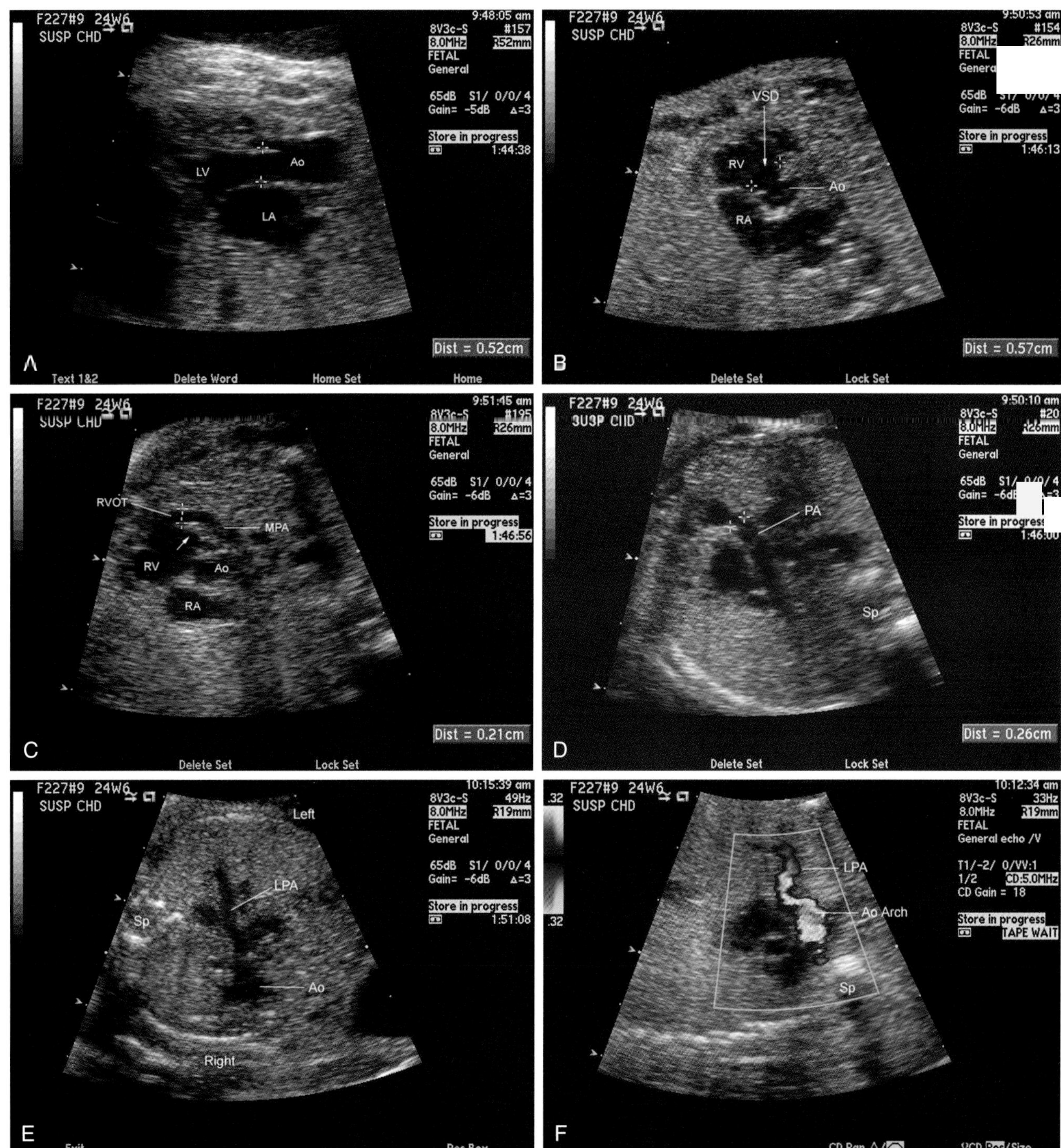

Case 10-3. **(A)** Long-axis view angled cephalad demonstrates a large aorta (Ao) and no obvious evidence in this view for a second vessel, the pulmonary artery. LA, left atrium; LV, left ventricle. **(B)** Short-axis view demonstrates a large ventricular septal defect (VSD). The infundibular septum is very thickened and malaligned anteriorly. RA, right atrium; RV, right ventricle. **(C)** A bit more anterior angulation reveals a very small right ventricular outflow tract (RVOT), impinged upon by a very hypertrophied conal/infundibular septum. Arising from the heart is small main pulmonary artery (MPA). **(D)** Further angling cephaled reveals a small MPA and the RPA rising. PA, pulmonary artery; Sp, spine. **(E)** The origin of the left pulmonary artery (LPA) from a ductus arteriosus arising from the underside of the arch. This is a transverse cut through the chest at the level of the origin of the ductus arteriosus. The descending aorta (Ao) is seen in cross-section and the ductus arteriosus is seen in continuity with the LPA entering into the left lung parenchyma. **(F)** Image of the aortic arch (Ao arch) giving rise to the ductus arteriosus perfusing the isolated left pulmonary artery (LPA).

11

Tetralogy of Fallot with Pulmonary Atresia

Amanda Shillingford

Key Echocardiographic Features

- Large malalignment type of ventricular septal defect.
- Single semilunar valve, that of the aorta, arising from the heart.
- No antegrade flow into the pulmonary artery from the heart
- Atretic "platelike" pulmonary valve may be seen or there may be no visible pulmonary valve at all.
- Main pulmonary artery segment may be present and small or completely absent.
- Branch pulmonary arteries are typically small and may be too small to image and adequately visualize on fetal echocardiography.
- Sources of pulmonary blood flow from the aorta, ductus arteriosus, and/or aortopulmonary collaterals should be investigated.
- Ductus arteriosus may be absent.

Anatomy and Anatomical Associations

Tetralogy of Fallot with pulmonary atresia (TOF/PA) is a severe form of tetralogy of Fallot (TOF), in which the pathway out of the right ventricle across the pulmonary valve is fully sealed (atretic) (Figure 11-1). Although, in many ways, it is similar to TOF with pulmonary stenosis, this subtype of TOF is unique because the prenatal findings, management, and prognosis can be quite different.[1] Anatomically, there is a large malalignment ventricular septal defect (VSD) in conjunction with an aorta that overrides the ventricular septum. There can be platelike valvar atresia, in which the valve alone is fused, or complete infundibular atresia with the entire subpulmonic region sealed. A main pulmonary artery segment may or may not be present, and oftentimes, just a remnant thread represents the main pulmonary artery. The branch pulmonary arteries and distal pulmonary arterial bed are often abnormal. The aorta is larger than normal.

Postnatally, a great deal of variability exists in the origin and distribution of the pulmonary arteries. The branch pulmonary arteries may be supplied by a single ductus arteriosus (DA) and, in most cases, are confluent. Although rare, bilateral ducti can occur with each supplying a single branch pulmonary artery, resulting in discontinuous branch pulmonary arteries. Collateral arterial vessels from the aorta to the pulmonary arteries, referred to as *major aortopulmonary collateral arteries (MAPCAs)*, typically arise from the distal aortic arch or thoracic aorta, but they can also originate from the aortic arch vessels or abdominal aorta (Figure 11-2). Any number of collaterals can be present (typically two to six) with numerous patterns of distribution into the lungs. The size of the collaterals within a single patient can vary as well. Furthermore, the aortopulmonary collateral vessels are residual structures from cardiac development and not intended to serve the same role as a true pulmonary artery. This results in significant abnormalities of these vessels, including diffuse hypoplasia and multiple areas of stenosis.[2] Ductal-dependent pulmonary arteries and MAPCAs can be present in the same patient. As in TOF with pulmonary stenosis, TOF/PA can be associated with other cardiac abnormalities, including coronary artery anomalies, common atrioventricular canal defect, and heterotaxy syndrome.

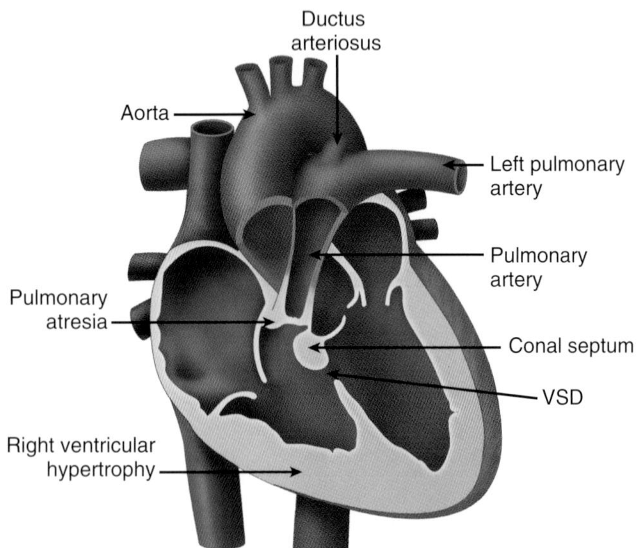

Figure 11-1. Tetralogy of Fallot with pulmonary atresia.

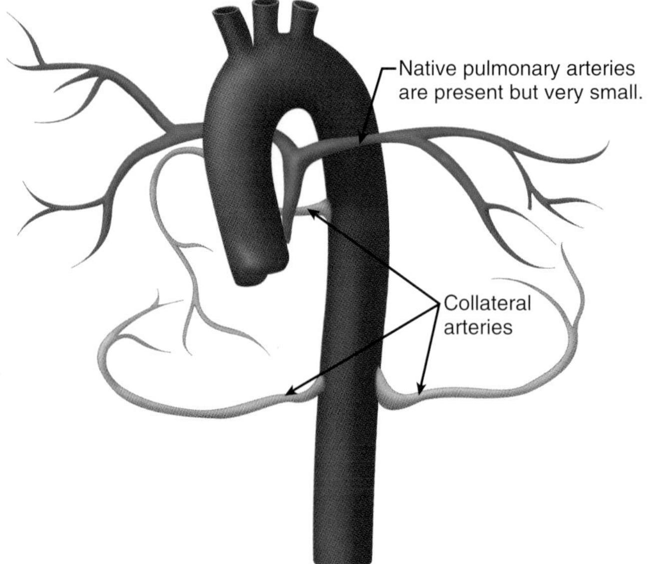

Figure 11-2. Collateral arteries feeding the pulmonary circulation.

Frequency, Genetics, and Development

TOF/PA accounts for 20% of all forms of TOF and occurs in 0.07 per 1000 live births.[2] Extracardiac abnormalities are found in one quarter to one half of all infants with TOF/PA with microdeletion of chromosome 22q11 (22q11del) being the most common chromosomal abnormality.[2,3] 22q11del is present in 90% of patients with DiGeorge syndrome, a genetic disorder associated with multiple extracardiac issues including palatal deformities, feeding and speech difficulties, thymic hypoplasia leading to immunodeficiency and hypocalcemia, varying degrees of developmental, cognitive, and psychological deficits, facial dysmorphism, and renal abnormalities.[4] The incidence of 22q11del in TOF/PA has been reported as high as 40% and is more frequent in the presence of MAPCAs and hypoplastic branch pulmonary arteries.[5] Associated thymic aplasia or a right aortic arch increases the risk of having 22q11del. Other associated genetic conditions include VACTERL (vertebral abnormalities, anal atresia, cardiac abnormalities, tracheoesophageal fistula and/or esophageal atresia, renal agenesis and dysplasia, and limb defects) association, CHARGE (coloboma, heart disease, atresia choanae, retarded growth and retarded development and/or central nervous system anomalies, genital hypoplasia, and ear anomalies and/or deafness) association, Alagille syndrome, and trisomy 21. The precise genetic etiology of TOF/PA remains undefined and, thus far, parallels the mutations described in TOF with pulmonary stenosis.[6]

The development of collateral vessels and an abnormal pulmonary vasculature are what make TOF/PA such a unique anomaly. There is not only the cardiac anomaly of TOF but also a profound change in the makeup of the lung—in essence, a congenital anomaly of the vessels of the lung in association. Early in cardiac development, the lungs normally receive dual blood supply from branches of the dorsal aorta as well as branches from the sixth aortic arches. As normal cardiac development progresses, the branches from the dorsal aorta involute and the branches of the sixth aortic arch enlarge to give rise to main and branch pulmonary arteries. In the absence of antegrade flow across a pulmonary valve as in TOF/PA, normal pulmonary vascular development is interrupted, resulting in the creation of abnormal blood flow patterns to the lungs from the DA or MAPCAs.

Prenatal Physiology

The fetus with TOF/PA is not expected to have significant hemodynamic problems that affect fetal well-being. Atrial level right-to-left shunting is no different than normal. A large VSD allows unrestrictive right-to-left shunting and the combined ventricular cardiac outputs of both right and left ventricle are ejected into the aorta. Pulmonary blood flow is supplied by a DA or collateral vessels originating from the aorta. The fetal lungs receive only approximately 15% to 20% of the combined cardiac output, and therefore, significant hypoplasia or stenoses of the pulmonary vessels may not be evident until the postnatal period when pulmonary blood flow increases significantly. Other physiological features are similar to TOF with pulmonic stenosis. Polyhydramnios and intrauterine growth restriction is common in TOF/PA when associated with 22q11del.[3]

Prenatal Management

Several studies have documented that the degree of right ventricular outflow tract obstruction observed in midgestation can progress, with moderate stenosis advancing to pulmonary atresia by late gestation. Therefore, serial fetal echocardiography is recommended.[7] Identification of whether pulmonary blood flow is supplied by the DA or collateral vessels is important, although origins of all MAPCAs and destination within the lung can be difficult to precisely delineate.

TOF/PA can be categorized into two general subtypes. In the first type, there is platelike pulmonary valvar atresia, a well-formed infundibulum, and a well-formed main pulmonary artery. In this type, the branch pulmonary arteries are typical of what is seen in TOF with pulmonary stenosis, and they are relatively well formed. MAPCAs in this scenario are unusual, and pulmonary blood flow is supplied by the DA. In the second type, there is more profound right ventricular outflow tract atresia, with infundibular and muscular atresia. In this scenario, the main pulmonary can be quite small or absent. MAPCAs are often present and need to be searched for with rigor on fetal echocardiography. A careful search of the ascending and descending aorta to the level beneath the diaphragm using color Doppler imaging should be undertaken. One should look for anomalous vessels arising from the aorta, diving into the lung parenchyma. Pulse Doppler interrogation of these vessels will reveal an arterial waveform.

Because of the high prevalence of associated extracardiac abnormalities, every fetus should have a comprehensive obstetrical ultrasound scan. As in TOF, absent thymus and a right aortic arch increase the risk of 22q11del. Karyotype analysis via chorionic villus sampling or amniocentesis is strongly recommended. Prognosis and counseling will be affected if extracardiac abnormalities are present.

Postnatal Physiology

The neonatal presentation of the newborn with TOF/PA is quite variable and is very much dependent upon the sources of pulmonary blood flow present. A variety of clinical scenarios are possible. As the fetus transitions to postnatal life, pulmonary vascular resistance decreases, resulting in an increase in pulmonary blood flow. The first spontaneous respiration after delivery activates a cascade pathway to signal closure of the DA, a process that may take hours to weeks to complete. In the immediate postnatal period as the DA is open, the infant with TOF/PA may appear quite well without obvious cyanosis or respiratory distress. However, once the DA closes, profound hypoxemia can occur, especially in the subtype in which no collateral vessels are present. Severe hypoxemia can also occur in the newborn absent a DA, but with MAPCAs in which there are significant stenoses and diffuse hypoplasia. Furthermore, cyanosis can develop over time in infants with only moderate hypoplasia or stenoses of collateral vessels at birth, but in whom a mismatch in supply and demand develops as the pulmonary blood flow demands increase with somatic growth. Alternatively, if a persistent large DA remains patent or an abundance of MAPCA vessels are present, ironically, despite having pulmonary atresia, there can be an excessive amount of pulmonary blood flow with pulmonary overcirculation and the development of heart failure symptoms during the first months of life.

The physical examination of a newborn with TOF/PA reveals the second heart sound is single because no pulmonary valve is present. A continuous murmur is appreciated in the presence of a patent DA, and multiple continuous murmurs will be auscultated throughout the lung fields in the case of MAPCAs.

Postnatal Management

In TOF/PA, a vessel originating from the underside of the aortic arch, perfusing the pulmonary arteries, may be the DA or a collateral vessel. Distinguishing between the two can be difficult, because the former will respond and remain patent with infusion of prostaglandin but the latter will not. Because it is difficult to differentiate, it is recommended that every infant with TOF/PA have a prostaglandin (PGE) infusion initiated after delivery until a complete postnatal evaluation is performed. Transthoracic echocardiography is an excellent modality of defining the intracardiac anatomy as well as the aortic arch and proximal branch pulmonary arteries (if present). However, identification of the precise origin and course of MAPCA vessels can be challenging, particularly when vessels arise from the distal thoracic or abdominal aorta. Some investigators have demonstrated that the smaller the branch pulmonary arteries on echocardiography, the greater the likelihood of there being collateral vessels present.[8] At our center, our practice has been to obtain further imaging beyond echocardiography to assess for all sources of pulmonary blood flow, when there is muscular pulmonary atresia or very small branch pulmonary arteries. Cardiac catheterization has been the gold standard, but reliable images have been acquired with computed tomography angiography and magnetic resonance imaging as well.[9] If there is platelike valvar atresia and relatively good size branch pulmonary arteries, echocardiography alone should suffice in the evaluation. However, even in this subtype, a collateral is rarely identified. If so, further imaging modalities beyond echocardiography are applied, because the presence of one collateral may indicate the presence of more, if not searched for carefully.

A PGE infusion should be maintained until information is obtained as to the origins and sources of pulmonary blood flow. If pulmonary blood flow originates predominantly from collateral vessels, PGE is not necessary and can be discontinued. Management of congestive heart failure symptoms due to excessive pulmonary blood flow may be necessary, but this does not usually occur in the first few postnatal days.

The surgical management of TOF/PA is evolving, and a great deal of controversy continues regarding the optimal management. In patients with TOF/PA associated with good-sized confluent branch pulmonary arteries and no evidence of significant flow contribution from collateral vessels, surgical repair consists of closure of the VSD and creation of a connection between the right ventricle and the pulmonary arteries utilizing either the transannular patch technique as used in TOF with pulmonary stenosis or a conduit made from homograft or synthetic material that does not have growth potential. Good results utilizing this approach with outcomes similar to that of TOF with pulmonary stenosis have been reported.[10] Some institutions advocate initial palliation with a Blalock-Taussig shunt followed by a complete repair at 6 to 12 months of age.[11] Stenting the DA in the cardiac catheterization has also been utilized as a palliative procedure with good results.[12] Placement of a right ventricle–to–pulmonary artery conduit in early childhood necessitates that at least one additional surgical procedure (and probably more than one) will be required during a lifetime in order to upsize the conduit as the child grows.

Surgical management of TOF/PA with MAPCAs is much more complicated because of the extreme variability of the collateral vessels. Collaterals often have a tortuous course into the lungs and can even connect with true pulmonary arteries, resulting in dual supply of lung segments. As a result, surgical management is primarily linked to the distribution and anatomy of the collateral vessels and whether true pulmonary arteries are present. The general concept has been to surgically "unifocalize" as many collateral vessels as possible together with the native pulmonary arteries in order to create a confluence. Unifocalization has been described as a multi-stage approach or a single-stage approach. A conduit is placed from the right ventricle to the confluence, and the VSD is closed in order to achieve distinct pulmonary and systemic circulations. Oftentimes, the true pulmonary arteries are extremely small and, hence, benefit from a staged approach in which blood flow is increased through a shunt, a small conduit, or direct connection to the aorta in order to promote growth. Unifocalization with conduit placement and VSD closure can then take place at a later point in time.[13,14] Because of the inherent abnormalities of the collateral vessels and risk for later stenoses, some centers now advocate recruiting only the native pulmonary arteries, even if severely hypoplastic, since these vessels have a greater growth potential.[15] Catheter interventions for balloon angioplasty of stenosed pulmonary arteries and placement of stents are common after surgery. In some cases, MAPCAs provide a balanced pulmonary circulation or the distribution of the vessels is so abnormal that surgical management is deemed futile. These patients may report limited symptoms in childhood and early adulthood, but they rarely live beyond their third decade.[16]

Outcomes

In general, surgical outcomes for TOF/PA are less favorable than TOF with pulmonary stenosis but largely depend on the architecture of pulmonary blood flow supply. Patients with platelike pulmonary atresia, well-formed pulmonary arteries, and no MAPCAs have outcomes that are very good and approximate that seen in TOF with pulmonary stenosis. Patients with MAPCAs, however, have worse outcomes, but there is variability within this group. Recent reports of TOF/PA with MAPCAs reveal a 3-year survival of 80% and 10-year survival of 71%.[13,14] Re-intervention rates are high, with over half of the patients requiring a catheter or surgical intervention within 5 years.[14] Patients with TOF/PA can encounter long-term issues associated with a conduit and chronic pulmonary insufficiency, including exercise intolerance, right ventricular dilation with failure, and arrythmias.[17,18]

Imaging Essentials and Important Points

- Identify a large VSD and enlarged aorta overriding the ventricular septum.
- Using color Doppler imaging and pulse wave imaging determine whether there is evidence for forward antegrade flow across the pulmonary outflow.
- Assess the nature of the right ventricular outflow tract obstruction with attention to the presence or absence of an infundibular chamber, valvar platelike atresia, and main pulmonary artery segment.
- Assess branch pulmonary artery size and determine whether they are confluent.
- If the main pulmonary artery is present, determine whether there is retrograde flow from a patent DA. The DA will typically insert into the junction between the right and the left branch pulmonary arteries. In a fetus with a left aortic arch, a left-sided DA arises from the underside of the aortic arch, and a right-sided DA arises from the base of the left innominate artery. In a right aortic arch, a left-sided DA arises from the base of the left innominate artery and a right-sided DA arises from the underside of the aortic arch.
- Evaluate the aortic arch looking for collateral (MAPCAs) vessels arising. Search along the transverse as well as descending aorta to the level just beneath the diaphragm. Remember that the smaller the branch pulmonary arteries, the more likely you are to have MAPCAs vessels.
- Assess aortic arch sidedness.
- Assess for the presence of thymus tissue.

References

1. O'Leary PW, Mair DD, Edwards WD, Julsrud PR, Puga FJ, Goldmuntz E. Pulmonary atresia and ventricular septal defect. In Allen HD, Gutsegal HD, Clark EB, Driscoll DJ, eds. *Moss and Adams' Heart Disease in Infants, Children, and Adolescents*. 6th ed. Philadelphia: Lippincott Williams & Wilkins; 2001:864-879.
2. Ferencz C, Rubin JD, McCarter RJ, et al. Congenital heart disease: prevalence at livebirth. The Baltimore-Washington Infant Study. *Am J Epidemiol*. 1985;121:31-36.
3. Kaguelidou F, Fermont L, Boudjemline Y, Le BJ, Batisse A, Bonnet D. Foetal echocardiographic assessment of tetralogy of Fallot and post-natal outcome. *Eur Heart J*. 2008;29:1432-1438.
4. Goldmuntz E. DiGeorge syndrome: new insights. *Clin Perinatol*. 2005;32:963-978.
5. Chessa M, Butera G, Bonhoeffer P, et al. Relation of genotype 22q11 deletion to phenotype of pulmonary vessels in tetralogy of Fallot and pulmonary atresia–ventricular septal defect. *Heart*. 1998;79:186-190.
6. Bruneau BG. The developmental genetics of congenital heart disease. *Nature*. 2008;451:943-948.
7. Hornberger LK, Sanders SP, Sahn DJ, et al. In utero pulmonary artery and aortic growth and potential for progression of pulmonary outflow tract obstruction in tetralogy of Fallot. *J Am Coll Cardiol*. 1995;25:739-745.
8. Mackie AS, Gauvreau K, Perry SB, del Nido PJ, Geva T. Echocardiographic predictors of aortopulmonary collaterals in infants with tetralogy of Fallot and pulmonary atresia. *J Am Coll Cardiol*. 2003; 41:852-857.
9. Boshoff D, Gewillig M. A review of the options for treatment of major aortopulmonary collateral arteries in the setting of tetralogy of Fallot with pulmonary atresia. *Cardiol Young*. 2006;16: 212-220.
10. Hirsch JC, Mosca RS, Bove EL. Complete repair of tetralogy of Fallot in the neonate: results in the modern era. *Ann Surg*. 2000;232: 508-514.
11. Fraser CD Jr, McKenzie ED, Cooley DA. Tetralogy of Fallot: surgical management individualized to the patient. *Ann Thorac Surg*. 2001; 71:1556-1561.
12. Gewillig M, Boshoff DE, Dens J, et al. Stenting the neonatal arterial duct in duct-dependent pulmonary circulation: New techniques, better results. *J Am Coll Cardiol*. 2004;43:107-112.

13. Amark KM, Karamlou T, O'Carroll A, et al. Independent factors associated with mortality, reintervention, and achievement of complete repair in children with pulmonary atresia with ventricular septal defect. *J Am Coll Cardiol.* 2006;47:1448-1456.
14. Reddy VM, McElhinney DB, Amin Z, et al. Early and intermediate outcomes after repair of pulmonary atresia with ventricular septal defect and major aortopulmonary collateral arteries: experience with 85 patients. *Circulation.* 2000;101:1826-1832.
15. Brizard CP, Liava'a M, d'Udekem Y. Pulmonary atresia, VSD and MAPCAs: Repari without unifocalization. *Semin Thorac Cardiovasc Surg Pediatr Card Surg Ann.* 2009;12:139-144.
16. Marelli AJ, Perloff JK, Child JS, Laks H. Pulmonary atresia with ventricular septal defect in adults. *Circulation.* 1994;89:243-251.
17. Samman A, Schwerzmann M, Balint OH, et al. Exercise capacity and biventricular function in adult patients with repaired tetralogy of Fallot. *Am Heart J.* 2008;156:100-105.
18. Gatzoulis MA, Balaji S, Webber SA, et al. Risk factors for arrhythmia and sudden cardiac death late after repair of tetralogy of Fallot: a multicentre study. *Lancet.* 2000;356:975-981.

CASES

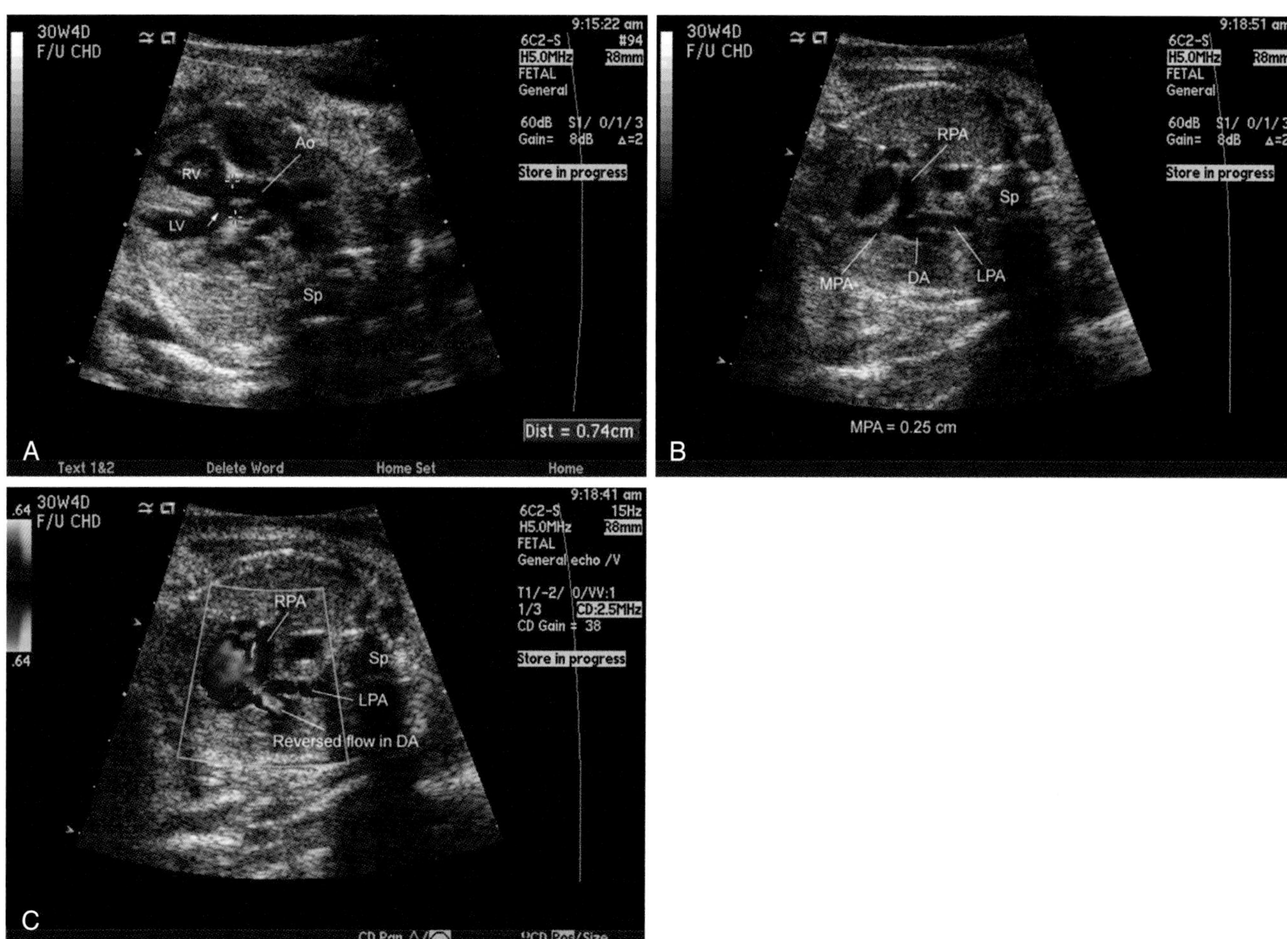

Case 11-1. **(A)** Long-axis view of the heart reveals evidence of a large ventricular septal defect *(arrow)*. The aorta (Ao) is quite large and at 30 weeks' gestation measures over 7 mm. The aorta is seen overriding the right (RV) and left (LV) ventricles. Sp, spine. **(B)** Angling toward the great vessels reveals the main pulmonary artery (MPA) to be relatively small. This is a case of pulmonary atresia; however, there is an MPA segment that comes down to the base of the heart. We also see the right pulmonary artery (RPA), left pulmonary artery (LPA), and ductus arteriosus (DA). **(C)** Color Doppler imaging reveals blood flow in the RPA, LPA, and DA. There is no antegrade flow across the MPA. All pulmonary blood flow in this case depends upon retrograde and reversed flow from the DA. Notice the blood flow in the DA is *red,* toward the transducer, and the LPA is perfused in a retrograde manner from the DA and is *blue.* Flow in the RPA is seen toward the transducer and is *red.*

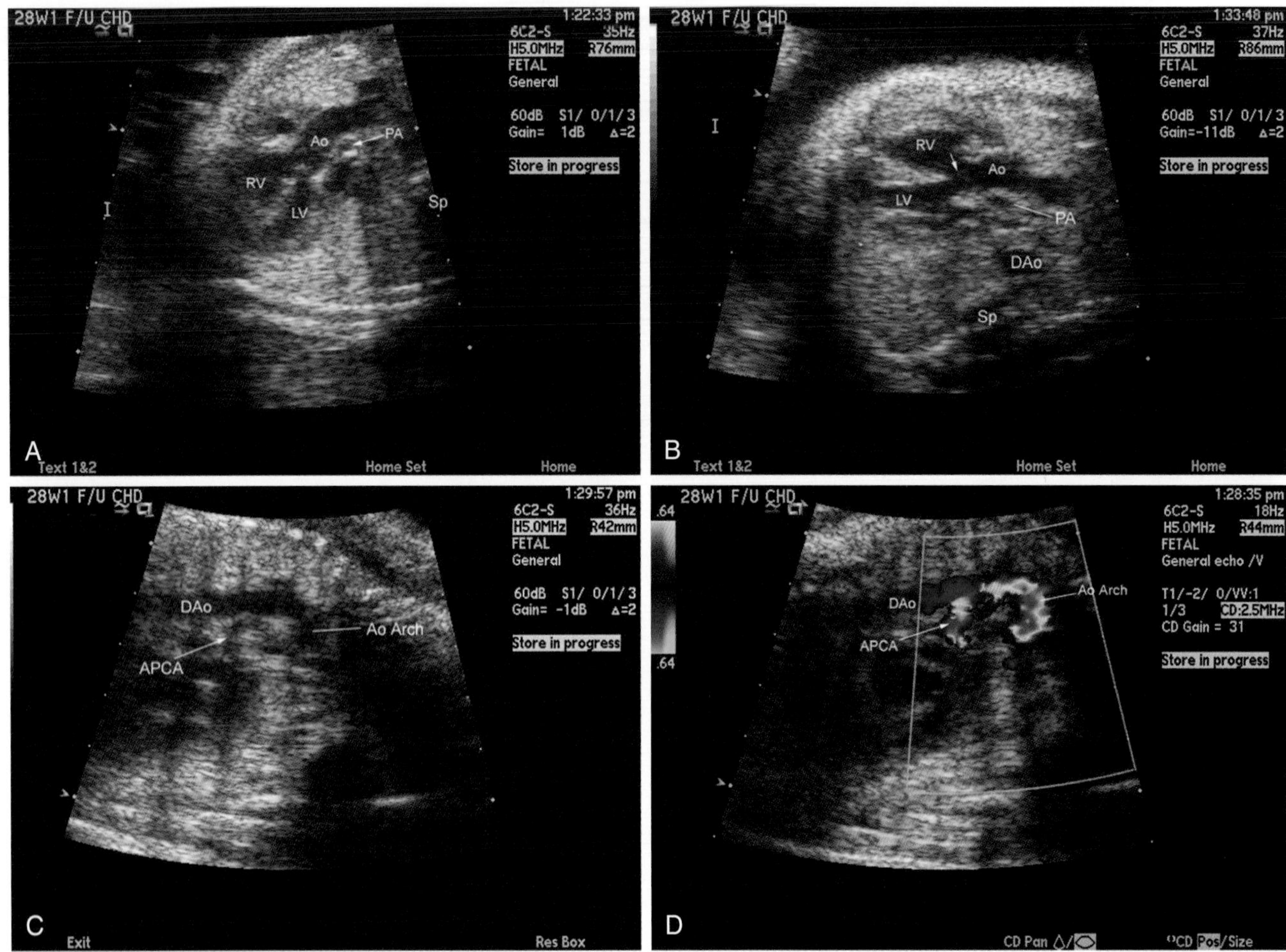

Case 11-2. **(A)** Apical view of the heart angled superiorly reveals one large great vessel. This is the aorta (Ao) and it is overriding the ventricular septum. There is a large ventricular septal defect. There is a hint of a small pulmonary artery (PA) next to and to the left of the aorta. **(B)** Long-axis view demonstrates large ventricular septal defect with overriding aorta, with a small PA adjacent to the aorta but without any evidence of patent connection to the heart. **(C)** View of the distal aortic arch (Ao Arch) and the descending aorta (DAo) reveals a hint of an aortopulmonary collateral artery (APCA). This is arising much lower from the arch than would be expected for a DA. **(D)** Color Doppler imaging demonstrates a large APCA vessel originating from the DAo and perfusing the lung.

12

Tetralogy of Fallot with Absent Pulmonary Valve Syndrome

Amanda Shillingford

Key Echocardiographic Features

- Large malalignment type of ventricular septal defect
- Large overriding aorta
- Rudimentary, primitive pulmonary valve tissue with both stenosis and severe insufficiency
- Massively dilated, aneurysmal proximal branch pulmonary arteries
- Dilated right ventricular outflow tract and right ventricle
- Right ventricular systolic dysfunction, possible
- Absence of the ductus arteriosus (unless rare case of discontinuous left pulmonary artery arising from ductus arteriosus)

Anatomy and Anatomical Associations

Tetralogy of Fallot with absent pulmonary valve syndrome (TOF/APVS) is a rare variant of tetralogy of Fallot (TOF) in which the pulmonary valve leaflets are extremely underdeveloped resulting in severe pulmonary insufficiency and aneurysmal dilation of the main and branch pulmonary arteries.[1] The entity of absent pulmonary valve leaflet syndrome can exist in association with an intact ventricular septum, but is discussed elsewhere. In TOF/APVS, a large malalignment ventricular septal defect (VSD) is present, as well as an overriding aorta, and some degree of pulmonary stenosis. Malalignment of the conal septum may be difficult to appreciate because of the right ventricle, subpulmonary, infundibular, and pulmonary artery dilation. In the position of the pulmonary valve annulus, there is a thickened gelatinous ring of tissue that gives rise to very abnormal rudimentary leaflets. The pulmonary valve annulus is usually hypoplastic, but not to the same degree as seen in standard TOF. The pulmonary valve is completely incompetent, resulting in severe pulmonary insufficiency. The main pulmonary artery and branch pulmonary arteries are markedly dilated (Figure 12-1). Because the branch pulmonary arteries are adjacent to the airways, these vessels can cause significant compression of the bronchi. In addition, studies have shown that the pulmonary arterioles in TOF/APVS exhibit peculiar branching patterns with dilated proximal and hypoplastic distal vessels in addition to the appearance of coiling. The abnormal vessels further cause impingement on the intraparenchymal bronchi and inhibit alveolar growth.[2] The right ventricle is markedly dilated, and tricuspid regurgitation is common related to annular dilation. The ductus arteriosus is almost always absent in TOF/APVS, except in rare cases in which there is discontinuity between the pulmonary arteries and the ductus arteriosus connects to a discontinuous left pulmonary artery.[3]

TOF/APVS has been associated with several other cardiac abnormalities, including anomalous origin of the branch pulmonary arteries, coarctation of the aorta, and total anomalous pulmonary venous return.[4,5]

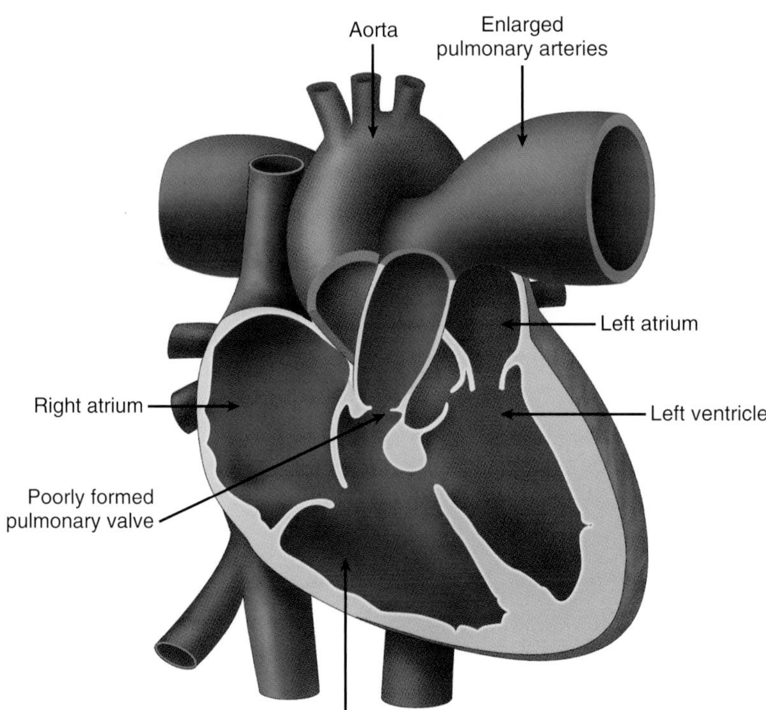

Figure 12-1. No ductus arteriosus.

Frequency, Genetics, and Development

TOF/APVS accounts for approximately 3% to 6% of all cases of TOF.[6,7] Limited data are available in the literature regarding the genetic etiology.[8] Microdeletion of chromosome 22q11, which is present in 90% of patients with DiGeorge syndrome, is identified in 21% to 38% of patients with TOF/APVS without any specific correlation to aortic arch sidedness.[9,10] Sporadic cases of other chromosome abnormalities have been reported in the literature,[5,9,11] although these are more common in the presence of absent pulmonary valve with an intact ventricular septum.

Two main theories exist regarding the developmental abnormality resulting in TOF/APVS. In the first, because the pulmonary valve is always structurally very abnormal in this disorder, it suggests an original primary error in signaling leading to improper formation of the pulmonary valve and severe pulmonary insufficiency. If a ductus arteriosus were to be present, survival would not be possible according to this argument. The presence of a ductus arteriosus in the fetus with severe pulmonary insufficiency would seriously affect systemic perfusion because flow through such a ductus arteriosus would be retrograde, stealing from the systemic circulation and becoming part of the regurgitant flow across the pulmonary valve. It is believed that in such a scenario, fetuses suffer early demise, which may explain why a ductus arteriosus is almost always absent in TOF/APVS.[3] A second proposed theory suggests that congenital agenesis of the ductus arteriosus is primary, which in the presence of a select group of susceptible TOF, results in altered pulmonary artery flow hemodynamics and impairs normal development of the pulmonary valve and pulmonary arteries.[2]

Increased nuchal translucency in the first trimester has been noted in 40% of fetuses with TOF/APVS without a specific association with chromosomal abnormalities.[9]

Fetal Physiology

Regardless of the events prompting abnormal pulmonary valve formation and absence of the ductus arteriosus, the prenatal manifestations of TOF/APVS pertain to severe pulmonary insufficiency, right ventricular dilation, and markedly dilated pulmonary arteries. In the setting of severe pulmonary insufficiency, stroke volume from the right ventricle is elevated with potential progression to right ventricular dysfunction. Moreover, in the absence of a ductus arteriosus, blood ejected out of the right ventricle is fully delivered to the pulmonary circulation and the pulmonary arteries must withstand significant increases of blood volume. Progression of pulmonary artery dilation from mid to late gestation has been documented, suggesting that vascular remodeling is a dynamic process in this anomaly.[7] Both left and right ventricular dysfunction can be impaired in the fetus, based on qualitative inspection of systolic shortening and measures of myocardial performance index and Doppler flow reversal in the umbilical artery.[12] The prenatal course is not based on the pulmonary aspect of the disease, but on the cardiac aspects, and in particular, the impact of severe pulmonary insufficiency on right ventricular performance. Because there is a large VSD, progressive volume loading of the right ventricle will ultimately affect the left ventricle as well. There is a high prevalence of fetal demise in TOF/APVS, which is associated with preceding fetal hydrops.[13]

Fetal lung development, both vascular and airway, is abnormal and related to a combination of bronchi compression from dilated pulmonary arteries and right ventricle, as well as inhibition of appropriate alveolar multiplication related to aberrant branching patterns of the bronchioles.[2]

Prenatal Management

Fetuses with TOF/APVS have a high incidence of fetal demise, but to date, there are no available prenatal interventions to improve outcomes. Serial echocardiography should be performed in all fetuses to assess for signs of ventricular failure and hydrops, although the options are limited unless the fetus is near term and delivery can be performed safely. Counseling with families should include the possibility of fetal demise as well as the risk of abnormal lung development and airway compromise, which can affect postnatal prognosis. Unfortunately, neither the degree of pulmonary insufficiency nor any other variables have been found to prognosticate for the degree of lung disease present in the fetus with TOF/APVS. Each fetus should undergo a comprehensive obstetrical fetal anatomy ultrasound, and karyotype evaluation is strongly recommended.

Postnatal Physiology

The clinical presentation of fetuses that survive to term is variable. Upon delivery, the pulmonary vascular resistance decreases after the infant takes the first breath. A drop in pulmonary vascular resistance may promote forward flow into the pulmonary arteries, achieving adequate levels of oxygenation. The pulmonary annular hypoplasia is generally not significant enough to cause severe right ventricular outflow obstruction. In the absence of respiratory symptoms related to lung disease, these infants will follow a clinical course similar to standard TOF and undergo elective surgical repair before 6 months of age. However, approximately half of newborns with TOF/APVS present with severe respiratory symptoms due to either compression of the bronchi from the severely dilated pulmonary arteries or abnormal alveolar development.[14] These infants can be quite ill and may require urgent surgical intervention.

The physical examination reveals varying levels of hypoxemia and often tachypnea and respiratory distress. A prominent "to-and-fro" murmur is appreciated along the left sternal border, representing a harsh systolic component due to flow across the hypoplastic pulmonary annulus (and increased stroke volume) and a low-pitched diastolic component representing insufficiency. Hepatic enlargement may be present in the setting of right ventricular dysfunction.[5]

Postnatal Management

Any fetus with a diagnosis of TOF/APVS should be delivered at a tertiary care center where urgent intensive care is available since the clinical severity of the postnatal course can be difficult to predict and is dependent upon the degree of bronchial compression and lung disease. Prostaglandin infusion is not necessary because there typically is no ductus arteriosus present at birth. Patients with TOF/APVS are at risk for hypercyanotic spells due to changes in systemic vascular resistance and suddenly increased right-to-left shunting. Intubation and sedation may be required to stabilize the infant. Medical therapies to increase systemic vascular resistance and decrease pulmonary vascular resistance may also be necessary. Placing the infant in a prone position may alleviate respiratory symptoms by "lifting" the dilated pulmonary arteries off the airways and relieving the pulmonary arterial compression of the bronchi. The infant should be monitored closely in the first postnatal days as the physiology can change markedly as the pulmonary vascular resistance decreases. Evaluation of the extent of airway compression and parenchymal involvement may be performed using computed tomography or magnetic resonance imaging.[15]

A stable infant without respiratory distress and acceptable arterial oxygen saturations can be discharged home after a period of observation in the hospital with close follow-up by a pediatric cardiologist. The principle of surgical correction for this group is closure of the VSD, augmentation of the right ventricular outflow tract, and usually some element of size reduction and suspension of the pulmonary arteries in such as manner so as to reduce airway impingement. The timing of surgery for TOF/APVS in these patients mirrors the philosophy of standard TOF adopted by the individual institution. Another more radical strategy is to remove the entire native main pulmonary artery and proximal branch pulmonary and replace the sections with homograft.[16] A more recent modification has been to perform a "Lecompte maneuver" in which the pulmonary arteries are divided and translocated anterior to the aorta and away from the bronchus.[17]

Outcomes

The overall outcome for patients with TOF/APVS is less favorable than other forms of TOF, but it is largely based on the degree of airway compression and lung disease present. The rate of fetal demise is high in this population. In particular, when there is evidence for ventricular dilation and dysfunction, half of the newborns will experience significant respiratory compromise. Operative mortality in patients presenting with respiratory symptoms, however, is as high as 50%.[18] Overall, multiple centers have reported 10-year survival rates of 79% to 87%.[15,18] Finally, patients with TOF/APVS also face long-term morbidities similar to the standard TOF population, including chronic pulmonary insufficiency, right ventricular failure, and exercise intolerance.

Imaging Essentials and Important Points

- Identify a large VSD and anterior malalignment of the conal septum.
- Two-dimensional assessment of the pulmonary valve reveals dysplastic "nubbins" of rudimentary leaflets, which do not coapt. At times, there may be no leaflets at all, simply a "napkin ring" type narrowing in the region of the pulmonary valve where a valve should be but none exists.
- Although the pulmonary annulus will be smaller than the aortic annulus, there will not be much subpulmonary or infundibular narrowing in TOF/APVS.
- Color Doppler imaging across the right ventricular outflow tract will reveal severe pulmonary insufficiency. The peak velocity of flow across the pulmonary valve will be increased as the volume of flow due to the regurgitant fraction is markedly increased.
- The branch pulmonary arteries can be quite large, even as large as the right atrium itself. The appearance of massively dilated right and left branch pulmonary arteries sitting atop a compressed heart is referred to as the Mickey Mouse ears sign.
- Search for a ductus arteriosus; however, in most cases, it will typically be absent, unless the branch pulmonary arteries are discontinuous, in which case the ductus will be perfusing the isolated pulmonary artery.
- Assess for arch sidedness.
- Look for thymus tissue.

Imaging Essentials and Important Points—cont'd

- Assessment of overall heart size and individual ventricular size and systolic function are important and have prognostic implications for fetal survival.
- The degree of pulmonary vascular or airway disease present cannot be determined in the fetus with TOF/APVS. Hence, counseling after diagnosis of this disorder is a challenge. Distinguishing between the fetus who will have a good outcome similar to standard TOF but have mild reactive airway disease versus the fetus who will have life-threatening respiratory failure and poor outcome cannot be made based on fetal echocardiographic factors, to date.

References

1. Zucker N, Rozin I, Levitas A, Zalzstein E. Clinical presentation, natural history, and outcome of patients with the absent pulmonary valve syndrome. *Cardiol Young*. 2004;14:402-408.
2. Rabinovitch M, Grady S, David I, et al. Compression of intrapulmonary bronchi by abnormally branching pulmonary arteries associated with absent pulmonary valves. *Am J Cardiol*. 1982;50:804-813.
3. Emmanoulides GC, Thanopoulos B, Siassi B, Fishbein M. "Agenesis" of ductus arteriosus associated with the syndrome of tetralogy of Fallot and absent pulmonary valve. *Am J Cardiol*. 1976;37:403-409.
4. Jeewa A, Mann GS, Hosking MC. Tetralogy of Fallot with absent pulmonary valve and obstructed totally anomalous pulmonary venous connection. *Cardiol Young*. 2007;17:551-553.
5. Gutgesell HP, Goldmuntz E. Congenital absence of the pulmonary valve. In Allen HD, Gutsegall HP, Clark EB, Driscoll DJ, eds. *Moss and Adams' Heart Disease in Infants, Children, and Adolescents*. 6th ed. Philadelphia: Lippincott Williams & Wilkins; 2001:903-909.
6. Rao BN, Anderson RC, Edwards JE. Anatomic variations in the tetralogy of Fallot. *Am Heart J*. 1971;81:361-371.
7. Lev M, Eckner FA. The pathologic anatomy of tetralogy of Fallot and its variations. *Dis Chest*. 1964;45:251-261.
8. Goldmuntz E. DiGeorge syndrome: new insights. *Clin Perinatol*. 2005;32:963-978.
9. Galindo A, Gutierrez-Larraya F, Martinez JM, et al. Prenatal diagnosis and outcome for fetuses with congenital absence of the pulmonary valve. *Ultrasound Obstet Gynecol*. 2006;28:32-39.
10. Boudjemline Y, Fermont L, Le Bidois J, Lyonnet S, Sidi D, Bonnet D. Prevalence of 22q11 deletion in fetuses with conotruncal cardiac defects: a 6 year prospective study. *J Pediatr*. 2001;138:520-524.
11. Tansatit M, Kongruttanachok N, Kongnak W, et al. Tetralogy of Fallot with absent pulmonary valve in a de novo derivative chromosome 9 with duplication of 9p13 → 9pter and deletion of 9q34.3. *Am J Med Genet A*. 2006;140:1981-1987.
12. Inamura N, Kado Y, Nakajima T, Kayatani F. Left and right ventricular function in fetal tetralogy of Fallot with absent pulmonary valve. *Am J Perinatol*. 2005;22:199-204.
13. Moon-Grady AJ, Teitel DF, Hanley FL, Moore P. Ductus-associated proximal pulmonary artery stenosis in patients with right heart obstruction. *Int J Cardiol*. 2007;114:41-45.
14. Kirshbom PM, Kogon BE. Tetralogy of Fallot with absent pulmonary valve syndrome. *Semin Thorac Cardiovasc Surg Pediatr Card Surg Annu*. 2004;7:65-71.
15. Alsoufi B, Williams WG, Hua Z, et al. Surgical outcomes in the treatment of patients with tetralogy of Fallot and absent pulmonary valve. *Eur J Cardiothorac Surg*. 2007;31:354-359.
16. Kirshbom PM, Jaggers JJ, Ungerleider RM. Tetralogy of Fallot with absent pulmonary valve: simplified technique for homograft repair. *J Thorac Cardiovasc Surg*. 1999;118:1125-1127.
17. Hraska V, Kantorova A, Kunovsky P, Haviar D. Intermediate results with correction of tetralogy of Fallot with absent pulmonary valve using a new approach. *Eur J Cardiothorac Surg*. 2002;21:711-714.
18. Norgaard MA, Alphonso N, Newcomb AE, Brizard CP, Cochrane AD. Absent pulmonary valve syndrome. Surgical and clinical outcome with long-term follow-up. *Eur J Cardiothorac Surg*. 2006;29(5):682-687.

CASES

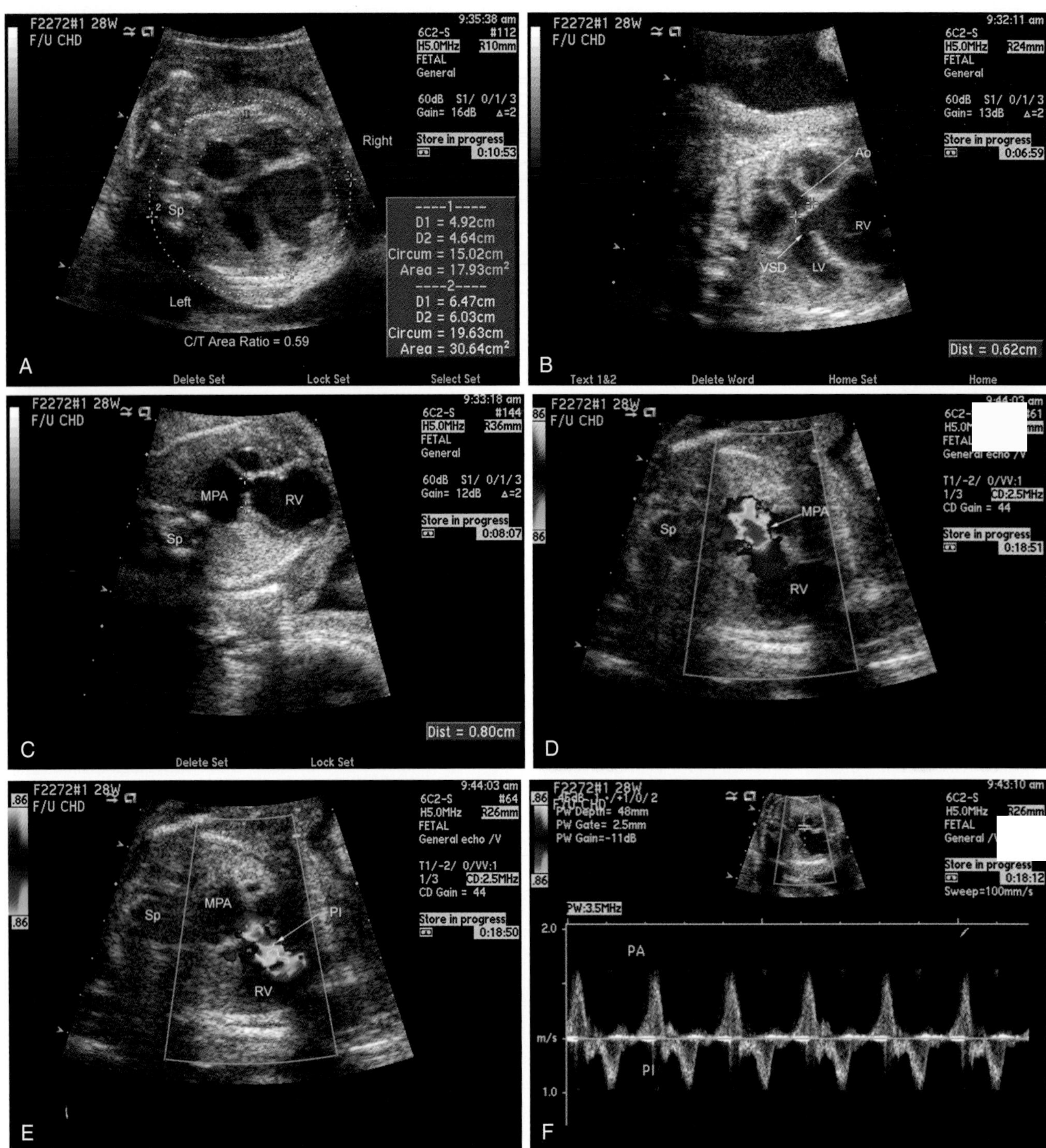

Case 12-1. (**A**) Four-chamber view of the heart shows severe cardiomegaly. The apex of the heart is pointing severely leftward and at a right angle to the plane of the spine (Sp), suggesting that the axis of the heart is abnormal. In addition, the right ventricle is markedly dilated in proportion to the left. Overall cardiothoracic area ratio is approximately 60%. (**B**) There is marked discrepancy in size between the right (RV) and the left (LV) ventricle with a dilated RV. Severe regurgitation into the RV is causing it to be markedly dilated and dysfunctional. The *arrow* points to a malalignment type ventricular septal defect (VSD). The aorta (Ao) overrides the ventricular septum. (**C**) Image of the right ventricular outflow tract in the long axis. The infundibulum and subpulmonary region within the RV is dilated. The pulmonary annulus is not very hypoplastic because it measures 8 mm at 28 weeks' gestation. There is evidence for rudimentary but nonfunctioning pulmonary valve leaflet tissue. The main pulmonary artery (MPA) is markedly dilated. (**D**) Color flow across the MPA reveals turbulence of flow during *systole* as blood is ejected. (**E**) In *diastole,* blood regurgitates back from the dysplastic and abnormal pulmonary valve into the dilated right ventricular outflow chamber. This reflects severe pulmonary insufficiency (PI). (**F**) Spectral display of Doppler flow imaging reveals both systolic and diastolic flow across the MPA. Flow below the baseline reflects PI.

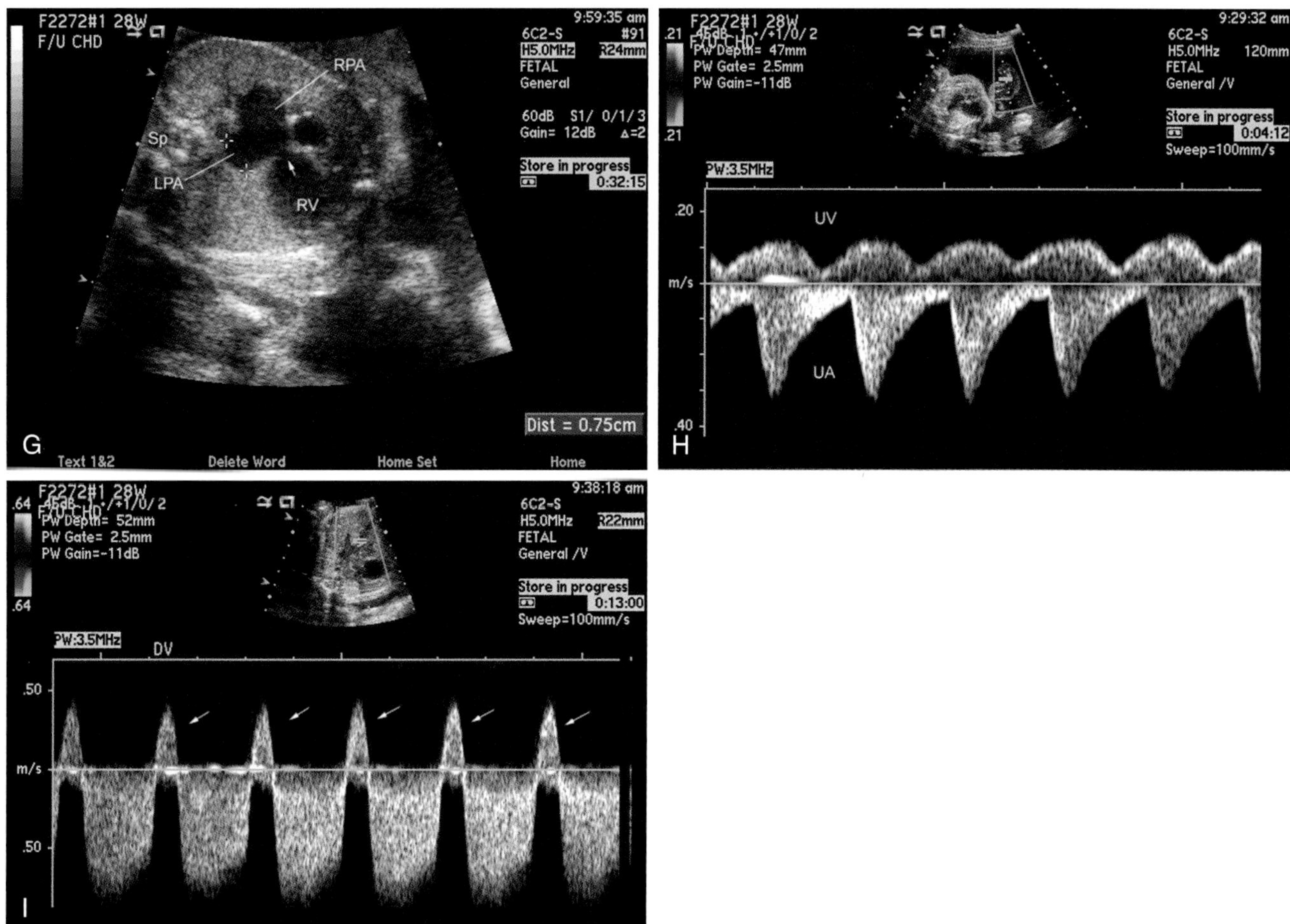

Case 12-1, cont'd (G) Two-dimensional image reveals the classic finding of severely dilated proximal branch pulmonary arteries. The *arrow* points to the "pinching-in" of the region of the pulmonary valve annulus and the very rudimentary pulmonary valve tissue that is present. Distal to the valve, the MPA and proximal branches are quite dilated. In this case, the degree of regurgitation was severe and angled predominantly toward the RV causing right ventricular dilation and right ventricular dysfunction. LPA, left pulmonary artery; RPA, right pulmonary artery. **(H)** Doppler interrogation of the umbilical cord demonstrates pulsations in the umbilical vein (UV) as seen above the baseline. There is a decrease in forward flow in the UV during ventricular diastole, as judged by the timing of systolic flow in the umbilical artery (UA). This decrease in umbilical venous forward flow is due to elevated right ventricular compliance and may also be a consequence of transmission of impedance to forward flow during diastole when the tricuspid valve is open, this in the presence of severe pulmonic insufficiency. **(I)** Doppler imaging in the ductus venosus (DV) reveals reversal of flow with atrial contraction as demonstrated by the *arrows*. This is a reflection of the severely abnormal compliance of the RV and diastolic dysfunction, also possibly related to the severe PI.

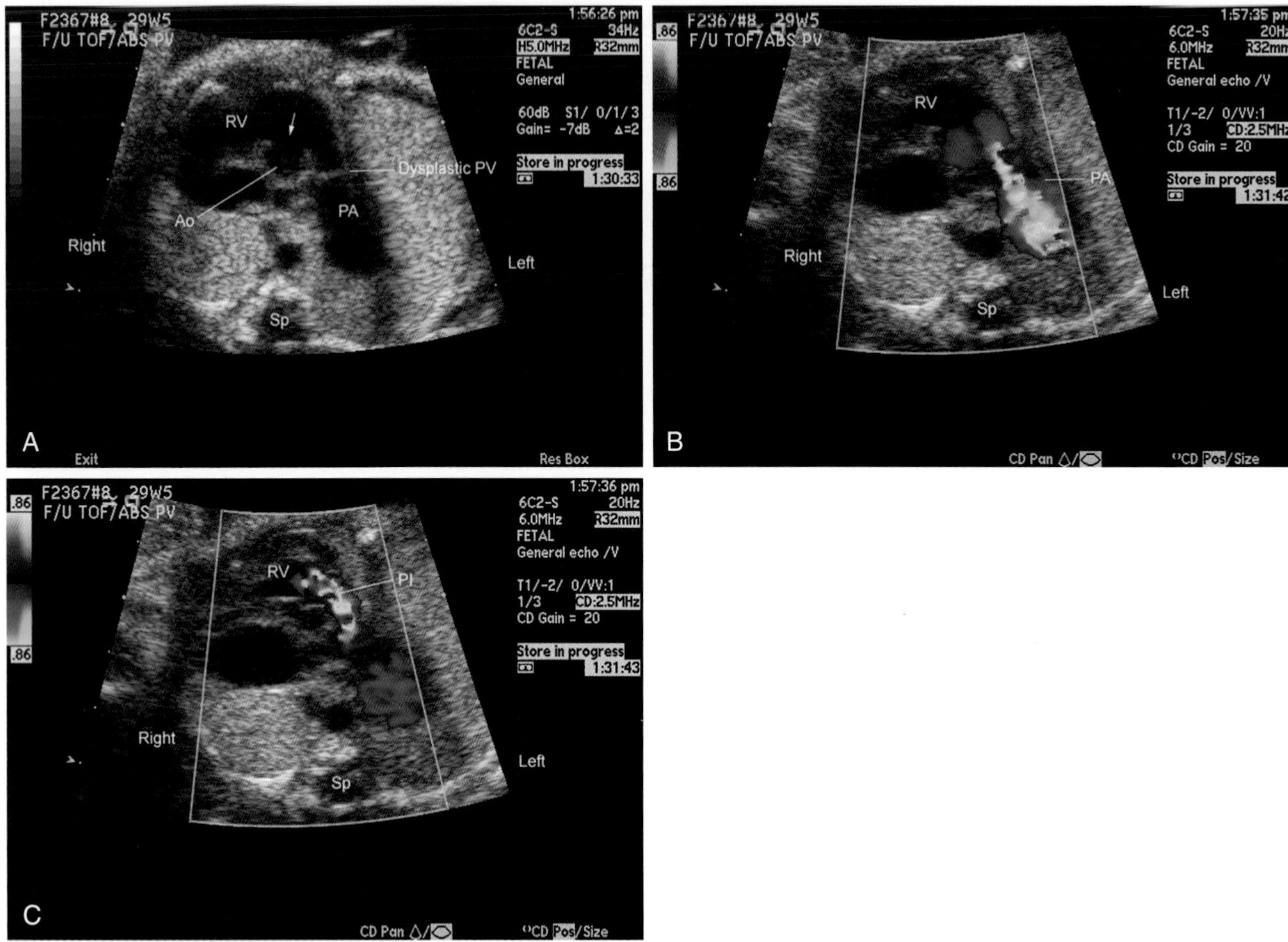

Case 12-2. **(A)** Short-axis view of a fetus with tetralogy of Fallot and dysplastic pulmonary valve (PV). Notice the typical findings of more classic tetralogy of Fallot in which there is anterior malalignment of the infundibular septum and a large VSD. A rudimentary dysplastic PV is present. The pulmonary artery (PA) is severely dilated. Ao, aorta; RV, right ventricle; Sp, spine. **(B)** Color flow imaging in *systole* reveals turbulence of flow across the right ventricular outflow tract and a dilated MPA. **(C)** Color flow in *diastole* reveals severe pulmonary insufficiency (PI) with blood regurgitating back into the infundibulum and right ventricular cavity.

13

Malalignment of Conal Septum with Arch Obstruction

Shobha Natarajan

Key Echocardiographic Features

- Position of the conal septum in relation to the ventricular septum and size of the ventricular septal defect created
- Degree of posterior deviation of the conal septum and size of the left ventricular outflow tract
- Aortic annulus diameter and presence or absence of aortic valvar stenosis
- Size of the left ventricle (typically normal)
- Mitral valve size and anatomy (typically normal)
- Size and caliber of the ascending aorta, transverse aorta, and aortic isthmus
- Presence or absence of coarctation of the aorta or interruption of the aortic arch
- Identification of the branching of the aortic arch and the origin of the upper extremity and head vessels
- Identification of the presence or absence of thymic tissue in the anterior mediastinum

Anatomy and Anatomical Associations

The conal or infundibular septum is the superior-anterior portion of the ventricular septum. It separates the aortic and pulmonary outlets. Abnormal development can result when there is deviation of the conal septum posteriorly in relation to the remainder of the muscular septum. This posterior malalignment situates the conal septum across the left ventricular outflow tract (LVOT). A ventricular septal defect (VSD) coexists with this posterior malalignment (Figure 13-1). This VSD can be located in the membranous, outlet, or muscular septum and is referred to as a *posterior malalignment ventricular septal defect (PMVSD)*. Such VSDs are almost always large and do not undergo spontaneous closure. In hearts with normally related great vessels, the VSD can be related more to the pulmonary artery and some degree of override of the pulmonary artery over the ventricular septum can be seen.

Depending on the degree of deviation of the conal septum into the LVOT, a PMVSD can be associated with narrowing of the subaortic region and decreased growth of the aortic valve. Thus, obstruction can be noted at the subvalvar or valvar level. In rare cases, posterior malalignment is associated with aortic atresia.[1] In addition, a PMVSD can be associated with various degrees of aortic

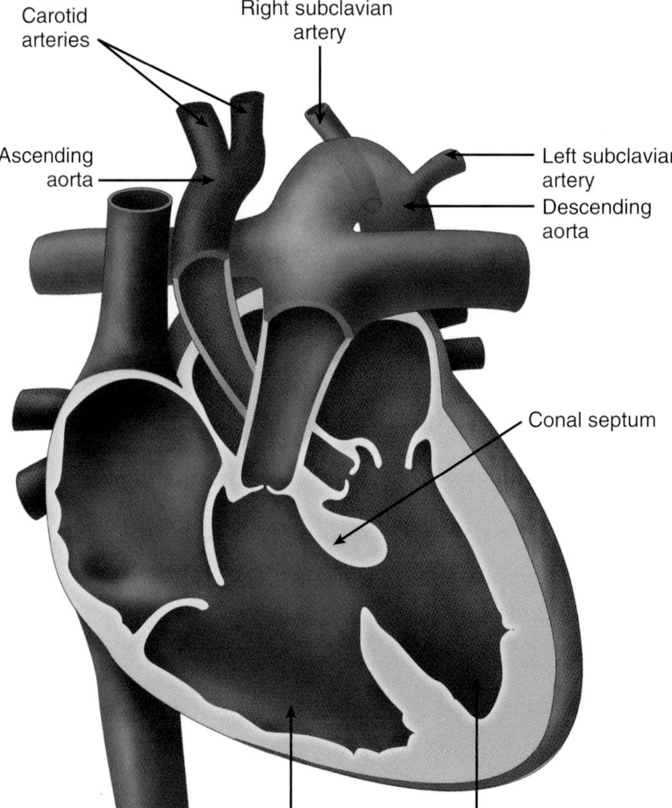

Figure 13-1. Posterior malalignment of conal septum and interrupted aortic arch type B.

arch obstruction, including aortic arch hypoplasia, coarctation of the aorta, and interrupted aortic arch (IAA).

IAA is a complete absence of the connection between the ascending and the descending aorta. The classification of IAA is as follows, working from the distal end to the proximal end of the aortic arch[2]:

- Type A: the interruption is distal to the left subclavian artery.
- Type B: the interruption is between the left common carotid and the left subclavian arteries.
- Type C: the interruption is between the innominate and the left common carotid arteries.

Type A interruptions can be associated with aortopulmonary window[3] and type C interruptions are extremely rare.

Type B interruptions are more common than type A and are commonly associated with a PMVSD and subaortic obstruction. Bicommissural aortic valve is often seen with these defects. Arch sidedness and arch vessel abnormalities such as right aortic arch with aberrant right subclavian artery can also be associated with PMVSD with or without aortic arch obstruction and marks a higher probability of a deletion in chromosome 22q11 in those patients.[4]

Frequency, Genetics, and Development

PMVSD is more often associated with IAA (93%) than with coarctation of the aorta (47%).[5] Twenty-four percent of patients with PMVSD have a normal aortic arch.[6] The incidence of IAA is 0.019 per 1000 live births and accounts for 1% of all congenital heart disease.[7]

Genetic factors have been linked to the development of PMVSD and type B IAA. Type B IAA is considered a conotruncal defect because of the abnormal ventricular septal development and abnormal aortic arch formation. As with other conotruncal defects, namely, tetralogy of Fallot and truncus arteriosus, IAA type B is found in patients with deletion of chromosome 22q11. In fact, deletions involving chromosome 22q11 are seen in 57% of patients with type B IAA and 33% of patients with PMVSD.[4] Interestingly, 22q11 deletions are more common in patients with associated vascular anomalies such as right aortic arch, aberrant right or left subclavian artery, aorticopulmonary collaterals, or absent/discontinuous branch pulmonary arteries.[4] DiGeorge, velocardiofacial, and conotruncal anomaly face syndromes all involve chromosome 22q11 deletions. Extracardiac manifestations of these syndromes include hypoplasia/aplasia of the thymus and/or parathyroid glands, hypocalcemia, palatal abnormalities, learning disabilities, and facial dysmorphism. The strong association of PMVSD and IAA with this chromosomal abnormality lends evidence for the genetic origin of abnormalities involving the infundibular septum and conotruncus. The significantly increased prevalence of chromosome 22q11 deletion in IAA type B indicates that this particular cardiac defect has a different developmental origin from the other types of interruptions and from simple coarctation of the aorta.

Embryological factors may also explain the development of PMVSD and IAA. The branchial arterial system in the embryo undergoes significant change during development that involves regression of particular segments and growth of other segments into portions of the aorta and pulmonary arteries. In IAA of all types, certain parts of the branchial arch system involute and the corresponding arch segment fails to form.

Lastly, reduced blood flow to the aorta may explain the development of aortic arch obstruction. PMVSD can create significant obstruction that reduces blood flow through the LVOT and aorta. Blood flow is directed preferentially to the pulmonary valve through the ductus arteriosus to the descending aorta, leaving the aortic arch and isthmus with reduced blood flow compared with normal. This reduced blood flow is thought to prevent normal growth of the aortic arch and produce various forms of obstruction.

The heterogeneity of aortic arch obstruction and the variety of intracardiac defects make it difficult to propose a unifying etiology for PMVSD and aortic arch obstruction. For instance, greater than 90% of patients with IAA type B have PMVSD versus 50% of patients with type A interruption.[8] Therefore, there may be a difference in etiologies between these subtypes. Genetic differences make it more likely that IAA type B is due to a primary developmental defect rather than a flow-related etiology related to the PMVSD. It is important to take these developmental, genetic, and physiological factors into consideration when evaluating the fetus and counseling families regarding these particular congenital heart abnormalities.

Fetal Physiology

Significant LVOT obstruction in the presence of a PMVSD reduces the blood flow across the aortic valve. Reduced forward flow across the aortic valve then reduces the percentage of combined cardiac output that traverses the aortic arch and isthmus. The majority of the combined cardiac output is now directed across the pulmonary valve to the ductus arteriosus and into the descending aorta. Because more left ventricular blood traverses the pulmonary valve, the oxygen content of the pulmonary arteries and of the descending aorta is higher than normal, but this change does not have a clinically noticeable impact on the development of the pulmonary vasculature or on lower body metabolism.

Because of the unrestrictive VSD, flow into the left ventricle (LV) is maintained. Therefore, unless there is mitral valve obstruction, LV growth continues and the LV is typically of normal size and is viable as a systemic ventricle. The right ventricle (RV) may be dilated due to the (1) increased flow from the VSD and (2) aortic arch obstruction.

In utero, flow across a VSD is usually bidirectional. An exclusive left-to-right shunt across the VSD suggests significant LVOT obstruction. In addition to alteration of flow across the VSD, LVOT obstruction may cause the shunt across the patent foramen ovale to be bidirectional. However, continuous left-to-right shunting across the foramen ovale is not expected and, if present, should raise concerns about the mitral valve or compliance of the LV.

Prenatal Management

Unlike other forms of aortic arch obstruction, the fetus with PMVSD and arch obstruction may not have LV-RV size discrepancy because of the associated VSD and ability for the ventricle to fill and have normal flow into it and out. Therefore, the standard four-chamber view is not likely to be abnormal unless there is mitral valve pathology or severe aortic valve hypoplasia/atresia. Angling anterior from the four-chamber view toward the LVOT will demonstrate the VSD, posterior malalignment of the infundibular septum, and encroachment of conal septum upon the subaortic region and the valve annulus. Assessment for the presence of subvalvar or valvar narrowing can be made with two-dimensional imaging. Doppler assessment may not detect LVOT obstruction in the presence of a large VSD with a left-to-right shunt. Angling further anteriorly will demonstrate the pulmonary valve and assessment of size discrepancy between the two outflow tracts can be made. The degree of pulmonary valve override of the VSD and the proportion of VSD shunt into the aorta versus the pulmonary artery can be determined. Angling further superiorly from the four-chamber view will visualize the great vessels in short axis and allows further assessment of size discrepancy between the great arteries. Normally, in this three-vessel view, the pulmonary artery is larger than the aorta and in turn, the aorta is larger than the right superior vena cava (RSVC). In the presence of a PMVSD and aortic arch obstruction, the aorta is significantly smaller than the pulmonary artery and the RSVC, which is easily demonstrated in the three-vessel view.

In the long-axis echocardiographic views, the LVOT, the degree of posterior malalignment, and the degree of LVOT narrowing are ideally assessed in an orthogonal plane to the four-chamber view. The direction of VSD shunt can be assessed in this plane where the color Doppler beam is parallel to flow. Normally, there is a bidirectional shunt across a VSD in utero. In the presence of LVOT obstruction, the shunt may be predominantly left to right. The ventricular septum should be scanned in its entirety by two-dimensional and color Doppler imaging to detect additional VSDs, keeping in mind that it may be difficult to detect additional VSDs in the setting of a large PMVSD.

Short-axis echocardiographic views of the heart can demonstrate a bicuspid aortic valve depending on the clarity of acoustic windows. The VSD is demonstrated in yet a different plane. A short-axis view of the mitral valve enables demonstration of structural abnormalities of the valve in the setting of mitral stenosis.

Intracardiac findings of LVOT obstruction, large VSD (especially in the presence of posterior malalignment of the conal septum), or aorta–pulmonary artery size discrepancy should prompt a full assessment of the aortic arch. Posterior malalignment of the conal septum should raise suspicion for arch hypoplasia, coarctation of the aorta, or type B IAA. A large mid-muscular VSD or LV-RV size discrepancy should raise the possibility of type A or C aortic interruption. Aortopulmonary window can be seen with type C interruption.

A long-axis view of the aortic arch will demonstrate the site of the interruption. In type B interruption (between the carotid and the subclavian arteries), the ascending aorta travels superiorly (or cranially) and does not arch back posteriorly. The subclavian artery is usually seen arising from the descending aorta just past the ductal insertion. It is easy to mistake the ductal arch for an aortic arch. Therefore, care must be taken to confirm that head and neck vessels arise from the arch before identifying it as the aortic arch versus the ductal arch. Arch sidedness may be assessed by angling superiorly from the three-vessel view. If the ductal and/or aortic arch connects to the descending aorta to the right of the spine, it is a right aortic arch. Arch-sidedness abnormalities, arch vessel anomalies, and the absence of thymic tissue should heighten suspicion for deletion of chromosome 22q11.

It is important to obtain serial fetal cardiology evaluations throughout the pregnancy because LVOT obstruction can be progressive over time. Parental counseling should include a discussion of possible genetic syndromes, including 22q11 deletion. Chorionic villous sampling or amniocentesis is recommended and important because an associated genetic syndrome can alter the prognosis of these cardiac defects. If there is ductal-dependent circulation, plans must be made to deliver in a center that can administer prostaglandin at birth to maintain ductal patency until a definitive neonatal surgical intervention can be made.

The essential question in PMVSD and arch obstruction is whether or not the LVOT will have the potential to accommodate a complete cardiac output across it. Hence, serial measurement of the narrowest portion of the LVOT in the long-axis view of the heart is important. Currently, there are no specific guidelines for measurements at different gestational ages that can predict one way or the other for adequacy or inadequacy of the size of the LVOT. Nevertheless, we have found that at our center, full-term neonates of at least 3 kg will do well with closure of VSD and arch repair if they have a measured LVOT of at least 4 mm in diameter. We have extrapolated from this experience to say that the fetus diagnosed in the second trimester with LVOT measuring at least 3 mm will likely have a bit more growth and have an adequate-sized LVOT at birth. Conversely, the presence of an LVOT measured in the third trimester that is less than 3 mm in diameter may reflect an inadequate LVOT for which an alternate surgical strategy beyond VSD closure and arch repair should be employed (see later).

Postnatal Physiology

For a PMVSD, the postnatal physiology depends on the degree of malalignment and LVOT obstruction. Mild posterior malalignment usually does not produce significant outflow tract obstruction in the neonatal period. The neonate undergoes the normal circulatory changes associated with birth and the PMVSD has the physiology of a left-to-right shunt with increased pulmonary blood flow once the pulmonary vascular resistance decreases.

Severe outflow tract obstruction and hypoplasia of the aortic valve is usually associated with aortic arch obstruction. In IAA, perfusion of the descending aorta is dependent on the ductus arteriosus. In the presence of a large VSD, pulmonary artery pressure reaches systemic levels. The combination of aortic arch obstruction and subvalvar and/or aortic valve obstruction imposes a high afterload on the LV. Therefore, a left-to-right shunt develops at the VSD communication as blood takes the pathway of least resistance through the VSD into the pulmonary circulation. The volume load from the left-to-right shunt in combination with pressure load on the LV results in the early development of heart failure, despite adequate lower body perfusion from the ductus arteriosus. Lower body (postductal) oxygen content and saturation may be only slightly lower than upper body (preductal) saturation because of the significant intracardiac left-to-right shunt.

In the ensuing hours to several days, as the ductus arteriosus constricts, pulmonary vascular resistance decreases and there is preferential flow through the communication to the pulmonary circulation versus the lower body. Increased pulmonary venous return elevates left atrial pressure and severe heart failure develops with respiratory distress and hepatomegaly. In addition, ductal constriction reduces blood flow to the lower body. Reduced systemic oxygen delivery results in metabolic acidosis. End-organ damage such as renal and liver failure ensues. Without medical and surgical intervention, newborns with PMVSD and IAA do not survive beyond the first few weeks of life.

Postnatal Management

If serial prenatal imaging demonstrates significant LVOT obstruction or IAA, prostaglandin infusion should be administered at birth to maintain patency of the ductus arteriosus and ensure adequate systemic perfusion.

Administration of 100% oxygen may be detrimental in the setting of PMVSD and IAA. Oxygen dilates the pulmonary vascular bed and will increase the shunt into the pulmonary circulation and accelerate the development of heart failure. Increased partial pressure of oxygen (PO_2) also constricts the ductus arteriosus, which is the predominant source of systemic perfusion.

Patients with significant arch obstruction and LVOT obstruction will need surgical intervention in the neonatal period. In the recent past, the surgical approach was to repair the aortic arch and place a pulmonary artery band to limit pulmonary blood flow from the PMVSD in the neonatal period and repair the VSD later in life. Early experience with single-stage repair that included aortic arch repair and VSD closure in the neonatal period resulted in up to a 65% early mortality rate.[9] In the current era with improved prenatal diagnosis and perioperative management, one-stage repair of VSD closure and repair of the arch has become the standard of care in most large centers, with excellent outcomes.

LVOT obstruction clearly complicates the repair and is a risk factor in early mortality. There are risks to relieving subaortic obstruction with muscle or infundibular resection and patients can have significant morbidity and mortality from postoperative residual LVOT obstruction. Preoperative echocardiographic measurements including absolute subaortic diameter, subaortic diameter Z-score, subaortic diameter indexed to body surface area, and LVOT cross-sectional area have all been shown to be predictors of postoperative LVOT obstruction. Problems in reliability and reproducibility have made it absolutely difficult to predict outcomes using these measurements.[10,11]

Newborns assessed as having critically small LVOTs that will not accommodate a normal cardiac output but yet have normal-sized LV undergo an alternate strategy. Utilizing the VSD as a newly created LVOT, one can close the VSD through an interventricular baffle to the pulmonary artery, anastomose the pulmonary artery to the aorta, reconstruct and repair the arch, and place a conduit from the RV to the branch pulmonary arteries. Although this approach demands further surgery because future conduit replacement will be required, results are quite satisfactory.[12]

Outcomes

In one single-center study, 119 consecutive patients were included with IAA.[13] Of the 30 patients in the later birth cohort, 5-year survival was 83%. Freedom from re-intervention on the aortic arch was 60% at 5 years.[13] In a multi-institutional study including over 450 neonates who underwent repair of IAA, 16-year survival was 59% with improving outcomes in patients born in the later cohort. Risk factors for death include lower birth weight, younger age at repair, type B IAA, smaller size of the VSD, and the presence of subaortic narrowing. Procedural risk factors included failure to address LVOT obstruction at the time of repair and use of subaortic muscle resection to address subaortic narrowing. After 16 years, 28% underwent re-interventions for recurrent aortic arch obstruction. Thirty-four percent had undergone an initial LVOT procedure as part of the IAA repair. Among this subgroup, after 16 years, 37% had died and 28% had undergone a second procedure.[14] Other studies have reported lower morbidity and mortality (13%) in the subgroup undergoing subaortic resection at birth with more favorable outcome.[15] Genetic abnormalities can adversely affect prognosis.

Imaging Essentials and Important Points

- Assess the LVOT in the four-chamber view angled anteriorly to view the VSD and the degree of posterior malalignment of the conal septum into the LVOT.
- Assess the LVOT in the long-axis view of the heart with measurements made of the narrowest part of the subaortic region as well as the aortic annulus. A measurement of 3 mm or greater in the third trimester suggests that the LVOT may be sufficient for a surgical strategy that will consist of VSD closure and arch repair.
- Compare the diameter of the aortic valve to the pulmonary valve to obtain a sense of the degree of aortic valve hypoplasia. A ratio of less than 0.5 between aortic and pulmonic valve indicates aortic hypoplasia. A small aortic annulus in this manner further suggests the possibility of an inadequate LVOT.
- There are no definitive data on prenatal cut-off values for adequacy of the size of the LVOT; hence, counseling of families at initial diagnosis can be difficult. It is our habit to inform families of the possibility of the need for a more complicated postnatal surgical strategy, if the LVOT measures less than 4 mm in the third trimester.
- Investigate the direction of shunt across the VSD.
- Search for any additional VSDs.
- Assess for the aortic valve leaflet morphology.
- Two-dimensional assessment of ascending aorta, aortic arch, and isthmus, including diameter measurements, arch sidedness, and branching abnormalities should be performed.
- Doppler assessment of aortic arch, noting continuous or turbulent flow in the aorta indicative of obstruction.
- Evaluate for other levels of left-sided obstruction, including the anatomy and size of the mitral valve as well as size of the LV.
- Note the presence or absence of thymus.

References

1. Freedom RM, Bain HH, Esplugas E, Dische R, Rowe RD. Ventricular septal defect in interruption of aortic arch. *Am J Cardiol.* 1977;39: 572-582.
2. Celoria GC, Patton RB. Congenital absence of the aortic arch. *Am Heart J.* 1959;58:407-413.
3. Braunlin E, Peoples WM, Freedom RM, Fyler DC, Goldblatt A, Edwards JE. Interruption of the aortic arch with aorticopulmonary septal defect. An anatomic review. *Pediatr Cardiol.* 1982;3:329-335.
4. Goldmuntz E, Clark BJ, Mitchell LE, et al. Frequency of 22q11 deletions in patients with conotruncal defects. *J Am Coll Cardiol.* 1998;32:492-498.
5. Kreutzer J, Van Praagh R. Comparison of left ventricular outflow tract obstruction in interruption of the aortic arch and in coarctation of the aorta, with diagnostic, developmental, and surgical implications. *Am J Cardiol.* 2000;86:856-862.
6. Kitchiner D, Jackson M, Malaiya N, et al. Morphology of left ventricular outflow tract structures in patients with subaortic stenosis and a ventricular septal defect. *Br Heart J.* 1994;72:251-260.
7. Van Praagh R, Bernhard WF, Rosenthal A, Parisi LF, Fyler DC. Interrupted aortic arch: surgical treatment. *Am J Cardiol.* 1971;27: 200-211.
8. Chin AJ, Jacobs ML. Morphology of the ventricular septal defect in two types of interrupted aortic arch. *J Am Soc Echocardiogr.* 1996;9: 199-201.
9. Menahem S, Rahayoe AU, Brawn WJ, Mee RB. Interrupted aortic arch in infancy: a 10-year experience. *Pediatr Cardiol.* 1992;13: 214-221.
10. Apfel HD, Levenbraun J, Quaegebeur JM, Allan LD. Usefulness of preoperative echocardiography in predicting left ventricular outflow obstruction after primary repair of interrupted aortic arch with ventricular septal defect. *Am J Cardiol.* 1998;82:470-473.
11. Geva T, Hornberger LK, Sanders SP, Jonas RA, Ott DA, Colan SD. Echocardiographic predictors of left ventricular outflow tract obstruction after repair of interrupted aortic arch. *J Am Coll Cardiol.* 1993;22:1953-1960.
12. Gruber PJ, Fuller S, Cleaver KM, et al. Early results of single-stage biventricular repair of severe aortic hypoplasia or atresia with ventricular septal defect and normal left ventricle. *J Thorac Cardiovasc Surg.* 2006;132:260-263.
13. Oosterhof T, Azakie A, Freedom RM, Williams WG, McCrindle BW. Associated factors and trends in outcomes of interrupted aortic arch. *Ann Thorac Surg.* 2004;78:1696-1702.
14. McCrindle BW, Tchervenkov CI, Konstantinov IE, et al. Risk factors associated with mortality and interventions in 472 neonates with interrupted aortic arch: a Congenital Heart Surgeons Society study. *J Thorac Cardiovasc Surg.* 2005;129:343-350.
15. Suzuki T, Ohye RG, Devaney EJ, et al. Selective management of the left ventricular outflow tract for repair of interrupted aortic arch with ventricular septal defect: management of left ventricular outflow tract obstruction. *J Thorac Cardiovasc Surg.* 2006;131: 779-784.

CASES

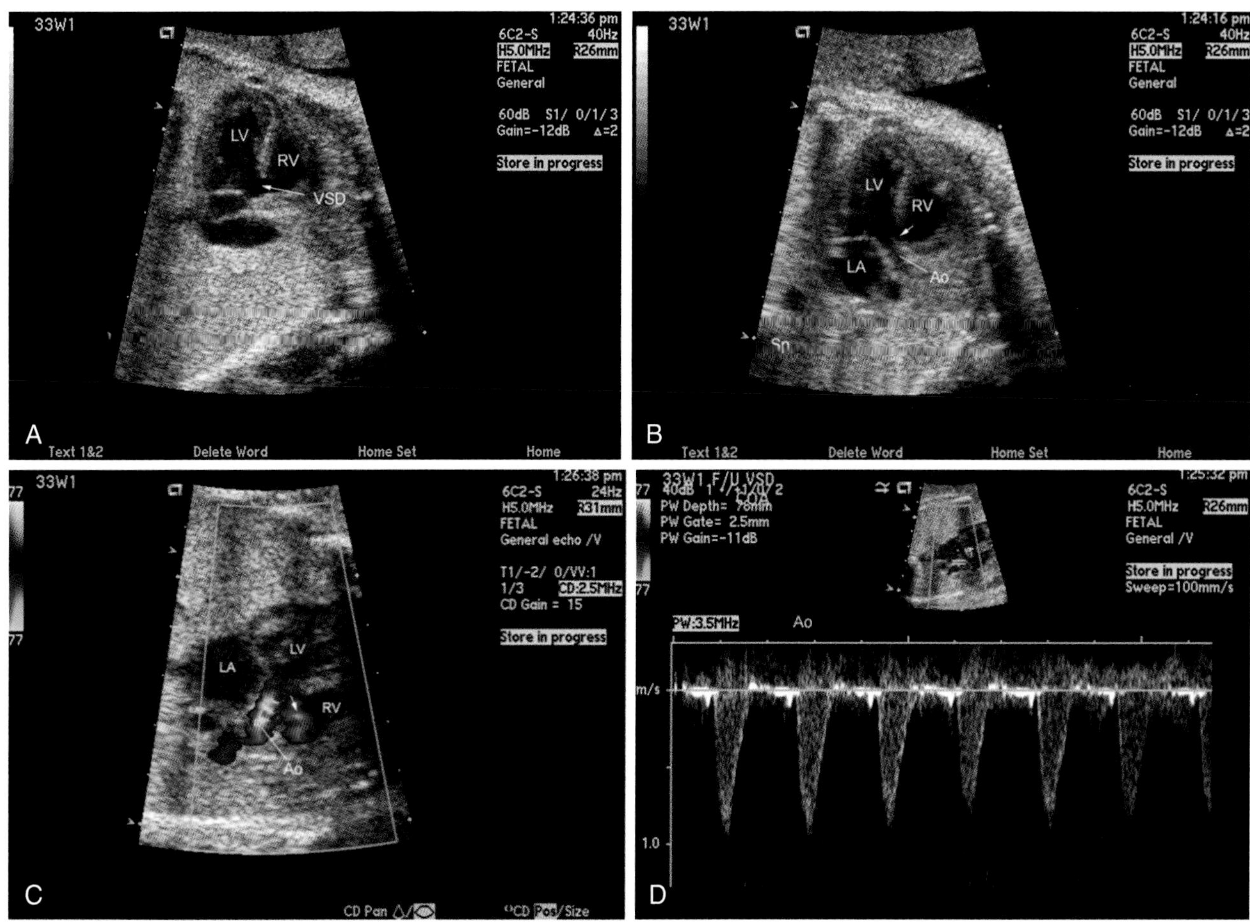

Case 13-1. (A) Apical view demonstrates the left (LV) and right (RV) ventricles and the presence of a large ventricular septal defect (VSD). In this view, the conal septum is not visualized, hence, this VSD cannot be confidently distinguished between a conoventricular or a malalignment type. (B) Anterior angulation toward the left ventricular outflow tract demonstrates the borders of the VSD *(arrow)* and the deviation of the conal septum leftward and posteriorly. Ao, aorta; LA, left atrium; Sp, spine. (C) Color flow demonstrates flow across the narrowed left ventricular outflow tract into the ascending aorta and flow across the VSD from left to right. (D) Although there is narrowing of the subaortic region due to conal deviation, Doppler flow in the Ao remains laminar because the volume of flow across this region is difficult to predict in the face of a large VSD with large left-to-right flow across it. *Continued*

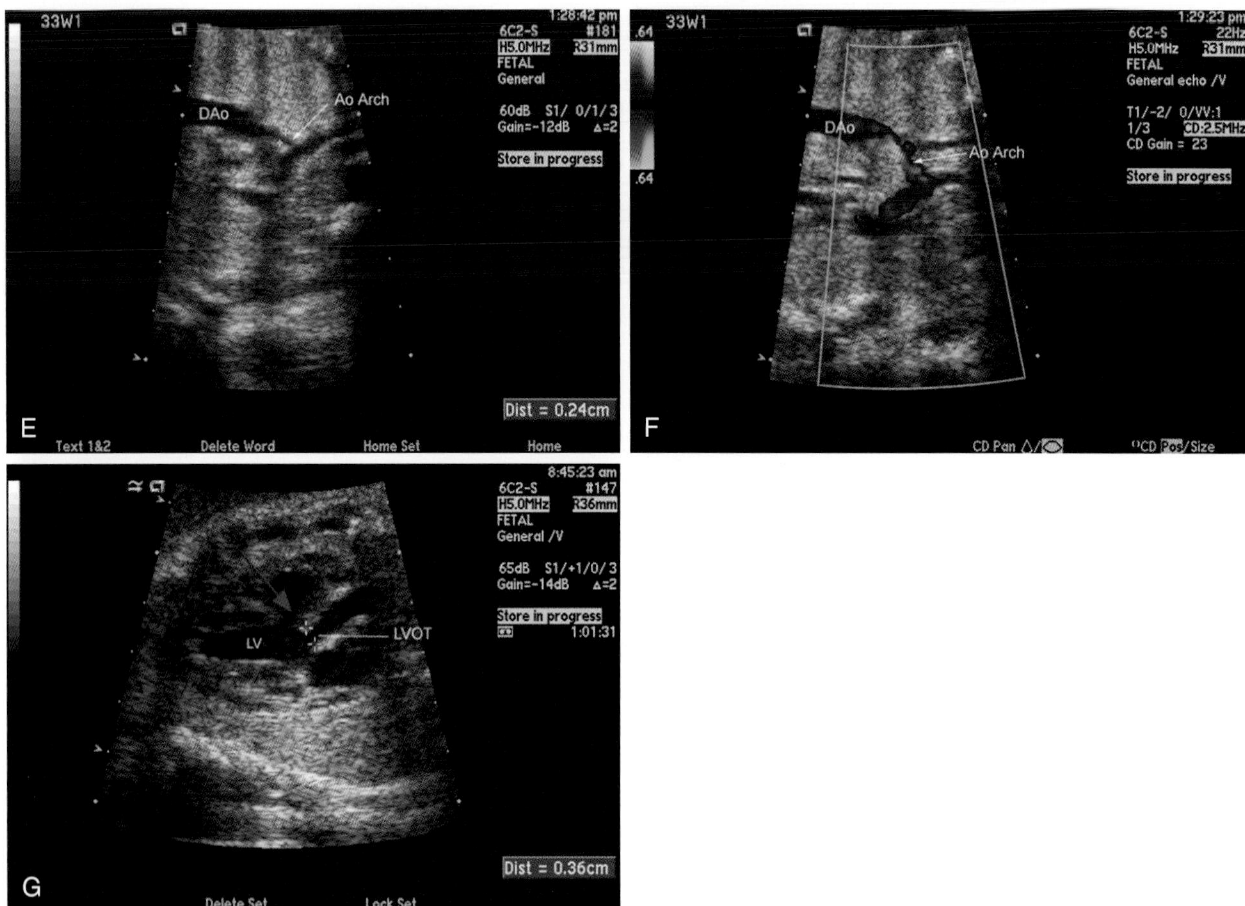

Case 13-1, cont'd **(E)** As is commonly associated with the posterior conal malalignment type of VSD, this fetus at 33 weeks demonstrates marked aortic isthmul hypoplasia and coarctation of the Ao. DAo, descending aorta. **(F)** There is antegrade flow present across this arch, which has both an element of transverse arch hypoplasia and a coarctation of the Ao. **(G)** Long-axis view is one of the most important in this anomaly in order to assess the degree of posterior conal deviation and the limiting dimensions for forward flow into the Ao. Note that at 33 weeks, this fetus has a narrowest narrow subaortic left ventricular outflow tract (LVOT) diameter of 3 to 4 mm *(red arrow)*, which is considered the lower limit of acceptability for adequacy to allow for a full complement of cardiac output after birth.

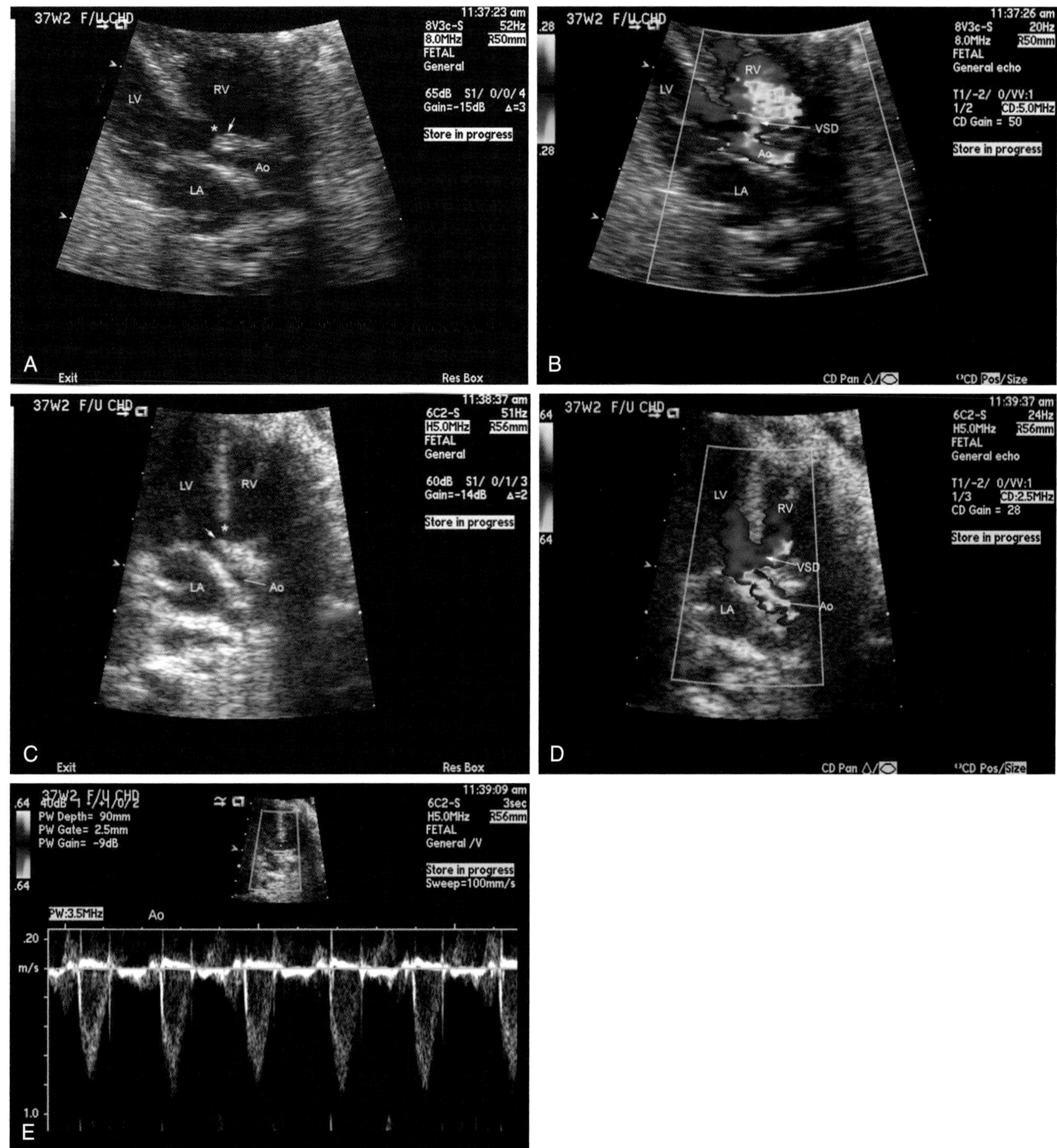

Case 13-2. **(A)** Long-axis view of the same fetus as in Case 13-1, but now evaluated 4 weeks later at 37 weeks' gestation. Note the increased thickness in the conal septum *(arrow)*, and the left ventricular outflow tract (LVOT) measures 2 to 3 mm in diameter. This suggests a high likelihood of inability to use the native LVOT as part of the repair. Hence, either enlargement of the region via conal resection, enlargement of the entire outflow tract and aortic annulus via a Konno procedure, or utilization of the ventricular septal defect (VSD) as part of a "new" LVOT by baffling the VSD to the pulmonary valve and performance of a "pulmonary artery–to–aorta (Ao) anastomosis" with right ventricle (RV)–to–pulmonary artery conduit (Yasui repair) should be considered. LA, left atrium; LV, left ventricle. **(B)** Long-axis view with color reveals antegrade flow into a narrowed subaortic region and flow left to right across the malalignment type of VSD. **(C)** Apical view with anterior angulation demonstrates the normal-sized LV and mitral valve, but a narrowed subaortic region due to conal leftward deviation *(arrow)*. **(D)** Color flow demonstrates antegrade flow into the ascending Ao and left-to-right flow across the VSD. The VSD diameter is larger than the diameter of the subaortic region. **(E)** Doppler interrogation across the aortic valve with laminar flow. The presence of laminar flow across the narrowed region cannot be interpreted as predicting unobstructed flow after repair, because currently in the presence of a large VSD, much blood is shunted away from the narrowed region. Dimensional measures are more reliable in predicting adequacy of the left ventricular outflow pathway, with less than 4 mm being the lower limit of adequacy. In this case, counseling to the family would include discussion about the possibility of a more complex operation than just simple VSD closure and arch repair.

14

Transposition of the Great Arteries

Michael D. Quartermain

Key Echocardiographic Features

- Presence or absence of great vessels crossing as they course just above the heart.
- Relationship of the great vessels to each other as they arise from the heart.
- Relative size of the great vessels—is the pulmonary artery larger than the aorta by approximately 25%, as is expected in transposition of the great arteries?
- Presence or absence of ventricular septal defects.
- Presence or absence of left or right outflow tract obstruction.
- Presence or absence of semilunar valve stenosis.
- Presence or absence of a patent ductus arteriosus with shunting from the pulmonary artery to the descending aorta.
- Ductus arteriosus is typically smaller than in normally related great vessels.
- Ductal and aortic arches appear as running parallel in their course in the superior mediastinum.
- Atrial septal defect and redundancy of the septum primum.

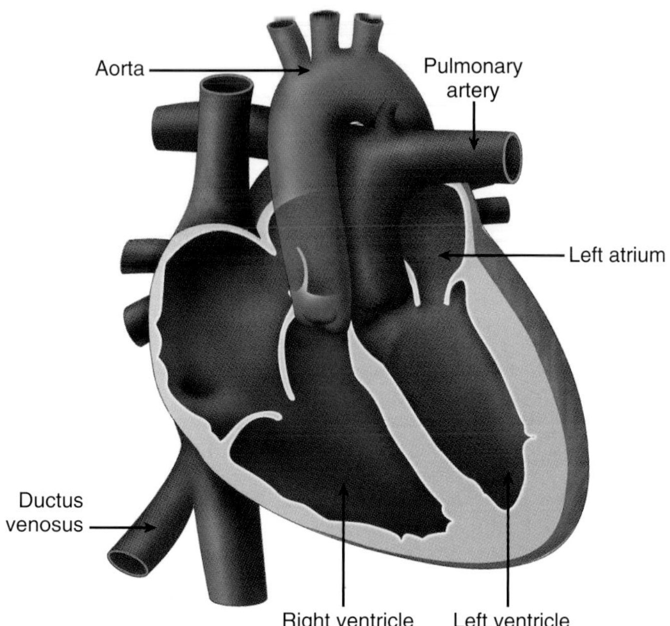

Figure 14-1. Illustration of transposition of the great arteries with the aorta arising from the right ventricle anterior and rightward to the pulmonary artery, which arises from the left ventricle.

Anatomy and Anatomical Associations

Transposition of the great arteries (TGA) is a congenital anomaly in which the aorta arises from the right ventricle and the pulmonary artery from the left ventricle, creating discordance in the ventricular-arterial relationship. In the normal heart, the aorta is posterior and rightward arising from the left ventricle and the pulmonary artery sits anterior and leftward arising from the right ventricle. In the most common form of TGA, the aorta is anterior and rightward with concordant atrioventricular relationships and normal D-looping of the ventricles. The conus is subaortic in TGA, as opposed to subpulmonic in normal, and there is fibrous continuity of the mitral and pulmonary valves in TGA, unlike fibrous continuity between the mitral and the aortic valves in the normal (Figure 14-1).[1] This common form of transposition is referred to as D-TGA and is the focus of this chapter. TGA can occur in more complex settings such as single-ventricle lesions, heterotaxy, and L-looped hearts. These complex forms of TGA are discussed in their respective chapters.

Associated lesions are common in fetuses with D-TGA and are important to identify in order to reliably predict postnatal stability and suitability for specific surgical strategies after birth. Approximately 50% of fetuses with D-TGA will have an intact ventricular septum and no associated cardiac defect other than a patent foramen ovale and a patent ductus arteriosus.

Frequency, Genetics, and Development

The incidence of D-TGA is approximately 2.5 per 10,000 live births and remains one of the more common causes of cyanotic congenital heart disease (CHD).[2] There is a strong male predominance that accounts for 60% to 70% of live D-TGA births. At this time, there is no known causative genetic abnormality associated with D-TGA Most frequently, there is a normal karyotype and extracardiac abnormalities are relatively unusual in this form of CHD.

The developmental abnormalities that lead to D-TGA remain unknown. One of the more common theories relates to abnormal embryonic development of the normal anterior and leftward subpulmonary conus. This theory suggests that abnormal resorption of the subpulmonary conus with abnormal persistence of subaortic conus leads to the migration of the great vessels to their abnormal, discordant locations. A second theory focuses on abnormal spiraling of the primitive truncus arteriosus as the cause of a rightward and anterior aorta originating from the right ventricle.

Prenatal Physiology

The hemodynamic alterations in the fetus with D-TGA are tolerated well and are compatible with excellent fetal survival rates. There is usually normal growth and development with the fetus reaching term and of generous birth weight. In the fetus with D-TGA, the patency of the foramen ovale and the ductus arteriosus allows for mixing of circulations and maintenance of adequate oxygenation and a normal cardiac output. Nonetheless, there are alterations in blood flow that have the potential to affect the fetus with D-TGA. Normally, highly oxygenated blood in the umbilical vein has preferential return from the ductus venosus directed across the foramen ovale into the left side of the heart. The left ventricle and pulmonary arteries receive blood with a relatively high oxygen concentration. As well, deoxygenated blood from the superior vena cava is preferentially directed across the tricuspid valve to the right ventricle. This pattern is a natural strategy deemed to provide the most vital organs that are normally perfused by the left ventricle—the heart and brain—with the greatest degree of oxygenated blood. In the normal fetus, the right ventricle ejects into the descending aorta via the ductus arteriosus. In D-TGA, the right ventricle ejects into the ascending aorta, supplying blood with a lower oxygen concentration to the head and neck vessels compared with a fetus with normal ventricular-arterial relationships. Animal studies in fetal lambs have demonstrated a partial pressure of oxygen (PO_2) of approximately 18 mm Hg in the ascending aorta in D-TGA, which is significantly less than the values of 25 to 28 mm Hg seen in normal fetuses.[3] The full extent of these alterations is not fully understood in the human fetus; however, it is safe to assume that cerebral oxygenation in the human fetus with TGA may not be normal.

Prenatal Management

TGA is commonly missed on prenatal scanning. The four-chamber view will appear normal and the diagnosis of this critical heart defect requires inspection of the great vessels arising from the heart. Training and experience of obstetricians and perinatologists who perform imaging will increase the diagnosis and improve outcome. Normally related great vessels will cross in space as scanning of the heart moves cephalad and superiorly—the larger pulmonary artery will be seen arising from the right ventricle and crossing over the more posterior aorta arising from the left ventricle. The appreciation of this relationship takes time; however, it should be performed in every fetus that presents for evaluation. In D-TGA, the great vessels arise from the heart in parallel and do not cross.

When the diagnosis of D-TGA is made in a fetus, it is important to identify the presence of associated intracardiac anomalies. Similar to other forms of CHD, there is an indication for analysis of the fetal chromosomes and an obstetrical ultrasound to evaluate for extracardiac anomalies. This allows the caretaker to accurately counsel families in regard to potential suitability for an arterial switch operation, the optimal postnatal treatment, and provide information regarding outcomes and survival rates. It is important to mention the potential need for postnatal balloon atrial septostomy (BAS), which is necessary in approximately 20% to 40% of neonates with D-TGA. This procedure is done in order to improve the mixing of oxygenated and deoxygenated blood at the level of the atria and improve overall arterial saturation. At our center, we serially evaluate the fetus with D-TGA every 4 weeks to monitor for restriction at the foramen ovale and ductus arteriosus. This also allows for surveillance of ventricular function and fetal growth and to document progression of any associated defects such as pulmonary stenosis or coarctation of the aorta.

The status of the foramen ovale and the ductus arteriosus are two key structures that predict postnatal stability. Restriction at either structure will limit mixing between the circulations and put the fetus at risk for hemodynamic compromise and severe hypoxemia after separation from the placenta. Careful evaluation of the atrial septum and ductus arteriosus should be performed in every fetus with D-TGA.[4]

Predicting the need for urgent postnatal BAS based on prenatal data, however, is very challenging. In the fetus, the flap of the foramen ovale will almost always bow right to left into the left atrium; however, with birth and an increase in pulmonary venous return, left atrial pressure rises and the flap of the foramen ovale may close, causing impaired atrial level mixing and severe hypoxemia. In order to attempt to predict *postnatal* atrial level restriction based on *prenatal* atrial findings, we have developed an index that describes the degree of redundancy of the atrial septum, with the theory being that the greater the atrial redundancy, the less likely it will become restrictive once left atrial pressures rise after birth. The atrial septal excursion ratio (ASE ratio) is obtained in the four-chamber view. It is a measure of the ratio of the maximum excursion of the flap of the foramen ovale leftward toward the free wall of the left atrium from the anchored portion of the septum divided by the diameter of the left atrium from septum to free wall (Figure 14-2). The greater this ratio, the less likely there should be a need for urgent BAS. In a recent review, we found that no fetus with a ratio greater than 0.5 required urgent BAS at birth (unpublished data).

Assessment of the ductus arteriosus involves direct inspection and Doppler flow interrogation. In D-TGA, the ductus arteriosus is typically smaller than normal. Whereas in normal, the ductus arteriosus carries blood from the dominant right ventricle through the pulmonary artery to the descending aorta, in D-TGA, it is carrying a smaller quantity of blood from the left ventricle through the pulmonary artery to the descending aorta. Furthermore, it has been proposed that, as the left ventricle is receiving a higher degree of oxygenated blood that is then ejected into the pulmonary artery, the ductus arteriosus is witnessing a higher than normal degree of oxygenated blood, which may cause ductal constriction. This may pose a serious problem, in particular during the third trimester, when ductal sensitivity to higher levels of oxygenation may increase because the fetus is closer to term.[5] Ductal constriction, even mild, may lead to

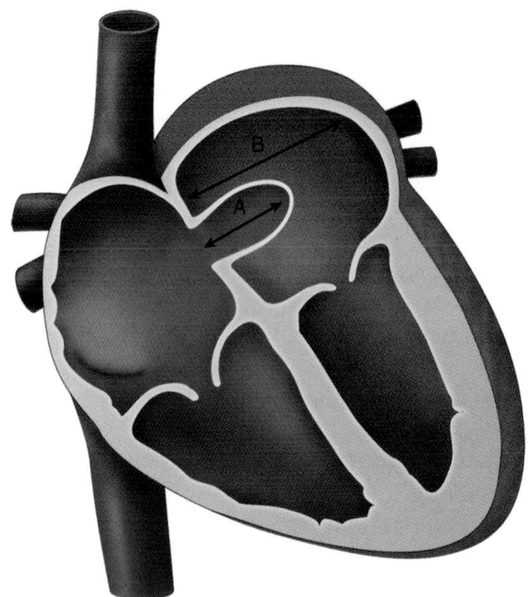

Figure 14-2. Calculation of the atrial septal excursion (ASE) ratio, an estimate of atrial septal redundancy that may help predict postnatal atrial restriction in transposition of the great arteries and the need for urgent postnatal balloon atrial septostomy. ASE ratio = a/b, where a is the maximal excursion length of septum primum and b is the left atrial diameter, both obtained in the four-chamber view in the same plane.

alterations in flow patterns to the lung with an increase in blood volume and an increase in the level of oxygenation of blood delivered to the developing pulmonary vasculature relative to normal. This may explain why there is an increased likelihood of developing pulmonary hypertension in D-TGA because the pulmonary vasculature may be different than normal. Visual inspection of flow on color Doppler across the ductus arteriosus as well as assessment of ductal pulsatility index on pulse wave imaging are important. In our view, the pulsatility index of the ductus arteriosus should in general be higher than 1.8. Hence, an ASE ratio of less than 0.5 or a ductal pulsatility index of less than 1.8 raises suspicion of the likelihood for marked hypoxemia at birth. It should be noted that these are general guidelines used at our center to help aid in predicting those with D-TGA most in need for urgent postnatal care, but these criteria have not yet been rigorously or prospectively evaluated to date.

Does a prenatal diagnosis of D-TGA make a difference? Investigators compared 250 newborns with a postnatal diagnosis of D-TGA to 68 fetuses diagnosed prenatally. There were statistically significant differences in multiple outcomes including age at admission, need for mechanical ventilation, preoperative metabolic acidosis, preoperative and postoperative mortality that were all worse in the postnatally diagnosed group.[6] Unlike many other forms of complex CHD, D-TGA is fairly unique because there is potential for hemodynamic compromise and need for urgent intervention immediately at birth. Therefore, in all fetuses diagnosed with D-TGA, a planned delivery at a referral center with neonatal and cardiology specialists is the optimal form of care. This allows for a controlled delivery and rapid transfer of the neonate to the intensive care unit for assessment of oxygenation, initiation of prostaglandin infusion, and confirmation of the diagnosis by transthoracic echocardiography.

Postnatal Physiology

In transposition physiology at birth, there can be severe hypoxemia and profound cyanosis because the pulmonary artery saturation is greater than the aortic saturation. The pulmonary and systemic circulations run in *parallel* rather than in *series*. Systemic venous blood returns to the right atrium and transverses the tricuspid valve to enter the right ventricle and finally is ejected in the aorta. Pulmonary venous blood returns to the left atrium, crosses the mitral valve, and is ejected by the left ventricle to the pulmonary artery.

As the fetus is separated from the placenta, the lungs take over the role of oxygenation. It is imperative that normal lung function is present and that oxygenated blood returning to the heart must have unobstructed access to the systemic circulation. In D-TGA, this can occur only through persistence of fetal channels (patent foramen ovale or patent ductus arteriosus) or through a ventricular septal defect (VSD) if present. If the normal separation of the left and right sides of the heart by closure of the foramen ovale or closure of the ductus arteriosus occurs in the fetus with D-TGA, severe hypoxemia and metabolic acidosis will result.

After separation from the placenta, the main physiological abnormality is a deficiency of oxygen supply to the tissues. The postnatal circulation and the degree of cyanosis depend on the status of the foramen ovale and ductus arteriosus in combination with associated abnormalities such as a VSD or pulmonary stenosis.

The neonate with D-TGA and a VSD will have increased volume of mixing with shunting into the pulmonary circulation. This will allow for higher arterial saturations but can lead to unrestrictive pulmonary blood flow and heart failure if not recognized in the newborn period. The presence of severe pulmonary stenosis in the neonate with D-TGA is usually seen in association with a VSD. This form of left ventricular outflow obstruction leads to shunting across the VSD from the left to the right ventricle. Pulmonary blood flow is usually maintained by the patent ductus arteriosus. The systemic arterial saturation in these fetuses is reduced but usually not to the point of severe cyanosis and metabolic acidosis.

Postnatal Management

As previously stated, fetuses with D-TGA require delivery at a medical center equipped with the facilities and staff to handle the potential dramatic hemodynamic changes after separation from the placenta. After delivery, umbilical lines are placed with initiation of prostaglandin infusion in order to maintain ductal patency. Aggressive correction of metabolic acidosis, hypoglycemia, and electrolyte abnormalities is important. A complete transthoracic echocardiogram is performed when the neonate is clinically stable to allow for confirmation of the prenatal diagnosis and identification of any associated anomalies and to document patency of the foramen ovale and ductus arteriosus and direction of shunting.

Neonates with inadequate mixing of systemic and pulmonary circulations experience severe hypoxemia and metabolic acidosis. These will often require mechanical ventilation with sedation, paralysis, and inotropic support for stabilization. Neonates with severe hypoxemia and restrictive atrial septum require urgent BAS. In this procedure first described by Dr. William Rashkind, a balloon-tipped catheter is advanced from the femoral or umbilical vein through the inferior vena cava and right atrium and across the foramen ovale. The balloon is inflated in the left atrium and rapidly pulled across the atrial septum. The rupture of septum primum creates a larger atrial communication, improves mixing from left atrium to right, and increases the arterial saturation.[7] The septostomy can be performed in the intensive care unit under the guidance of echocardiography or in the catheterization laboratory. After successful BAS, prostaglandin infusion can often be discontinued and the neonate extubated from mechanical ventilation to await surgical intervention.

Surgical repair of D-TGA will usually occur in the first 2 weeks of life while the left ventricle is still naturally prepared to undertake the task of systemic perfusion. Definitive neonatal repair is the preferred option and has been possible since the arterial switch procedure was first reported in 1975 by Jatene and coworkers.[8] In this procedure, the great vessels are transected and the pulmonary artery is brought anterior and the aorta posterior. The great vessels are then reanastomosed to the appropriate ventricle, pulmonary artery to right ventricle and aorta to left ventricle. The coronary arteries are transferred as buttons from the native aorta to the native pulmonary artery (neo-aorta) (Figure 14-3). This allows for near "anatomic correction" with the return of the great arteries to their normal anterior-posterior positions.

In the fetus with D-TGA with VSD, the surgery is not as urgent but should be performed in the first 1 to 2 months of life before the development of pulmonary vascular disease. In the presence of D-TGA with VSD and left ventricular outflow tract obstruction, the Rastelli procedure remains a viable option if the native pulmonary valve is not suitable in the neo-aortic position. This procedure is accomplished by closing the VSD to the aorta and placement of a right ventricle–to–pulmonary artery conduit.[9]

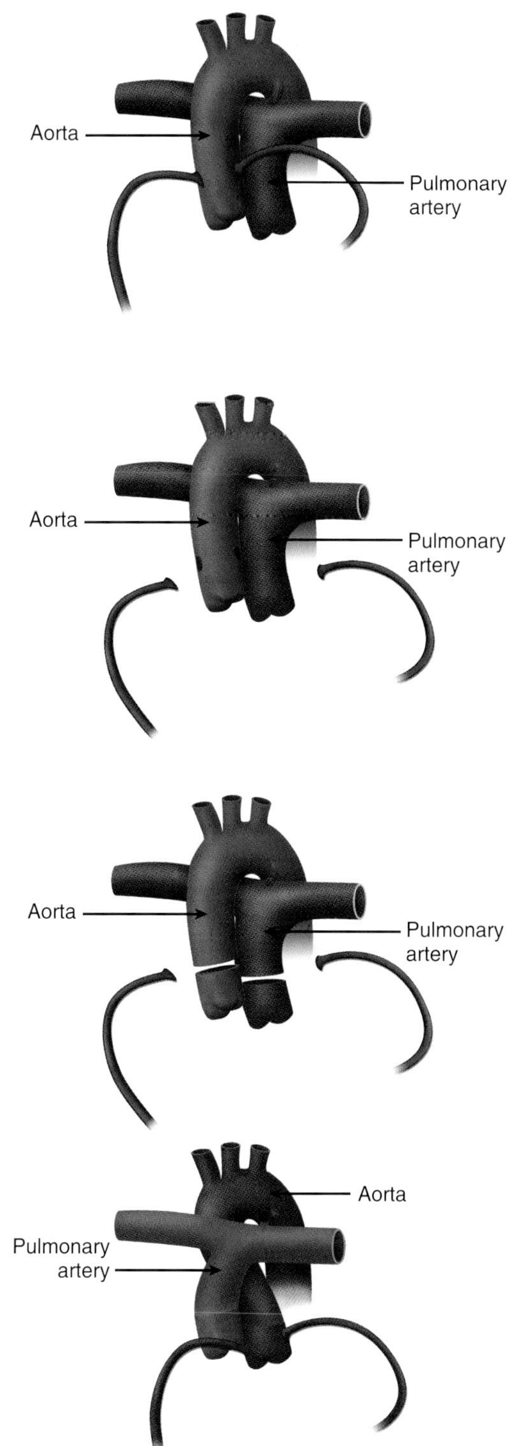

Figure 14-3. Coronary translocation in the arterial switch operation. The great vessels are transected and the coronary arteries are removed as "buttons" of tissue from the aorta. The great vessels are reconnected with the pulmonary artery to the native aortic root and the aorta to the native pulmonary artery root with translocation of the coronary arteries to the aorta. Note that the position of the proximal branch pulmonary arteries is now anterior to and drapes over the aorta.

Outcomes

The natural history of untreated D-TGA is dismal—50% of infants will die within 1 month and 90% by 1 year of life if left untreated.[10] Surgical repair with the arterial switch operation has excellent results.[11] Current statistics from experienced centers report less than 5% mortality for the arterial switch procedure for D-TGA. Risk factors include prematurity, genetic abnormalities, associated cardiac lesions, and late repair (>2 wk of life). Short-term complications are usually due to obstruction of the coronary arteries after translocation or significant bleeding from suture lines. The most common intermediate-term complication is development of supravalvar pulmonary stenosis because the pulmonary arteries are draped in front of the aorta during the arterial switch procedure. This is often amenable to balloon dilation in the catheterization laboratory. Another finding late after the arterial switch is neo-aortic (native pulmonary valve) dilation and regurgitation. The neo-aortic root has been shown to dilate and mild neo-aortic insufficiency is common but progression to moderate or severe is rare.[12] Exercise testing has demonstrated preserved cardiopulmonary function after the arterial switch operation[13] and significant arrhythmias are rare.[14] Most commonly, these children have excellent quality of life with normal school and activity levels. As our oldest patients who have undergone successful arterial switch operation begin to reach their third and fourth decades of life, questions will arise as to the competence of the coronary artery circulation. The impact of neonatal surgical manipulation of the coronary arteries on the development of atherosclerotic coronary artery disease is yet unknown but will become evident in the coming years.

Imaging Essentials and Important Points

- TGA is very commonly missed during the prenatal assessment. Practice and comfort in assessing the crossing relationship of normally related great vessels is important before one can identify the abnormal absence of crossing vessels. Parallel emergence of the pulmonary artery and aorta from the fetal heart with absence of crossing in space and side-by-side great vessels strongly suggests a conotruncal anomaly, which most likely will be D-TGA.
- Look for associated anomalies such as VSD and left ventricular outflow tract obstruction.
- Assess the relative size of the right and left ventricle to each other because ventricular hypoplasia can be seen in TGA.
- Inspect the septum with special attention to the conal septum. The conal septum may be malaligned in the presence of TGA. With posterior malalignment, there will be pulmonary stenosis; with anterior malalignment, there will be subaortic stenosis and the potential for arch obstruction such as coarctation of the aorta.
- Inspect the atrial septum. Assessment of the degree of atrial septal redundancy via the ASE ratio may help in predicting postnatal restriction and the need for urgent BAS. An ASE ratio of less than 0.5 should raise suspicion for possible atrial level restriction and may predict the need for urgent BAS.
- Inspect the ductus arteriosus for color flow across and measure the pulsatility index via Doppler echocardiography. A low pulsatility index (<1.8) suggests restriction and should raise suspicion for possibility of postnatal hypoxemia and development of pulmonary hypertension.
- The ductal and aortic arches often appear in parallel in the mediastinum in TGA. The aortic arch is typically positioned superiorly over the ductal arch and can appear smaller, especially in the isthmus region. This does not necessarily imply the presence of a coarctation, but is a normal expected finding in TGA.
- Coronary anatomy plays a role in performance of the arterial switch operation. However, determining coronary anatomy in the fetus is extremely challenging and should be left for the postnatal assessment.

References

1. Van Praagh R. Transposition of the great arteries: history, pathologic anatomy, embryology, etiology and surgical considerations. *Cardiac Surg*. 1991;5:7-82.
2. Botto LD, Correa A, Erickson DJ. Racial and temporal variations in the prevalence of heart defects. *Pediatrics*. 2001;107:e32.
3. Rudolph AM. *Congenital Diseases of the Heart: Clinical-Physiological Considerations*. 2nd ed. Amonk, NY: Futura Publishing Company, 2001.
4. Rudolph AM. Aortopulmonary transposition in the fetus: speculations on pathophysiology and therapy. *Pediatr Res*. 2007;61: 375-380.
5. Maeno YV, Kamenir SA, Sinclair B, van der Velde ME, Smallhorn JF, Hornberger LK. Prenatal features of ductus arteriosus constriction and restrictive foramen ovale in D-transposition of the great arteries. *Circulation*. 1999;99:1209-1214.
6. Bonnet D, Coltri A, Butera G, et al. Detection of transposition of the great arteries in fetuses reduces neonatal morbidity and mortality. *Circulation*. 1999;99:916-918.
7. Rashkind WJ, Miller WW. Creation of an atrial septal defect without thoracotomy. A palliative approach to complete transposition of the great arteries. *JAMA*. 1996;196:991.
8. Jatene AD, Fontes VF, Paulista PP, et al. Anatomic correction of transposition of the great vessels. *J Thorac Cardiovasc Surg*. 1976; 72:364-370.

9. Rastelli GC, Wallace RB, Ongley PA. Complete repair of transposition of the great arteries with pulmonary stenosis. A review and report of a case corrected by using a new surgical technique. *Circulation*. 1969;39:83.
10. Liebman J, Cullum L, Belloc NB. Natural history of transposition of the great arteries. Anatomy and birth and death characteristics. *Circulation*. 1969;40:237.
11. Wernovsky G, Mayer JE, Jonas RA, et al. Factors influencing early and late outcome of the arterial switch operation for transposition of the great arteries. *J Thorac Cardiovasc Surg*. 1995;109:289-302.
12. Schwartz ML, Gauvreau K, del Nido P, et al. Long-term predictors of aortic root dilation and aortic regurgitation following the arterial switch operation. *Circulation*. 2004;110(suppl 2):128.
13. Mahle WT, McBride MG, Paridon SM. Exercise performance after the arterial switch operation for D-transposition of the great arteries. *Am J Cardiol*. 2001;87:753.
14. Rhodes LA, Wernovsky G, Keane JF, et al. Arrhythmias and intracardiac conduction after the arterial switch operation. *J Thorac Cardiovasc Surg*. 1995;109:303.

CASES

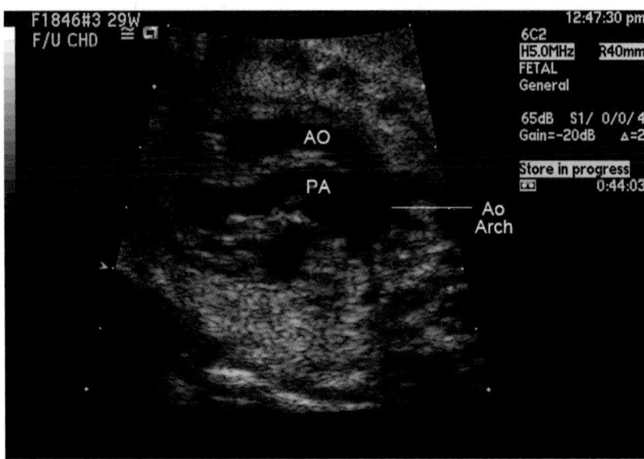

Case 14-1. Long-axis view demonstrates that both great vessels, the aorta (AO) and the pulmonary artery (PA), arise in parallel. There is no crossing of the aorta and PA above the heart. Both the left ventricular outflow tract and the right ventricular outflow tract are seen well and the aorta and PA arise in parallel and travel in parallel in the mediastinum. Although, in this view, one cannot tell whether the vessel coming off the left ventricle bifurcates, there appears to be a head vessel coming off the great vessel superiorly, suggesting that it is the aorta and that we are seeing the proximal part of the aortic arch (Ao Arch).

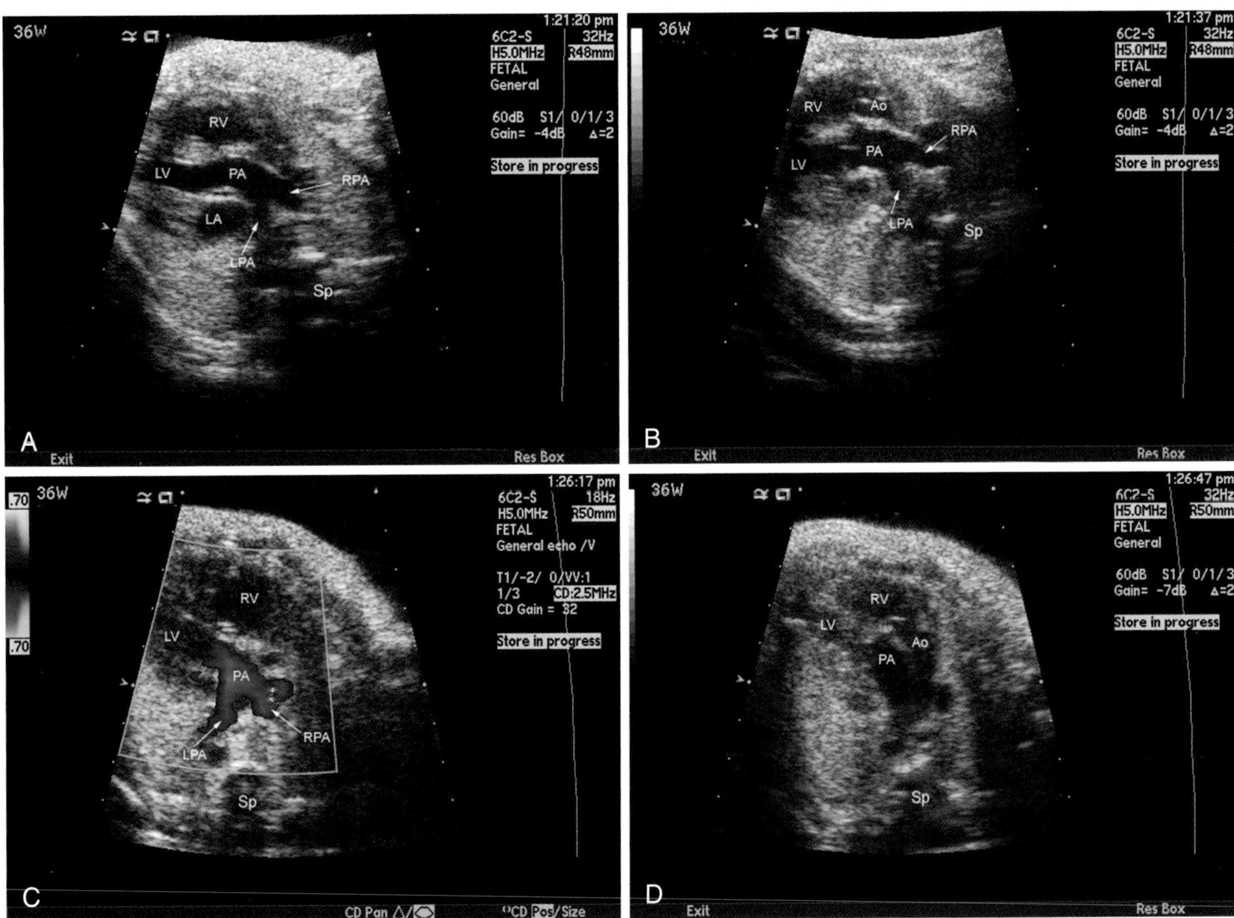

Case 14-2. **(A)** Long-axis view of the left ventricle (LV) demonstrates a great vessel arising that branches quite early in its course into the right (RPA) and left (LPA) pulmonary arteries, hence, confirming the presence of transposition of the great arteries. LA, left atrium; PA, pulmonary artery; RV, right ventricle; Sp, spine. **(B)** Further cephalad imaging reveals the presence of the two semilunar valves, the aortic (Ao) and the pulmonary; the aortic arises from the RV and the PA arises from the LV. The branching of the PAs is seen both right and left. **(C)** Imaging with color Doppler flow demonstrates that the vessel coming off the LV bifurcates early into branch pulmonary arteries (RPA and LPA); hence, the PA arises from the LV. **(D)** When looking just at the great arteries as they arise from the heart, the PA and aorta are in parallel and do not appear to cross.

Continued

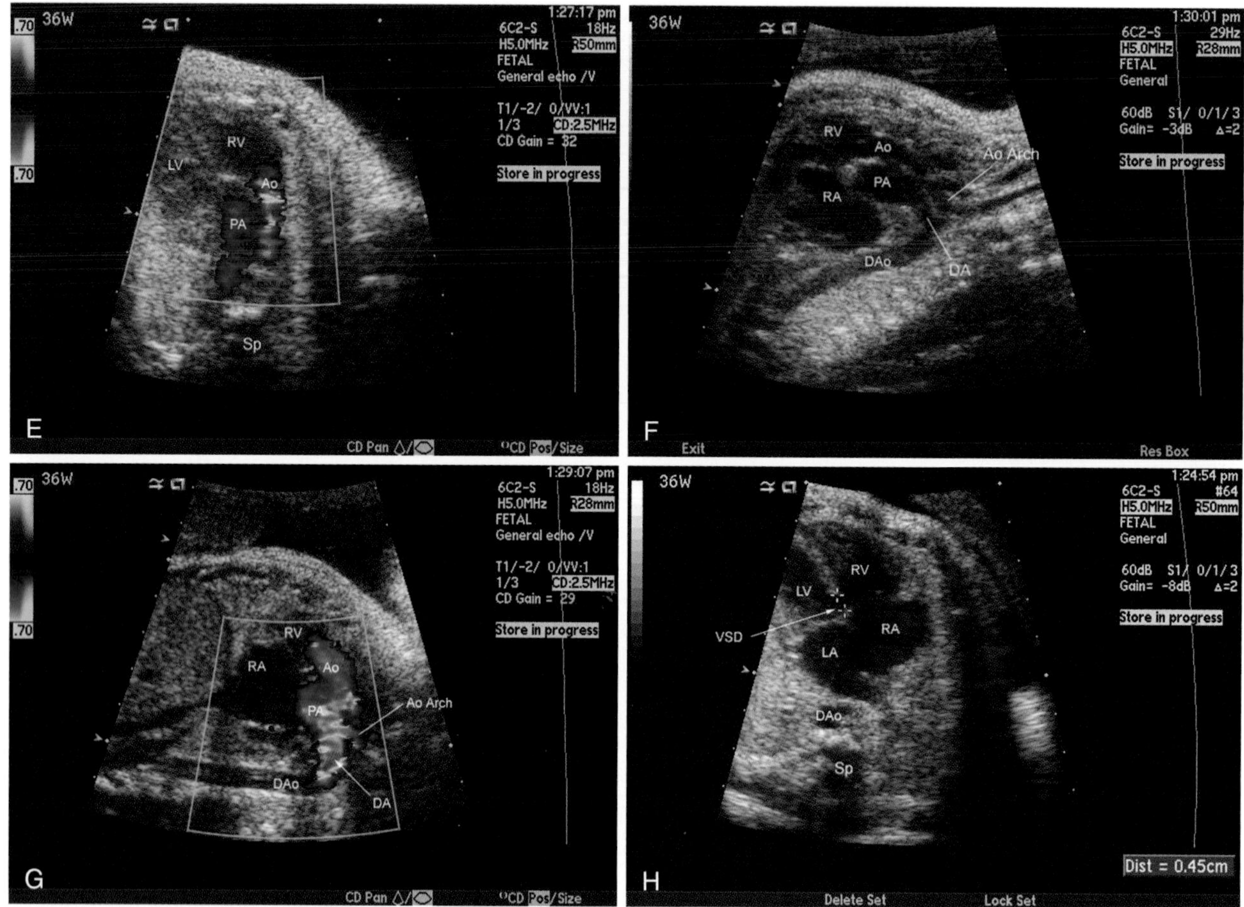

Case 14-2, cont'd **(E)** Application of color flow onto the previous image demonstrates *blue color* suggesting flow away from the transducer and the parallel position of the great vessels as they arise from the heart. **(F)** This view demonstrates the great vessels and the aortic (Ao) and ductal (DA) arches. There is an interesting relationship between the arches in the fetus with transposition of the great arteries. The aortic arch (Ao Arch) is superior and runs in parallel with the DA. It almost appears as if it is lying on top of the DA, and typically, in transposition of the great vessels, one can visualize both arches in the same plane, as seen here. Both arches connect with the descending aorta (DAo). **(G)** Color flow imaging demonstrates the Ao Arch overlying the DA. The isthmus portion of the Ao Arch sometimes appears small because it is situated just above the entry site of the ductus arteriosus into the DAo. **(H)** Demonstration of a conoventricular ventricular septal defect (VSD) in this fetus with transposition of the great arteries. Despite the presence of this VSD, one should consider starting prostaglandin infusion at birth to allow for maximal exchange of blood between the two circulations, in order to optimize oxygenation at birth.

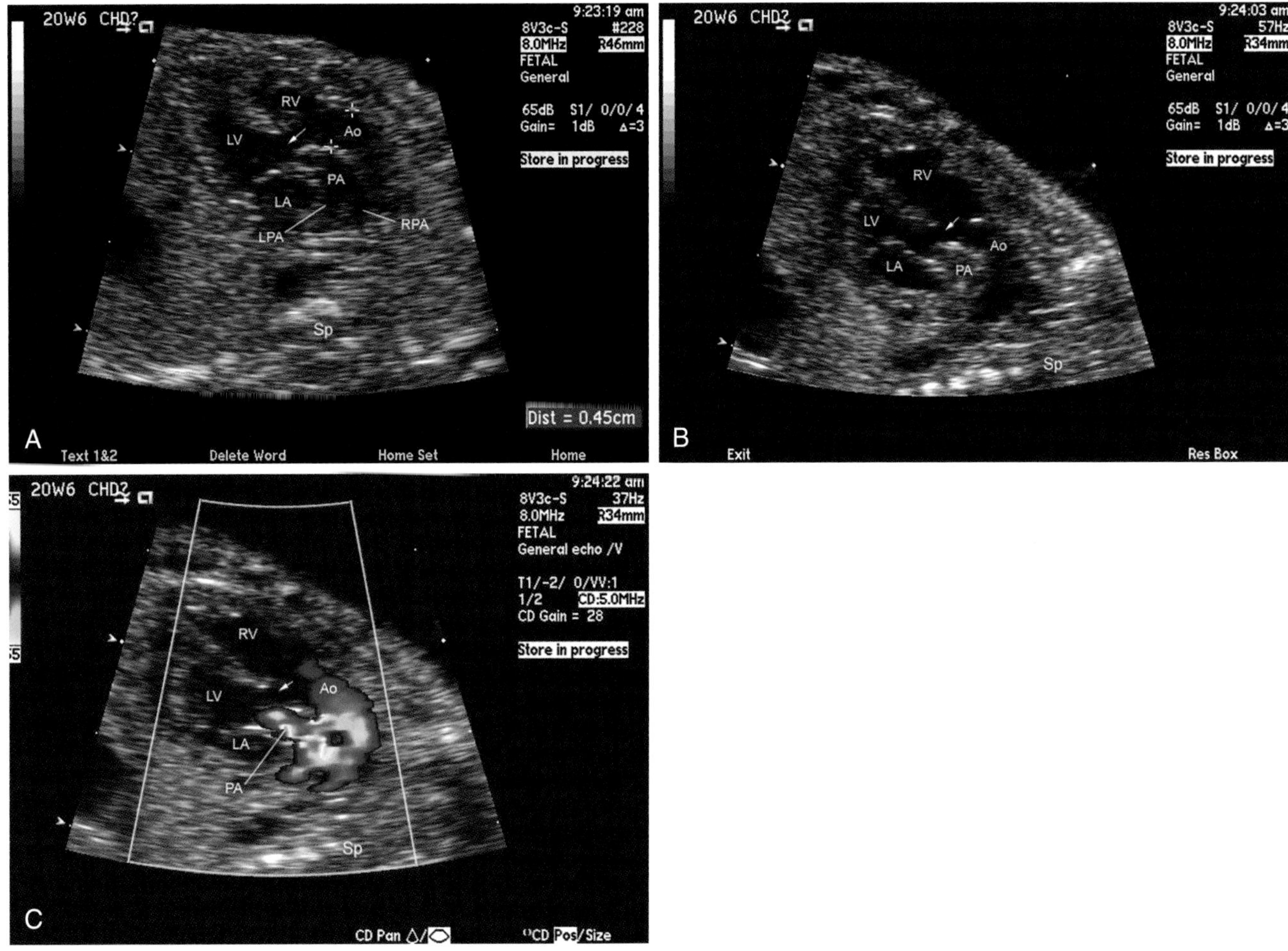

Case 14-3. **(A)** A fetus with transposition of the great arteries and posterior malalignment of the infundibular septum causing subpulmonary stenosis and left ventricular outflow tract obstruction. The *arrow* points to the VSD and just beneath it is the posteriorly malaligned conal septum. The vessel arising from the LV is the PA, and it is obstructed just beneath its origin from the heart. **(B)** Further cephalad imaging reveals posterior malalignment of the infundibular septum causing subpulmonic stenosis and the aorta arising from the RV. **(C)** Color flow imaging reveals a narrowed left ventricular outflow tract with the PA arising from the LV and the aorta arising from the RV. The *arrow* points to the VSD.

15

Corrected Transposition of the Great Arteries

Shobha Natarajan

Key Echocardiographic Features

- Position of the morphological right ventricle on the left, giving rise to the aorta, and the morphological left ventricle on the right, giving rise to the pulmonary artery.
- Left-sided tricuspid valve abnormalities such as "Ebstein-like" appearance, valve thickening, dysplasia, and/or valvar insufficiency.
- Presence or absence of ventricular septal defects.
- Right-sided left ventricular outflow tract obstruction as either subpulmonic or pulmonary valve stenosis.
- Left-sided right ventricular hypoplasia and possible hypoplasia of the aorta or coarctation of the aorta.
- In the presence of a large ventricular septal defect, straddling or overriding of the atrioventricular valves.
- Conduction disorders, heart block (look for bradycardia or asynchrony between contraction of the atria and ventricles).

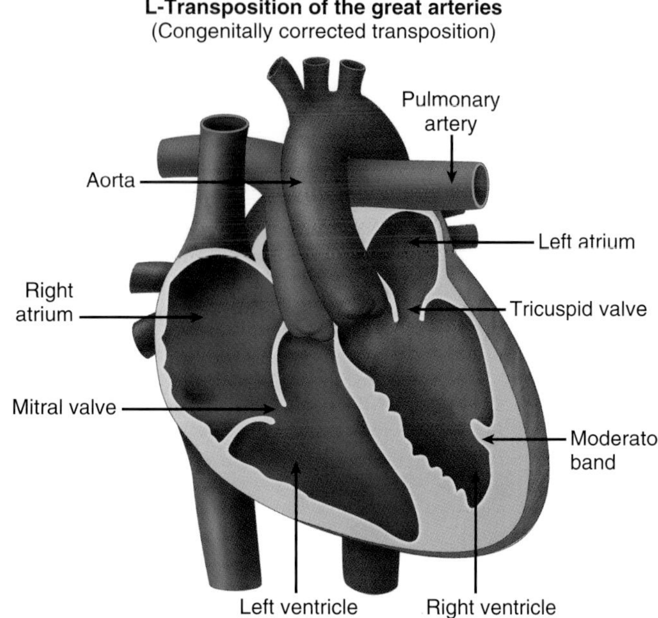

Figure 15-1. L-Transposition of the great arteries.

Anatomy and Anatomical Associations

Corrected transposition of the great arteries (cTGA) is a cardiac defect in which there is atrioventricular (AV) discordance and ventriculoarterial concordance.[1] What this means is as follows.

In the setting of atrial situs solitus, the right atrium connects via the mitral valve to a right-sided morphological left ventricle, which then ejects into the pulmonary artery. In turn, the left atrium connects via the tricuspid valve to the left-sided morphological right ventricle, which ejects into the aorta. If one defines "transposition of the great arteries" as the aorta arising from the right ventricle and the pulmonary artery from the left ventricle, this condition is achieved in cTGA. However, because the ventricles, not the great vessels, are switched, in effect, the systemic venous return (deoxygenated blood) makes its way to the lungs via the right atrium–to–left ventricle–to–pulmonary artery connection and the pulmonary venous return (oxygenated blood) makes its way to the body via the left atrium–to–right ventricle–to–aorta connection (Figure 15-1). There is "physiological correction" because the normal pathways of deoxygenated blood to the lungs and oxygenated blood to the body persist in the correct manner.

In cTGA, the aorta is anterior and leftward of the pulmonary artery. The cardiac segments are as follows: atrial situs solitus (S), L-ventricular loop (L), L-transposition of the great arteries (L) or {S,L,L} in the Van Praagh nomenclature. cTGA can also occur in the setting of atrial situs inversus with levocardia or with mirror-image dextrocardia. The segments in these arrangements are situs inversus, D-loop ventricles, and D-transposition of the great arteries {I,D,D}.

Only approximately 10% of cTGA occurs in isolation; this defect is most often associated with other intracardiac abnormalities. Dextrocardia or mesocardia is present in 25% of patients.[2] Atrial situs inversus is found in 3% to 5%. Ventricular septal defect (VSD) is the most common association, present in 70% to 80% of cases of cTGA. The majority of these defects involve the membranous septum owing to the misalignment of the atrial and ventricular septa usually seen in cTGA. They are often large and extend anteriorly.

Autopsy studies have shown over 90% of cases of cTGA are associated with anomalies of the tricuspid valve.[3,4] Approximately 25% patients with cTGA have an Ebstein-like malformation of the left-sided tricuspid valve where the septal leaflet is significantly displaced below the level of the annulus.[5] Other tricuspid valve anomalies include dysplastic leaflets and straddling across the VSD. These anomalies can result in significant tricuspid regurgitation.

Right-sided left ventricular or pulmonary outflow tract obstruction occurs in 40% to 50% of patients with cTGA and is usually found at the subvalvar level as a result of fibrous tissue protruding into the outflow tract. Pulmonary atresia is found in 15% of patients.[3,4] Less commonly, mitral valve abnormalities occur in 10%[6] and right ventricular outflow tract obstruction and aortic arch obstruction are present in 13%.[3]

Patients with cTGA also have abnormalities in their conduction system. The sinoatrial node is in the normal position. However, the AV node with its conducting bundle is situated anteriorly in the interatrial septum, on the right side. In some patients, there is an additional, hypoplastic AV node found in the normal posterior position.[7] It has been shown that dual AV nodes are most often found in cTGA patients with significant AV septal misalignment.[8] The abnormal positioning of the AV node and the fibrosis noted in this elongated node explain the relatively high percentage of AV block and other arrhythmias found in patients with cTGA.[7]

In cTGA with L-looped ventricles, the left main coronary artery arises from the anterior-rightward facing sinus and the right coronary artery arises from the posterior-facing sinus. Coronary anomalies are rare in cTGA when compared with D-transposition of the great arteries.

Frequency, Genetics, and Development

cTGA occurs in approximately 0.03 per 1000 live births[2] and accounts for less than 1% of all congenital heart disease. Clearly, a multifactorial etiology must be considered. Environmental factors have been documented in some cases.[9] Epidemiology studies have demonstrated the recurrence risk in siblings of patients with congenital heart disease to be approximately 1% to 3%. One study involving 102 patients specifically with cTGA demonstrated a recurrence risk of congenital heart defects in 5% of their siblings.[10] More recent molecular studies have given important consideration to gene abnormalities involved in congenital heart defects, but specific gene abnormalities in cTGA have yet to be reported.[11]

As early as day 15 of human embryological development, the heart field begins as a crescent-shaped group of cells. By day 21, the heart is a long tube with the sinus venosus on one pole and the conotruncus on the other. Normally, the tube loops to the right (D-looping) to ensure the proper positioning of the right and left ventricles. In cTGA, the tube loops to the left (L-looping). This abnormal looping, in turn, disturbs the normal process by which the conotruncus septates, twists, and rotates to ensure normal ventricular-arterial connections.[11]

Fetal Physiology

In fetuses with cTGA and no other significant associated defects, the physiology is equivalent to a normal fetal circulation. cTGA with a VSD results in fetal physiology similar to that of an isolated VSD. Bidirectional shunting is usually seen in utero. The presence of unidirectional shunt indicates outflow tract obstruction contralateral to the direction of shunting. Significant pulmonary or aortic outflow tract obstruction in the setting of cTGA may result in a ductal-dependent circulation. Fetuses generally tolerate obstruction well in utero as long as the ductus arteriosus is widely patent.

In cTGA, the left ventricle situated on the right side takes on the task of dominant perfusion through ejection into the ductus arteriosus to the descending aorta, and the right ventricle situated on the left performs the task of perfusion into the aorta and head and neck vessels. This shifting of duties between the ventricles is well tolerated in the fetus, without consequence, as long as the AV valves function well.

Fetuses with cTGA and an Ebstein-like malformation of the tricuspid valve may develop significant tricuspid valve regurgitation. The resulting increase in atrial pressure can lead to fetal hydrops with cardiomegaly, decreased ventricular shortening, pericardial and pleural effusions, and arrhythmias. Severe hydrops fetalis in this scenario commonly leads to fetal demise. If these fetuses survive, they are at high risk of significant complications after birth. In addition, there are reports of severe tricuspid valve regurgitation leading to decreased forward flow through the aorta in fetal life and the development of aortic arch obstruction.

As high as 20% of fetuses with cTGA have varying degrees of AV block and associated bradycardia.[12] Heart block may be present at the first prenatal evaluation or develop over gestation. Rarely, supraventricular tachycardia has been noted.[12]

Prenatal Management

The fetal echocardiogram demonstrates the cardiac segmental anatomy, AV discordance, transposition of the great arteries, and the presence of the associated anomalies outlined previously.[12,13]

After the right and left side of the fetus is established, a cross-sectional view of the abdomen will aid in the determination of situs by noting on which side of the spine the aorta and the inferior vena cava lie. If the aorta is to the right and the inferior vena cava is to the left of the spine, situs inversus is present.

A cross-sectional view of the chest with the four chambers of the heart in view will demonstrate the position of the heart within the chest (levocardia, mesocardia, or dextrocardia). Usually, in this view of the heart when imaging posteriorly at the level of the inflows, atrial situs can be confirmed by visualization of pulmonary vein connections to the left atrium. In turn, the connection of the left atrium to the morphological right ventricle can be seen in this view (features of the right ventricle include the presence of a moderator band, coarse trabeculations, triangular-shaped cavity, and a more apically displaced tricuspid valve with direct attachments to the ventricular septum), confirming the ventricular looping abnormality in cTGA. A sweep of the ventricular septum from posterior to anterior may also reveal significant VSDs.

Morphologic assessment of the tricuspid valve by two-dimensional imaging and color Doppler interrogation for regurgitation can be performed in this view. Details of mitral valve morphology can also be obtained. An anterior sweep from this four-chamber view to the level of the great vessels confirms the ventricular-arterial discordance and will demonstrate parallel exit of the great vessels with the aorta anterior and to the left of the pulmonary artery in the setting of normal atrial situs. Assessment of outflow tract obstruction and the mechanism of obstruction (valvar, subvalvar muscle or membrane, accessory AV valve tissue) may be determined in this view. In the setting of severe outflow tract obstruction, an element of ventricular hypoplasia may be present. Ventricular size discrepancy can be appreciated in this four-chamber view.

The abnormal great vessel relationship and the size of the great vessels relative to each other can also be confirmed using the three-vessel view. From the four-chamber view, a sweep superiorly moving leftward normally demonstrates cross-sectional views of the right superior vena cava, followed by the aorta, followed by the pulmonary artery in order from posterior and rightward to anterior and leftward (Figure 15-2A). In cTGA in such a sweep, the right superior vena cava is followed by the pulmonary artery, which is situated posterior, and then the aorta, which is situated anterior and leftward to the pulmonary artery (see Figure 15-2B). Usually, the aorta is slightly smaller than the pulmonary artery. If the aorta is the same size or larger, this discrepancy may indicate pulmonary outflow obstruction. Often, the direction of flow in the ductus arteriosus can be assessed in this view along with the branch pulmonary artery size.

A short-axis view of the ventricles can demonstrate significant VSDs. Color Doppler interrogation may reveal unidirectional shunting, which is a marker for outflow tract obstruction. Straddling or override of the AV valve should also be determined. This view can also confirm the abnormal ventricular looping by confirming the posterior position of the right ventricle.

Other important details include aortic and ductal arch views, the bicaval view to confirm systemic venous connections, and delineation of interatrial septal communication(s).

Once the anatomy of cTGA is confirmed, rhythm should be assessed. Pulse Doppler and M-mode interrogation aid in determination of heart rate and AV association to rule out heart block.

In the setting of significant tricuspid valve regurgitation and/or AV block, signs of hydrops fetalis should be sought after including ventricular shortening abnormalities, pleural or pericardial effusions, ascites, abnormal flow patterns in the ductus venosus and umbilical vein, and arrhythmias.

Counseling of the family should involve the need for serial assessment during gestation for the progression of tricuspid valve regurgitation, outflow tract obstruction, and rhythm issues, in particular. Depending on the associated defects, medical/surgical management and long-term prognosis can also be gauged and discussed.

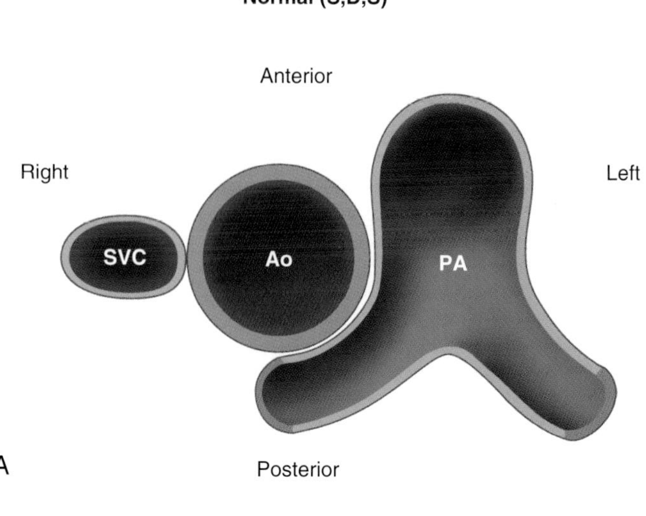

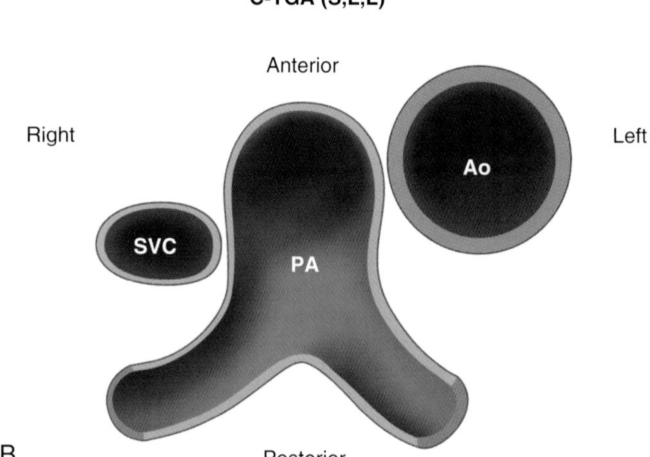

Figure 15-2. **A,** Normal relationship of the great vessels in a heart with the cardiac segments {S,D,S}. The pulmonary artery is the most anterior great vessel. **B,** Relationship of the great vessels one to the other in corrected transposition cardiac segments {S,L,L}. The aorta is the most anterior great vessel.

Postnatal Physiology

Postnatal physiology of cTGA depends on the associated defects. Although there is AV and ventriculoarterial discordance, systemic venous blood flows to the pulmonary circulation and pulmonary venous blood flows to the systemic circulation in the normal manner. Therefore, patients with isolated cTGA have relatively normal cardiovascular physiology after birth.

Those patients with cTGA and VSD may experience physiology similar to that of an isolated VSD with normal cardiac segments and may present with heart failure from increased pulmonary blood flow in infancy if the defect is large enough.

Patients who have associated pulmonary outflow tract obstruction may present with decreased pulmonary blood flow and cyanosis as the ductus arteriosus closes if there is significant obstruction. If there is a large VSD, the physiology is similar to that of tetralogy of Fallot. Neonates with significant, ductal-dependent aortic outflow tract obstruction or aortic arch obstruction can present with low cardiac output.

The subsets of patients with cTGA that tend to be sickest in the neonatal period are those with significant tricuspid valve abnormalities and severe regurgitation. Because the tricuspid valve in cTGA is the systemic AV valve, if there is severe regurgitation, these infants may present with elevated pressures in the lungs and have low cardiac output.

Predicting who will have significant postnatal tricuspid regurgitation in the fetus with cTGA can be difficult. If the valve appears structurally normal and there is no regurgitation on fetal echocardiography, the valve is likely to perform well after birth. However, a structurally abnormal valve that has even only mild regurgitation as a fetus may manifest hemodynamically significant regurgitation after birth. The change in loading conditions of increased preload secondary to increased pulmonary venous return and increased afterload as a consequence of elimination of the low-resistance placenta can negatively affect the competence of a structurally abnormal systemic tricuspid valve.

Postnatal Management

Patients who have ductal-dependent pulmonary or systemic circulation will need to have prostaglandin therapy initiated after birth. Depending on the degree of pulmonary outflow tract obstruction, a catheter- or surgical-based valvotomy, a left ventricle–to–pulmonary artery conduit, or an aortopulmonary shunt will be needed. Similarly, systemic outflow tract obstruction will also need to be relieved. If one ventricle is hypoplastic or if one of the AV valves straddles across a VSD, single-ventricle palliation may need to be undertaken.

Severe tricuspid (systemic) valve regurgitation may be initially managed with medication such as those that reduce systemic afterload to promote forward flow through the right ventricle out the aorta and diuretic therapy to reduce fluid accumulation in the lungs due to elevated left atrial pressure. If this management fails to improve the regurgitation, some patients may undergo pulmonary artery banding. Banding is thought to change the geometry of the interventricular septum, alter the mechanics of tricuspid valve function, and reduce the systemic AV valve regurgitation. It may also improve regurgitation by reducing the amount of pulmonary blood flow and, hence, right ventricular volume.[14,15]

Patients can also have significant morbidity related to the development of varying degrees of AV block. In some neonates, the bradycardia may be so profound or the baby so unstable as to warrant early placement of a pacemaker.

In the long term, patients with a VSD, if symptomatic, may undergo banding of the pulmonary artery or a conventional surgical approach with VSD closure, leaving the right ventricle to support the systemic circulation. Some patients with cTGA will also need tricuspid valvuloplasty or replacement in the long term.

Another, more recent surgical approach to cTGA is to undergo an "anatomical" repair, otherwise referred to as a "double-switch" procedure. In this surgery, an atrial switch procedure (the Senning or Mustard procedure) and either an arterial switch or, in the setting of significant pulmonary (or left ventricular) outflow tract obstruction, a Rastelli procedure (baffle closure of the VSD to the aorta with placement of a right ventricle–to–pulmonary artery conduit) are performed. This repair reroutes the blood flow patterns twice and enables the left ventricle to receive pulmonary venous blood and eject it into the systemic circulation. Occasionally, this procedure is preceded by pulmonary artery banding in order to train the left ventricle to pump against a higher resistance.

Outcomes

In cTGA, long-term survival into adulthood is reported.[16] However, outcomes will vary significantly depending on the severity of the associated defects. Heart block can be present in fetal life but can develop spontaneously at any point in life, even in adulthood. It occurs in 20% to 30% of patients with cTGA, with a higher prevalence in those with an intact ventricular septum.[17] The risk of natural spontaneous-onset AV block in cTGA continues at a rate of approximately 2%/yr.[17] Even in the absence of significant associated defects and prior interventions, natural history studies have shown a high rate of systemic right ventricular dysfunction in the long term.[5] Factors that compound systemic right ventricular dysfunction are tricuspid valve regurgitation, heart block with significant bradycardia, and ventricular pacing with discordant ventricular contraction. In addition, myocardial blood flow is reported to be compromised in unoperated patients with cTGA even in the absence of symptoms.[18]

In one report of 123 patients with cTGA, 119 underwent an intracardiac repair (VSD closure, tricuspid valve procedure, or Fontan operation). The overall 1-, 5-, 10-, and 15-year survivals after intracardiac procedures were 84%, 75%, 68%, and 61%, respectively. The worst outcome was in those who underwent tricuspid valve surgery and the best outcome was in the Fontan subgroup.[19] Almost 50% of patients who underwent intracardiac repair developed systemic right ventricular dysfunction in the long term, and approximately 25% of patients developed heart block after their procedure.[19]

The problems with the right ventricle supporting the systemic circulation and with progressive systemic (tricuspid valve) AV valve regurgitation have led to the consideration of anatomical repair (double-switch), which enables the left ventricle to support the systemic circulation. Some studies have shown promising intermediate outcomes with this double-switch procedure.[20,21] Long-term outcomes have not shown to be significantly different from traditional surgical approaches in some series.[22] Although right ventricular function and tricuspid valve regurgitation improve, there are reports of progressive left ventricular dysfunction after anatomical repair, especially in those who are pacemaker-dependent and those who required training of the left ventricle with pulmonary artery banding.[23,24] Further investigation needs to delineate which patients are the best candidates for the double-switch procedure and to determine appropriate timing of the intervention and follow-up strategies for this population.

Imaging Essentials and Important Points

- The fetus with cTGA may exhibit levocardia or dextrocardia; hence, careful determination of cardiac position and situs is key.
- Ventricular looping can be determined based on identification of the morphological features of the ventricles and their position in the chest.
- The aorta is very anterior and leftward in cTGA and situs solitus. It can be difficult to image because it can sit just behind the sternum.
- Investigate for the presence of VSDs and left ventricular (pulmonary) outflow tract obstruction.
- In the four-chamber view, pay careful attention to the left-sided tricuspid valve because it may appear like a true Ebstein's anomaly, with apical displacement of the septal leaflet, or more commonly, have an "Ebstein-like" appearance with multiple apically displaced chordal attachments, tethering of the valve, dysplasia of the leaflets, and other abnormalities.
- Assess for heart rate and rhythm, with particular attention to the presence of synchrony between atrial and ventricular contraction.
- Inspect the mitral valve for possible abnormalities.
- Check for obstruction of aortic valve and aortic arch, which will likely not be present when there is pulmonary stenosis.

References

1. Anderson RC, Lillehei CW, Lester RG. Corrected transposition of the great vessels of the heart: a review of 17 cases. *Pediatrics.* 1957;20:626-646.
2. Allan HD, Driscoll DJ, Shaddy RE, Feltes TF. *Moss and Adams' Heart Disease in Infants, Children, and Adolescents: Including the Fetus and Young Adult.* Philadelphia: Lippincott Williams & Wilkins; 2008.
3. Rutledge JM, Nihill MR, Fraser CD, Smith OE, McMahon CJ, Bezold LI. Outcome of 121 patients with congenitally corrected transposition of the great arteries. *Pediatr Cardiol.* 2002;23:137-145.
4. Allwork SP, Bentall HH, Becker AE, et al. Congenitally corrected transposition of the great arteries: morphologic study of 32 cases. *Am J Cardiol.* 1976;38:910-923.
5. Graham TP Jr, Bernard YD, Mellen BG, et al. Long-term outcome in congenitally corrected transposition of the great arteries: a multi-institutional study. *J Am Coll Cardiol.* 2000;36:255-261.
6. Penny DJ, Somerville J, Redington AN. Echocardiographic demonstration of important abnormalities of the mitral valve in congenitally corrected transposition. *Br Heart J.* 1992;68:498-500.
7. Anderson RH, Becker AE, Arnold R, Wilkinson JL. The conducting tissues in congenitally corrected transposition. *Circulation.* 1974; 50:911-923.
8. Hosseinpour AR, McCarthy KP, Griselli M, Sethia B, Ho SY. Congenitally corrected transposition: size of the pulmonary trunk and septal malalignment. *Ann Thorac Surg.* 2004;77:2163-2166.
9. Kuehl KS, Loffredo CA. Population-based study of L-transposition of the great arteries: possible associations with environmental factors. *Birth Defects Res A Clin Mol Teratol.* 2003;67:162-167.
10. Piacentini G, Digilio MC, Capolino R, et al. Familial recurrence of heart defects in subjects with congenitally corrected transposition of the great arteries. *Am J Med Genet A.* 2005;137:176-180.
11. Srivastava D, Olson EN. A genetic blueprint for cardiac development. *Nature.* 2000;407:221-226.
12. Chiappa E, Micheletti A, Sciarrone A, Botta G, Abbruzzese P. The prenatal diagnosis of, and short-term outcome for, patients with congenitally corrected transposition. *Cardiol Young.* 2004;14: 265-276.
13. Sharland G, Tingay R, Jones A, Simpson J. Atrioventricular and ventriculoarterial discordance (congenitally corrected transposition of the great arteries): echocardiographic features, associations, and outcome in 34 fetuses. *Heart.* 2005;91:1453-1458.
14. Poirier NC, Mee RB. Left ventricular reconditioning and anatomical correction for systemic right ventricular dysfunction. *Semin Thorac Cardiovasc Surg Pediatr Card Surg Annu.* 2000;3:198-215.
15. Jahangiri M, Redington AN, Elliott MJ, Stark J, Tsang VT, de Leval MR. A case for anatomic correction in atrioventricular discordance? Effects of surgery on tricuspid valve function. *J Thorac Cardiovasc Surg.* 2001;121:1040-1045.
16. Beauchesne LM, Warnes CA, Connolly HM, Ammash NM, Tajik AJ, Danielson GK. Outcome of the unoperated adult who presents with congenitally corrected transposition of the great arteries. *J Am Coll Cardiol.* 2002;40:285-290.
17. Huhta JC, Maloney JD, Ritter DG, Ilstrup DM, Feldt RH. Complete atrioventricular block in patients with atrioventricular discordance. *Circulation.* 1983;67:1374-1377.
18. Hauser M, Bengel FM, Hager A, et al. Impaired myocardial blood flow and coronary flow reserve of the anatomical right systemic ventricle in patients with congenitally corrected transposition of the great arteries. *Heart.* 2003;89:1231-1235.
19. Hraska V, Duncan BW, Mayer JE Jr, Freed M, del Nido PJ, Jonas RA. Long-term outcome of surgically treated patients with corrected transposition of the great arteries. *J Thorac Cardiovasc Surg.* 2005; 129:182-191.
20. Imamura M, Drummond-Webb JJ, Murphy DJ Jr, et al. Results of the double switch operation in the current era. *Ann Thorac Surg.* 2000;70:100-105.
21. Devaney EJ, Charpie JR, Ohye RG, Bove EL. Combined arterial switch and Senning operation for congenitally corrected transposition of the great arteries: patient selection and intermediate results. *J Thorac Cardiovasc Surg.* 2003;125:500-507.
22. Shin'oka T, Kurosawa H, Imai Y, et al. Outcomes of definitive surgical repair for congenitally corrected transposition of the great arteries or double outlet right ventricle with discordant atrioventricular connections: risk analyses in 189 patients. *J Thorac Cardiovasc Surg.* 2007;133:1318-1328, 1328.e1-1328.e4.
23. Bautista-Hernandez V, Marx GR, Gauvreau K, Mayer JE Jr, Cecchin F, del Nido PJ. Determinants of left ventricular dysfunction after anatomic repair of congenitally corrected transposition of the great arteries. *Ann Thorac Surg.* 2006;82:2059-2065; discussion 2065-2066.
24. Quinn DW, McGuirk SP, Metha C, et al. The morphologic left ventricle that requires training by means of pulmonary artery banding before the double-switch procedure for congenitally corrected transposition of the great arteries is at risk of late dysfunction. *J Thorac Cardiovasc Surg.* 2008;135:1137-1144, 1144.e1-1144.e2.

CASES

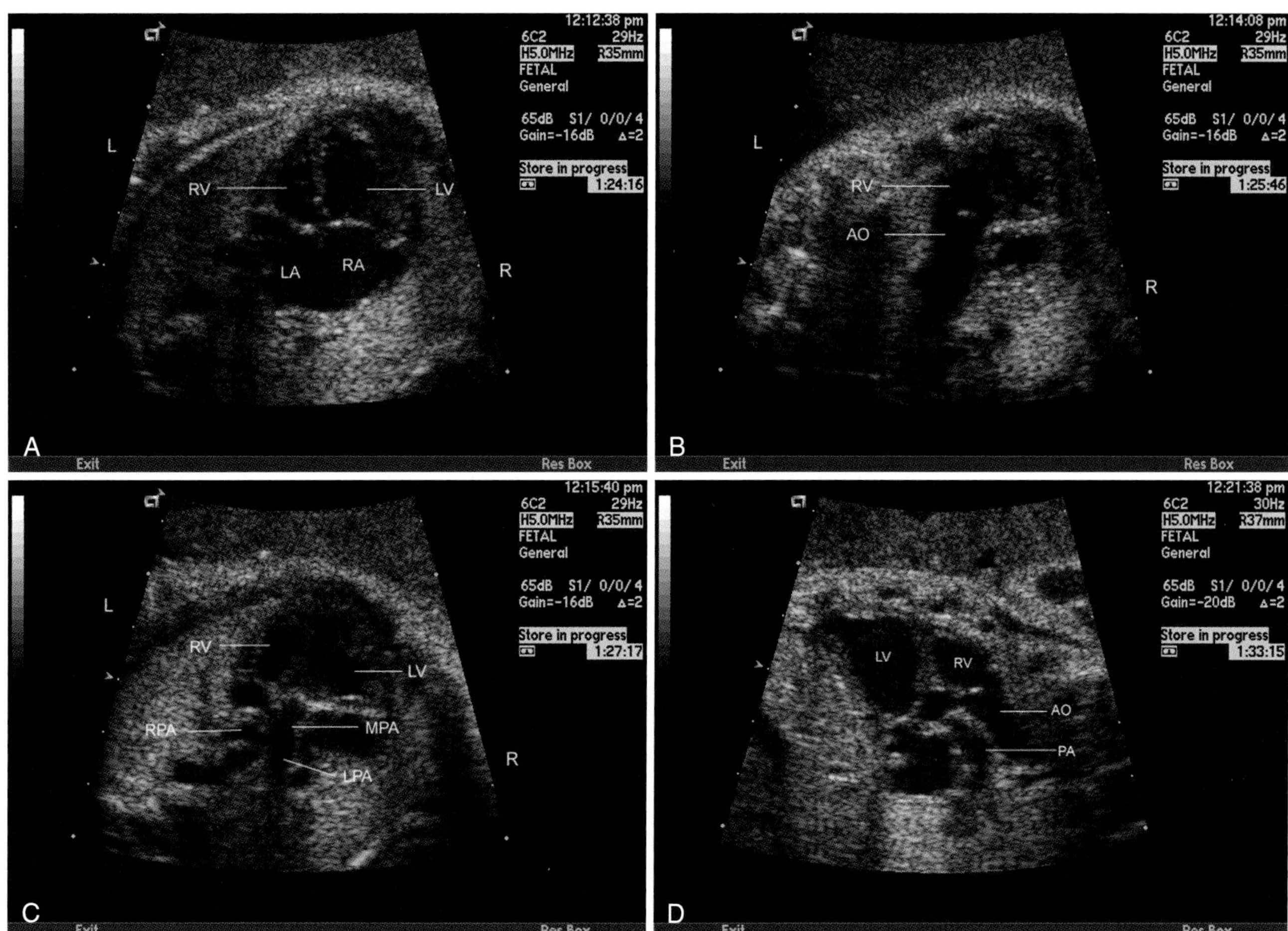

Case 15-1. (A) The morphological right ventricle is on the left side of the chest and the morphological left ventricle is on the right. The atria, left and right are on the left and right side, respectively. Note the atrium on the left has an appendage, which appears to be of left atrial morphology, and the atrium on the right has a broad-based appendage of right atrial morphology. (B) Anterior and superior angulation demonstrates the aorta (Ao) arising very leftward, but from the morphological right ventricle. (C) The main pulmonary artery (MPA) arises from the left ventricle. There is subpulmonic crowding. (D) Long-axis view angled superiorly and slightly leftward demonstrates the aorta arising from the right ventricle anteriorly and the smaller pulmonary artery behind it. There is subpulmonic stenosis in this case of corrected transposition.

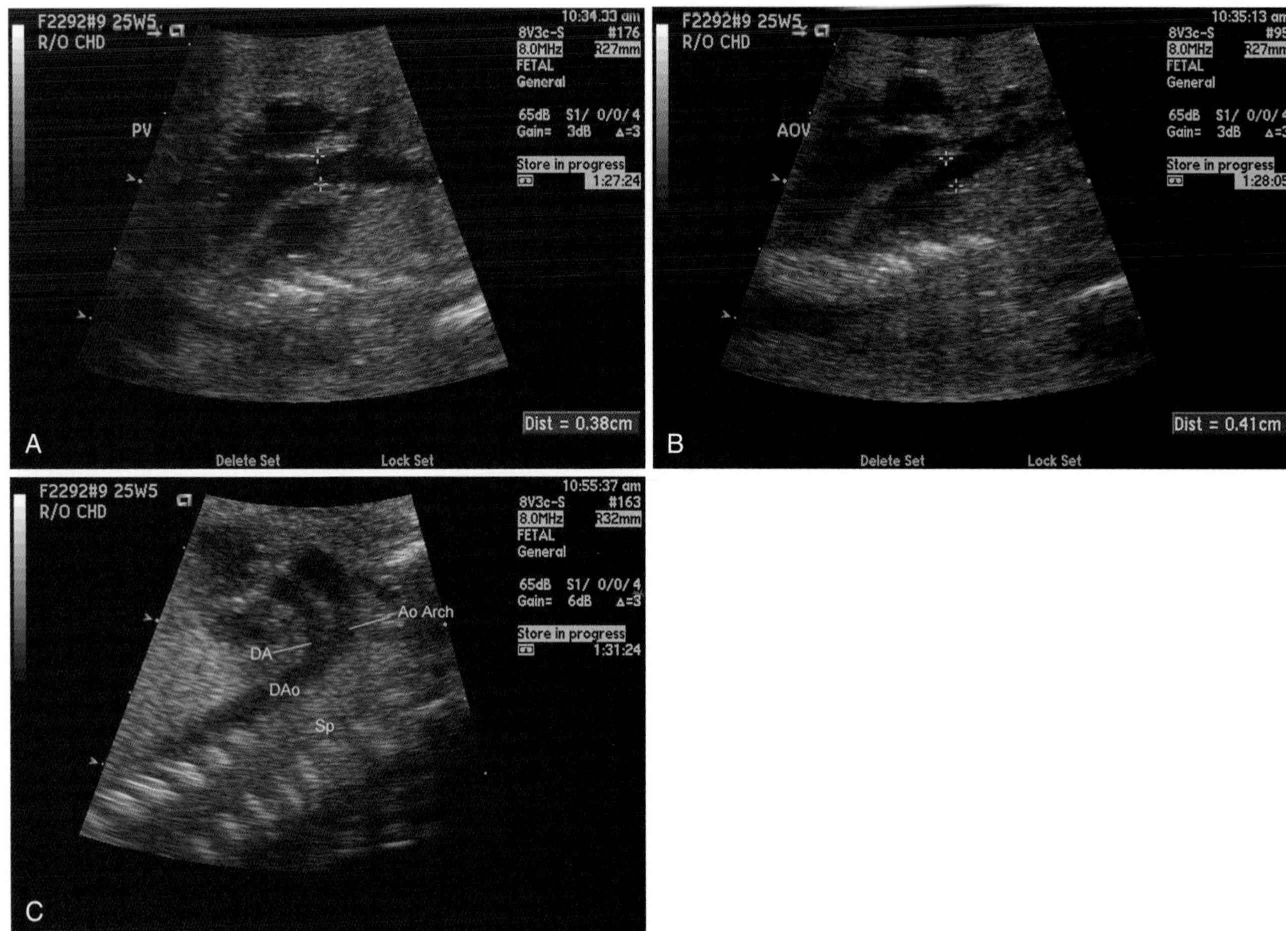

Case 15-2. **(A)** The ventricle on this fetus' right side has a smooth-walled septal surface and looks morphologically like a left ventricle (LV); however, it is giving rise to a vessel that bifurcates into the pulmonary artery (PA). Hence, this is a case of corrected transposition of the great vessels. **(B)** The aorta arises from the RV situated on the left. **(C)** The aortic arch (Ao Arch) and ductal arch (DA) travel in parallel as they course toward the descending aorta.

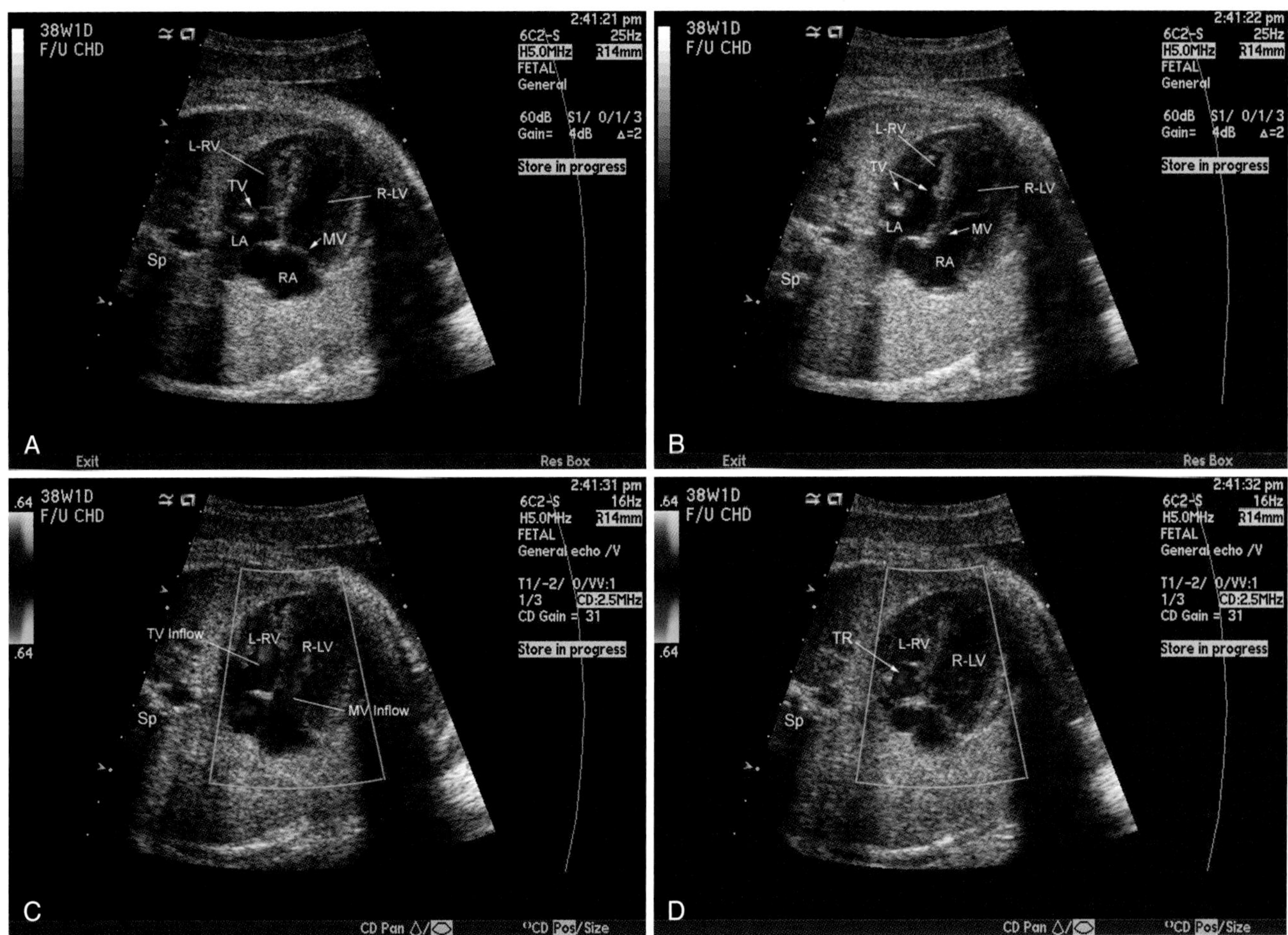

Case 15-3. **(A)** Four-chamber view of a corrected transposition of the great arteries with an abnormal, Ebstein's left-sided tricuspid valve. The atrioventricular valves are closed, as this is ventricular systole. Note the prominent moderator band on the septal surface of the left-sided right ventricle and the smoother septal surface of the right-sided left ventricle. Also note the plane of the tricuspid valve when closed is apically displaced relative to the plane of the mitral valve annulus. The atrial septum separating the right atrium (RA) from the left atrium (LA) is bowing right-to-left, in the normal fashion. **(B)** Same view, but now in ventricular diastole with the atrioventricular valves open. Note the marked apical displacement of the septal leaflet attachment of the left-sided tricuspid valve and how uneven it is with the attachment of the lateral aspect of the tricuspid valve. This is an Ebstein's malformation of this left-sided tricuspid valve. The mitral valve attaches normally at the crux of the heart. **(C)** Color flow during diastole across the ventricular inflows. Note how the color inflow jet starts much more apically in the ventricle on the left-sided right ventricle than on the right-sided left ventricle, further demonstrating the presence of an Ebstein's malformation of the left-sided tricuspid valve. **(D)** Mild left-sided tricuspid valve regurgitation. The *arrow* points to the blue jet of tricuspid regurgitation. Although only mild at this point in time, such valves may become more regurgitant with time as postnatal physiology alters loading conditions on the right ventricle.

16

Double-Outlet Right Ventricle

Michael D. Quartermain

Key Echocardiographic Features

- Origin of the great vessels from the right ventricle.
- Relationship of the great vessels to each other (aorta is typically to the right of the pulmonary artery).
- Identify the location of the ventricular septal defect in relation to the great vessels as either subpulmonic or subaortic.
- Identify the presence or absence of pulmonic or aortic outflow obstruction.
- If there is pulmonic outflow obstruction, identify the direction of shunting across the ductus arteriosus.
- If there is aortic outflow obstruction, assess the aortic arch for possible coarctation of the aorta or interruption of the aortic arch.

Anatomy and Anatomical Associations

Double-outlet right ventricle (DORV) is a type of congenital heart disease in which both great arteries arise from the right ventricle (RV).[1] More specifically, it is a ventriculoarterial alignment that occurs when both the aorta and the pulmonary artery are positioned at least 50% over the RV, and there is a lack of aortic–mitral annular fibrous continuity.

DORV is not a single, specific abnormality but, rather, defines an anatomical relationship that encompasses a wide spectrum of different congenital heart defects with varying physiologies. A ventricular septal defect (VSD) almost always accompanies DORV and is the only path out of the left ventricle (LV). DORV can be classified into different subtypes based on the location of the VSD: (1) DORV with subaortic VSD, (2) DORV with subpulmonic VSD, and (3) DORV with a double, or uncommitted, VSD. The first two types are the most common and are discussed here. DORV with an atrioventricular canal type VSD can be a type of DORV with uncommitted VSD and typically occurs in heterotaxy syndrome; this is addressed in another chapter. DORV with mitral hypoplasia and associated left ventricular hypoplasia can also occur; this is discussed separately in Chapter 22.

Variations in the relationship of the VSD to the great vessels are determined based on the three-dimensional spatial relationship between the plane of the ventricular septum and the position of the great vessels to the septum and to each other. The relative position of the vessels is in turn dependent upon the presence and amount of conus muscle underneath. Whereas, in the normal heart, there is no subaortic conus and only subpulmonary conus, in DORV, there can be conus beneath one or both great vessels to varying degrees, lifting and positioning the great vessels over the ventricular septum and VSD, creating the different great vessel–to–VSD relationships that exist. Furthermore, the position of the conal septum and its deviation and malalignment away from the plane of the muscular septum contribute to the development of sub–great vessel narrowing (subpulmonary narrowing in the subaortic VSD type DORV; subaortic narrowing in the subpulmonic VSD type of DORV).

The VSD–to–great vessel relationship determines the nature of the defect that is seen. VSD position determines where the outflow of the LV and blood exiting the LV will be directed (Figure 16-1). The VSD is classified as *subaortic* when it is more closely related to the aortic valve. In such cases, left ventricular outflow is directed into the aorta and pulmonary stenosis is common. The physiology and clinical manifestations are similar to that of a simple VSD, if there is no pulmonic stenosis, or similar to tetralogy of Fallot (TOF), if there is pulmonic stenosis. Common associated anomalies in DORV with subaortic VSD include pulmonary stenosis, atrial septal defects, mitral valve abnormalities, and left superior vena cava to coronary sinus.

The VSD is classified as *subpulmonic* when it is more closely associated with the pulmonary valve. In such cases, left ventricular outflow is directed into the pulmonary artery. The physiology and clinical manifestations are similar to that of transposition of the great arteries (TGA) because oxygenated blood from the LV is ejected into the pulmonary circulation. Common associated anomalies in DORV with subpulmonic VSD include aortic arch hypoplasia, coarctation of the aorta, and left superior vena cava to coronary sinus. The conal (infundibular) septum may be malaligned beneath the aorta causing variable degrees of subaortic narrowing. In a particular form of DORV with subpulmonic VSD, called the "Taussig-Bing" anomaly, there is bilateral conus underneath both great vessels, the aorta and pulmonary artery are side by side, and there is arch hypoplasia, or coarctation of the aorta.[2]

In DORV in general, the aorta is almost always more rightward than normal and the relative arrangement is for the great vessels to lay more side by side than usual. As such, coronary artery anomalies with aberrant insertion may occur. Furthermore, a rightward-positioned aorta is associated with the rare anomaly of leftward "juxtaposition of the atrial appendages." In this condition, the right atrium is its normal position; however, the right atrial appendage is positioned over on the left next to the left atrial appendage.

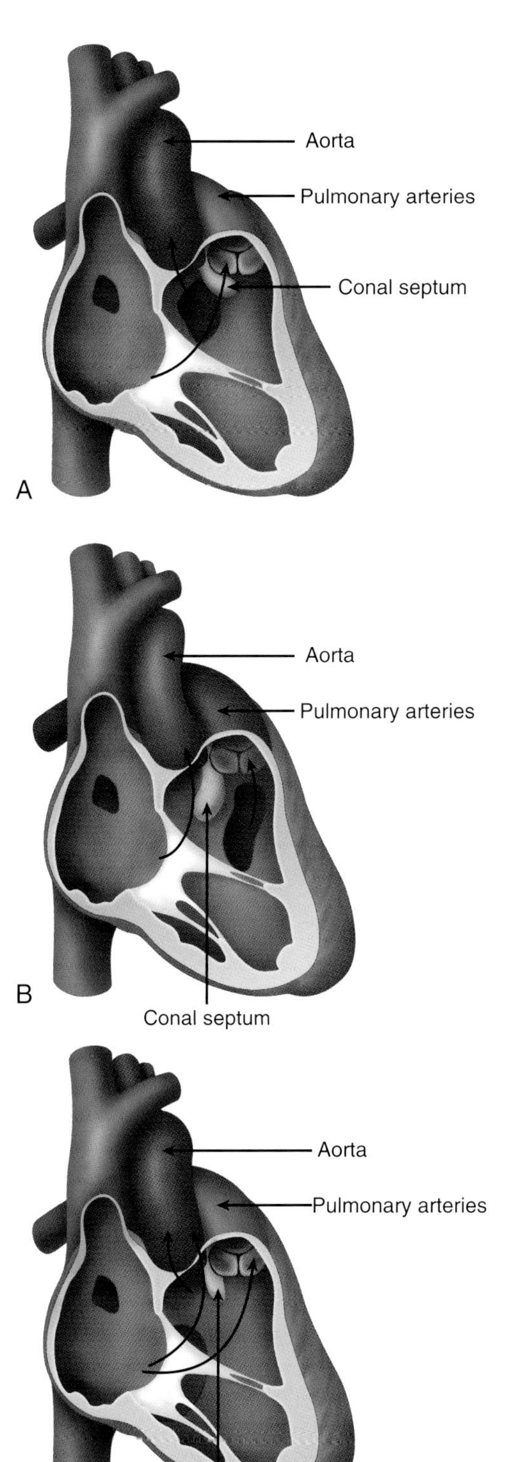

Figure 16-1. Variability in double-outlet right ventricle based on the position of the ventricular septal defect (VSD) to the great vessels. **(A)** The VSD is subaortic; hence, blood from the left ventricle is directed through the VSD and streams into the aorta. There is usually subpulmonic narrowing as shown due to conal septal deviation and often pulmonary valve and pulmonary artery stenosis. The postnatal physiology is similar to tetralogy of Fallot. **(B)** The VSD is subpulmonic; hence, blood flow from the left ventricle is directed through the VSD and streams into the pulmonary artery. In this case, there is often subaortic narrowing due to conal septal deviation beneath the aortic valve. Commonly, there can be associated aortic hypoplasia and coarctation of the aorta. **(C)** The VSD is uncommitted to any specific great vessel and there is no obstruction to any great vessel. Right and left ventricular blood mixes with relatively equal quantities streaming to the aorta and pulmonary artery. Postnatal physiology for such lesions is typically that of a large VSD.

Frequency, Genetics, and Development

The incidence of DORV is approximately 0.2 per 1000 live births with the subaortic defect being the most common form, occurring approximately 50% of the time.[3,4] To date, no specific genetic abnormality is associated with DORV. The developmental abnormalities that lead to DORV are likely related to a failure of the normal rotation of the conus with persistence of both great vessels from the RV.

Prenatal Physiology

The hemodynamic alterations in the fetus with DORV are usually mild and well tolerated. Oxygenated blood from the placenta returns to the left heart across the foramen ovale and will course across the VSD to the ascending aorta if there is a subaortic VSD and into the pulmonary artery if there is a subpulmonic VSD.

In the subaortic VSD type, when mild pulmonary stenosis is present, antegrade flow is ejected by the RV into the pulmonary circulation and antegrade flow through the ductus arteriosus to the descending aorta. If the pulmonary stenosis is severe, blood supply to the developing lungs is derived from the aorta via retrograde flow across the ductus arteriosus. Severe pulmonic stenosis will also divert blood away from the pulmonary artery and the ascending aorta will carry more of the combined cardiac output, but at slightly lower oxygen saturation.

In the subpulmonic VSD type, the physiology is similar to that of TGA. The combination of (1) right-to-left shunted atrial-derived blood and (2) small amount of pulmonary venous return that traverses the mitral valve is ejected out of the LV, through the VSD, into the pulmonary circulation with the predominance of it directed to the ductus arteriosus and descending aorta. If there is marked conal septal deviation beneath the aortic valve, there may be limitation of blood flow into the aorta, which may explain why many such fetuses exhibit arch hypoplasia and coarctation of the aorta.

Prenatal Management

Imaging of DORV involves careful evaluation of the position of the great vessels in relation to the ventricles and the ventricular septum.[5] The great vessels will arise from the heart parallel to each other and will not cross in space.[6] In the four-chamber view, angling anteriorly, one will see a VSD; further anterior and superior angling will reveal the origin of the great vessels. On two-dimensional imaging, the relationship of the VSD to the great vessels can be determined. In subaortic VSD, the aorta is positioned rightward but adjacent to and just above the VSD. Another way to confirm presence of a subaortic VSD is in fact to identify absence of the ability to "connect" VSD flow with the pulmonary artery in any plane because the conal septum gets in the way of any such visual connection. In subpulmonic VSD, the pulmonary artery will commonly appear to straddle the ventricular septum. Sometimes, it is difficult to distinguish whether in fact the pulmonary artery is 50% over the RV or the LV, the former being DORV, the latter TGA with VSD.

Color Doppler imaging will further indicate the direction of flow exiting the LV via the VSD. Oftentimes, a stream of color flow will be seen in a single plane exiting the VSD directed into either the aorta or the pulmonary artery. This is best determined in the four-chamber or long-axis views.

In cases of DORV with subaortic VSD with pulmonary stenosis, one must predict whether there will be ductal-dependent pulmonary blood flow and the need for prostaglandin (PGE) infusion in the immediate newborn period. Guidelines to those for TOF can be used. If the narrowest diameter of the pathway to the pulmonary circulation is less than half the diameter of the aorta, this should raise suspicion of the possible need for supplemental pulmonary blood flow through ductal perfusion and the need for PGE infusion at birth.

In cases of DORV and subpulmonic VSD, the pulmonary artery will be relatively large and analysis of the subaortic region and aortic arch are indicated. The degree of conal deviation beneath the aorta can be appreciated in the long-axis views. The aortic annulus should be assessed and measured, as should the ascending and transverse aorta, because the severity of hypoplasia of the aorta will dictate the postnatal surgical strategy.

If pulmonary stenosis or abnormalities of the aorta have been identified, it is recommended to serially evaluate the fetus to monitor for progression. DORV is considered a form of conotruncal anomaly; therefore, there is indication for analysis of the fetal chromosomes and an obstetrical ultrasound to evaluate for extracardiac anomalies.

Postnatal Physiology

In the newborn with DORV and subaortic VSD, the postnatal physiology and clinical course depend on the presence of associated lesions such as pulmonary stenosis and the relationship of the systemic to the pulmonary artery resistance. When there is little or no pulmonary stenosis, the physiology is similar to that for a VSD. There is no cyanosis but there can be mild respiratory symptoms from increased pulmonary blood flow with later development of heart failure symptoms. In cases with pulmonary stenosis, the clinical picture is similar to TOF. There are varying degrees of cyanosis depending on the severity of outflow obstruction. In cases of severe pulmonary stenosis or atresia, a patent ductus arteriosus is required to maintain adequate oxygen saturation.

In cases of DORV with subpulmonic VSD, the predicted postnatal physiology of TGA is present. It is indicated to start PGE at birth regardless of the subaortic or arch anatomy, with ductal patency being important to allow for adequate mixing between the circulations in order to promote proper oxygenation. Occasionally, such neonates may require a balloon atrial septostomy in order to optimize mixing between the circulations. If there is significant arch narrowing, the neonate may manifest a picture of "reverse cyanosis" in which the upper extremity is cyanosed while the lower extremity remains relatively pink. This is caused by the streaming of blood flow as oxygenated blood is delivered via the LV through the subpulmonic VSD into the pulmonary artery. Because there is critical arch obstruction, the relatively pink oxygenated blood in the pulmonary artery is ejected into the ductus arteriosus to the descending aorta, while the ascending aorta receives antegrade, relatively deoxygenated blood from the aorta and RV.

Postnatal Management

The postnatal management of DORV depends on the presence of associated intracardiac anomalies. Multiple surgical approaches are available depending on the precise anatomical findings. A complete postnatal transthoracic echocardiogram is performed to allow for confirmation of the prenatal diagnosis and to identify more subtle anatomical abnormalities, such as unusual coronary patterns.

In DORV with subaortic VSD, it is important to identify the precise location of the VSD and its potential for baffle closure to the aorta as well as the severity and location of pulmonary stenosis if present. In the neonate with DORV, an unrestrictive subaortic VSD, and no pulmonary stenosis, the clinical course is similar to an isolated VSD. These newborns can electively undergo repair, which is performed by creating an intraventricular tunnel that channels left ventricular blood through the VSD to the aorta.[4] If the VSD is suspected to be smaller than the aorta, it can be surgically enlarged. When pulmonary stenosis and TOF-like features are present, if adequate oxygen saturations are maintained after ductal closure, elective repair is performed in the first few months of life. When anatomically possible, a complete repair is performed that consists of baffling the VSD to the aorta with resection of RV muscle bundles and reconstruction of the pathway to the pulmonary artery to relieve obstruction. Similar to TOF repair, a transannular patch or an RV–to–pulmonary artery conduit may be necessary to completely relieve the subpulmonic obstruction.

In DORV with subpulmonic VSD, the optimal strategy for repair is to close the VSD and perform an arterial switch operation. Once the arterial switch is performed, left ventricular outflow across the VSD is directed into the "new" aorta, previously the pulmonary artery. If there is arch obstruction, this is relieved through arch augmentation and/or coarctation repair. Subaortic narrowing due to conal septal deviation can be a challenge to address, depending upon its severity. Following the arterial switch, subaortic narrowing will now become subpulmonic narrowing. This can be addressed either via resection of conal septal tissue, or if the aortic, now "new" pulmonic annulus is small, a transannular patch can be applied. Occasionally, the aorta is atretic with severe aortic hypoplasia. In such cases, a more complex operation can be performed involving a pulmonary artery–to–aortic anastomosis, arch augmentation, and intraventricular baffle closure of VSD to the pulmonary artery with placement of a RV–to–pulmonary artery conduit.[7]

Outcomes

Outcomes for DORV are variable and depend on the subtype, the presence of additional defects, and the surgical procedure undertaken. Outcome for DORV with subaortic VSD is excellent. In uncomplicated baffle closure of the VSD to the aorta, survival rates of 95% have been shown at 15 years.[8,9] Survival for repair of DORV with subaortic VSD and pulmonary stenosis are also excellent and similar to that seen in TOF repair. Because an intraventricular baffle is necessary to close the VSD to the aorta, late baffle obstruction and development of subaortic narrowing can occur owing to restriction at the rim of the VSD or deposition of fibrous material. Patients who have undergone surgical repair of DORV with subaortic VSD generally have a good quality of life. Reoperation for residual VSD, pulmonary stenosis, conduit revision when used, or development of subaortic VSD baffle obstruction occurs in approximately one third of patients. If a transannular patch is used across the pulmonary valve in order to relieve pulmonary stenosis, long-term chronic pulmonary insufficiency may cause RV dilation and dysfunction, similar to that seen in repaired TOF.

Outcome for DORV with subpulmonic VSD is somewhat less favorable, because surgical management is much more complicated and variable. Overall, in a recent report, survival can be as high as 85% at 15 years.[10] Residual subpulmonary stenosis due to residual conal septal obstruction can occur, as can arch obstruction in patients with the Taussig-Bing anomaly.[11] Similar to TGA after arterial switch operation, the native pulmonary valve, or "neo-aortic" valve can develop insufficiency with root dilation. Early survival is based on center experience. The long-term adult outcomes for this complex anomaly are not yet fully described.

Imaging Essentials and Important Points

- Identify the origin of the aorta and the pulmonary artery as arising from the RV.
- Identify the anatomical location of the VSD in relation to the great vessels.
- Use color flow imaging to help define the association between the VSD and the great vessels.
- Identify the presence or absence of obstruction to the pulmonary or aortic outflows.
- In general, as a rule of thumb, the association of the VSD and its flow to one particular great vessel suggests that the other great vessel will get "short-changed" and will have an element of obstruction. For example, if there is DORV and subaortic VSD, there will be associated pulmonary obstruction; if there is DORV and subpulmonic VSD, there will be associated aortic obstruction.
- Measure the narrowest diameter of the pathways that are obstructed. An obstructed pathway to the pulmonary artery that has a diameter measurement less than 0.5 that of the aortic annulus might suggest serious pulmonary obstruction and the possible need for supplementary blood flow after birth via initiation of PGE to promote ductal patency.
- DORV is distinguished from TGA in the following manner: in both anomalies, the aorta arises from the RV, but in DORV, the pulmonary artery is greater than 50% positioned over the RV whereas in TGA, the pulmonary artery is greater than 50% positioned over the LV.
- Similar to TGA, the great vessels will arise from the heart in a parallel manner, and they will NOT cross in space above the heart as is seen in normal fetuses.
- DORV with subpulmonic VSD will have the postnatal physiology of TGA and, therefore, should be managed as such to include initiation of PGE infusion at birth to maintain ductal patency and mixing. Delivery at a center that can manage possible marked cyanosis and hemodynamic instability is essential.

References

1. Mahle WT, Martinez R, Silverman N, Cohen MS, Anderson RH. Anatomy, echocardiography, and surgical approach to double outlet right ventricle. *Cardiol Young*. 2008;18(suppl 3):39-51.
2. Van Praagh R. What is the Taussig-Bing malformation? *Circulation*. 1968;38:445-449.
3. Botto LD, Correa A, Erickson JD. Racial and temporal variations in the prevalence of heart defects. *Pediatrics*. 2001;107:E32.
4. Sridaromont S, Ritter DG, Feldt RH, Davis GD, Edwards JE. Double-outlet right ventricle. Anatomic and angiocardiographic correlations. *Mayo Clin Proc*. 1978;53:555-577.

5. Gelehrter S, Owens ST, Russell MW, van der Velde ME, Gomez-Fifer C. Accuracy of the fetal echocardiogram in double-outlet right ventricle. *Congenit Heart Dis*. 2007;2:32-37.
6. Allan LD. Sonographic detection of parallel great arteries in the fetus. *AJR Am J Roentgenol*. 1997;168:1283-1286.
7. Rychik J, Murdison KA, Chin AJ, Norwood WI. Surgical management of severe aortic outflow obstruction in lesions other than the hypoplastic left heart syndrome: use of a pulmonary artery to aorta anastomosis. *J Am Coll Cardiol*. 1991;18:809-816.
8. Brown JW, Ruzmetov M, Okada Y, Vijay P, Turrentine MW. Surgical results in patients with double outlet right ventricle: a 20-year experience. *Ann Thorac Surg*. 2001;72:1630-1635.
9. Gomes MM, Weidman WH, McGoon DC, Danielson GK. Double-outlet right ventricle without pulmonic stenosis. Surgical considerations and results of operation. *Circulation*. 1971;43:I31-I36.
10. Rodefeld MD, Ruzmetov M, Vijay P, Fiore AC, Turrentine MW, Brown JW. Surgical results of arterial switch operation for Taussig-Bing anomaly: is position of the great arteries a risk factor? *Ann Thorac Surg*. 2007;83:1451-1457.
11. Alsoufi B, Cai S, Williams WG, et al. Improved results with single-stage total correction of Taussig-Bing anomaly. *Eur J Cardiothorac Surg*. 2008;33:244-250.

CASES

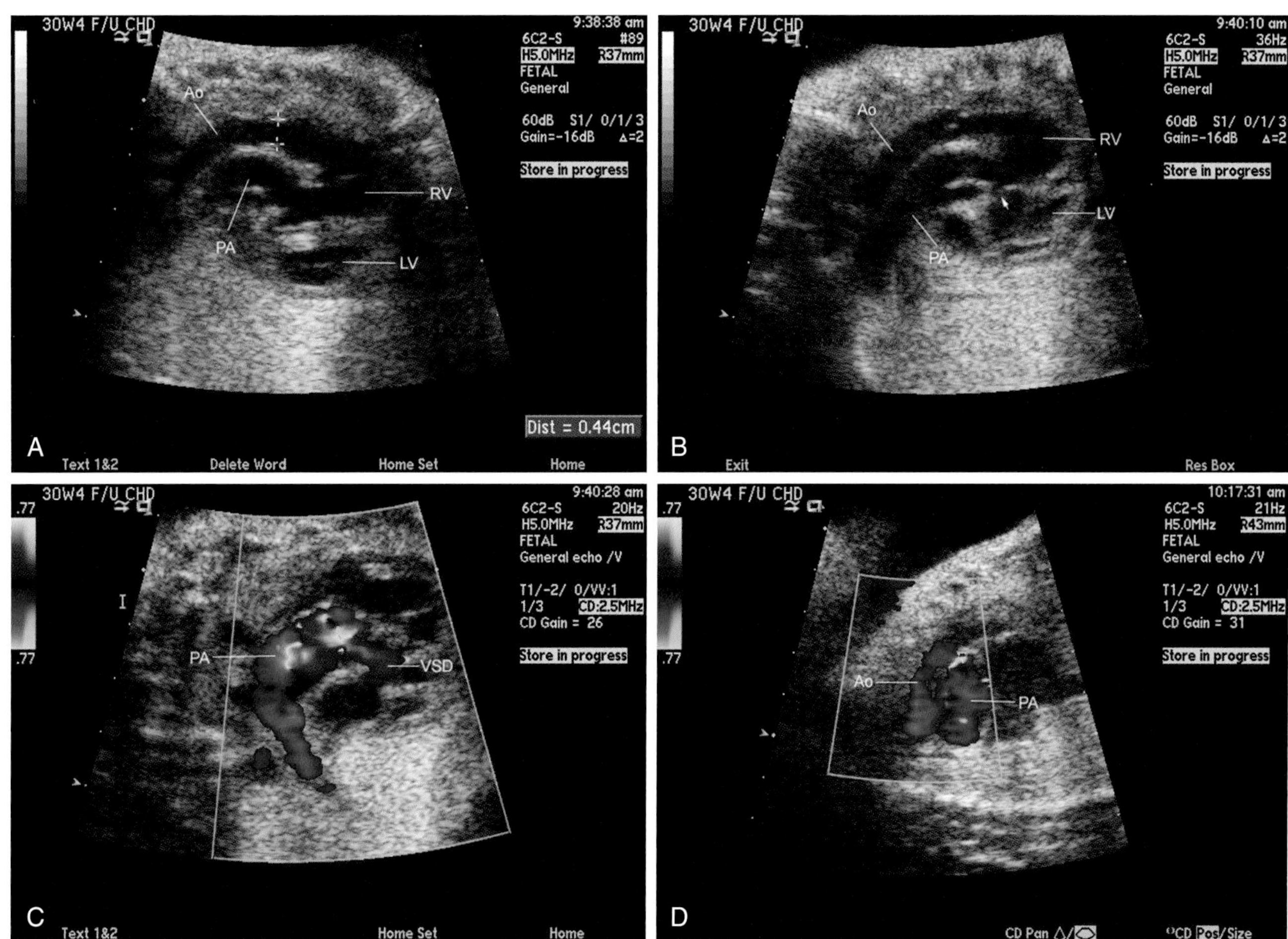

Case 16-1. **(A)** In this fetus with double-outlet right ventricle (DORV), the two great vessels arise directly from the right ventricle (RV). They are of relatively equal size. Ao, aorta; LV, left ventricle; PA, pulmonary artery. **(B)** Angling superiorly, two vessels arising from the RV and travel in parallel. The Ao is more rightward and anterior and the PA is more leftward and slightly posterior. One can begin to see evidence of a ventricular septal defect as identified by the *arrow.* **(C)** Color flow imaging demonstrates the presence of a ventricular septal defect (VSD) as identified by the red jet. The jet emerges from the LV and traverses through the VSD and into the PA; hence, this is a DORV with subpulmonary VSD. **(D)** More cephalad angling with color flow imaging demonstrates parallel vessels emerging from the heart.

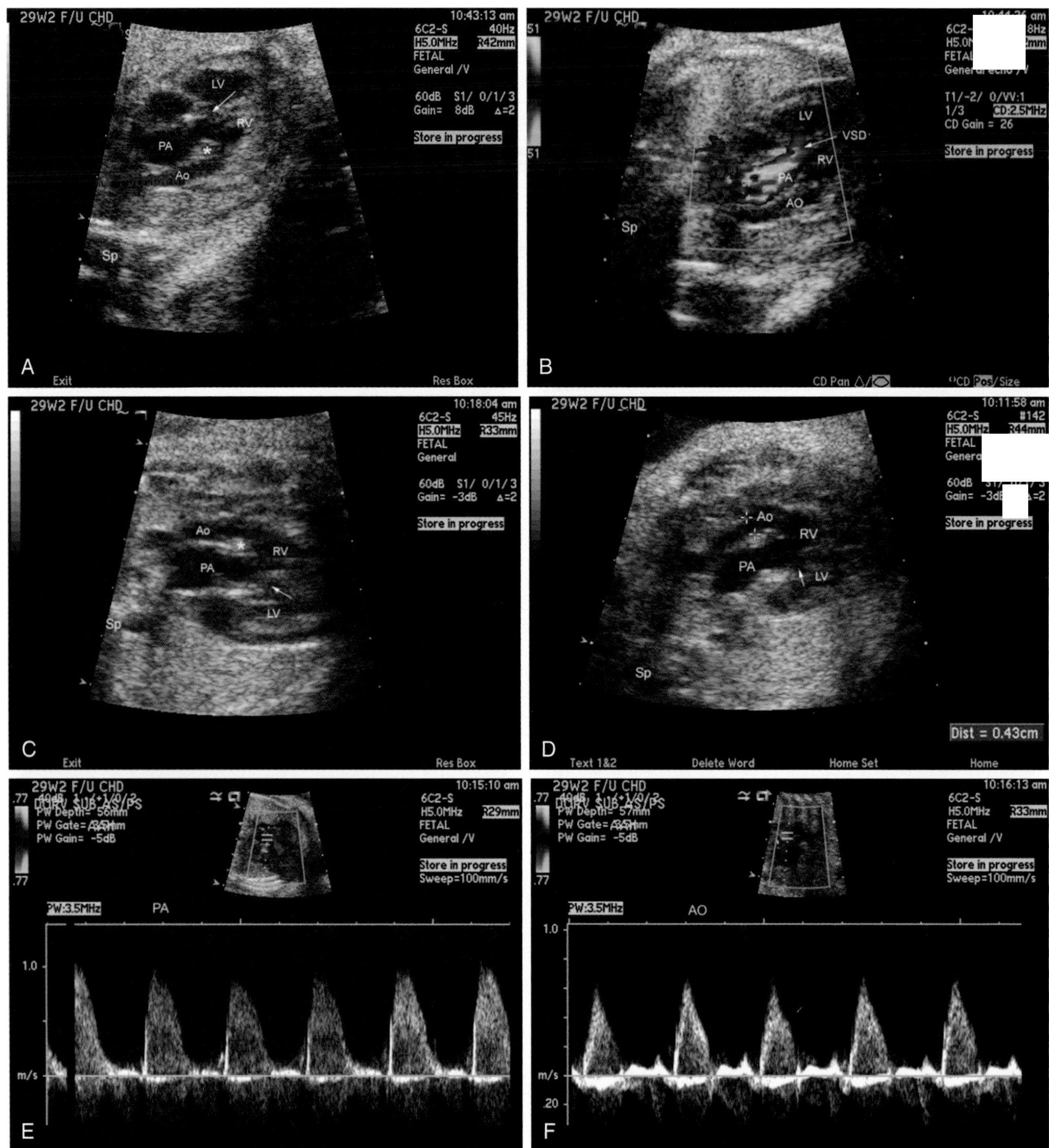

Case 16-2. (A) Image of a fetus with DORV. The *arrow* points to the VSD. The *star* demonstrates the position of the infundibular/conal septum, which is anteriorly malaligned and partially obstructing the subaortic region. The VSD is located just beneath the PA; this reflects a subpulmonic VSD type of DORV. Sp, spine. (B) Color flow imaging demonstrates flow across the VSD. One can see flow continuity between the cavity of the LV, the VSD, and flow into the PA. This demonstrates a subpulmonic type VSD. Notice the conal septum sitting beneath the aorta, which prevents VSD flow from reaching the subaortic and aortic region. This particular configuration is important because it has implications for postoperative management. In DORV, one will try to baffle the VSD to a great vessel. The intent would be to direct left ventricular flow to the aorta; however, because of this particular configuration, and with the septal defect being subpulmonic, it is not possible to baffle the LV to the aorta directly. Hence, an arterial switch operation placing the aorta onto the site of the PA and closure of the VSD to the newly positioned aorta is the option of choice. (C) Long-axis view of the heart demonstrates the substantial difference in size between the PA and the aorta. The *arrow* points once again to the VSD, which is subpulmonic in nature. The *star* demonstrates the infundibular septum, which is narrowing the outflow tract pathway to the aorta. Often, such patients will also have abnormalities distal to the subaortic narrowing such as a coarctation of the aorta or an interruption of the aortic arch. (D) Image focusing on the subaortic region and the position of the VSD. (E) Doppler flow pattern in the PA reveals laminar flow but with an increased velocity up to 1 m/sec reflecting a somewhat increased volume of blood flow relative to normal. (F) Doppler flow pattern in the aorta (AO) reveals somewhat diminished peak velocity. Notice the rapid upstroke and altered deceleration slope, which reflects an aspect of dynamic subaortic narrowing because, during systole, there is diminution in diameter of the outflow tract secondary to the conal position and hypertrophy.

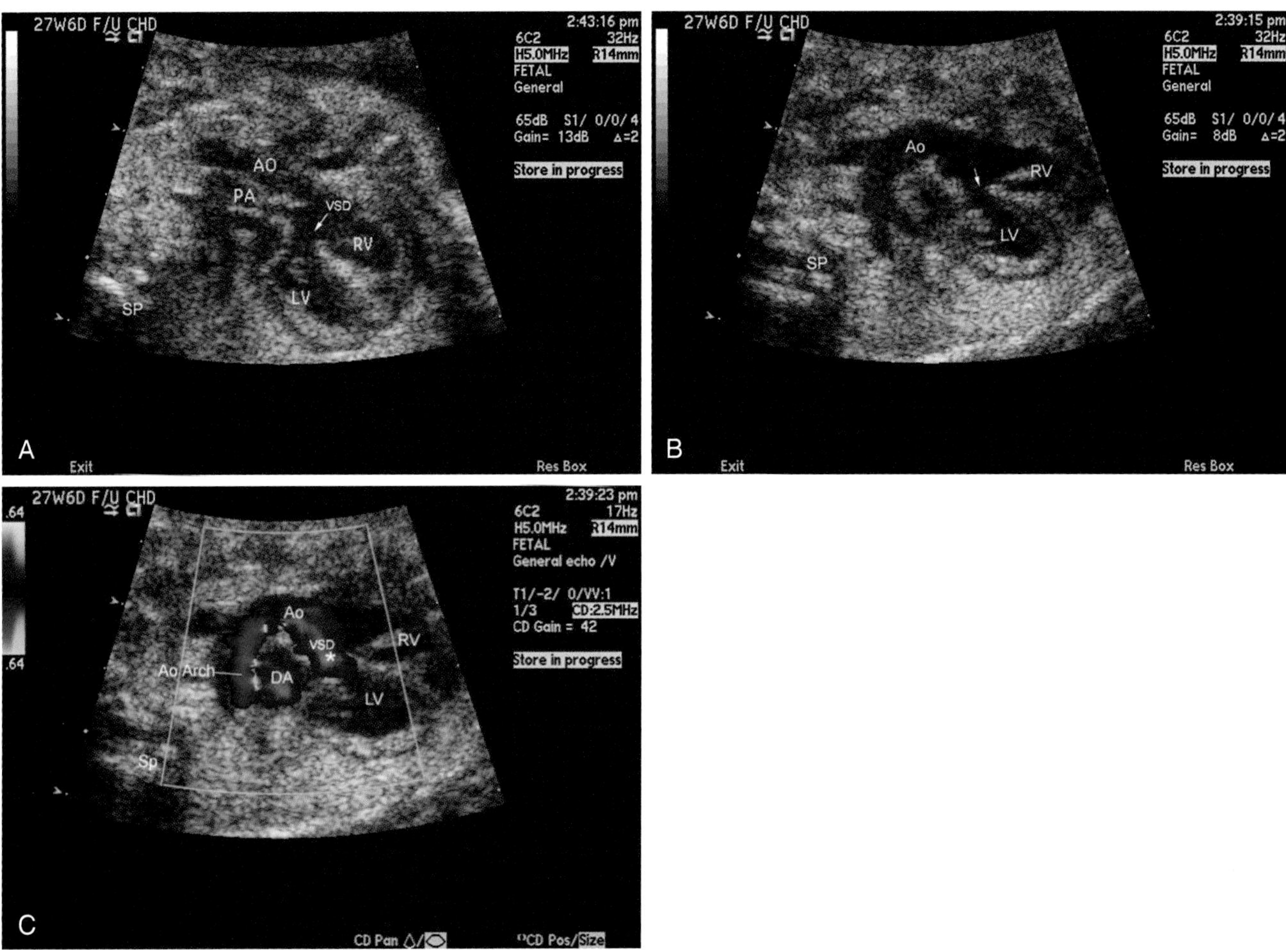

Case 16-3. **(A)** Demonstration of a DORV with a large VSD (*arrow*). It is difficult to say in this cut as to whether this is a subaortic or subpulmonic VSD; however, the aorta (AO) appears larger than the PA, suggesting a subaortic defect. **(B)** More rightward and superior angulation demonstrates the VSD (*arrow*) to be positioned directly beneath the aorta; hence, this is a subaortic VSD type of DORV. SP, spine. **(C)** Color flow imaging further highlights the subaortic nature of this VSD as the flow exits the LV and is directed into the aorta (Ao), which arises from the RV. Note the retrograde (*red*) flow in the ductus arteriosus (DA), suggesting the presence of pulmonic stenosis as is typically the case in a subaortic VSD type of DORV. The physiology and flow patterns in this anomaly are similar to that in tetralogy of Fallot. Ao Arch, aortic arch.

17

Truncus Arteriosus

Amanda Shillingford

Key Echocardiographic Features

- One great vessel and one semilunar valve arising from the heart.
- Origin of the branch pulmonary arteries from the trunk—from a single main pulmonary artery? Independently from the sides of the trunk?
- Commonly, no ductus arteriosus is present, unless the branch pulmonary arteries are discontinuous, in which case, the branch pulmonary artery not connected to the trunk is perfused by a ductus arteriosus.
- Large ventricular septal defect beneath the large single great vessel arising from the heart.
- Function of the truncal valve—is there stenosis or insufficiency?
- Aortic arch sidedness.
- Continuity or interruption of the aortic arch.

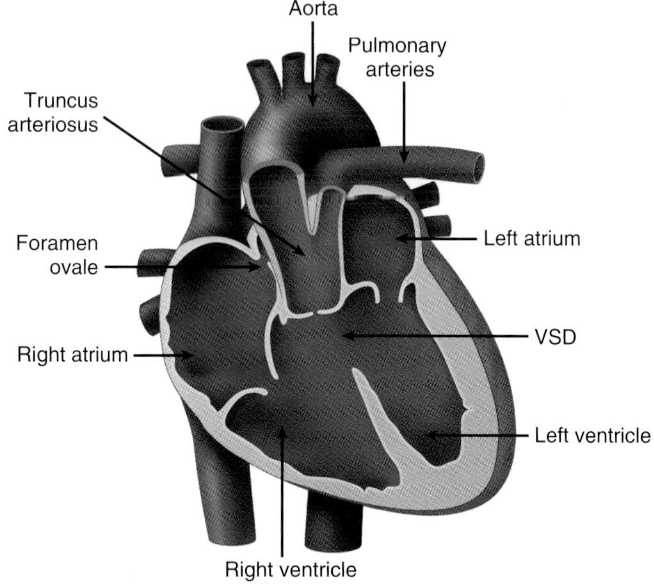

Figure 17-1. Truncus arteriosus.

Anatomy and Anatomical Associations

Truncus arteriosus (TA) is a conotruncal malformation of the heart. The embryologic *conotruncus* consists of the muscularized conus or conal septum and the adjacent *truncus arteriosus,* which gives rise to the outflow tracts. Early in development, the *conotruncus* originates from the primitive right ventricle but then shifts leftward over the forming ventricular septum. To complete normal development, septation of the *truncus arteriosus* must occur followed by rotation of the outflow tracts giving rise to a left ventricle-to-aorta relationship and a right ventricle-to-pulmonary artery relationship. In TA, septation does not occur properly, leaving a single arterial trunk that originates from both ventricles and gives rise to the aortic arch, at least one pulmonary artery, and at least one coronary artery. The arterial trunk almost always sits over a large ventricular septal defect (VSD), which exists because of a deficiency of the conal septum (Figure 17-1).

TA occurs in several forms described in two main classification schemes. Collett and Edwards[1] proposed a classification system in 1949 based on the origin of the pulmonary arteries. A type I TA occurs when a short main pulmonary artery trunk originates from the proximal trunk and gives rise to the branch pulmonary arteries. In type II TA, the branch pulmonary arteries arise separately from the arterial trunk but are close in proximity. In type III TA, the branch pulmonary arteries arise separately but are further away from one another. Type IV TA was originally described as pulmonary arteries originating from the descending aorta, but this anatomical variant is now considered to be a form of tetralogy of Fallot with pulmonary atresia. Van Praagh and Van Praagh[2] proposed a modified scheme in 1965 (Figure 17-2). A type AI is identical to the Collett and Edwards type I with a main pulmonary artery arising from the arterial trunk. Type AII includes all cases in which the branch pulmonary arteries arise separately from the proximal trunk regardless of the distance between them. Type AIII includes cases in which one pulmonary artery, usually the right, arises from the proximal trunk, and the contralateral lung is supplied by a pulmonary artery arising more distally either from the aortic arch or from a collateral vessel. Type AIV is TA associated with an interrupted aortic arch. In this type, a

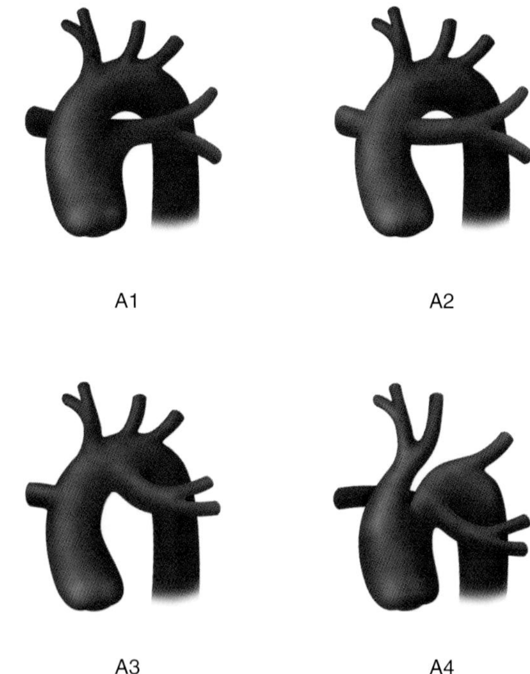

Figure 17-2. Truncus arteriosus classification.

large common trunk gives rise to (1) a main pulmonary artery that bifurcates into both branch pulmonary arteries, (2) an ascending aorta that gives rise to head and neck vessels, and (3) a patent ductus arteriosus that connects to the descending aorta. Types AI and AII are the most common variants, followed by type AIV then AIII.[3]

There is a single semilunar truncal valve in TA. This common truncal valve is often abnormal with thickened, dysplastic leaflets and is in fibrous continuity with the mitral valve. The truncal valve may have multiple leaflets, reflecting its developmental origins and potential for differentiation into the aortic and pulmonic valves, which failed to occur. A trileaflet truncal valve is most common, followed by a quadrileaflet and a bileaflet, or bicuspid, variant.[4,5] Significant stenosis or regurgitation is common and can affect clinical presentation and prognosis. A ductus arteriosus is absent in Van Praagh type AI and AII, but is always present in type AIV, and can be present in type AIII because a pulmonary artery can originate from the ductus arteriosus. Coronary artery abnormalities are frequent, with a single coronary artery the most common variant.[3,6] Other cardiac associations include aberrant origin of the arch vessels, right aortic arch, and a left superior vena cava.[5] Intracardiac abnormalities such as hypoplasia of an atrioventricular valve and ventricular hypoplasia have been reported in association with TA, but these are exceedingly rare.

Frequency, Genetics, and Development

TA is an uncommon anomaly, accounting for 1% to 2% of all forms of congenital heart disease. Extracardiac anatomic anomalies and chromosomal abnormalities exist in nearly one half of patients with TA.[7,8] The most common genetic abnormality is microdeletion of chromosome 22q11 (22q11 del). This is the chromosome abnormality identified in 90% of patients with DiGeorge syndrome and is associated with multiple extracardiac defects such as palatal abnormalities; feeding and speech difficulties; thymic hypoplasia leading to immunodeficiency and hypocalcemia; varying degrees of developmental, cognitive, and psychological deficits; facial dysmorphism; and renal and skeletal abnormalities. Congenital heart disease is estimated to occur in 75% to 80% of patients with 22q11 del; the most common cardiac defects noted are abnormalities of conotruncal formation, including tetralogy of Fallot, interrupted aortic arch, and truncus arteriosus.[9] Over one third of patients with TA have been identified to have 22q11 del, and 50% of cases with an associated interrupted aortic arch (Van Praagh type AIV) have 22q11 del.[10,11] The molecular and genetic causes specific to the formation of TA are still mostly unknown, although studies have demonstrated that abnormalities of neural crest cell migration play an important role.[12]

Prenatal Physiology

In TA, the normal fetal flow patterns are disrupted. In the normal fetal heart, the left ventricle and aorta have higher oxygen content due to right-to-left streaming of ductus venosus flow across the atrial septum. The presence of a large VSD allows intracardiac mixing of the blood returning to the right heart, and with only one outlet in existence, the blood in the pulmonary circulation has the same oxygen content as the blood in the systemic circulation. In general, the fetus tolerates this environment quite well. However, significant abnormalities of the truncal valve can result in fetal distress in TA because the common arterial trunk is the only exit from the heart. Stenosis and regurgitation of the truncal valve tend to occur mutually within the same patient, typically, in the setting of a markedly dysplastic valve.[8] In such cases, the fetus can develop ventricular dilation, heart failure, and hydrops.

If the pulmonary arteries are discontinuous as in TA Van Praagh type AIII, the pulmonary vasculature of the lung that is not attached to the main trunk may have relatively limited blood flow in comparison with the pulmonary vasculature of the lung that is directly receiving blood flow from the trunk. Such disparity in flow between the lungs may cause differences in pulmonary vascular development, which may be problematic after birth.

Intrauterine growth retardation is commonly present in the fetus with TA and is associated with 22q11del.[13]

Prenatal Management

Fetal echocardiographic imaging will detail all elements of the anatomy. The four-chamber view may appear normal because the right and left ventricles and atrioventricular valves are of normal size and structure. A single great vessel with a single semilunar valve will be seen originating from the heart, with a large VSD beneath. The greatest challenge in TA is identifying the origin and course of the branch pulmonary arteries. The pulmonary artery origins should be identified in every patient in order to appropriately classify the type of TA and determine whether postnatal prostaglandin therapy should be initiated. The base of the trunk should be identified in either long- or short-axis view and a slow, careful sweep cephalad should reveal the origin of the pulmonary arteries. Alternatively, if not found in this manner, a reverse search back from "lung-to-trunk" may be helpful. By identifying the branch pulmonary artery in the lung parenchyma using color Doppler imaging, one can track the branch pulmonary artery vessel back to the heart and trace its origin from the trunk.

The differential diagnosis of TA includes tetralogy of Fallot with pulmonary atresia. In the latter, a separate main pulmonary artery trunk can be identified, even if there is no flow into it. In TA, at least one of the branch pulmonary arteries is seen arising from the trunk, whereas in tetralogy of Fallot with pulmonary atresia, no pulmonary artery arises directly from the aorta without an interposed ductus arteriosus or collateral vessel (see Chapter 11).

In the absence of severe truncal valve abnormalities or extracardiac abnormalities, the fetus with TA is usually stable. Serial fetal echocardiography studies are recommended to delineate the morphology and competency of the truncal valve and, if abnormalities are present, to monitor for signs of heart failure or hydrops. Color Doppler flow across the valve as well as pulse Doppler will allow an estimate of the degree of regurgitation or stenosis present.

Given the high frequency of extracardiac abnormalities in the TA population, a comprehensive obstetrical fetal anatomy ultrasound should be performed in every fetus, and an assessment of karyotype is strongly recommended. Counseling of families regarding the operative course and prognosis will be linked to these findings. Families should also be aware that there is the risk of fetal demise when there are truncal valve abnormalities.

Postnatal Physiology

The newborn with TA has a significant amount of mixing of the pulmonary and systemic circulations. Mixing of the venous returns takes place at the ventricular level due to the large VSD, and mixing further take place at ejection into the common trunk. Owing to this intracardiac mixing, the ratio of pulmonary blood flow to systemic flow is determined by the relative resistances of the two vascular beds. Thus, during the immediate postnatal period when pulmonary vascular resistance is still elevated, a newborn with TA (and without significant truncal valve abnormalities or ductal dependent flow) may have a mild degree of hypoxemia and otherwise balanced pulmonary and systemic circulation. However, over the next several weeks as the pulmonary vascular resistance continues to drop, pulmonary blood flow increases. Hypoxemia will resolve, and the infant will develop signs of congestive heart failure such as tachycardia, tachypnea, diaphoresis, and poor feeding. If left unaddressed, pulmonary vascular obstructive disease can develop early in TA as compared with other lesions with large left-to-right shunts.[4]

There are some patients with TA who, relatively early in the first few days of life, exhibit an interesting and dangerous phenomenon. Due to a precipitous drop in pulmonary vascular resistance, there can be torrential run-off into the pulmonary vasculature creating a steal from the systemic circulation. Such patients may be unstable and exhibit very wide pulse pressure and hypotension. Systemic steal can also cause mesenteric vascular supply insufficiency leading to gut ischemia and the development of necrotizing enterocolitis. Renal insufficiency can also occur in this scenario. These complications can increase the surgical risks for the patient.

In Van Praagh type AIII, one branch pulmonary artery can originate from a ductus arteriosus. Similarly, in Van Praagh type AIV, the descending aorta is supplied by a large ductus arteriosus. These infants are at risk for significant hemodynamic compromise in the event of ductal closure, and therefore, prostaglandin therapy should be initiated immediately upon delivery.

In patients with significant truncal valve stenosis or regurgitation, congestive heart failure symptoms due to chronic volume and pressure overload may develop early. Moreover, truncal valve stenosis is a risk factor for death.[13] Although rare, some patients with TA may have stenosis of the origin of the branch pulmonary vessels and may not develop pulmonary overcirculation, but exhibit cyanosis.[4]

The physical examination of patients with TA depends on the status of the truncal valve and the amount of pulmonary blood flow present. Peripheral pulses are prominent and bounding with a widened pulse pressure. A systolic thrill may be appreciated, as well as a single loud second heart sound. An ejection click may be heard after the first heart sound and has been shown to correlate with maximal opening of the truncal valve. A loud pandiastolic murmur can be auscultated at the lower left sternal border. A diastolic murmur may be heard near the apex due to increased flow across the mitral valve. If significant truncal valve regurgitation is present, a more prominent diastolic murmur will be appreciated.[4]

Postnatal Management

In the absence of significant truncal valve disease or ductal dependency, the infant with TA is often stable after delivery. In Van Praagh types AI and AII, there is no ductus arteriosus, so prostaglandin should not be initiated. A prostaglandin infusion should be offered in cases in which a ductus arteriosus is present, as in Van Praagh types AIII and AIV, for perfusion of the isolated lung in the former and the systemic circulation in the latter.

In the past, infants without ductal dependent flow were routinely discharged home and managed medically for congestive heart failure symptoms with a plan for elective repair at several weeks or months of age. However, this strategy has fallen out of favor, in particular because it is difficult to predict who will develop the scenario of torrential pulmonary overcirculation and its sequelae as stated previously. In the current era, most centers perform complete repair in the neonatal period with good results.[3,5]

A complete repair involves closure of the VSD and removal of the branch pulmonary arteries from the common arterial trunk with commitment of the common arterial trunk to the left ventricle and conduit from the right ventricle to the pulmonary artery. In Van Praagh types AII and AIII, the branch pulmonary arteries are brought together as a confluence, and a conduit is placed between the right ventricle and the pulmonary arteries. Since the first surgical repair of TA in 1967, numerous modifications of the surgical technique have been offered, and as for all surgery for congenital heart disease, techniques continue to improve for the better.[14]

The type of material used for the right ventricle-to-pulmonary artery conduit has varied from aortic or pulmonary homograft to xenograft (bovine or porcine) valved conduits. No currently available conduits have the ability to grow with the patient, and therefore, all neonatal conduits must be upsized and changed at some point in later childhood and almost certainly again in adulthood. This obligates the neonate with TA to multiple heart operations throughout life. In addition, the truncal valve when now utilized as the aortic valve after repair is not developmentally normal and is at risk for developing insufficiency over time.[4] Finally, patients with a Van Praagh type AIV undergo aortic arch repair for interruption and are at risk for late narrowing and need for re-intervention.

Outcomes

Overall, surgical outcomes for TA have improved significantly, and several centers report early surgical mortality after neonatal repair as 3% to 5% and survival at 6 years as high as 93%.[3,5] Patients with significant truncal valve disease or an interrupted aortic arch are at higher risk for mortality and complications.[3,15] A report from the Congenital Heart Surgeons Society[16] pooled results from 33 institutions that performed surgical repair on patients with TA type AIV between 1987 and 1997. Hospital survival was only 44% in this group of 50 patients.[16] However, in another single center experience of 16 patients who underwent repair for TA Van Praagh type AIV, 12.5% mortality was found at a median follow-up of 18 years.[17]

Patients with TA are at risk for a number of morbidities and the need for multiple re-interventions. Almost 50% of neonates will need the right ventricle-to-pulmonary artery conduit replaced by 5 years and 70% by 10 years.[3,5] In one recent study of TA repair between 1986 and 2003, the need for truncal valve (neo-aortic) re-intervention was nearly 20% at 5 years.[15] There is a correlation between significant truncal valve insufficiency at neonatal presentation and the need for early re-intervention.[15] Finally, the presence of a right ventricle-to-pulmonary conduit places the patient at similar risks as described in the tetralogy of Fallot population, including chronic pulmonary insufficiency, right ventricular dilation and failure, exercise intolerance, and arrhythmias.

Imaging Essentials and Important Points

- Identify a large VSD and a single large great artery arising from the heart, positioned over the ventricular septum.
- A true TA gives rise to the aortic arch, at least one pulmonary artery, and at least one coronary artery (the coronary will likely not be visualized in the fetus).
- At least one pulmonary artery arises proximal on the common arterial trunk in TA—if the first pulmonary artery does not originate until one sees the aortic arch or descending aorta, the diagnosis is likely tetralogy of Fallot with pulmonary atresia and not TA.
- In a Van Praagh type AI TA, the main pulmonary artery trunk may be very short and originates very proximal on the common arterial trunk.
- In a Van Praagh type AII TA, the branch pulmonary arteries can arise very close together or further apart and more posterior, but still proximal on the common arterial trunk.
- A ductus arteriosus will only be seen in a Van Praagh type AIV TA or in a type AIII TA if the ductus arteriosus gives rise to the second pulmonary artery.
- Evaluate the appearance of the truncal valve and assess the truncal valve for insufficiency and stenosis.
- Assess aortic arch sidedness.
- In the setting of significant truncal valve stenosis or insufficiency, evaluate the fetus for signs of ventricular dysfunction and hydrops.
- In type AIV TA, the interruption usually occurs after the left carotid artery.
- Assess for thymic tissue, because its absence may suggest the presence of DiGeorge's syndrome (22q11 deletion).

References

1. Collett RW, Edwards JE. Persistent truncus arteriosus: a classification according to anatomic types. *Surg Clin North Am.* 1949;29: 1245-1270.
2. Van Praagh R, Van Praagh S. The anatomy of common aorticopulmonary trunk (truncus arteriosus communis) and its embryologic implications. A study of 57 necropsy cases. *Am J Cardiol.* 1965;16: 406-425.
3. Thompson LD, McElhinney DB, Reddy M, Petrossian E, Silverman NH, Hanley FL. Neonatal repair of truncus arteriosus: continuing improvement in outcomes. *Ann Thorac Surg.* 2001;72: 391-395.
4. Mair DD, Edwards WD, Julsrud PR, Seward JB, Danielson GK, Goldmuntz E. Truncus arteriosus. In Allen HD, Gutsegall HP, Clark EB, Driscoll DJ, eds. Moss and Adams' Heart Disease in Infants, Children, and Adolescents. 6th ed. Philadelphia: Lippincott Williams & Wilkins; 2001:910-923.

5. Kalavrouziotis G, Purohit M, Ciotti G, Corno AF, Pozzi M. Truncus arteriosus communis: early and midterm results of early primary repair. *Ann Thorac Surg*. 2006;82:2200-2206.
6. de la Cruz MV, Cayre R, Angelini P, Noriega-Ramos N, Sadowinski S. Coronary arteries in truncus arteriosus. *Am J Cardiol*. 1990;66: 1482-1486.
7. Ferencz C, Rubin JD, McCarter RJ, et al. Congenital heart disease: prevalence at livebirth. The Baltimore-Washington Infant Study. *Am J Epidemiol*. 1985;121:31-36.
8. Volpe P, Paladini D, Marasini M, et al. Common arterial trunk in the fetus: characteristics, associations, and outcome in a multicentre series of 23 cases. *Heart*. 2003;89:1437-1441.
9. Goldmuntz E. DiGeorge syndrome: new insights. *Clin Perinatol*. 2005;32:963-967.
10. Goldmuntz E, Clark BJ, Mitchell LE, et al. Frequency of 22q11 deletions in patients with conotruncal defects. *J Am Coll Cardiol*. 1998;32:492-498.
11. Volpe P, Marasini M, Caruso G, et al. 22q11 deletions in fetuses with malformations of the outflow tracts or interruption of the aortic arch: impact of additional ultrasound signs. *Prenat Diagn*. 2003;23:752-757.
12. Hutson MR, Kirby ML. Neural crest and cardiovascular development: a 20-year perspective. *Birth Defects Res C Embryo Today*. 2003; 69:2-13.
13. Duke C, Sharland GK, Jones AM, Simpson JM. Echocardiographic features and outcome of truncus arteriosus diagnosed during fetal life. *Am J Cardiol*. 2001;88:1379-1384.
14. McGoon DC, Rastelli GC, Ongley PA. An operation for the correction of truncus arteriosus. *JAMA*. 1968;205:69-73.
15. Henaine R, Azarnoush K, Belli E, et al. Fate of the truncal valve in truncus arteriosus. *Ann Thorac Surg*. 2008;85:172-178.
16. Konstantinov IE, Karamlou T, Blackstone EH, et al. Truncus arteriosus associated with interrupted aortic arch in 50 neonates: a Congenital Heart Surgeons Society study. *Ann Thorac Surg*. 2006;81: 214-222.
17. Bohrta L, Hussein A, Fricke T, et al. Surgical repair of truncus arteriosus associated with interrupted aortic arch: long term outcomes. *Ann Thorac*. 2011;91:1473-1478.

CASES

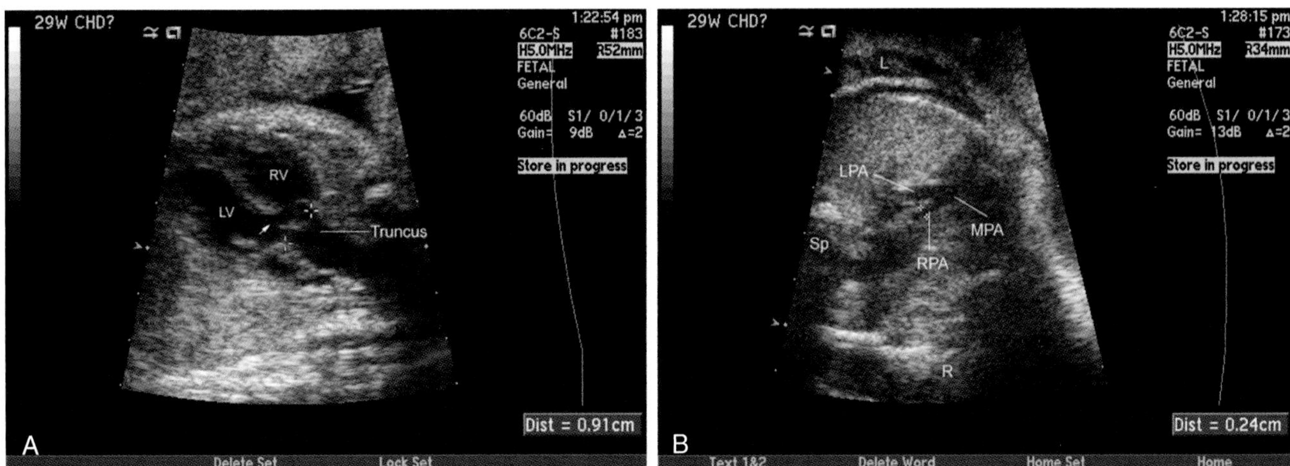

Case 17-1. **(A)** Long-axis view of the right (RV) and left ventricle (LV). There is a single large great vessel arising from the heart, which is a common trunk (truncus). The *arrow* points to the ventricular septal defect. **(B)** Posterior and cephalad angulation demonstrates the origin of the main pulmonary artery (MPA) and right (RPA) and left (LPA) branches. Because an MPA segment is present, this is a type I truncus arteriosus. Sp, spine.

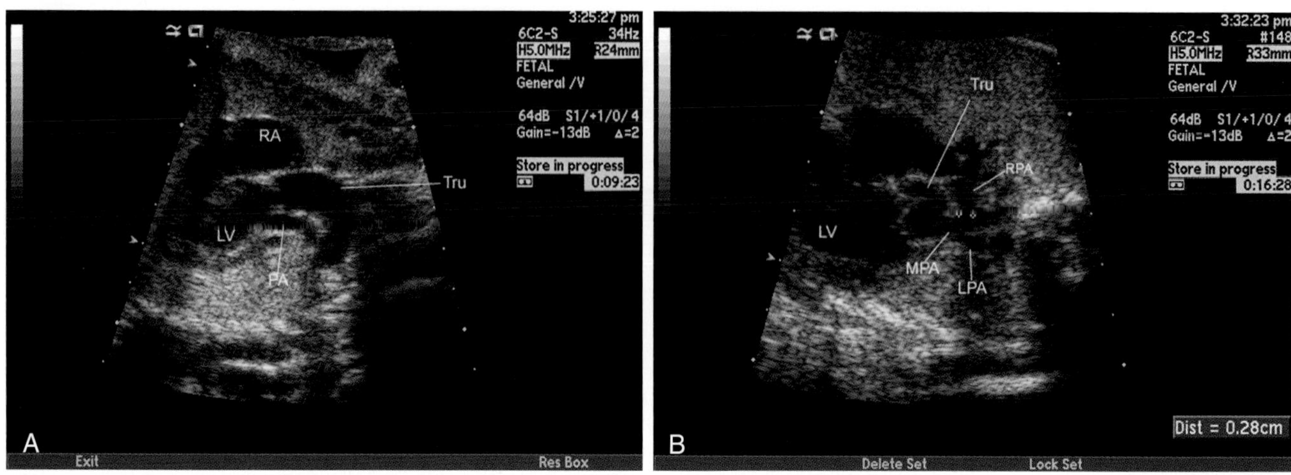

Case 17-2. **(A)** Truncus arteriosus (Tru) with a well-formed main pulmonary artery (MPA) segment (PA). **(B)** Slight posterior angulation demonstrates the MPA and the origins of the left (LPA) and right (RPA) pulmonary arteries. LV, left ventricle.

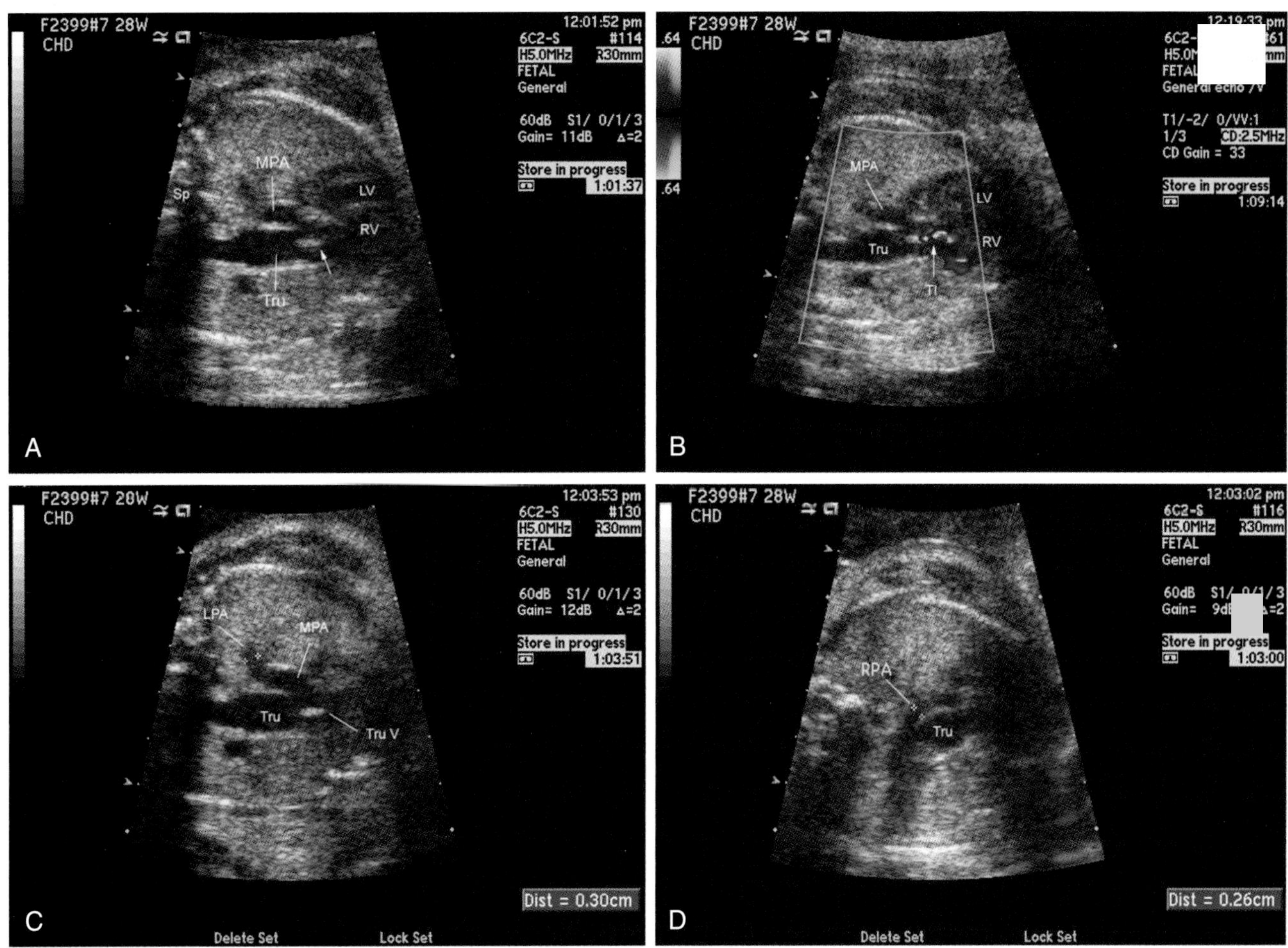

Case 17-3. **(A)** Truncus arteriosus type I (Tru) with main pulmonary artery segment (MPA). The *arrow* points to a thickened truncal valve. LV, left ventricle; RV, right ventricle; Sp, spine. **(B)** Mild truncal valve insufficiency (TI) is noted. **(C)** The left pulmonary artery (LPA) arises from the MPA and trunk in an unobstructed manner. The LPA measures 3 mm in diameter, which is of good size at 28 weeks' gestation. TruV, truncal valve. **(D)** The right pulmonary artery (RPA) measures 2.6 mm in diameter.

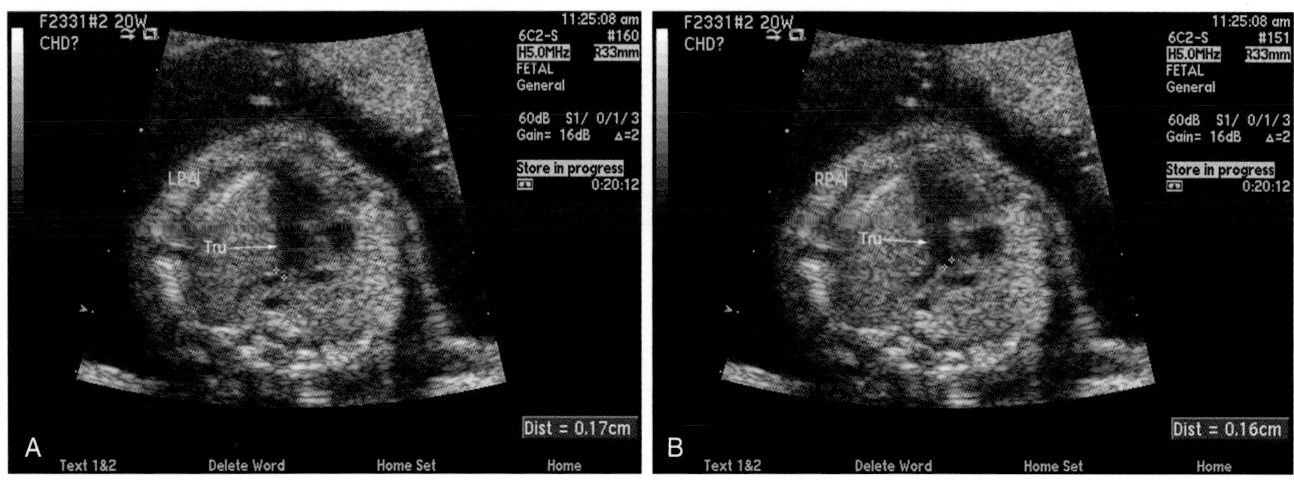

Case 17-4. **(A)** Truncus arteriosus type II (Tru) with the branch pulmonary arteries arising directly from the trunk without a main pulmonary artery. This image demonstrates the left pulmonary artery (LPA) arising directly from the side of the trunk. **(B)** Origin of the right pulmonary artery (RPA) from the side of the common trunk.

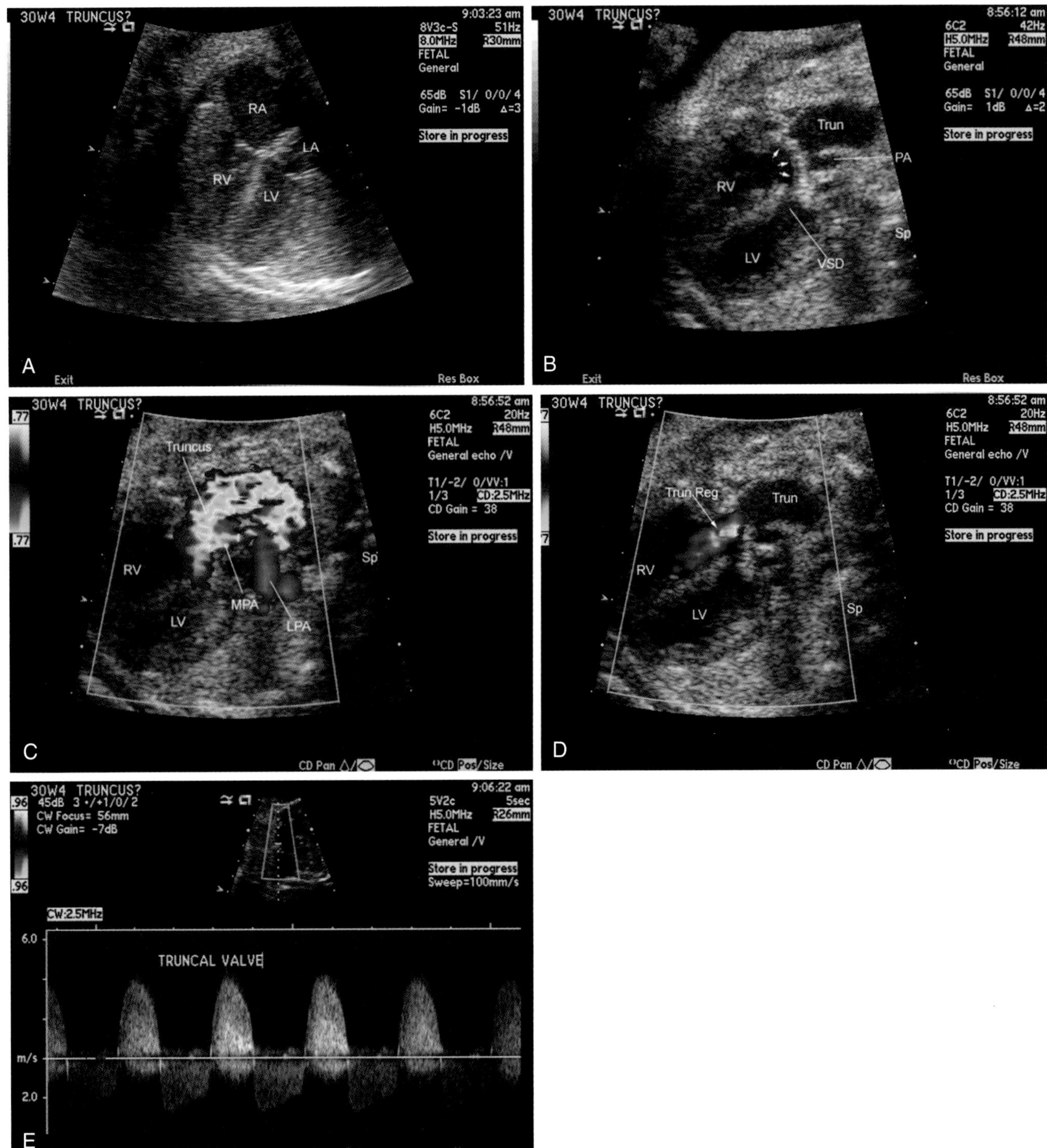

Case 17-5. **(A)** Four-chamber view of a fetus with truncus arteriosus and an abnormal, stenotic and regurgitant truncal valve. Note the abnormally thickened right ventricle (RV) and dilated right atrium (RA). LA, left atrium; LV, left ventricle. **(B)** The *arrows* point to a doming abnormally thickened, stenotic truncal valve (Trun). Both the pulmonary artery (PA) and the systemic artery arise from a single great vessel with a common semilunar valve. Sp, spine; VSD, ventricular septal defect. **(C)** Color image in systole shows turbulent flow distal to the stenotic truncal valve with color also filling the main pulmonary artery (MPA) and left pulmonary artery (LPA). **(D)** Color image in diastole demonstrates severe truncal valve (Trun) regurgitation. The regurgitant color jet (Trun Reg) is wide and is greater than 50% of the diameter of the Trun. **(E)** Spectral Doppler tracing of truncal valve stenosis and regurgitation. Continuous wave Doppler interrogation across the truncal valve demonstrates a peak systolic velocity of 4 m/sec (peak instantaneous gradient of 64 mm Hg). There is also evidence of truncal regurgitation (flow below the baseline).

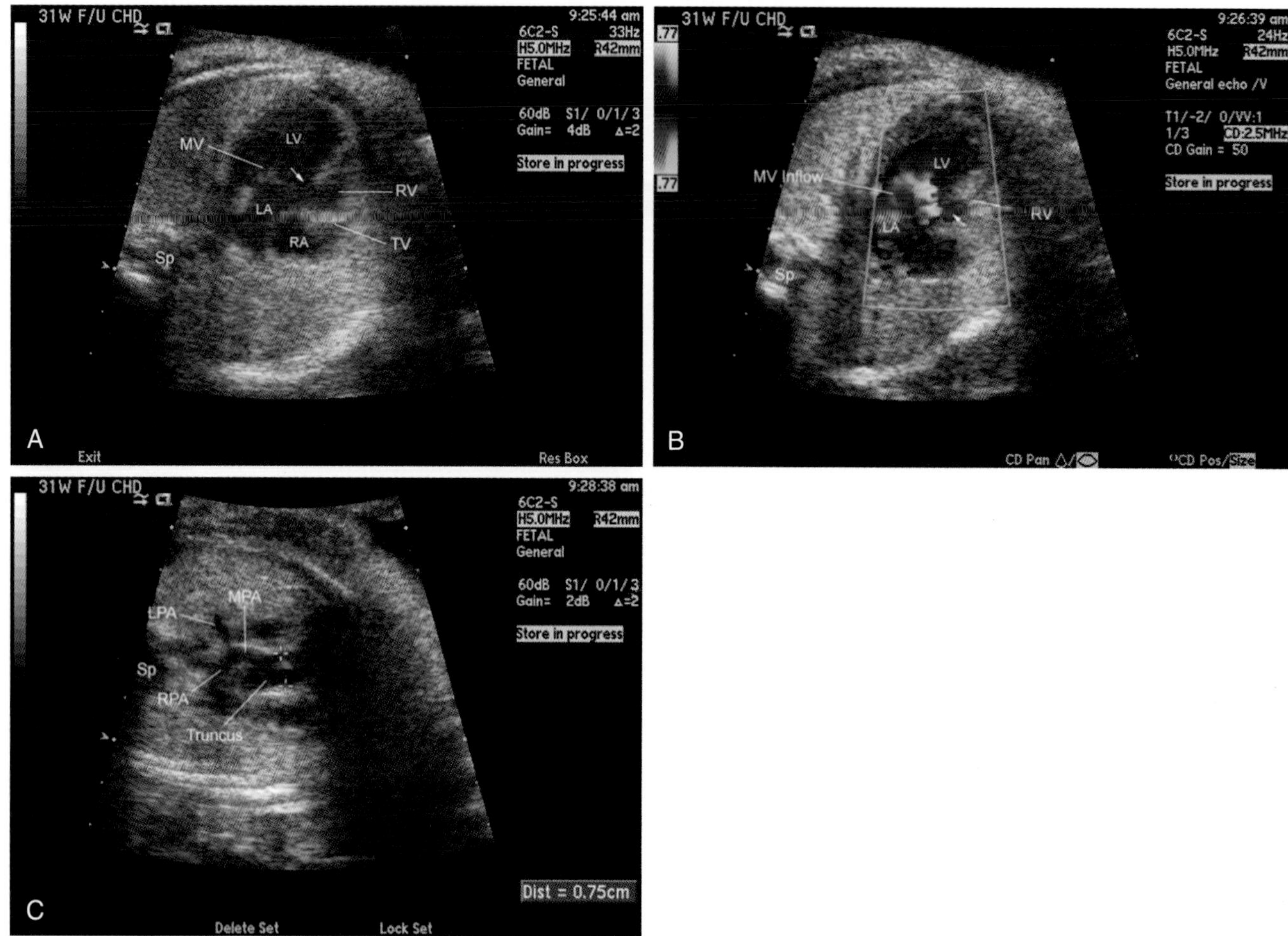

Case 17-6. **(A)** Four-chamber view of an unusual case of truncus arteriosus and tricuspid atresia. The right ventricle (RV) is small and communicates with the left ventricle (LV) via a ventricular septal defect *(arrow)*. The region of the tricuspid valve (TV) is atretic. LA, left atrium; MV, mitral valve; RA, right atrium. **(B)** Color imaging demonstrates inflow across the MV into the dilated LV; however, there is no atrioventricular valve inlet into the RV. The *arrow* points to the VSD leading into the hypoplastic RV. **(C)** Cephalad angulation reveals the common trunk with a main pulmonary artery (MPA) segment giving rise to the branch pulmonary arteries. LPA, left pulmonary artery; RPA, right pulmonary artery; Sp, spine.

18

Aortopulmonary Window

Jennifer Glatz

Key Echocardiographic Features

- Connection between the pulmonary artery and the aorta above the level of the two semilunar valves.
- The window is typically large.
- Commonly seen in association with other anomalies such as interruption of the aortic arch, coarctation of the aorta, and tetralogy of Fallot.

Anatomy and Anatomical Associations

An *aortopulmonary window (APW)* is a communication, or natural connection, between the ascending aorta and the main pulmonary artery. The presence of two semilunar valves distinguishes this anomaly from a truncus arteriosus. Both semilunar valves are normal in position (except when APW is in the presence of other malformations such as tetralogy of Fallot). The pulmonary artery and the aorta are typically contiguous at the defect (Figure 18-1). Generally, the connection occurs between the left margin of the ascending aorta and the right margin of the pulmonary artery. The defect is typically quite large and may be located a variable distance from the semilunar valves. A *simple APW* is defined as one without any significant associated anomalies, defects not requiring repair (such as a right aortic arch), or defects requiring a minor or simple repair (patent ductus arteriosus, atrial septal defect). A *complex APW* is one that occurs with another complex anomaly such as interruption of the aortic arch, tetralogy of Fallot, or anomalous origin of the coronary arteries. A variety of classification systems have been developed based on location and anatomical variations.[1-4]

Coexisting cardiac anomalies have been reported in 17% to 77% of patients with an APW.[3,5-7] Kutsche and Van Mierop[5] reviewed 249 patients with an APW and found 52% of the patients had an associated congenital cardiovascular anomaly. The most common anomalies were type A interruption of the aortic arch or severe coarctation of the aorta (13%). Other reported lesions included a right aortic arch (9%), bicuspid aortic valve, ventricular septal defect (VSD), tetralogy of Fallot (6%), anomalous origin of the coronary arteries from the pulmonary trunk (5%), atrial septal defect, pulmonary valve stenosis, tricuspid valve atresia, and aortic valve atresia or stenosis. After birth a persistent patent ductus arteriosus has been reported in approximately 12%.[8] Complete transposition of the great arteries and APW has also been reported.[9] Berry's syndrome consists of a distal APW, interrupted aortic arch, and aortic origin of the right pulmonary artery.[10] Other extracardiac malformations have also been reported including anomalies of the musculoskeletal, central nervous, renal, pulmonary, and gastrointestinal systems.[11] VATER (vertebral defects, imperforate anus, tracheoesophageal fistula, and radial and renal dysplasia) and VACTERL (vertebral abnormalities, anal atresia, cardiac abnormalities, tracheoesophageal fistula and/or esophageal atresia, renal agenesis and dysplasia, and limb defects) syndrome associations have also been reported in patients with APW.[5,11]

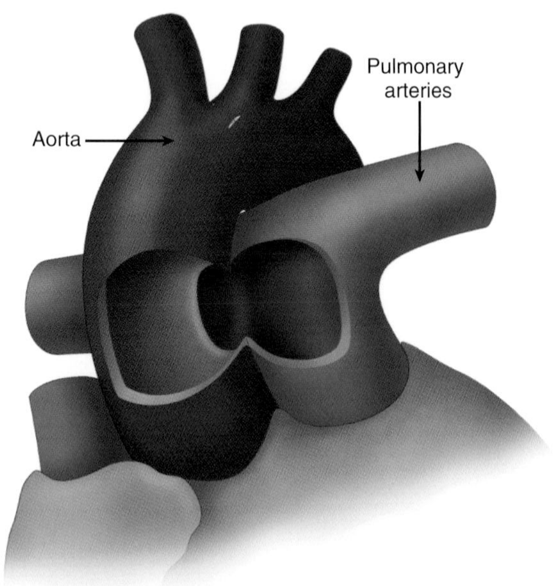

Figure 18-1. Aortopulmonary window.

Frequency, Genetics, and Development

APW is a rare congenital heart defect accounting for 0.2% to 0.6% of all congenital heart disease.[5] The female-to-male gender ratio for this defect is 1:3.

APW is caused by defective development of conotruncal ridges that normally grow to partition the aorta from the pulmonary artery.[5] The separation of the truncus arteriosus is incomplete or totally absent, leaving a persistent window between the aorta and the pulmonary artery. The aortopulmonary septum is formed by the two opposing truncal cushions that rapidly enlarge and fuse, dividing the truncus arteriosus into separate aortic and pulmonary channels. This division is influenced by cells that migrate from the neural crest. Removal of neural crest tissue results in other conotruncal abnormalities such as truncus arteriosus and transposition, but not APW, suggesting perhaps a different embryological origin.[12,13]

APW is not typically a hallmark for chromosomal abnormalities. Despite the fact that the anomalies are in the same region within the heart, an APW appears to be pathogenetically unrelated to other conotruncal malformations such as truncus arteriosus. There is no known causative genetic abnormality associated with APW.

Prenatal Physiology

APW has very little impact on the fetus owing to the high pulmonary vascular resistance associated with fetal circulation. The defect can be identified in utero by visualization of the large communication between the aorta and the pulmonary artery.[14] Flow patterns in the aorta, however, may be slightly altered. An APW can play the same role as a ductus arteriosus in the fetus, allowing for delivery of blood from the pulmonary artery to the aorta. Because the APW connects to the aorta more proximally than does the ductus arteriosus, the transverse aorta and isthmus may appear larger than normal because it receives antegrade flow from the left ventricle/ascending aorta as well as from the pulmonary artery via the APW. Because a greater degree of blood from the right ventricle is shunted to the aorta through the APW, the ductus arteriosus may be smaller than normal.

Prenatal Management

Prenatal diagnosis of APW is possible and has been described, although reports are limited.[14] Because the pulmonary artery and aorta are contiguous, adjacent structures at the site of the APW connection, it can be difficult to make the diagnosis because the tissue planes are quite thin and the region in question can have false drop-out.

The APW connection can be seen wherever bifurcation of the pulmonary arteries are best seen and wherever there is contiguity between the aorta and the pulmonary artery. The short-axis view in particular can be helpful because it best aligns the planes between the aorta and the pulmonary artery. By angling from a short-axis view cephalad into the mediastinum, the aortopulmonary septum can be visualized between the aortic root and the bifurcation of the pulmonary arteries.

Postnatal Physiology

Infants with a simple APW are hemodynamically stable and frequently asymptomatic in the early postnatal period and, therefore, do not require an urgent neonatal intervention. Following the typical hemodynamic alterations of early infancy, the heart often becomes enlarged owing to increased shunting across the defect from aorta to pulmonary artery and volume load. The pulmonary arteries may also become enlarged as a result of increased flow.

The timing to identification of APW is often based on the presence and type of associated lesions. Those with ductal-dependent lesions such as interruption of the aortic arch will present very early in infancy. Those patients with a moderate-sized isolated APW will commonly present with symptoms within the first few weeks of life.[1,2,12] These include signs of heart failure such as tachypnea, diaphoresis, and failure to thrive. Cyanosis is rare but can occur with bidirectional shunting through a large defect. On physical examination, there may be tachypnea, retractions, prominent right ventricular impulse, and bounding pulses (due to diastolic runoff). By auscultation, the second heart sound is accentuated and narrowly split. A prominent ejection click may also be heard in the pulmonic area.[12] A loud systolic ejection murmur at the left upper sternal border or a machinery-type murmur is present.[1] A thrill may be palpated. A middiastolic rumble may also be heard at the apex due to increased flow across the mitral valve. The anomaly may be confused with a patent ductus arteriosus. A large VSD and truncus arteriosus should also be considered in the differential diagnosis.

Postnatal Management

Medical management of this defect is limited because the definitive treatment is surgical. Operative repair should be performed early in life to avoid pulmonary vascular disease, which can occur as a result of the left-to-right shunt. Surgical techniques have included simple ligation, division and suture, trans-pulmonary artery closure, trans-window closure, and trans-aortic closure, and these may be performed with or without cardiopulmonary bypass.[15] The recommended approach for most patients is the trans-aortic patch closure utilizing cardiopulmonary bypass.[7,16] This transaortic approach allows for adequate exposure to the defect and access to correct the associated defects, such as arch anomalies. Although ligation seems to be a more simple procedure, it has been associated with incomplete closure of the defect, coronary artery injury, and distortion of the pulmonary artery. Reports of transcatheter closure of an APW have also been described with some success in patients in whom the size and location of the defect is amenable to device closure and in the absence of other coexisting anomalies.[17,18]

Outcomes

The prognosis of an APW depends on the associated cardiac malformations, age at operation, and presence of preoperative pulmonary vascular disease. Many of these risks are eliminated by the making of a prenatal diagnosis. The prognosis of an uncorrected APW is poor, with 40% of infants dying within the first year of life, and therefore, early surgical repair is essential.[7]

Many centers have reported successful outcomes for operative repair of an APW. Jansen and coworkers[19] reviewed their 37-year experience with 18 patients. They reported no early or late deaths after surgery with both primary and patch closure. In a recent series by Bhan and colleagues,[15] the hospital mortality for 21 infants was 13% for simple APW and 33% for complex APW. There were no reoperations or late deaths. McElhinney and associates[6] described their series of 24 patients all younger than 6 months of age, 12 of whom had a complex APW. There were no deaths for those with a simple APW. Two patients required re-intervention for pulmonary arterial narrowing at the anastomosis or patch site. Four (33%) of those with a complex APW died in the early postoperative period and another died 4 months after surgery. Re-intervention was required in 2 patients with arch interruption. Tkebuchava and coworkers[7] reported similar results with only 1 operative death and no late deaths in a total of 13 patients with an APW, giving an actuarial survival rate of 90%. In summary, the outcome for an isolated lesion repaired by trans-aortic approach before the development of pulmonary vascular disease is excellent.[6,7,16]

Subsequent operations are typically not required. Most of the late mortality is associated with pulmonary hypertension due to delayed repair, which should not occur when there is a prenatal diagnosis. Other possible morbidity and mortality is related to the associated cardiac lesions, in particular, interruption of the aortic arch.

Imaging Essentials and Important Points

- Unusual dilation of the aorta adjacent to the right pulmonary artery should raise suspicion of an APW.
- Diagnosis is confirmed by identifying a large communication between the proximal ascending aorta and the trunk of the pulmonary artery.
- A large APW may appear similar to a truncus arteriosus because the communication may give the impression of a single large vessel. APW is distinguished from truncus arteriosus by the presence of the two semilunar valves, aortic and pulmonic, in the former, with only a single truncal valve in the latter.
- Obtaining the correct plane to visualize the presence or absence of thin tissue between the aorta and the pulmonary artery can be tricky. False dropout in this region is common. The short-axis view with cephalad angulation can aid in best visualizing the aortopulmonary septum between the aortic root and the bifurcation of the pulmonary arteries.[20] Color Doppler flow may not be helpful because flow velocities across a large defect may be relatively low.
- Associated heart anomalies are common and should be searched for in all cases of APW.

References

1. Mori K, Ando M, Takao A, et al. Distal type of aortopulmonary window: report of 4 cases. *Br Heart J*. 1978;40:681-689.
2. Richardson JV, Doty DB, Rossi NP, Ehrenhaft JL. The spectrum of anomalies of aortopulmonary septation. *J Thorac Cardiovasc Surg*. 1979;78:21-27.
3. Ho SY, Gerlis LM, Anderson C, Devine WA, Smith A. The morphology of aortopulmonary window with regard to their classification and morphogenesis. *Cardiol Young*. 1994;4:146-155.
4. Jacobs JP, Quintessenza JA, Gaynor JW, Burke RP, Mavroudis C. Congenital Surgical Nomenclature and Database Project: aortopulmonary window. *Ann Thorac Surg*. 2000;69(suppl):S44-S49.
5. Kutsche LM, Van Mierop LH. Anatomy and pathogenesis of aorto-pulmonary septal defect. *Am J Cardiol*. 1987;59:443-447.
6. McElhinney DB, Reddy M, Tworetzsky W, Silverman NH, Hanley FL. Early and late results after repair of aorticopulmonary septal defect and associated anomalies in infants <6 months of age. *Am J Cardiol*. 1998;81:195-201.
7. Tkebuchava T, von Segesser LK, Vogt PR, et al. Congenital aortopulmonary window: diagnosis, surgical technique and long-term results. *Eur J Cardiothorac Surg*. 1997;11:293-297.
8. Neufeld HN, Lester RG, Adams P, Anderson RC, Lillehei CW, Edwards JE. Aorticopulmonary septal defect. *Am J Cardiol*. 1962;9:12-25.
9. Duca V, Sulliotti G, Maggio C, Corsello G. Transposition of the great arteries and aortopulmonary window in the same patient: clinical report and follow-up. *Pediatr Cardiol*. 2002;23:474-475.
10. Abbruzzese PA, Merlo M, Chiappa E, Bianco R, Ferrero F, Cappone CM. Berry syndrome, a complex aortopulmonary malformation: one stage repair in a neonate. *Ann Thorac Surg*. 1997;64:1167-1169.
11. Bagtharia R, Freedom RM, Yoo S. Aortopulmonary window. In Freedom R, Yoo S, Mikailian H, Williams W, eds. *The Natural and Modified History of Congenital Heart Disease*, 1st ed. Boston: Blackwell Publishing; 2004:237-240.
12. Blieden LC, Moller JH. Aorticopulmonary septal defect. An experience with 17 patients. *Br Heart J*. 1974;36:630-635.
13. Kirby ML, Gale TF, Stewart DE. Neural crest cells contribute to normal aorticopulmonary septation. *Science*. 1983;220:1059-1061.
14. Collinet P, Chatelet-Cheront C, de l'Aulnoit DH, Rey C. Prenatal diagnosis of an aorto-pulmonary window by fetal echocardiography. *Fetal Diagn Ther*. 2002;17:302-307.
15. Bhan A, Gupta M, Abraham S, Sharma R, Kothari S, Juneja R. Surgical experience of aortopulmonary window repair in infants. *Interact Cardiovasc Thorac Surg*. 2007;6:200-203.
16. Backer CL, Mavroudis C. Surgical management of aortopulmonary window: a 40-year experience. *Eur J Cardiothorac Surg*. 2002;21:773-779.
17. Trehan V, Nigam A, Tyagi S. Percutaneous closure of nonrestrictive aortopulmonary window in three infants. *Catheter Cardiovasc Interv*. 2008;71:405-411.
18. Naik GD, Chandra VS, Shenoy A, et al. Transcatheter closure of aortopulmonary window using Amplatzer device. *Catheter Cardiovasc Interv*. 2003;59:402-405.
19. Jansen C, Hruda J, Rammeloo L, Ottenkamp J, Hazekamp MG. Surgical repair of aortopulmonary window: thirty-seven years of experience. *Pediatr Cardiol*. 2006;27:552-556.
20. Rice MJ, Seward JB, Hagler DJ, Mair DD, Tajik AJ. Visualization of aortopulmonary window by two-dimensional echocardiography. *Mayo Clin Proc*. 1982;57:482-487.

CASES

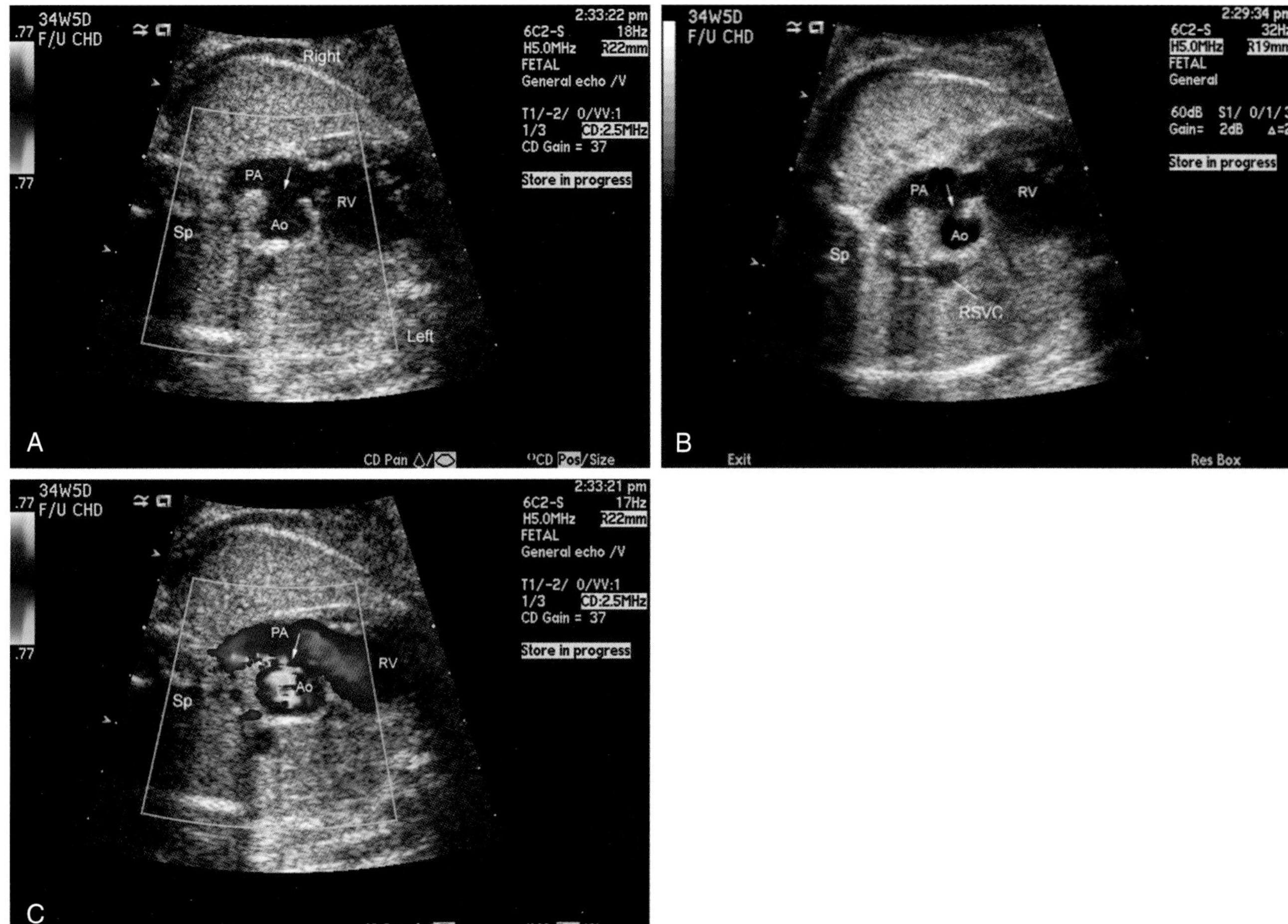

Case 18-1. **(A)** Fetus with a large aortopulmonary window. The *arrow* points to the aortopulmonary window connection. Ao, aorta; PA, pulmonary artery; RV, right ventricle; Sp, spine. **(B)** More superior angulation shows the relationship between the vessels in the mediastinum. The right superior vena cava (RSVC) is to the right and slightly posterior, the Ao is to the left of the RSVC, and the pulmonary artery is further to the left of the Ao. The *arrow* points to the aortopulmonary window. **(C)** The *arrow* points to color flow between the Ao and the PA through the communication of the aortopulmonary window.

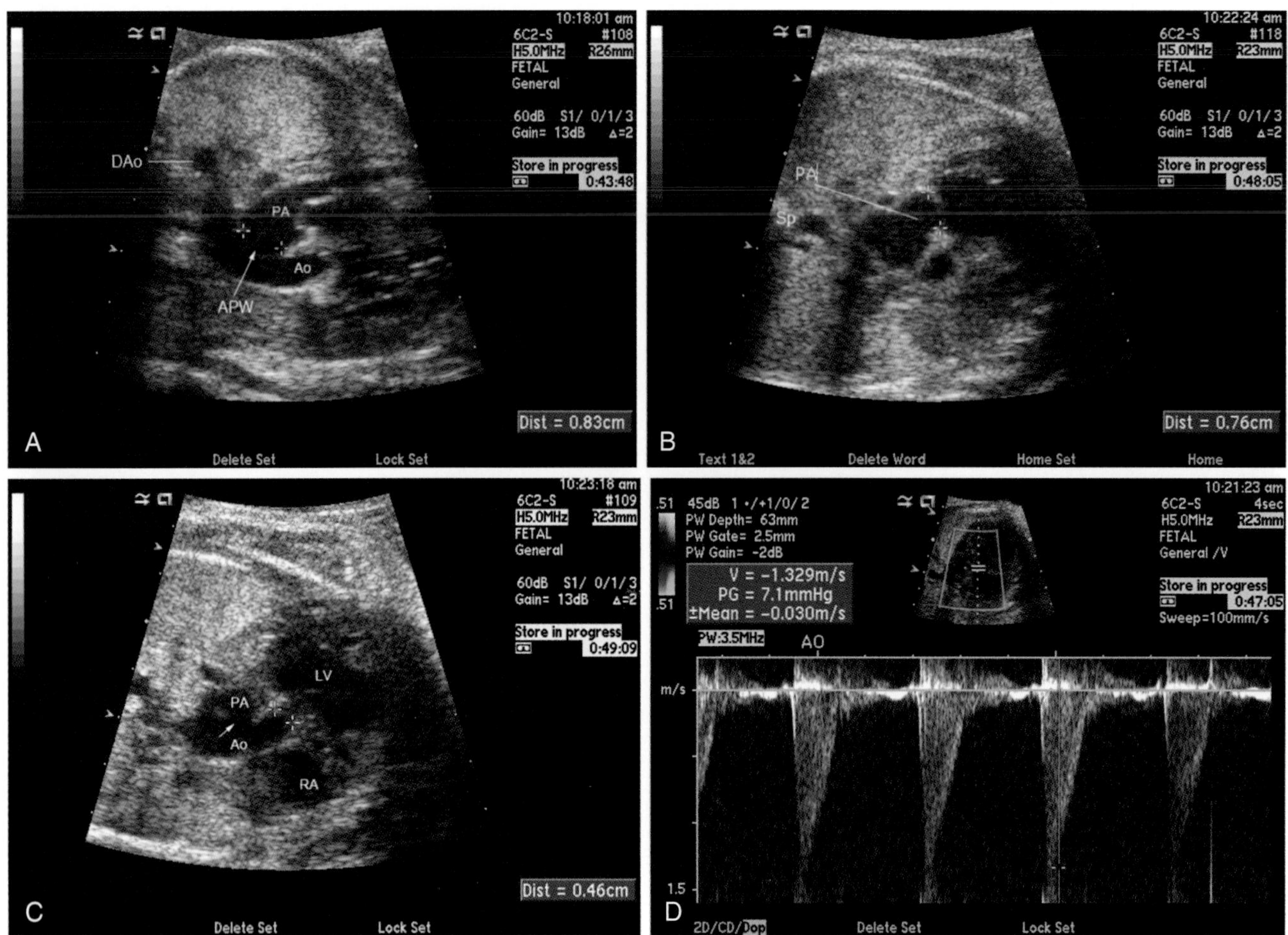

Case 18-2. **(A)** A large aortopulmonary window (APW; *arrow)* is seen in this unusual case of a fetus with aortic valve disease in addition to the APW. Ao, aorta; DAo, descending aorta; PA, pulmonary artery. **(B)** The pulmonary annulus measures 7.6 mm and the PA is quite large. **(C)** The aortic annulus measures approximately 4 to 5 mm and the aortic valve is narrowed. The *arrow* points to the APW. LV, left ventricle; RA, right atrium. **(D)** Pulse wave Doppler across the aortic valve reveals an increase in velocity and turbulence of flow. The peak velocity is approximately 1.3 m/sec.

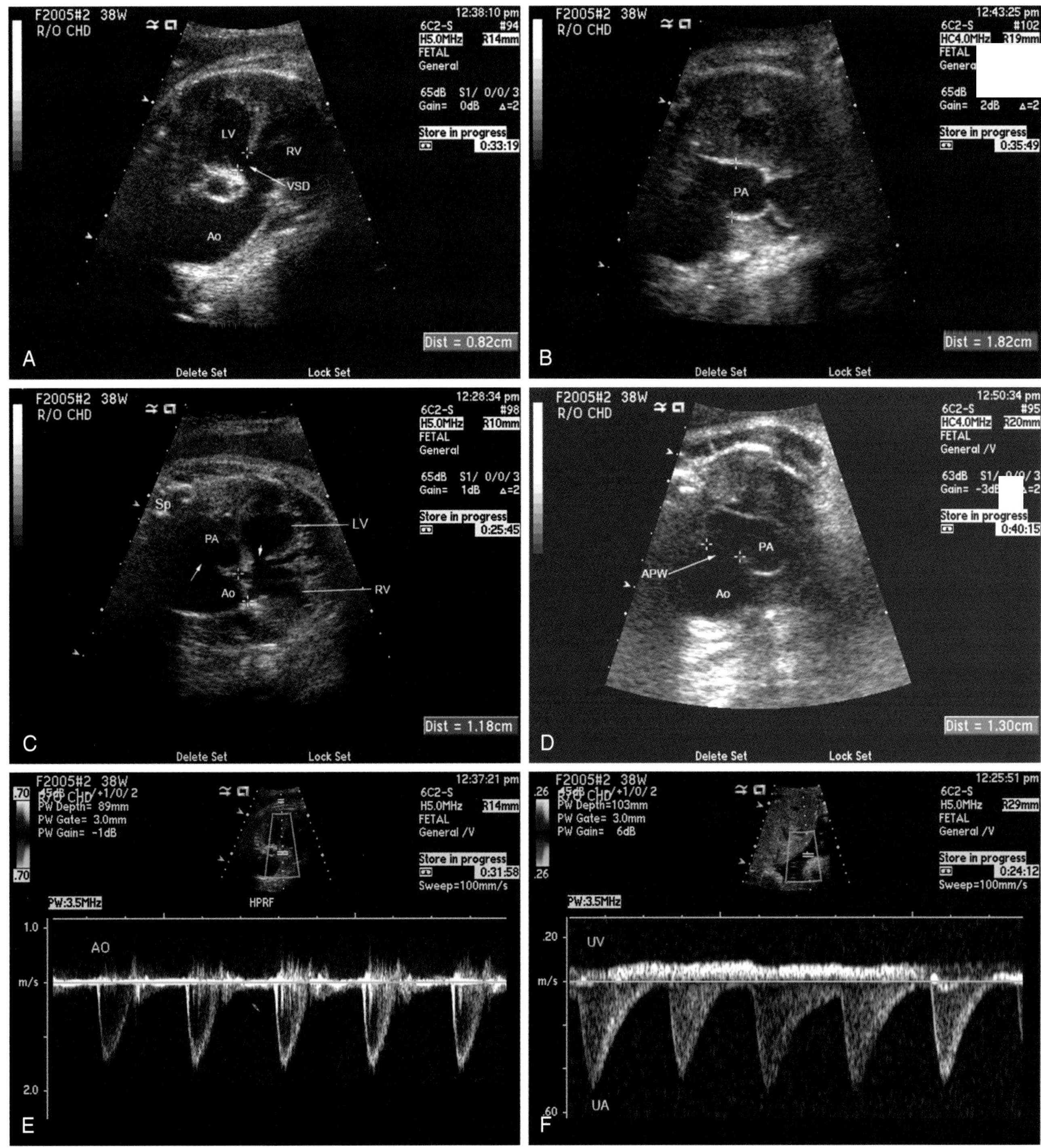

Case 18-3. **(A)** Unusual constellation of findings in a fetus at 38 weeks' gestation including ventricular septal defect (VSD), absent pulmonary valve leaflets, and a large aortopulmonary window. In this image, we see the large VSD and a markedly dilated ascending aorta (Ao). LV, left ventricle; RV, right ventricle. **(B)** A long-axis view of the main pulmonary artery (PA). This demonstrates absence of pulmonary valve leaflets. There is a "pinching in" at the region of where the semilunar valve leaflets should be; however, no leaflets are in place and free pulmonary insufficiency (severe regurgitation) was noted across this pulmonary valve. **(C)** The *long arrow* points to the large aortopulmonary window communication between the Ao and the PA. Both vessels are dilated. The VSD between the LV and the RV is seen, as designated by the *short arrow.* The heart is overall enlarged and there is dilation and hypertrophy of both the LV and the RV. Sp, spine. **(D)** View of the great vessels demonstrates the large aortopulmonary window (APW) communication. **(E)** Doppler flow across the aortic valve revealed slightly increased velocity but laminar flow suggesting no aortic stenosis. **(F)** Doppler sampling in the umbilical cord reveals normal umbilical venous flow; however, umbilical arterial flow reveals diminished diastolic velocity. In this fetus, this reflects a runoff pattern and a "steal" into the heart through the APW and through the incompetent, regurgitant PA because no pulmonary valve is present. UV, umbilical vein.

Continued

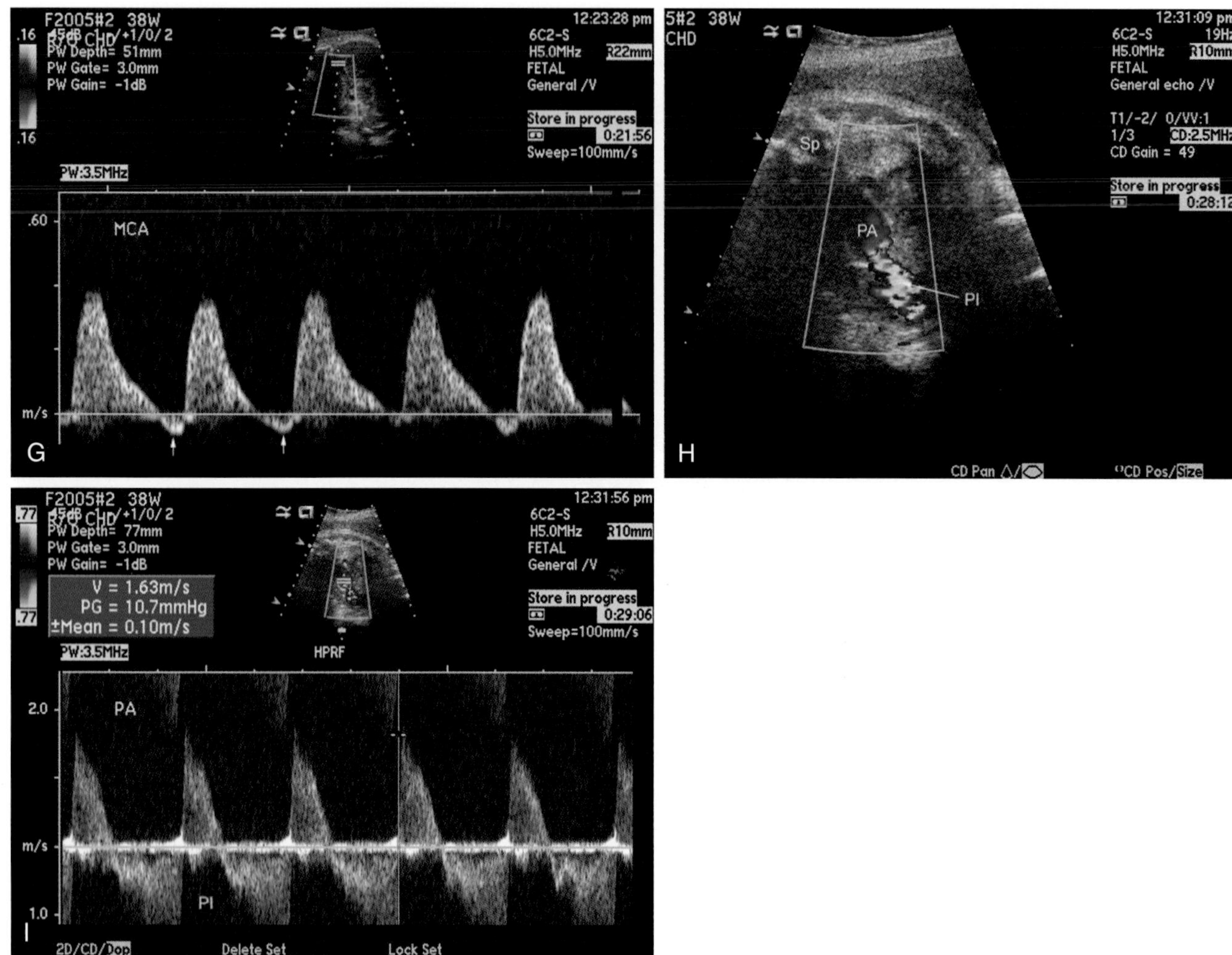

Case 18-3, cont'd (**G**) Sampling in the middle cerebral artery (MCA) demonstrates reversal of flow in diastole. This also reflects the "vascular steal" phenomenon taking place, as blood is being drawn retrograde in diastole from the cerebral vascular circulation into the Ao through the APW and into the regurgitant PA due to the absent pulmonary valve. (**H**) Color Doppler image of the PA demonstrates freely regurgitant pulmonary insufficiency (PI) back into the RV. (**I**) Pulse wave Doppler interrogation of the PA shows flow above the baseline antegrade in systole and retrograde flow below the baseline in diastole, indicating significant pulmonary regurgitation.

IV

Congenital Heart Anomalies: Left-Sided Heart Defects

19

Aortic Stenosis

David J. Goldberg and Deepika Thacker

Key Echocardiographic Features

- Thickened, doming aortic valve.
- Ascending aorta may be dilated in isolated aortic stenosis; however, aortic hypoplasia is common when aortic stenosis is seen in the presence of associated left ventricular anomalies.
- Measure aortic annulus diameter.
- Assess flow pattern across aortic valve looking for turbulence of flow and peak velocity in order to determine gradient.
- Assess for aortic insufficiency.
- Look for associated defects such as subaortic stenosis, mitral valve abnormalities.
- Assess left ventricular endocardium for "echo-brightness" suggesting endocardial fibro-elastosis.
- Assess left ventricular function.
- Aortic arch size and presence or absence of coarctation of the aorta.
- Shunting across the atrial septum (if right to left, there is normal left atrial and left ventricular compliance; if left to right, left atrial pressure and left ventricular compliance may be abnormal and may predict poor left-sided function and/or viability).

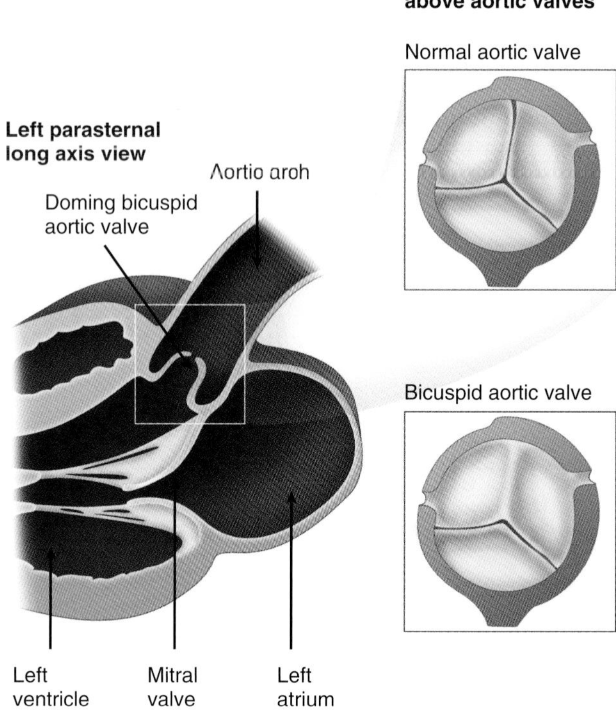

Figure 19-1. Aortic stenosis.

Anatomy and Anatomical Associations

Aortic stenosis (AS) is a disease in which egress from the left ventricle (LV) into the aorta is obstructed by an abnormality along the left ventricular outflow tract (LVOT). The obstruction can occur at any of three levels: the subvalvar region, across the aortic valve itself, or in the supravalvar region. The severity of AS is related to the degree of obstruction across the LVOT.

Discrete stenosis at the level of the aortic valve is the most common cause of LVOT obstruction.[1,2] Abnormal flow across a bicuspid aortic valve, a condition in which two of the coronary cusps fuse together, is a frequent finding in AS.[1,3] Other causes of valvar AS include abnormalities of the commissures between the aortic cusps, abnormalities of the leaflets themselves, or abnormalities of the valve annulus (Figure 19-1).

In the case of a bicuspid aortic valve, fusion may be complete or incomplete and the degree of obstruction may be inconsequential or may be so severe as to be of hemodynamic significance. The aortic valve is composed of leaflets or cusps, and commissures, or joining points/borders between the leaflets. There are three cusps, or leaflets, present in the aortic valve, designated based on their relationship to the origin of the coronary arteries—the right cusp (most anterior), the left cusp, and the noncoronary cusp (most posterior). Fusion of the right and left coronary cusps accounts for approximately 85% of bicuspid aortic valves.[4] Fusion of the right and noncoronary cusps is the next most common, whereas fusion of the left and noncoronary cusps is rare.

Single cups, unicuspid, or unicommissural aortic valves, although far less common than bicuspid aortic valves, are much more likely to present with significant obstruction early in life. These valves have only a slitlike opening along the unaffected commissure, causing a significant reduction in the effective cross-sectional orifice of the outflow tract. Another mechanism of obstruction is partial fusion of all three commissures. In these valves, there are no discrete aortic leaflets and the degree of obstruction is related to the size of the small central orifice as the leaflets attempt to separate and open during systole. Myxomatous aortic valves are unusual but may also be responsible for AS because the dysplastic nature of the leaflets prevents full excursion.[5] Hypoplasia of the aortic annulus is another potential cause of obstruction based on the inherent smallness of the outflow tract.[6] This either can occur with structurally normal valve leaflets or can be seen in association with valvar abnormality such as commissural fusion, as well.

Valvar AS is often found in isolation, although 20% of cases may have associated cardiac defects.[7] These commonly include ventricular septal defect, a patent ductus arteriosus, or coarctation of the aorta. Progressive aortic root dilation is a common finding in patients with bicuspid aortic valves.

Subvalvar AS is responsible for 8% to 20% of cases of congenital LVOT in infants and children.[8] It is often associated with the combination of a posteriorly malaligned infundibular septum and a ventricular septal defect. It may also be associated with mitral stenosis or left-sided obstructive lesions including coarctation of the aorta and interrupted aortic arch. Patients with complete common atrioventricular canals may have subaortic stenosis as a result of atrioventricular valve attachments obstructing LVOT.[9]

Secondary subaortic stenosis may complicate other forms of congenital heart disease. Patients with ventricular septal defects may develop subvalvar AS as a result of the development of a subaortic membrane. These are extremely rare in the fetus and newborn, and typically appear at approximately 2 to 3 years of age. Likewise, patients with hypertrophic cardiomyopathy may develop subvalvar AS as a result of asymmetrical septal hypertrophy.

Supravalvar AS is the least common type of AS and is most often associated with Williams' syndrome, which accounts for up to 50% of all cases.[10] Non-Williams syndrome defects in the elastin gene account for the vast majority of the remainder of supravalvar AS cases.[11]

Frequency, Genetics, and Development

Bicuspid aortic valve is the most common congenital cardiac abnormality found in the human species, with a prevalence of approximately 1.3%.[1] Most bicuspid aortic valves do not cause obstruction in childhood or adolescence, but the incidence of AS increases dramatically through adulthood as the bicuspid leaflets thicken and calcify.[12] It is estimated that AS as a whole accounts for approximately 4% of all congenital heart disease in the pediatric population.[1] For isolated AS, the male-to-female ratio is reported to be in the range of 3 : 1.[2]

Development of the aortic valve occurs early in gestation. The process begins after the aortopulmonary septum divides the bulbus cordis and the truncus arteriosus into two distinct vessels, the aorta and the pulmonary artery, at around 6 weeks of gestation. The aortic valve leaflets form from outpouchings of three subendocardial ridges near the orifice of the aortic valve. The subendocardial ridges go through a process of remodeling until they form the thin, pliable leaflets of the aortic valve. The three aortic cusps are attached to a fibrous ring at the valve annulus and, in normal development, are equal to each other in size. Alterations in the development of the aortic valve leaflets may result in valvar forms of AS.

The genetic basis for AS is likely multifactorial and is not completely delineated. Turner's syndrome (46 X,O) has been associated with AS as well as other forms of left-sided obstruction including coarctation of the aorta and hypoplastic left heart syndrome (HLHS).[13] The 11q terminal deletion disorder has also been associated with AS.[14] Other nonsyndromic forms of AS may be passed on in a familial manner, sometimes as a single, autosomal dominant mutation, or may be sporadic. When isolated AS occurs as part of a familial cluster, other left-sided obstructive lesions are often found in affected relatives.[15] Mutations in NOTCH-1 have been implicated as a specific genetic anomaly responsible for some cases of aortic valve malformations.[16]

Prenatal Physiology

In the fetus, isolated AS is well tolerated. Even in the case of HLHS, in which the LV does not develop into a normal-sized chamber, fetal growth and development is relatively unaffected. In the normal fetal circulation, the LV is responsible for pumping the small amount of pulmonary venous blood that returns from the lungs as well as the highly oxygenated blood that streams from the ductus venosus across the foramen ovale. These two blood pools represent 45% of total cardiac output and have the highest concentration of oxygen. The LV pumps this blood into the ascending aorta to the head and neck vessels, thereby supplying the brain and the coronary arteries with the most highly oxygenated blood in the fetus. In cases of AS, blood flow redistributes away from the LV such that it is responsible for a smaller amount of the overall cardiac output. Depending on the degree of stenosis, this may result in partial perfusion of the head and neck vessels in a retrograde manner from the right ventricle through the ductus arteriosus and into the aortic arch. This does not cause fetal distress, but the impact of mild alteration in the delivery of oxygen to the brain during fetal development is unknown.[17]

Prenatal Management

Depending upon the severity of AS, there may be an alteration in left ventricular compliance as the ventricle hypertrophies. There will then be less right-to-left shunting at the atria level, which will diminish left ventricular filling.

Upon echocardiographic evaluation, the direction of shunting at the atrial level should be assessed. In cases of isolated AS, but in which the LV is deemed to be adequate in size and makeup to function as the systemic ventricle, there will be the normal right-to-left direction of shunting, or bidirectional shunting. Evidence for left-to-right atrial level shunting suggests the possibility of an inadequate LV and present, or evolving, HLHS.

Echocardiography should assess the nature and velocity of flow across the aortic valve. In AS, the flow will be turbulent, nonlaminar flow. The peak systolic velocity will exceed 1.5 m/sec, but may not reach the very high levels seen after birth, because flow across the LV is limited and further distributed away from the LV in the presence of an abnormal aortic valve. Even in severe cases of AS, typical values for peak velocity reach 3 m/sec, but not much higher.

Investigation of the ascending aorta for the appearance of root dilation can help in the diagnosis of mild cases of bicuspid aortic valve. A complete assessment of the aortic arch for transverse arch hypoplasia and coarctation of the aorta is essential.

In prenatal life, the right ventricle is able to compensate for any amount of diminished output from the LV without affecting fetal growth and development. However, although AS does not affect global fetal growth, there is the potential for the arrest of fetal growth of the LV. In these cases, some centers have undertaken a strategy of intrauterine balloon dilation of the aortic valve to try to encourage left ventricular ejection to promote left ventricular growth (see discussion of hypoplastic left heart syndrome, earlier).[18]

Postnatal Physiology

After the closure of the ductus arteriosus, usually within the first 72 hours of life, the right ventricular contribution to systemic cardiac output is eliminated. The LV takes on the sole responsibility of pumping oxygenated blood returning from the lungs across the aortic valve and out to the body. In cases of mild or moderate AS, the obstruction may be well tolerated through the neonatal period and into childhood. However, in cases of severe or critical AS (*critical* is defined as requiring ductal support for systemic perfusion), neonatal intervention is often necessary to relieve the obstruction. Without early intervention, infants with severe or critical AS may present in shock and may not survive the neonatal period. Catheter-based balloon aortic valvuloplasty allows neonates to survive the neonatal period without surgery and may allow for the growth of an undersized LV.[19] Newborn infants with critical AS may, interestingly, not have a significantly high gradient across the aortic valve as blood is shunted away from the LV, and systemic perfusion occurs via the patent ductus arteriosus, shunting right to left (pulmonary artery to aorta) in systole.

Postnatal Management

For children who present with severe AS in the newborn period, defined as a gradient of greater than 70 mm Hg or with signs of left ventricular dysfunction or failure, or a newborn with critical AS in which the ductus arteriosus is needed to support the systemic circulation, a catheter-based balloon valvuloplasty is warranted to relieve the obstruction. Balloon dilation has a high success rate, but it is a blunt instrument and may cause valve distortion and significant aortic insufficiency.[19] Occasionally, surgical intervention is warranted. A commonly performed operation for the neonate or young child is the Ross procedure. In this operation, the aortic valve is removed and replaced by the native pulmonary valve, which becomes the "neo-aortic" valve. A homograft conduit is placed in the pulmonary position. Midterm results for the Ross procedure are encouraging, although aortic root dilation and neo-aortic insufficiency are common.[20] Even in the best case scenario, the Ross procedure should be considered as palliation. Many patients will require catheter-based conduit interventions or reoperation for plication of a dilated aortic root, replacement of the neo-aortic valve, or homograft replacement.[20]

Catheter-based balloon dilation is the standard first step in the approach to patients with AS outside of the neonatal period. According to the American College of Cardiology/American Heart Association (ACC/AHA) guidelines, intervention for AS is warranted in children and young adults if the peak-to-peak gradient as measured during a cardiac catheterization is greater than 60 mm Hg. If the patient wishes to participate in sports or to become pregnant, the guideline calls for intervention if the gradient is greater than 50 mm Hg. If a patient is symptomatic or has electrocardiographic changes with exercise testing, intervention should be performed if the gradient is greater than 50 mm Hg.[21]

Balloon dilation is a safe and effective tool but may not always be appropriate. If a patient demonstrates significant native aortic insufficiency, balloon dilation should not be performed. In these cases, the options include the Ross procedure or valve replacement with either a xenograft or a mechanical valve. For children who have not yet reached adolescence, the options are more limited. Currently, the available aortic mechanical valves are too large for the aortic position in small children. For these children, a Ross procedure can be safely performed and is the procedure of choice. Once a child approaches his or her adult size, xenografts and mechanical valves become more realistic options. Neither of these options is ideal. Xenografts do not have good durability in children and will inevitably require reoperation whereas mechanical valves require anticoagulation, which has its own profile of morbidity and mortality.[22]

Outcomes

The life expectancy for patients with AS is relatively good in comparison with other more complex forms of congenital heart disease, but is diminished compared with the population at large.[2] Some of the attrition is attributable to hemodynamic compromise and left ventricular failure as a result of severe or critical AS in the newborn period, and some is due to the deterioration of the aortic valve as the leaflets calcify over time. There is also an increased incidence of sudden death in patients with AS, particularly during exercise. The mechanism is presumably related to diminished coronary perfusion and an increase in myocardial oxygen demand creating a supply-demand mismatch and resultant myocardial ischemia.

Exercise limitations and guidelines have been established based on severity of disease as measured by gradient across the valve.[23,24]

Although, upon first glance, a simple anomaly, AS is not a disease that can be cured. In the modern era, catheter-based interventions and surgical valve replacements have improved the prognosis for many patients, but it is expected that lifelong scrutiny and the likelihood of multiple interventions will be required.

Imaging Essentials and Important Points

- The finding of turbulent, nonlaminar flow is more important than any actual peak velocity gradient across the aortic valve in identifying AS in the fetus.
- Normal velocity across the aortic valve is usually less than 1 m/sec. With increased volume of ejection under normal conditions, perhaps the velocity may be slightly higher but rarely will exceed 1.5 m/sec. Hence, a peak velocity greater than 1.5 m/sec suggests aortic valve stenosis. However, to confirm AS, this increased velocity should be seen in conjunction with turbulent, nonlaminar flow. The presence of an increased velocity across the aortic valve, but with laminar flow, should raise the suspicion of a disease causing an abnormal increase in output across the LV such as fetal anemia or arteriovenous malformation.
- Actual determination of the number of leaflets present and site of commissural fusion can be extremely challenging in the fetus with suspicion of AS. Typically, findings that hint toward a bicuspid valve include limited excursion in systole or thickening and increased echogenicity.
- The aortic annulus should be measured in the long-axis view with the ultrasound beam perpendicular to the LVOT, and a gestational age–matched Z-score value obtained in order to determine whether there is associated annular hypoplasia.
- Color Doppler flow across the aortic valve will demonstrate turbulence in the ascending aorta in the presence of significant AS. Pulse Doppler evaluation just above the aortic valve will reveal the peak velocity. An acute angle between the ascending aorta and the left ventricular septum can be seen in some cases, with an eccentric orifice across the aortic valve.
- Aortic root dilation alone may hint at the presence of a bicuspid aortic valve where there may be no gradient across. Abnormal dilation of the ascending aorta is not necessarily related to flow gradient and poststenotic dilatation, but may rather reflect an inherent pathological and histological abnormality of the ascending aorta associated with valvar AS.
- Assessment of the left ventricular cavity in AS is important because it can be either small or dilated. There can be thickening of the left ventricular myocardium or echo-brightness reflecting the presence of endocardial fibroelastosis.
- Severe mitral valve abnormalities can be seen in association with AS and are discussed separately.
- Arch hypoplasia or coarctation of the aorta can be seen in association with AS.

References

1. Hoffman JI, Kaplan S. The incidence of congenital heart disease. *J Am Coll Cardiol*. 2002;39:1890-1900.
2. Campbell M. The natural history of congenital aortic stenosis. *Br Heart J*. 1968;30:514-526.
3. Roberts WC. The congenitally bicuspid aortic valve. A study of 85 autopsy cases. *Am J Cardiol*. 1970;26:72-83.
4. Sabet HY, Edwards WD, Tazelaar HD, Daly RC. Congenitally bicuspid aortic valves: a surgical pathology study of 542 cases (1991 through 1996) and a literature review of 2,715 additional cases. *Mayo Clin Proc*. 1999;74:14-26.
5. Bharati S, Lev M. Congenital polyvalvular disease. *Circulation*. 1973;47:575-586.
6. Reeve R Jr, Robinson SJ. Hypoplastic annulus—an unusual type of aortic stenosis: a report of three cases in children. *Dis Chest*. 1964;45:99-102.
7. Braunwald E, Goldblatt A, Aygen MM, Rockoff SD, Morrow AG. Congenital aortic stenosis. I. Clinical and hemodynamic findings in 100 patients. II. Surgical treatment and the results of operation. *Circulation*. 1963;27:426-462.
8. Newfeld EA, Muster AJ, Paul MH, Idriss FS, Riker WL. Discrete subvalvular aortic stenosis in childhood. Study of 51 patients. *Am J Cardiol*. 1976;38:53-61.
9. Marasini M, Zannini L, Ussia GP, et al. Discrete subaortic stenosis: incidence, morphology and surgical impact of associated subaortic anomalies. *Ann Thorac Surg*. 2003;75:1763-1768.
10. Bruno E, Rossi N, Thuer O, Cordoba R, Alday LE. Cardiovascular findings, and clinical course, in patients with Williams syndrome. *Cardiol Young*. 2003;13:532-536.
11. Ewart AK, Jin W, Atkinson D, Morris CA, Keating MT. Supravalvular aortic stenosis associated with a deletion disrupting the elastin gene. *J Clin Invest*. 1994;93:1071-1077.
12. Ward C. Clinical significance of the bicuspid aortic valve. *Heart*. 2000;83:81-85.
13. Mazzanti L, Cacciari E. Congenital heart disease in patients with Turner's syndrome. Italian Study Group for Turner Syndrome (ISGTS). *J Pediatr*. 1998;133:688-692.
14. Grossfeld PD, Mattina T, Lai Z, et al. The 11q terminal deletion disorder: a prospective study of 110 cases. *Am J Med Genet A*. 2004;129A:51-61.
15. Wessels MW, Berger RM, Frohn-Mulder IM, et al. Autosomal dominant inheritance of left ventricular outflow tract obstruction. *Am J Med Genet A*. 2005;134A:171-179.
16. Garg V, Muth AN, Ransom JF, et al. Mutations in NOTCH1 cause aortic valve disease. *Nature*. 2005;437:270-274.
17. Kaltman JR, Di H, Tian Z, Rychik J. Impact of congenital heart disease on cerebrovascular blood flow dynamics in the fetus. *Ultrasound Obstet Gynecol*. 2005;25:32-36.
18. Tworetzky W, Wilkins-Haug L, Jennings RW, et al. Balloon dilation of severe aortic stenosis in the fetus: potential for prevention of hypoplastic left heart syndrome: candidate selection, technique, and results of successful intervention. *Circulation*. 2004;110:2125-2131.

19. McElhinney DB, Lock JE, Keane JF, Moran AM, Colan SD. Left heart growth, function, and reintervention after balloon aortic valvuloplasty for neonatal aortic stenosis. *Circulation*. 2005;111:451-458.
20. Pasquali SK, Shera D, Wernovsky G, et al. Midterm outcomes and predictors of reintervention after the Ross procedure in infants, children, and young adults. *J Thorac Cardiovasc Surg*. 2007;133: 893-899.
21. Bonow RO, Carabello BA, Chatterjee K, et al. ACC/AHA 2006 guidelines for the management of patients with valvular heart disease: a report of the American College of Cardiology/American Heart Association Task Force on Practice Guidelines (Writing Committee to Revise the 1998 guidelines for the management of patients with valvular heart disease) developed in collaboration with the Society of Cardiovascular Anesthesiologists endorsed by the Society for Cardiovascular Angiography and Interventions and the Society of Thoracic Surgeons. *J Am Coll Cardiol*. 2006;48:e1-148.
22. Turrentine MW, Ruzmetov M, Vijay P, Bills RG, Brown JW. Biological versus mechanical aortic valve replacement in children. *Ann Thorac Surg*. 2001;71(5 suppl):S356-S360.
23. Graham TP Jr, Driscoll DJ, Gersony WM, Newburger JW, Rocchini A, Towbin JA. Task Force 2: congenital heart disease. *J Am Coll Cardiol*. 2005;45:1326-1333.
24. Bonow RO, Cheitlin MD, Crawford MH, Douglas PS. Task Force 3: valvular heart disease. *J Am Coll Cardiol*. 2005;45:1334-1340.

CASES

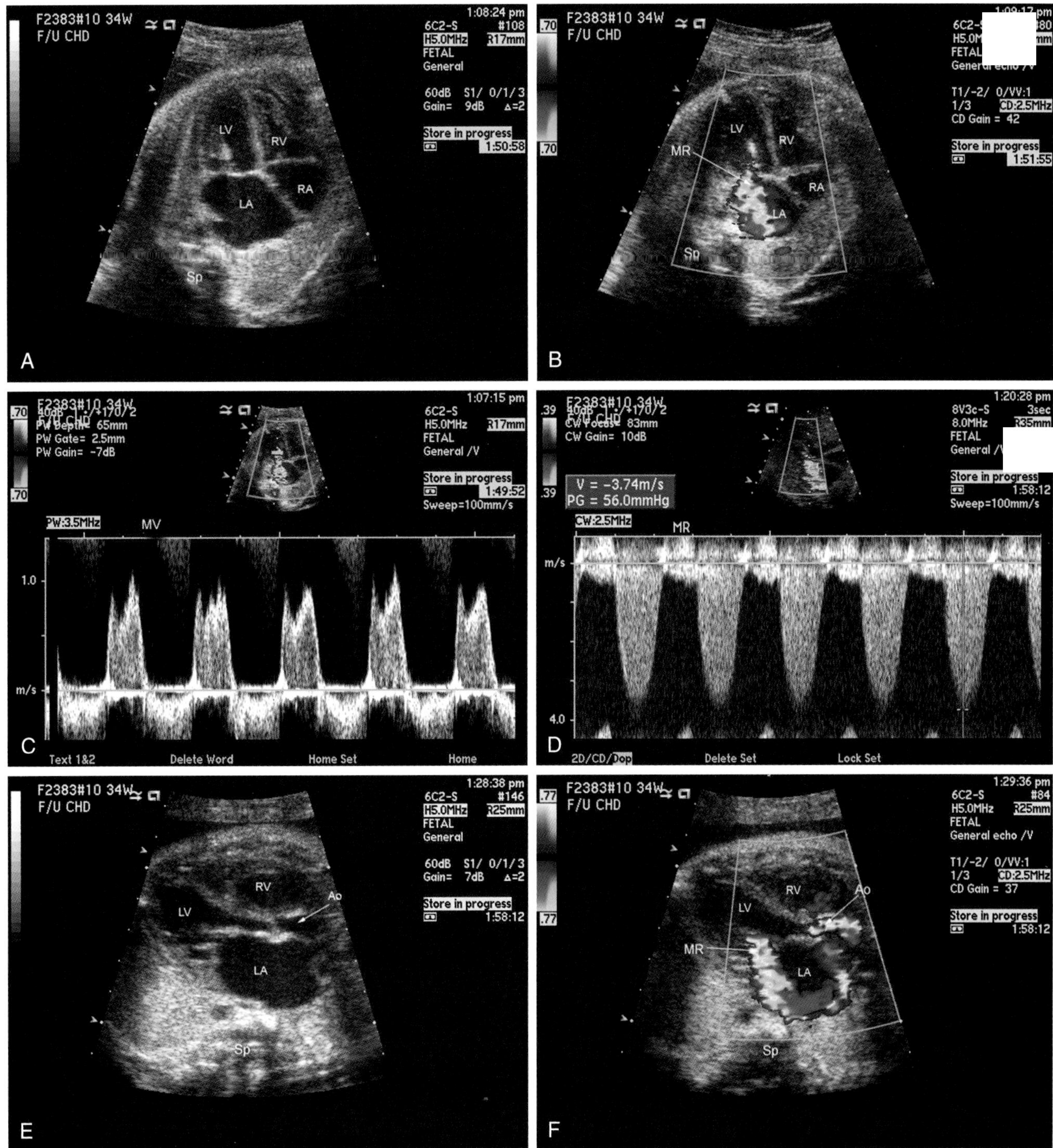

Case 19-1. (A) Four-chamber view of a fetus with aortic stenosis. The aortic valve is not seen in this view; however, the left ventricle (LV) and left atrium (LA) are slightly dilated. The mitral valve subleaflet apparatus appears echo-bright and thickened, suggesting a possible mitral valve anomaly. RA, right atrium; RV, right ventricle; Sp, spine. (B) Color Doppler imaging demonstrates severe mitral regurgitation (MR). (C) Pulse wave Doppler interrogation across the mitral valve with increased peak velocity over 1.0 m/sec. This may reflect increased volume of flow across the mitral valve (MV) in diastole due to the regurgitation. (D) Continuous wave Doppler estimate of the peak mitral regurgitant velocity is 3.7 m/sec. Hence, the estimated left ventricular pressure is approximately 56 mm Hg greater than the left atrial pressure. (E) Long-axis view of the LV. The aortic valve appears thickened. Ao, aorta. (F) Color Doppler imaging of long-axis view. There is turbulent flow just distal to the aortic valve suggesting stenosis. There is severe MR with a jet angled posteriorly toward the back of the LA.

Continued

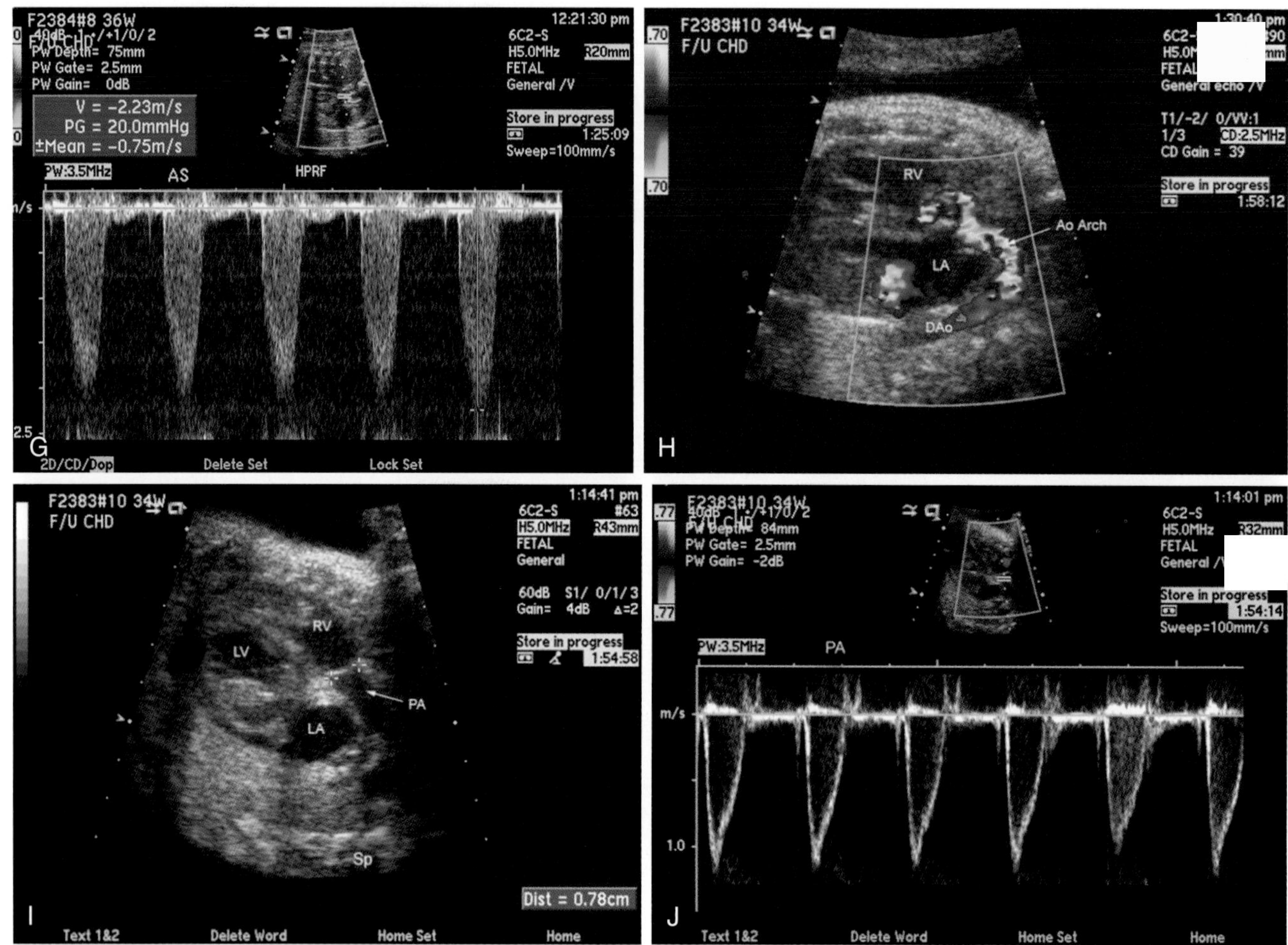

Case 19-1, cont'd (G) Pulse wave Doppler across the aortic valve demonstrates nonlaminar, turbulent flow with a peak velocity of 2.2 m/sec, with an estimate of 20 mm Hg peak instantaneous gradient from LV to ascending aorta. AS, aortic stenosis. **(H)** Color flow image of the aortic arch. There is turbulence secondary to the AS, which is transmitted distally into the transverse aortic arch (Ao arch). DAo, descending aorta. **(I)** Superior angling toward the right ventricular outflow tract. The pulmonary artery (PA) and pulmonary valve are demonstrated. **(J)** Pulse wave Doppler across the pulmonary valve. There is laminar flow, although the velocity is elevated at over 1 m/sec. This is likely due to decreased right-to-left shunting at the atrial level secondary to left-sided heart disease; as a consequence, there is an increase in right-sided flow across the pulmonary valve. PA, pulmonary artery.

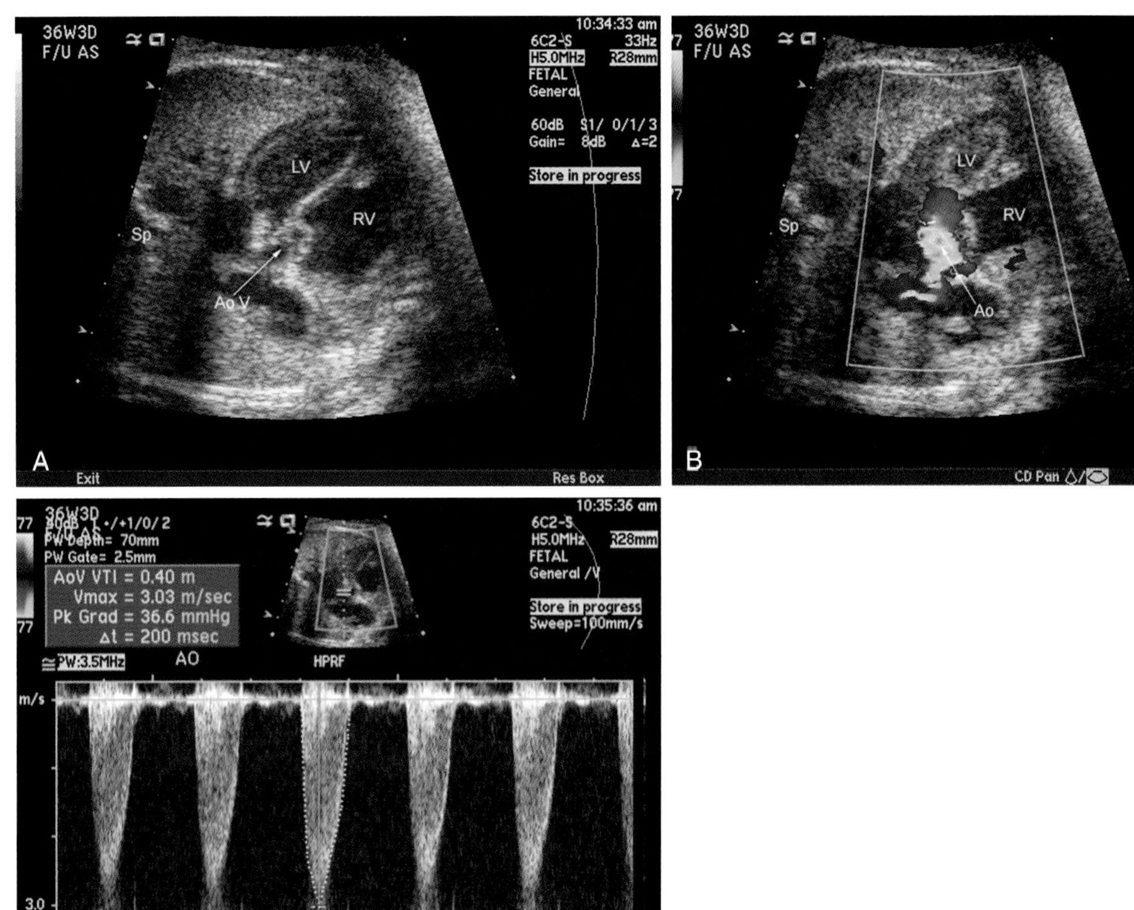

Case 19-2. **(A)** Thickened, stenotic aortic valve (Ao valve). LV, left ventricle; RV, right ventricle; Sp, spine. **(B)** Color flow across the stenotic Ao valve demonstrates turbulent flow in the ascending aorta (Ao). **(C)** Pulse Doppler interrogation across the stenotic Ao valve. There is turbulent flow and the peak velocity is over 3 m/sec, indicating a peak instantaneous gradient of 36 mm Hg.

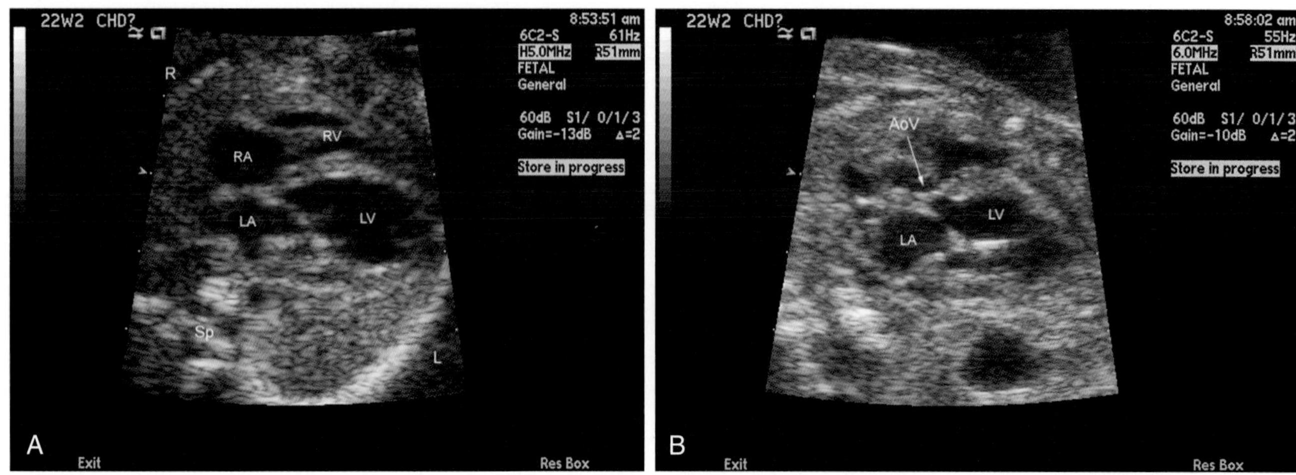

Case 19-3. **(A)** Left ventricle (LV) dilation with echo-brightness of the ventricular septum in a case of "critical" valvar aortic stenosis. LA, left atrium; RA, right atrium; RV, right ventricle. **(B)** Slight anterior angulation reveals the presence of a thickened and stenotic aortic valve (AoV).

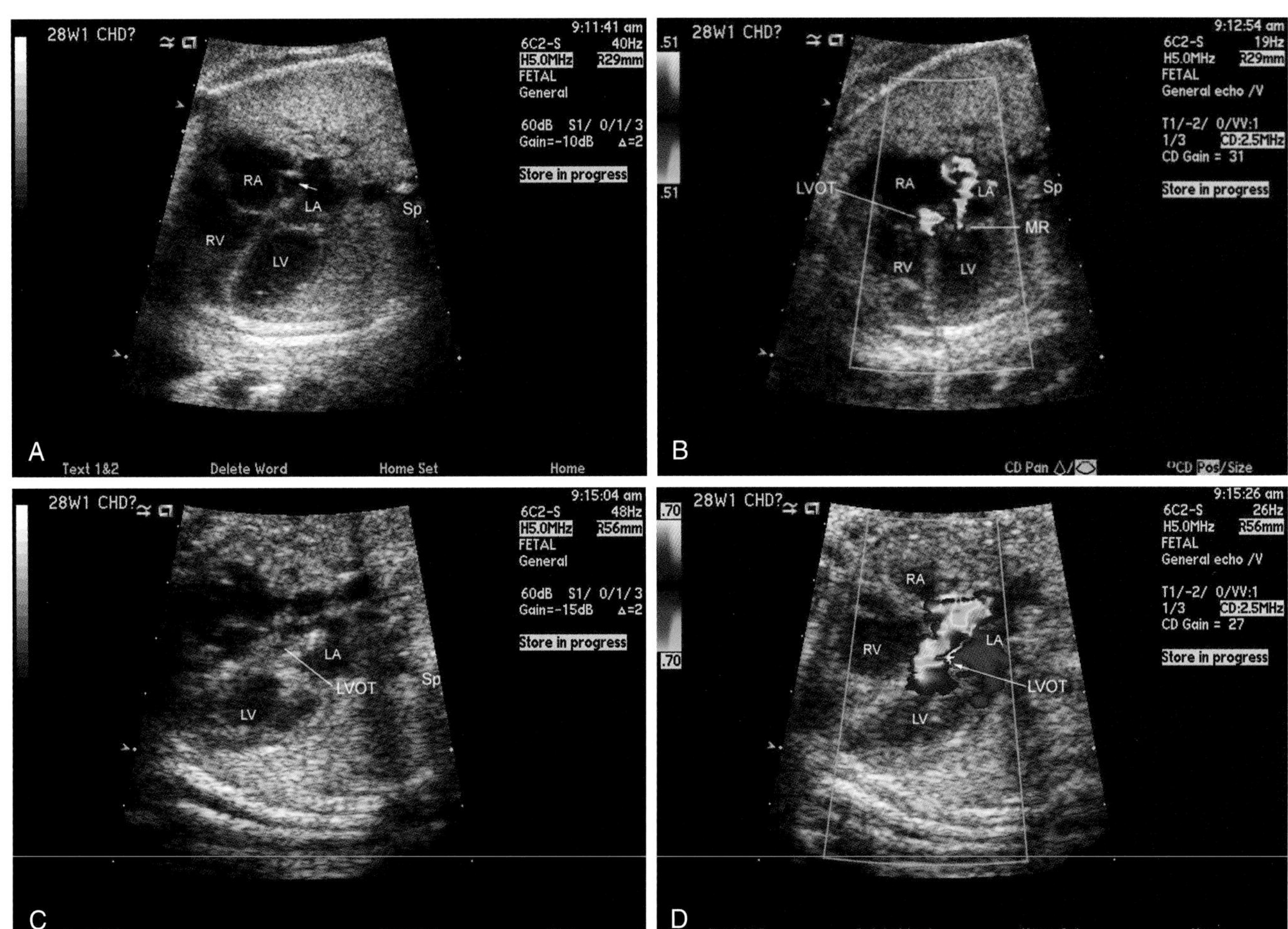

Case 19-4. (A) Four-chamber view with atrial septal bowing left to right. This fetus had evidence for bidirectional shunting at the atrial level, suggesting intermittent elevation in left atrium (LA) pressure, suggesting the presence of left-sided heart disease. LV, left ventricle; RA, right atrium; RV, right ventricle; Sp, spine. (B) During systole, there is mitral regurgitation (MR) and the presence of turbulence in the left ventricular outflow tract (LVOT) on color Doppler imaging. (C) Long-axis view of the LV demonstrates crowding of the LVOT and subaortic stenosis. (D) Color Doppler imaging with turbulence in the LVOT in this fetus with subaortic stenosis.

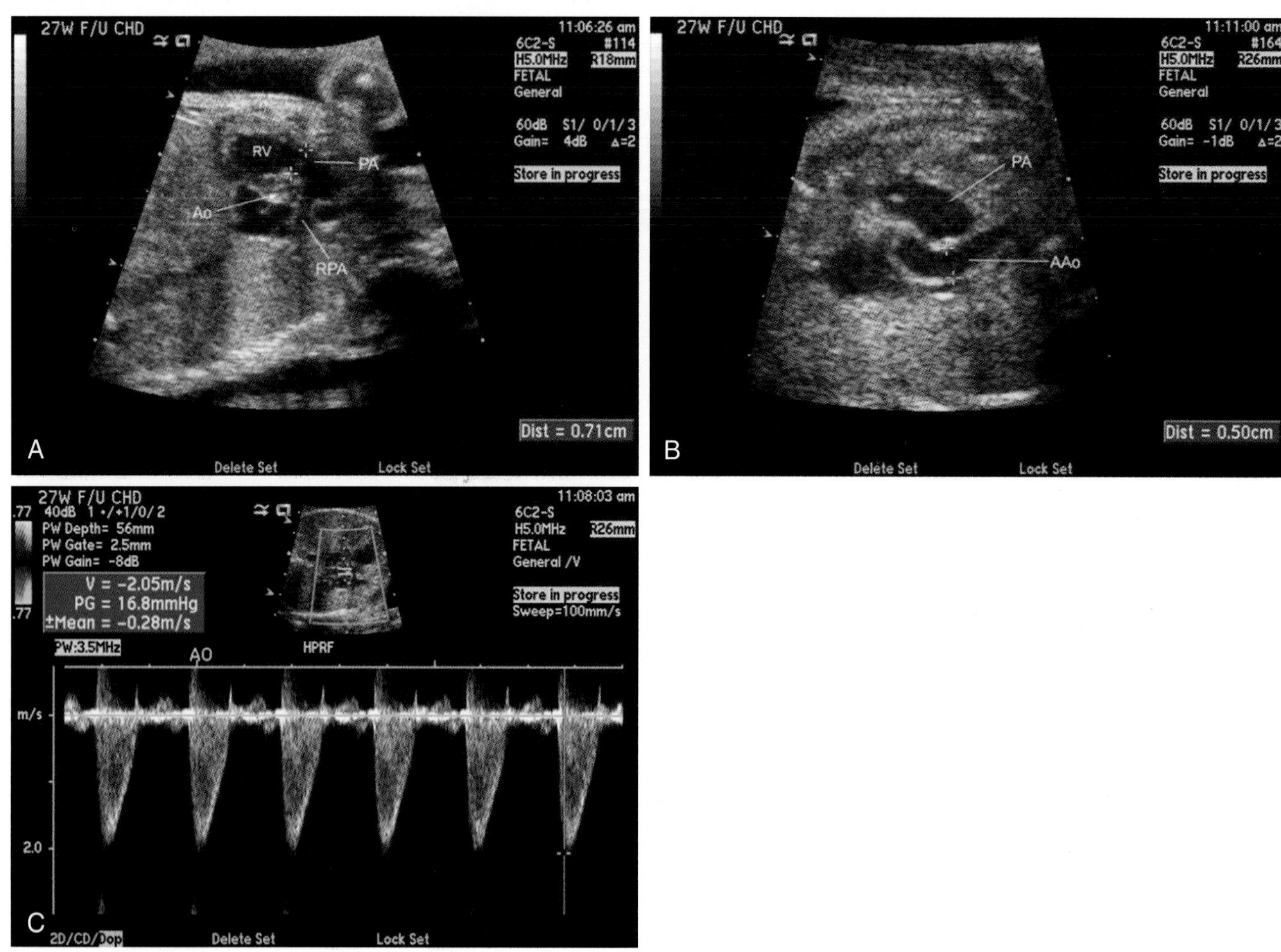

Case 19-5. **(A)** Short-axis view at the level of the aortic valve reveals a thickened, likely bicuspid aortic valve. Ao, aorta; PA, pulmonary artery; RPA, right pulmonary artery; RV, right ventricle. **(B)** Elongated view of the ascending aorta. Note the slight dilation of the ascending aorta (AAo) and loss of the normal "pinched-in" contour of the sinotubular junction. This type of mild dilation and alteration in ascending aortic architecture is common in those with a bicuspid aortic valve, even without significant gradient across. **(C)** There is a mild increase in peak velocity of flow across this bicuspid aortic valve.

20
Coarctation of the Aorta

Michael D. Quartermain

Key Echocardiographic Features

- Site of narrowing of the arch
- Associated anomalies such as aortic stenosis, subaortic narrowing, left ventricular hypoplasia, or ventricular septal defect
- Mitral valve size and function

Anatomy and Anatomical Associations

Coarctation of the aorta is a narrowing of the lumen of the aortic arch. There are two general types: (1) juxtaductal, or "adult-type" coarctation, is discrete narrowing at the isthmus, the region of the aortic arch distal to the take-off of the left subclavian artery, and (2) "infantile type," or tubular hypoplasia. In this form of aortic arch obstruction, there is long segment narrowing of the transverse arch and it is often associated with intracardiac defects.[1] Practically, most forms of coarctation seen in the perinatal period are a combination of these two, where there is an element of hypoplasia of the isthmus and then a discrete narrowing as one approaches the insertion into the ductal arch (Figure 20-1). Abdominal coarctation is a rare finding of narrowing of the descending aorta at the region beneath the diaphragm, commonly at the level of the renal arteries.

Anatomical associations are common in the fetus with aortic arch obstruction. One of the most common findings, and one that typically tips the fetal heart examiner off to the possibility of coarctation of the aorta, is left ventricle (LV)–to–right ventricle (RV) size discrepancy or disproportion, in which the LV cavity appears much smaller and the RV cavity much larger than expected. This disproportion is noted in the face of no ostensible mitral or aortic valve disease.

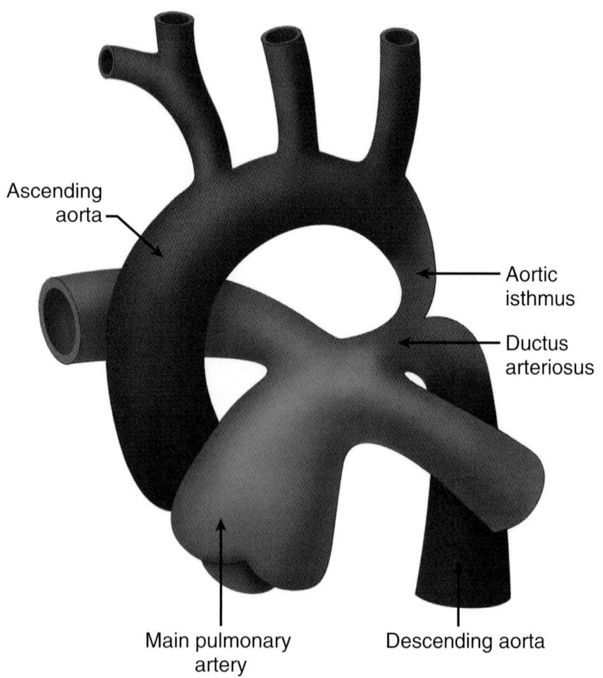

Figure 20-1. Coarctation of the aorta.

Ventricular septal defects are often present in coarctation and can be of the conal/infundibular posterior malalignment, conoventricular, or muscular type. Coarctation can occur in the setting of more complex cardiac lesions such as hypoplastic left heart syndrome (HLHS), complete atrioventricular canal, and transposition of the great arteries.

Frequency, Genetics, and Development

Coarctation of the aorta occurs in 0.3 per 1000 live births and accounts for 6% to 8% of infants with congenital heart disease.[2] As with other forms of left-sided obstructive lesions, coarctation occurs more frequently in males than in females. There is a known association with Turner's syndrome (45,XO) in both complete and mosaic forms. Coarctation occurs in 35% of patients who are affected by Turner's, and a documented familiar recurrence suggests a genetic substrate.

The precise developmental mechanism remains unknown, but two theories exist. The *hemodynamic theory* suggests that an associated defect such as a bicuspid aortic valve, or some other impetus, drives blood away from the developing LV and reduces the amount of flow in the ascending aorta and across the aortic arch.[3] This decrease in antegrade flow across the aortic arch leads to diminished growth and formation of a narrowed segment. In fact, the isthmus of the aorta normally receives the smallest proportion of cardiac output of any structure arising from the fetal heart. The LV ejects 40% of the entire fetal cardiac output; by the time flow reaches the isthmus after the head and neck vessels have been perfused, only 10% to 15% remains to cross the isthmus and join with the ductus arteriosus and descending aorta. Therefore, even a small reduction in aortic flow can have a substantial impact on the reduction of blood flow crossing the aortic isthmus. The *ductal tissue theory* suggests that actual ductal tissue migrates abnormally into the aortic arch and then constricts after ductal closure, leading to a coarctation.

Prenatal Physiology

In the normal fetal circulation, the dominant RV supplies output to the body via the ductus arteriosus. The left heart fills primarily via right-to-left shunting at the foramen ovale and the LV supplies output to the head and neck vessels, with only 10% to 15% of the fetal cardiac output traversing the aortic isthmus.[4] Therefore, the fetal aortic isthmus often normally appears relatively small with tapering at the region of ductal insertion.[5] Further abnormal narrowing in the isthmus as seen in coarctation is well tolerated in the fetus because the large ductus arteriosus allows for flow around any narrowed region, providing unobstructed perfusion to the body. There is typically normal growth and development, with the fetus reaching full term.

The region of the isthmus is quite interesting because it is the bridge between the cephalic and the subdiaphragmatic arterial circulations. Fouron[6] has written extensively about the importance of evaluation of the aortic isthmus through Doppler sampling. Analysis of flow patterns within the isthmus can provide a wealth of information concerning the relative resistances of the upper and lower fetal body, which change dramatically during periods of stress and unwellness (see Chapter 3).

Prenatal Management

When clear-cut, severe hypoplasia of the isthmus is seen on two-dimensional imaging, the diagnosis of coarctation is straightforward. However, because the aortic isthmus is normally a relatively small structure, in the presence of a normal large patent ductus arteriosus, the diagnosis can be quite challenging. LV-RV size discrepancy may suggest a coarctation; however, when looking at the isthmus, it may appear proportionately small but of good size relative to the LV and ascending aorta. Furthermore, LV-RV size discrepancy can be seen in a number of conditions besides coarctation of the aorta (Box 20-1). A left superior vena cava to the coronary sinus may theoretically impair filling of the LV by altering left atrial compliance and reducing right-to-left shunting at the foramen ovale. Interruption of the inferior vena cava with azygos continuation to the right superior vena cava results in a redirection of inferior vena caval flow because the normal streaming pattern across the foramen ovale caused by the inferior vena cava entering the floor of the right atrium is averted. The RV is dilated and can appear volume loaded in this condition because both inferior and superior venous return drains via the superior vena cava and is directed caudad across the tricuspid valve. Anomalies of pulmonary venous return, with connection and drainage away from the left atrium, may reduce LV filling and create the impression of a relatively underfilled LV. We have also seen situations in which LV-RV disproportion predicted the presence of a genetic syndrome or a neurological condition, without any venous anomaly or postnatal evidence for arch narrowing. Finally, there are cases of LV-RV size disproportion in which postnatal findings from a somatic, genetic, and cardiovascular perspective are completely normal.

Box 20-1 Conditions That May Cause the Appearance of Left Ventricle–Right Ventricle Size Disproportion with a Relatively Smaller than Normal–appearing Left Ventricle in the Fetus

- Coarctation of the aorta
- Bicuspid aortic valve
- Structural mitral valve disease resulting in limitation of flow across (e.g., mitral stenosis, supravalvar mitral ring)
- Left superior vena cava to the coronary sinus
- Interruption of the inferior vena cava with azygos continuation to the right superior vena cava
- Total anomalous pulmonary venous connection
- Partial anomalous pulmonary venous connection
- Genetic syndromes (e.g., Turner's syndrome)
- Central nervous system anomalies
- Normal fetus

Prenatal diagnosis of coarctation of the aorta is important because it has implications for immediate postnatal management and site of delivery. In order to better discriminate between LV-RV disproportion due to coarctation of the aorta versus other causes, a number of investigators have attempted to develop predictive criteria. First, it must be established whether one is dealing with the other end of the spectrum, in which there is a nonviable inadequate LV and HLHS. In HLHS, the LV cavity is quite small and dysmorphic in shape and appearance. One of the key diagnostic hallmarks is an associated continuous left-to-right shunt at the atrial level. This is not the condition we are speaking of when referring to the LV-RV size disproportion phenomenon in this chapter. In LV-RV size disproportion, the LV cavity appears small in its width and looks underfilled; however, it typically reaches greater than two thirds the distance toward the apex of the heart. Shunting at the atrial level is typically the normal right to left; however, it may be bidirectional. Parameters related to relative size of structures within the heart and great vessels as well as unique Doppler flow patterns have been described, which can help discriminate those that will require intervention for coarctation of the aorta after birth (Box 20-2).[7-12]

Gardiner and colleagues[9] looked at the utility of the three vessels and trachea view, in which the junction of the aortic isthmus and ductus arteriosus can be seen and measured as they join together into the descending aorta. A Z score measure of the aortic isthmus of less than −2 and an aortic isthmus–to–ductus arteriosus ratio of less than 0.74 reliably predict coarctation and the need for postnatal intervention. Normal values and Z score formulas for the aortic isthmus visualized in this view are published.[10] Most reliable was the finding of absence of growth of the aortic isthmus in those who had true coarctation. In other words, fetuses with LV-RV disproportion who had initial aortic isthmus Z score of less than −2 at first evaluation but demonstrated growth in the third trimester with Z score increasing to greater than −2 did not require postnatal intervention. Serial evaluation is, therefore, of tremendous value in this lesion.

Box 20-2 Echocardiographic Features That Suggest the Presence of Coarctation of the Aorta When There Is Left Ventricle–Right Ventricle Size Disproportion in the Fetus

- Visualization of a shelf, or discrete narrowing of the aorta in the region of the isthmus as it inserts into the ductal arch
- Visualization of continuous, persistent forward flow in the isthmus on color Doppler imaging
- Low-velocity persistent forward flow with low pulsatility index on pulse wave Doppler imaging
- Aortic isthmus Z score less than –2 on "three vessels and trachea" view
- Persistent absence of "catch-up" growth of the aortic isthmus, where serial measures continue to reveal aortic isthmus at Z score less than –2
- Isthmus-to-ductus arteriosus diameter ratio less than 0.74 on "three vessels and trachea" view
- Transverse aortic arch diameter measurement of less than 3 mm at greater than 30 weeks' gestation
- Aortic annulus-to-pulmonary annulus diameter measurement less than 0.6 in the outflow tract views
- Mitral valve–to-tricuspid valve annulus measurement in four-chamber view less than 0.6
- Main pulmonary artery–to-ascending aorta diameter ratio of greater than 1.6, when measured in the mediastinum
- Bidirectional shunting at the level of the atrial septum

Our group recently looked at factors that discriminate between true coarctation with need for postnatal intervention and those that did not, in a series of fetuses with LV-RV size discrepancy.[11] A smaller aortic annulus–to–pulmonary annulus diameter ratio, transverse aortic arch measurement of less than 3mm at 30 weeks' or greater gestation, and bidirectional shunting at the atrial level were findings that predicted for a true coarctation. Similar to Gardiner and colleagues' series, we found that absence of aortic isthmus growth over time was a strong predictor as well. In another study, a smaller ascending aorta–to–main pulmonary artery ratio also distinguished true coarctation from other causes of LV-RV size disproportion.[12]

Increased peak velocity, or a gradient across the aortic isthmus, will not be seen in the fetus with coarctation of the aorta. Unlike that seen in the infant or child, in the fetus with coarctation there is redistribution of blood flow away from the narrowing. So the effect of a narrowing such as a coarctation is a net reduction of flow across, not the generation of a pressure gradient. However, there can be severe cases of narrowing with a discrete shelf in which a continuous, phasic pattern of flow across the isthmus can be seen. Oftentimes, this can also be identified as continuous antegrade flow on color Doppler imaging, with persistence of color across the region seen throughout the cardiac cycle.

Similar to other forms of congenital heart disease, there is an indication for analysis of the fetal chromosomes and an obstetrical ultrasound to evaluate for extracardiac anomalies. Serial fetal echocardiography is also important, whether to document progression of left-sided disease in those with clear coarctation of the aorta or to predict the presence of a possible coarctation in those with LV-RV size disproportion.

In fetuses that are predicted to have postnatal arch obstruction, a planned delivery at a tertiary referral center with neonatal and cardiology specialists is recommended. This allows for a controlled delivery and transfer of the neonate to the intensive care unit for assessment of clinical status, initiation of prostaglandin infusion, and confirmation of the diagnosis by transthoracic echocardiography.

Postnatal Physiology

The postnatal physiology depends on the degree of obstruction and the presence of associated lesions. In the immediate postnatal period, the ductus arteriosus is usually patent and, therefore, there is no pressure gradient across the aortic arch. While the ductus arteriosus is open, upper and lower blood pressures are equal and the infant is asymptomatic. The ductus arteriosus begins to constrict in the first hours to days of life, closing from the pulmonary end first. It can take days to weeks for the aortic end to constrict at the level of the isthmus, which then causes narrowing of the lumen and obstruction to flow. This may explain why coarctation can present relatively late in infancy is some neonates. Once the ductus arteriosus closes, an increase in afterload to the neonatal myocardium results in myocardial dysfunction and cardiac failure.

The neonate with critical coarctation and transverse arch hypoplasia will present early with cyanosis, as the ductus arteriosus carrying desaturated blood from right side perfuses the lower extremities. Once the ductus arteriosus starts to close, there will be signs of impaired perfusion, hypotension, and acidosis because the entire cardiac output must now cross the narrowed region.

Postnatal Management

After delivery, intravenous access is obtained with initiation of prostaglandin infusion. A physical examination, chest x-ray, electrocardiogram, and arterial blood gas are performed. Correction of metabolic acidosis, hypoglycemia, and electrolyte abnormalities is important. A complete transthoracic echocardiogram is performed to allow for confirmation of the prenatal diagnosis and to identify any associated intracardiac defects. It is not uncommon to discontinue the prostaglandin infusion and follow blood pressure gradients and repeat an echocardiogram after ductal closure to clearly document the presence of arch obstruction.

In cases of LV-RV size discrepancy with suspected coarctation, but not confidently confirmed, one can undertake a course of careful scrutiny and observation in an intensive care unit setting. By not initiating prostaglandin therapy, and allowing for ductal closure to take place, serial blood pressure evaluation and echocardiography will allow for a correct diagnosis once natural ductal closure has taken place.

Coarctation presenting in infancy with evidence of a right-to-left shunt across the ductus arteriosus reflecting the need for ductal support of the systemic circulation or significant pressure gradient and symptoms of heart failure requires early treatment with repair. Surgical repair depends on the location of the obstruction and associated intracardiac lesions. If the coarctation is isolated to the region of the isthmus without other intracardiac defects, the repair can be successfully performed through a left lateral thoracotomy under the left axilla. This procedure can be done without the use of cardiopulmonary bypass. When extensive arch hypoplasia is present and coarctation is associated with other defects such as a large VSD, a median sternotomy is performed for a midline repair. Arch augmentation in this manner does require cardiopulmonary bypass.

A variety of techniques can be utilized, each with their individual advantages and disadvantages. The first repair of coarctation of the aorta was reported by Crafoord and Nylin in 1945[13] who performed a resection of the coarctation region with end-to end re-anastamosis of the aorta. To date, this procedure remains the technique of choice for repair of isolated coarctation. When extensive arch hypoplasia is present, material such as homograft patch can be used to augment the narrowed area and enlarge the overall dimensions of the aorta.

Outcomes

The morbidity and mortality rates for surgical repair of aortic arch obstruction vary depending on the age of correction, type of arch obstruction, associated intracardiac defects, and presence of genetic and extracardiac abnormalities. Mortality rates for repair of isolated coarctation in the neonate approach 0% at large centers but can be as high as 2% to 10% when additional lesions are present.[14,15] Postoperative complications include hypertension, recurrent laryngeal and phrenic nerve injury, and bleeding. Rarely, spinal cord ischemia and paralysis may occur; however, in the current era, these are quite uncommon.

Long-term follow-up is important for this group of patients to screen for persistent hypertension, residual coarctation as a consequence of scar tissue formation, and development of other forms of left-sided obstruction. Residual coarctation can occur in 10% to 15% of patients and typically requires balloon dilation angioplasty for successful relief.[16] Aneurysm formation at the site of coarctation repair can occur but is quite uncommon. Hypertension is a common long-term phenomenon after successful coarctation repair.[17] Of unclear etiology, it is believed to be due to developmental differences in fetal vascular receptor function, which persist despite successful relief of obstruction. Such hypertension can present in adolescence or young adulthood and may be an earlier manifestation of "essential hypertension," which is typically seen in the sixth or seventh decade of life. When hypertension is present, antihypertensive agents are used for control. Exercise stress testing should be performed regularly, because exaggerated blood pressure response to exercise can also be seen and may require management with antihypertensive agents or exercise restriction.

Nonetheless, the usual prognosis after successful repair of coarctation of the aorta is for an excellent quality of life with normal growth and development. Lifelong surveillance, however, is necessary to observe for residual arch gradients, hypertension, and aneurysm formation.

Imaging Essentials and Important Points

- Coarctation of the aorta in the fetus is a commonly missed diagnosis, with important implications. The neonate with coarctation may be completely asymptomatic until the ductus arteriosus closes, at which point hypotension, acidosis, and end-organ system damage can occur. Improving our diagnostic capabilities in making this diagnosis is of utmost importance.
- Suspicion of coarctation is most commonly manifest by the visualization of LV-RV size disproportion. Features listed in Box 20-2 should be carefully analyzed at initial evaluation and in a serial manner at subsequent evaluations.
- Coarctation in the presence of a large VSD will "equalize" volumes between the LV and the RV and size disproportion between the two ventricles will not be seen.
- Assessment of the aortic arch in both the long-axis arch views and a transverse view such as the three vessel and trachea view is of value.
- LV-RV size discrepancy in which the LV length is less than two thirds the distance toward the apex of the heart or in which there is continuous left-to-right shunting at the atrial level suggest important LV hypoplasia and the presence of HLHS.
- Look for venous anomalies, systemic and pulmonary, that may explain the presence of LV-RV size disproportion and give the false impression of a small isthmus.

References

1. Ho SY, Anderson RH. Coarctation, tubular hypoplasia, and the ductus arteriosus: histological study of 35 specimens. *Br Heart J.* 1979;41:268-274.
2. Botto LD, Correa A, Erickson DJ. Racial and temporal variations in the prevalence of heart defects. *Pediatrics.* 2001;107:e32.
3. Rudolph AM, Heymann MA, Spitznas U. Hemodynamic considerations in the development of narrowing of the aorta. *Am J Cardiol.* 1994;23:417-423.
4. Rudolph AM. *Congenital Diseases of the Heart: Clinical-Physiological Considerations.* 2nd ed. Armonk, NY: Futura Publishing; 2001.
5. Hornberger LK, Weintraub MB, Pesonen E, et al. Echocardiographic study of the morphology and growth of the aortic arch in the human fetus; observations related to prenatal diagnosis of coarctation. *Circulation* 1992;86:741-747.
6. Fouron JC. The unrecognized physiological and clinical significance of the fetal aortic isthmus. *Ultrasound Obstet Gynecol* 2003;22: 441-447.
7. Hornberger LK, Sahn SJ, Kleinman CS, Copel J, Silverman NH. Antenatal diagnosis of coarctation of the aorta: A multicenter experience. *JACC* 1994;23:417-423.
8. Berning RA, Silverman NH, Villegas M, Sahn DJ, Martin GR, and Rice MJ. Reversal of shunting across the ductus arteriosus or atrial septum in utero heralds severe congenital heart disease. *J Am Coll Cardiology* 1996;27:481-486.
9. Matsui H, Mellander M, Roughton M, Jicinska H, Gardiner HM. Morphological and physiological predictors of fetal aortic coarctation. *Circulation* 2008;118:1793-1801.
10. Pasquini L, Mellander M, Seale A, et al. Z-scores of the fetal aortic isthmus and duct: an aid to assessing arch hypoplasia. *Ultrasound Obstet Gynecol* 2007;29:628-633.
11. Quartermain MD, Cohen MS, Dominguez T, Tian Z, Donaghue DD, Rychik J. Left ventricle to right ventricle size discrepancy in the fetus: the presence of critical congenital heart disease can be reliably predicted *J Am Soc Echocardiogr* 2009;22:1296-1301.
12. Slodki M, Rychik J, Moszura T, Janiak K, Respondek-Liberska M. Measurement of the great vessels in the mediastinum could help distinguish true from false-positive coarctation of the aorta in the third trimester. *J Ultrasound Med* 2009;28:1313-1317.
13. Crafoord C, Nylin G Congenital coarctation of the aorta and its surgical treatment. *J Thorac Surg* 1945;14:347-352.
14. Corno AF, Botta U, Hurni M, et al. Surgery for aortic coarctation: a 30 year experience. *Eur J Cardiothorac Surg* 2001;20:1202-1205.
15. Wright GE, Nowak CA, Goldberg CS, et al. Extended resection and end-to-end anastamosis for aortic coarctation in infants: Results of a tailored surgical approach. *Ann Thorac Surg* 2005;80: 1453-1459.
16. Dodge-Khatami A, Backer CL, Mavroudis C. Risk Factors for recoarctation and results of reoperation: a 40 year review. *J Cardiac Surgery* 2000;15:369.
17. O'Sullivan J, Derrick G, Darnell R. Prevalence of hypertension in children after early repair of coarctation of the aorta. A cohort study using casual and 24 hour BP measurements. *Heart* 2002;88: 163-166.

CASES

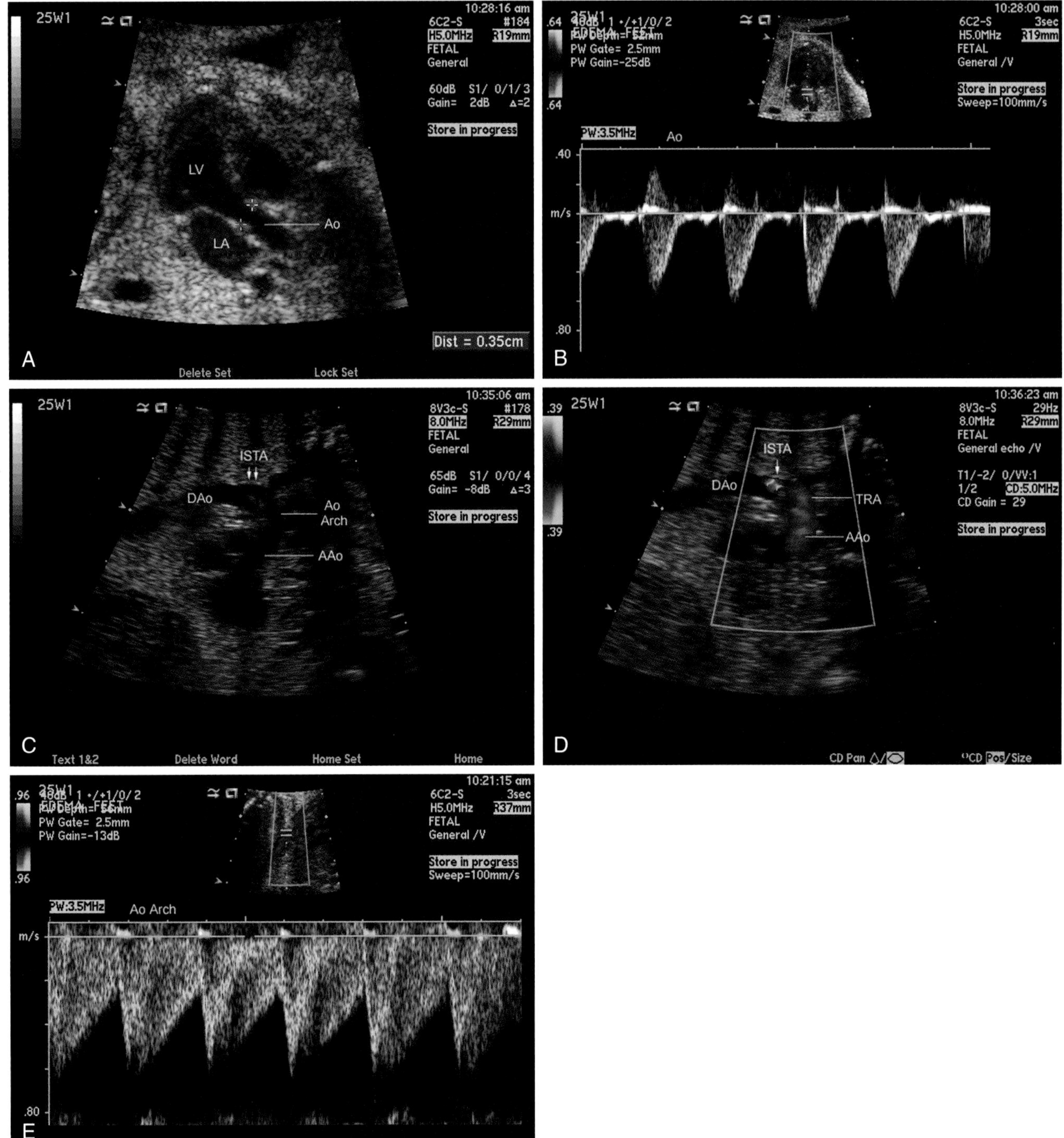

Case 20-1. **(A)** Long-axis view of the left ventricle (LV) demonstrates unobstructed outflow tract. The aortic annulus measures approximately 3 to 4 mm in diameter, which is normal for this gestational age at 25 weeks. Ao, aorta; LA, left atrium. **(B)** There is laminar flow across the aortic valve, indicating no aortic valve stenosis. **(C)** View of the aortic arch (Ao Arch) demonstrates coarctation of the aorta with hypoplasia (smallness) of the aortic isthmus (ISTA), the region in between the take-off of the left subclavian artery and the insertion of the ductus arteriosus into the descending aorta (DAo). AAo, ascending aorta. **(D)** Color Doppler imaging shows onset of turbulent flow at the ISTA as it inserts into the DAo. TRA, transverse arch. **(E)** Pulse wave Doppler interrogation of the narrowed coarctation region. Note the "saw-tooth" pattern indicating obstruction. The narrowing does not allow for the full complement of blood volume propelled into the area to be fully delivered in systole alone; hence, forward flow continues into diastole. This flow pattern is not a common finding in coarctation of the aorta in the fetus when there is a patent ductus arteriosus, but it is much more common in the neonate or older child. Nevertheless, when seen in fetal life, it is suggestive of significant narrowing.

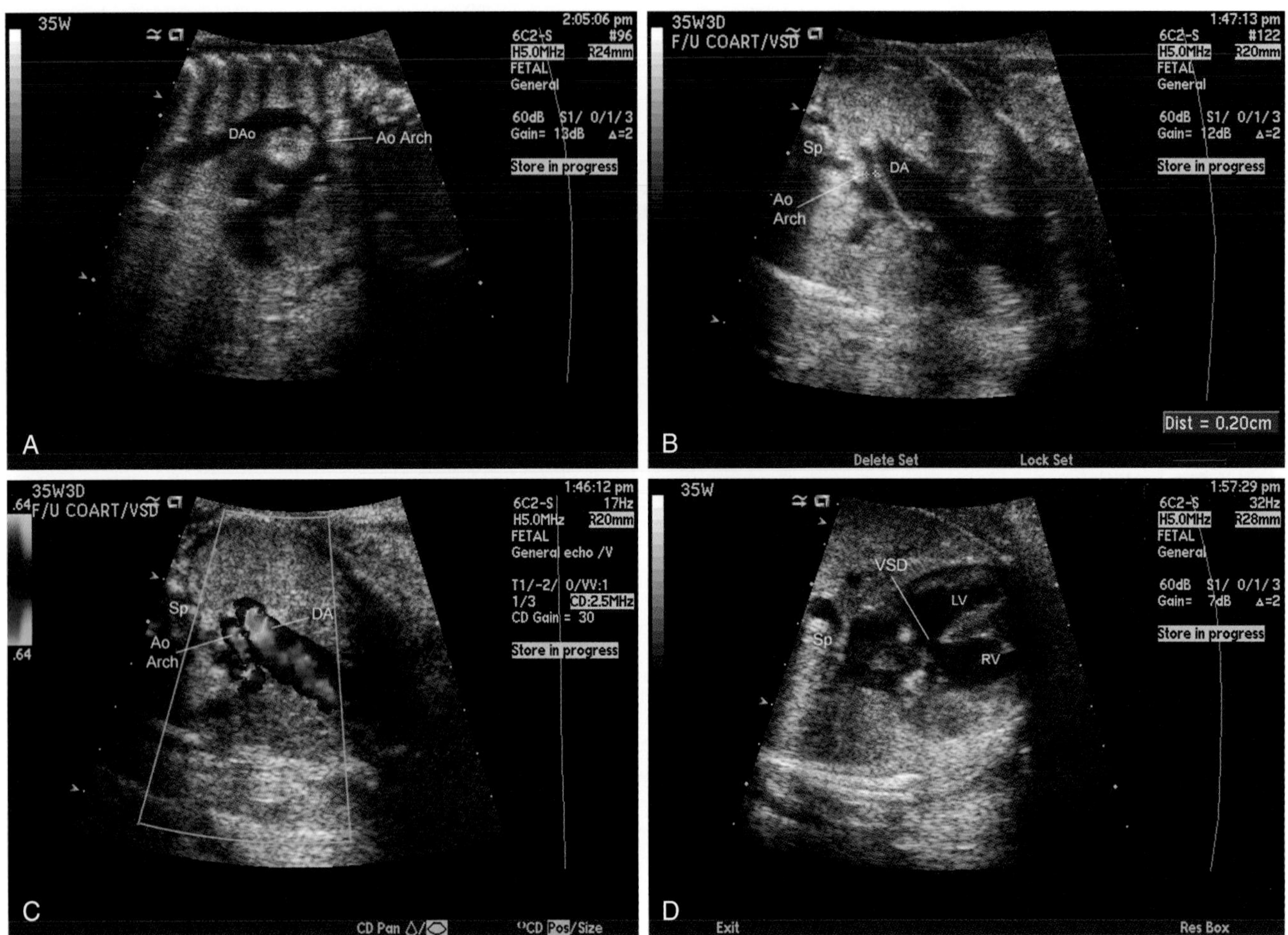

Case 20-2. **(A)** Arch view of a fetus with severe coarctation of the aorta. Note the substantial size discrepancy between the isthmus and the DAo. **(B)** This is a transverse view of the mediastinum at the level of the arches in the upper chest, above the level of the heart. The top of the ductal and aortic arches are seen. Note the substantial size discrepancy between the ductus arteriosus (DA) and the aortic arch (Ao arch). Sp, spine. **(C)** Color Doppler flow further demonstrates the marked size discrepancy between the ductal and aortic arches. **(D)** Imaging of the cardiac chambers reveals a large conoventricular ventricular septal defect (VSD) in addition to the coarctation of the aorta. RV, right ventricle.

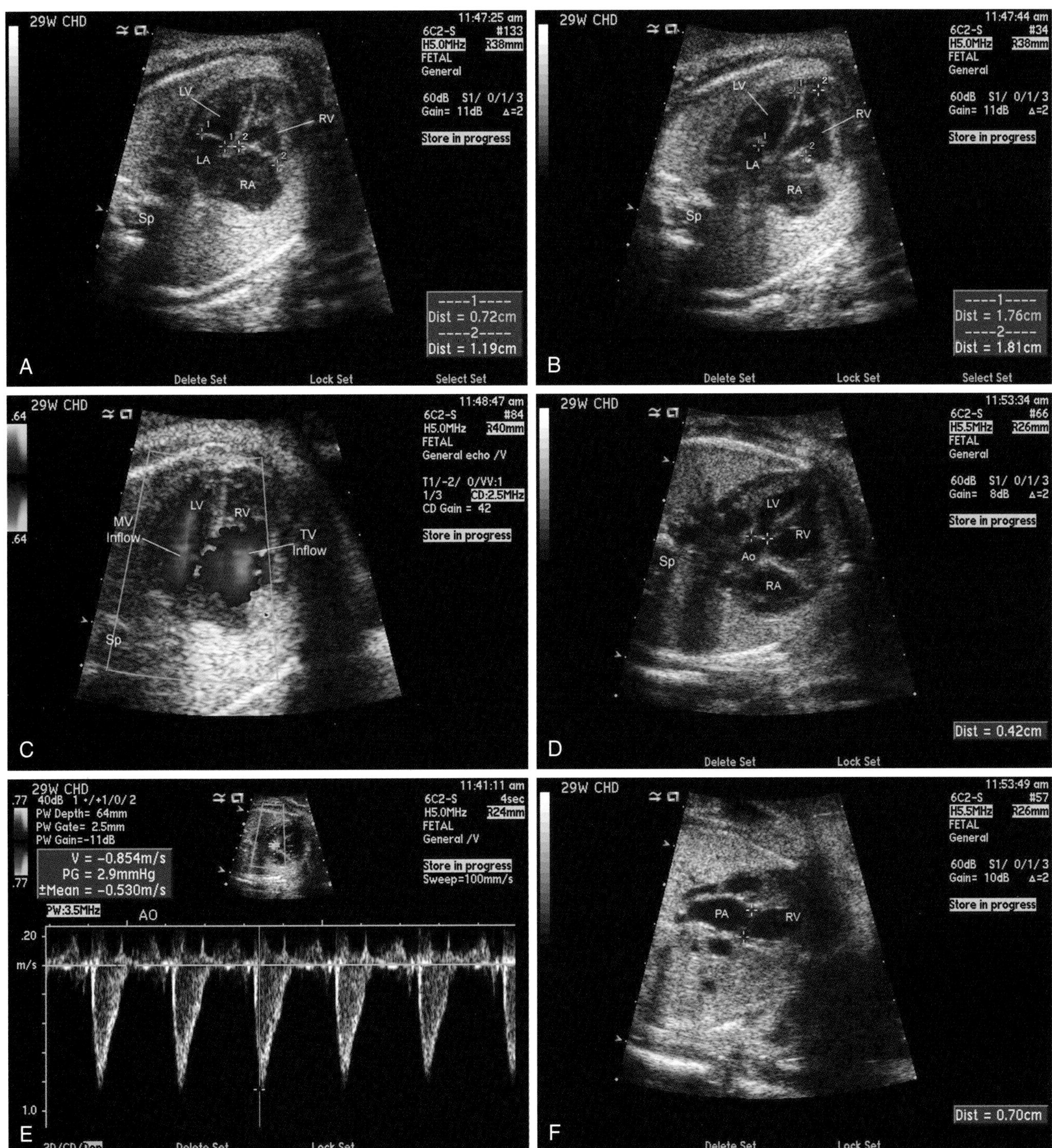

Case 20-3. **(A)** Size discrepancy between the RV and the LV with relative smallness of the left side is a common first indication of the possible presence of coarctation of the aorta. In this four-chamber view, the LV looks to be smaller than the RV to a greater degree than usual. Measurements of the mitral annulus (7.2 mm) and the tricuspid valve annulus (11.9 mm) reveal a ratio of approximately 0.6. Although the absolute value for the mitral valve annulus is not prohibitively small for this gestational age, the ratio reflects an element of unexpected size discrepancy. RA, right atrium. **(B)** Measurement of the LV and RV lengths reveal a ratio of slightly less than 1 : 1. **(C)** Color Doppler inflow suggests an element of unusual size discrepancy between the LV and the RV, with a somewhat smaller than expected left side. MV, mitral valve; TV, tricuspid valve. **(D)** Long axis of the LV. The aortic annulus measures 4.2 mm, which is low-normal size for 29 weeks' gestational age. **(E)** There is no evidence for aortic stenosis because the pulse wave Doppler flow pattern is laminar and with low-normal velocity. **(F)** The pulmonary artery (PA) annulus measures 7 mm; hence, the aortic-to-pulmonic annulus ratio is 0.6.

Continued

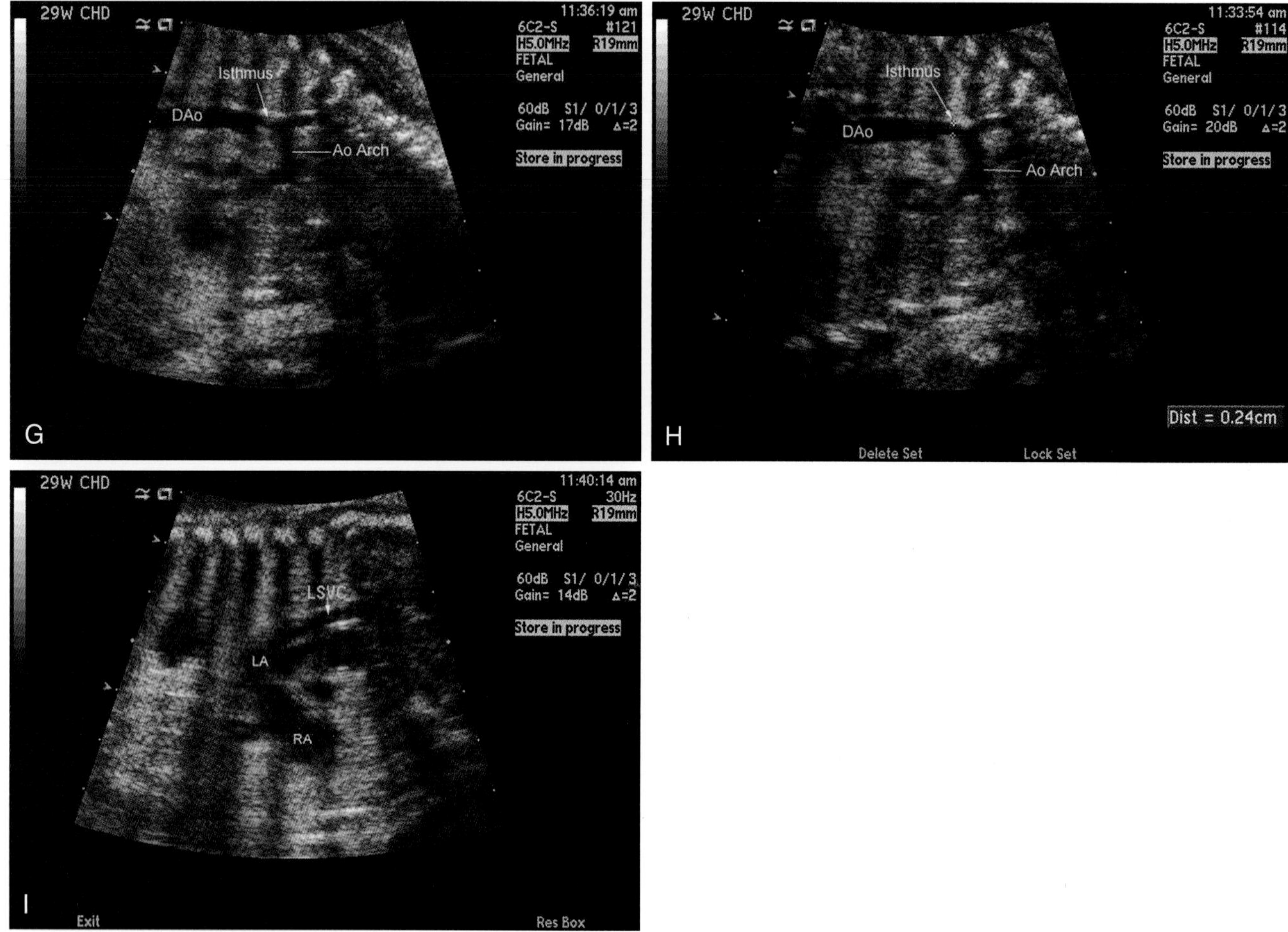

Case 20-3, cont'd **(G)** Imaging of the arch reveals hypoplasia of the isthmus and coarctation of the aorta. **(H)** The aortic isthmus measures 2.4 mm and remained less than 3 mm in diameter throughout the pregnancy. **(I)** Evidence for a left superior vena cava (LSVC) to coronary sinus. This is a common finding in the fetus with LV-to-RV size discrepancy and coarctation of the aorta.

21

Congenital Absence of Aortic Valve Leaflets

Jack Rychik

Key Echocardiographic Features

- Absence of competent aortic valve tissue at the site of the aortic annulus.
- Abnormally prominent pulsation of the ascending aorta.
- Abnormal dilation of the ascending aorta and/or head brachiocephalic vessels.
- Associated anomalies such as aortic arch obstruction and ventricular septal defect.
- Ventricular dysfunction.

Anatomy and Anatomical Associations

Congenital absence of the aortic valve leaflets is an extremely rare anomaly, with perhaps no more than two dozen reports in the literature.[1-4] Absence, or dysplasia, of the pulmonic leaflets is much more common and is seen with tetralogy of Fallot. In most instances of absent aortic valve leaflets, the only remnant of the aortic valve is a nonobstructive fibrous ridge.[3]

Absence of the aortic valve leaflets is typically not an isolated lesion. It is associated with conotruncal anomalies, ventricular septal defect, hypoplasia of the left ventricle, and dysplasia or aplasia of leaflets of the other semilunar, the pulmonic valve.[5] Absence of the aortic valve leaflets was first described in association with double-outlet right ventricle in a pathology specimen.[1] In a review of 15 cases of this anomaly, hypoplasia of the left heart was seen in 11 (73%), double-outlet right ventricle in 5 (33%), and aortic arch malformations in 6 (40%).[4]

Frequency, Genetics, and Development

Absence of the aortic valve leaflets is extremely rare. It is commonly associated with cystic hygroma, which may offer clues to the origin of this rare anomaly.[4] The relatively frequent association between absence of both the aortic and the semilunar valve leaflets has led some investigators to conclude that aplasia of the semilunar valve leaflets reflects an underdevelopment of the endocardial cushion swellings at the ventriculoarterial junction, rather than resulting primarily from an abnormality of septation of the outflow tracts.[6]

In one report, all seven cases were male, which suggests an X-linked process.[3] DiGeorge's syndrome has been reported in one case.[4]

Prenatal Physiology

Absence of a competent aortic valve results in severe aortic insufficiency. Severe aortic insufficiency affects the fetal circulation in a number of ways. In diastole, blood regurgitates back into the ventricle, which leads to a "steal" of blood flow away from the body organs and tissues. The heart dilates due to the volume load. Cardiomegaly and ventricular dysfunction ensue. Heart failure and fetal hydrops are common.[5,7] Placental insufficiency can occur as blood is diverted away during diastole. Survival under such conditions is unusual. Most fetuses with this anomaly succumb with fetal demise early in the first weeks of gestation, which may explain the rare nature of the anomaly.

Interestingly, the association with other anomalies may be protective. When seen with hypoplasia of the left ventricle, a stiff left ventricle with elevated end-diastolic pressure may limit the volume of regurgitation across the aortic valve, reducing the physiological effect of a perfusion steal.[8]

We recently saw a fetal case of absent aortic valve with ventricular septal defect and interruption of the aortic arch type C (interruption between the right subclavian artery and the left common carotid artery). Owing to the arch interruption, only the right arm and right common carotid were exposed to the deleterious physiological effects of severe aortic insufficiency because the remainder of the circulation was perfused by the right ventricle through the patent ductus arteriosus and a competent, normal pulmonary valve. This fetus survived to term and suffered sudden fetal demise at 38 weeks' gestation. We suspect that coronary insufficiency likely played a role in the fetal demise. As the left ventricle continued to dilate, there was a mismatch between coronary perfusion and myocardial demand, leading to myocardial ischemia and sudden death.

Prenatal Management

Absent aortic valve leaflets is essentially a lethal anomaly. The only reports of survival have been in association with hypoplasia of the left ventricle, in which the aorta is small.[8] In such cases, the degree of aortic insufficiency is not of great significance and may not seriously affect coronary perfusion. The essential aspect of prenatal management is making the correct diagnosis.

The fetal findings of absent aortic valve leaflets were first described in 1984 upon identification of pandiastolic reversal of flow in the descending aorta.[2] Today, direct inspection of the left ventricular outflow tract and ascending aorta will reveal absence of the thin normal leaflets of the aortic valve. The ascending aorta may be dilated as it receives an increased stroke volume with each beat. Prominent pulsations of the ascending and descending aorta are typical clues to the presence of this anomaly.

Color Doppler flow imaging will demonstrate severe aortic insufficiency with a wide jet of color flow returning into the left ventricle during diastole. This should be carefully distinguished from inflow across the mitral valve by appropriate angulation of the transducer. Pulse Doppler will demonstrate reversal of flow in the aorta. The more severe the aortic insufficiency, the more distal in the aorta the reversal will be seen. Diastolic reversal in the descending aorta is to be expected, with reversal in the umbilical artery an ominous sign and a substrate for likely fetal demise.

Associated anomalies such as absent pulmonary valve leaflets, conotruncal defects, and arch defects should be looked for. Karyotype assessment is essential because this rare anomaly may be associated with more pervasive genetic or chromosomal abnormalities.

Postnatal Physiology

Fetal demise is common, but some fetuses do survive to the neonatal period. Aortic insufficiency can worsen upon birth as overall vascular resistance is increased with removal of the low-resistance placental circulation. Hypotension, acidosis, and hypoxemia are to be expected.[3]

Postnatal Management

If the fetus survives to term, immediate postnatal surgical intervention in cases of hemodynamically severe aortic insufficiency may be helpful; however, there are no reports of such an undertaking. When absent aortic valve leaflets are seen in association with hypoplasia of the left ventricle, the volume of regurgitation is small and may not result in a substantial steal. A staged reconstructive approach using the Norwood operation leading to a single-ventricle palliation has been reported.[8] In this case, the aortic annulus was small and was left untouched during the reconstruction. The child has survived through Fontan operation as well, further suggesting that the degree of insufficiency is not of consequence, likely related to the "protective" hemodynamics of a small, stiff left ventricle.[9]

Outcomes

Overall survival for absent aortic valve leaflets is poor with hydrops, fetal demise, or early neonatal death occurring in the vast majority.

Imaging Essentials and Important Points

- Unusual and prominent pulsation of a dilated ascending or descending aorta is a clue to the presence of absent aortic valve leaflets.
- Unlike in absent pulmonary valve leaflets, in the absent aortic valve leaflets, no leaflet remnant is present. One may see only a small fibrous ridge or a completely smooth annulus at the site where the valve should be.
- The associated anomalies will dictate the hemodynamics, as in our unusual case of interrupted aortic arch. Owing to ductal perfusion of regions beyond the interruption, only the coronary circulation and the right common carotid artery were under the deleterious influences of severe aortic regurgitation. Nevertheless, in our case fetal demise likely occurred secondary to coronary insufficiency.
- Absence of the aortic valve leaflets in association with hypoplastic left heart syndrome may be amenable to staged reconstructive palliation with the Norwood operation, because the actual volume of aortic insufficiency and potential for blood steal are minimal.[9]

References

1. Toews WH, Lortscher RH, Kelminson LL. Double outlet right ventricle with absent aortic valve. *Chest*. 1975;68:381-382.
2. Bierman FZ, Yeh MN, Swersky S, Martin E, Wigger JH, Fox H. Absence of the aortic valve: antenatal and postnatal two-dimensional and Doppler echocardiographic features. *J Am Coll Cardiol*. 1984;3: 833-837.
3. Lin AE, Chin AJ. Absent aortic valve: a complex anomaly. *Pediatr Cardiol*. 1990;11:195-198.
4. Miyabara S, Ando M, Yoshida K, Saito N, Sugihara H. Absent aortic and pulmonary valves: investigation of three fetal cases with cystic hygroma and review of the literature. *Heart Vessels*. 1994;9:49-55.
5. Marek J, Skovranek J, Povysilova V. Congenital absence of aortic and pulmonary valve in a fetus with severe heart failure. *Heart*. 1996; 75:98-100.
6. Hartwig NG, Vermeij-Keers C, De Vries HE, Gittenberger-De Groot AC. Aplasia of semilunar valve leaflets: two case reports and developmental aspects. *Pediatr Cardiol*. 1991;12:114-117.
7. Eronen M, Heikkila P. Absent aortic and dysplastic pulmonary valves associated with ventricular septal defect in fetal hydrops. *Pediatr Cardiol*. 2003;24:400-402.
8. Harada Y, Takeuchi T, Satomi G, Yasukouchi S. Absent aortic valve: successful palliation in the neonate. *Ann Thorac Surg*. 1998;66: 935-936.
9. Hibino N, Harada Y, Hiramatsu T, Yasukochi S, Satomi G. Fontan operation for hypoplastic left heart syndrome with absent aortic valve. *J Thorac Cardiovasc Surg*. 2004;128:315-316.

CASE

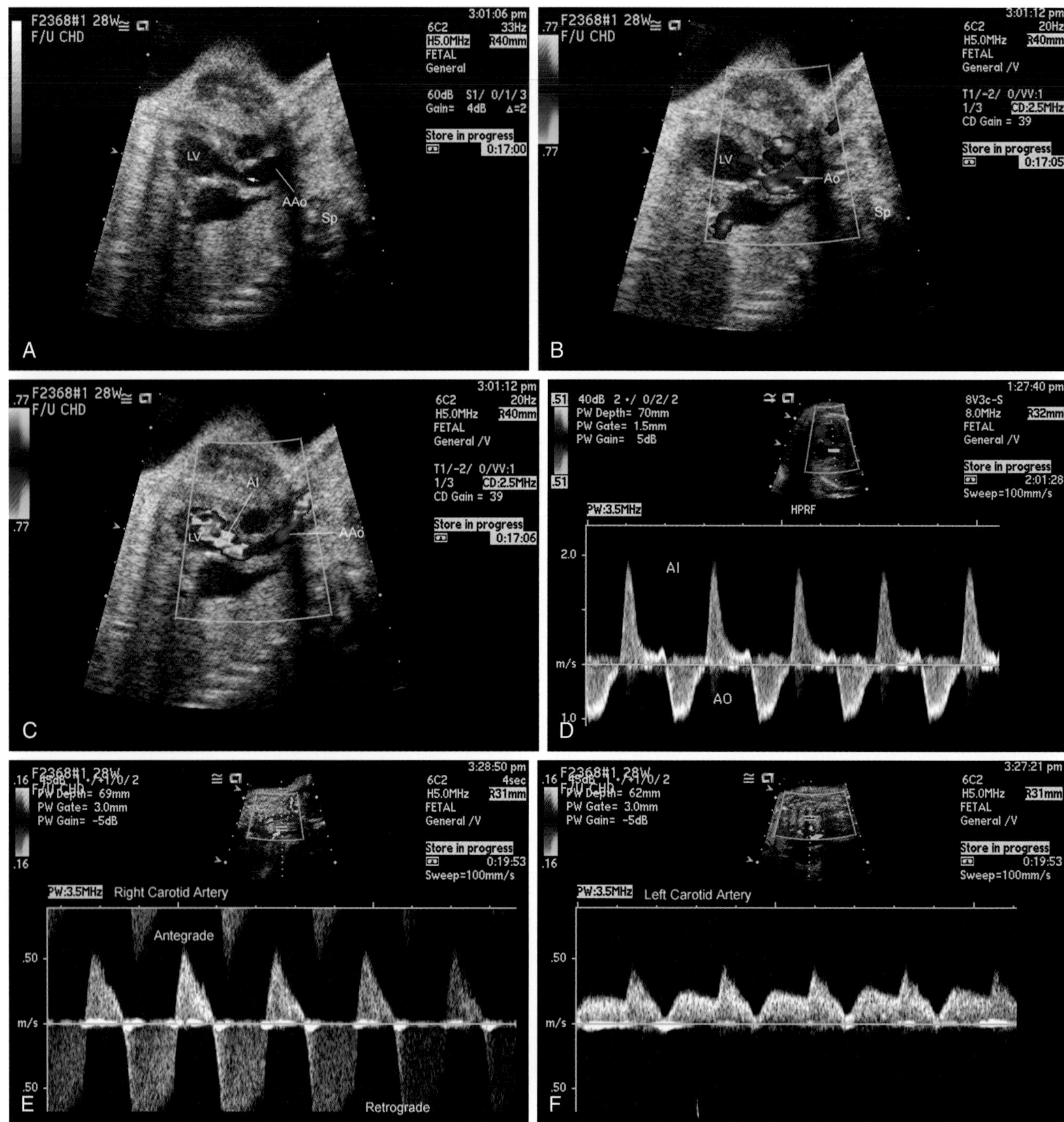

Case 21-1. **(A)** A rare case of absent aortic valve leaflet syndrome and interruption of the aortic arch type B (between the right innominate artery and the left carotid artery). The *arrow* points to the site where the aortic valve leaflets should be; however, they are absent. The ascending aorta (AAo) is dilated. LV, left ventricle; Sp, spine. **(B)** Flow during systole across the left ventricular outflow tract into the aorta (Ao). **(C)** Flow during diastole. There is a wide jet of aortic insufficiency (AI) into the cavity body of the LV. There is a blue jet in the AAo reflecting diastolic reversal back into the LV because no aortic valve leaflets are present. **(D)** Doppler flow in the AAo. There is laminar forward flow into the aorta during systole (flow below the baseline) and reversal of flow due to AI (above the baseline). **(E)** Because there is interruption of the aortic arch between the two carotids, the right carotid artery flow pattern is under the influence of the absent aortic valve leaflets. As a consequence, forward systolic flow is seen (above the baseline) as well as retrograde flow due to severe AI drawing blood back from the right carotid into the LV (below the baseline). **(F)** Flow pattern in the left carotid artery. There is antegrade flow in systole and also in diastole because this carotid arises distal to the interruption and is perfused via the ductus arteriosus. The antegrade flow in diastole is due to the impetus for forward flow due to connections at the circle of Willis. The degree of AI is so great that it is drawing blood forward from the left carotid to the right carotid at the circle of Willis; hence, diastolic flow is retrograde in the right carotid and antegrade in the left carotid both as a consequence of severe AI.

22

Hypoplastic Left Heart Syndrome

Jack Rychik

Key Echocardiographic Features

- Size and function of the left ventricle in comparison with the right ventricle.
- Direction of shunting at the atrial level (hypoplastic left heart syndrome is defined by inadequacy of the left-sided structures; hence, shunting at the atrial level in this anomaly is left to right).
- Presence and size of the mitral valve.
- Size of the aorta.
- Direction of shunting in the transverse aorta (retrograde in cases of aortic atresia or severe aortic stenosis).
- In cases of a patent mitral valve, the presence of coronary-cameral fistulae on color Doppler imaging of the small left ventricle.
- Anatomy of the atrial septum and patency of the foramen ovale.
- Pulmonary venous Doppler flow pattern as a reflection of adequate left atrial egress and an indirect gauge of possible restriction at the level of the atrial septum.
- Tricuspid valve function.
- Right ventricle function.

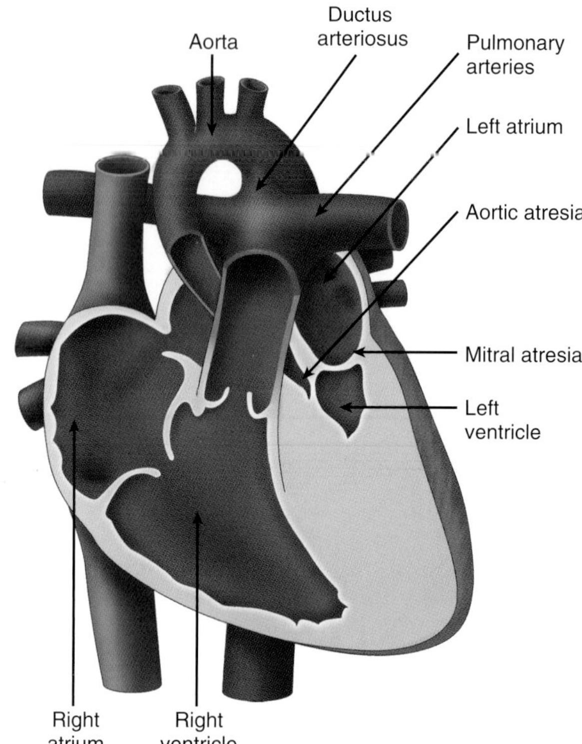

Figure 22-1. Hypoplastic left heart syndrome (HLHS) with mitral atresia and aortic atresia. There is no antegrade flow into the aorta; all flow into the aorta is retrograde via the ductus arteriosus. There is left-to-right shunting at the atrial level.

Anatomy and Anatomical Associations

Hypoplastic left heart syndrome (HLHS) is not a single specific anomaly, but rather, a term that refers to a constellation of congenital cardiac anomalies in which the left side of the heart is insufficient in makeup and/or size to perform the task of providing for perfusion of the systemic circulation.[1] The left ventricle (LV) may be nonviable as a provider of systemic perfusion owing to a spectrum of structural cardiac anomalies ranging from complete atresia of the mitral valve and aortic valves with no visible LV at all (Figure 22-1) to hypoplasia of the mitral valve and aortic valves with borderline small LV cavity (Figure 22-2).[2] Hypoplasia of the ascending aorta, aortic arch, and coarctation of the aorta are commonly seen as well.

Noncardiac anomalies including chromosomal abnormalities are seen in 28% of infants with HLHS on autopsy study.[3] Chromosomal abnormalities are seen in approximately 5% to 10% and include trisomy 13, trisomy 18, and Turner's syndrome (monosomy X).[4] One theory proposes a possible cause-and-effect relationship between the presence of large cystic hygroma as seen in Turner's syndrome and compression of the developing left-sided structures of the heart, in particular the aortic arch, resulting in left ventricular hypoplasia. Rarely, deletion of chromosome 22q11 can occur. Syndromes such as Smith-Lemli-Opitz, Holt-Oram, and the VACTERL (vertebral

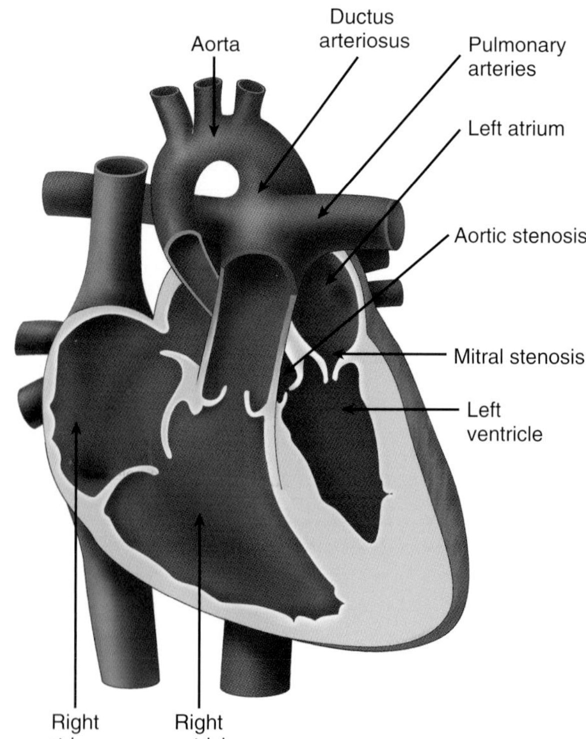

Figure 22-2. HLHS with mitral hypoplasia and aortic hypoplasia. Both mitral and aortic valves are patent; therefore, there is antegrade flow from the small left ventricle into the ascending aorta.

abnormalities, anal atresia, cardiac abnormalities, tracheoesophageal fistula and/or esophageal atresia, renal agenesis and dysplasia, and limb defects) association have been reported.

Identification of deficits in neurocognitive outcome of some children with HLHS after surgical palliation has prompted a more rigorous search for neuroanatomical differences in the infant brain with HLHS from those with a normal heart.[5–7] Subtle forms of cerebral dysgenesis such as an open cerebral operculum, micrencephaly (brain weight < 2 standard deviations below mean for age), and absence of the corpus collosum have been identified in newborns with HLHS at autopsy.[8] The precise relationship between these anatomical features and late neurocognitive outcome has not yet been established. Infants with HLHS are commonly small for gestational age, with data emerging that suggest the presence of microcephaly for gestational age as well.[9]

Frequency, Genetics, and Development

HLHS occurs in 0.26 per 1000 live births.[10] The precise incidence varies somewhat because the definition of the syndrome and the time period of analysis differ slightly from study to study. Of all the various forms of congenital heart disease, HLHS is one of the most commonly diagnosed before birth because it can be easily detected by simple four-chamber view of the heart with absence of visualization of two normal-sized ventricles. Of 385 fetuses examined prenatally at The Children's Hospital of Philadelphia (CHOP) with complex congenital heart disease requiring intervention between July 2002 and June 2005, 117 (30%) carried the diagnosis of HLHS. The recurrence risk for having another child with HLHS is relatively high in comparison with other forms of congenital heart disease and is 2% to 3%.[11] The risk of a family with one child with HLHS having another person in the family with any form of congenital heart disease is also relatively high at 13% to 14%.[12]

The developmental formation of HLHS is uncertain. There are no good animal models of HLHS, which has hampered our understandings of the origins of this anomaly. A number of theories exist. One is that poor development of the LV is a consequence of blood flow being diverted away from the left side of the heart early in development. The finding of abnormal atrial septal anatomy and restriction to flow found in so many patients suggests that perhaps limitation to right-to-left shunting, the primary source for filling of the LV in utero, may be the causative factor. With limited right-to-left shunting, there is less blood flow across the mitral and aortic valves; hence, the development of mitral, left ventricular, and aortic hypoplasia. Conversely, abnormal formation of the atrial septum may be secondary to an inability of the LV to fill for some other reason, perhaps altered compliance. Aortic stenosis may be the primary anomaly in some, with altered LV compliance and endocardial fibroelastosis limiting the filling capacity, resulting in poor growth. Alternatively, another theory holds to the view that none of these abnormalities are flow-derived one from the other, but rather, a series of associated, gene-signaled defects that occur simultaneously. The frequent occurrence of left- and right-sided valve dysplasia in HLHS probands and the increased prevalence of balloon aortic valvuloplasty in family members have influenced some investigators to conclude that HLHS is a severe form of valve malformation.[13]

Based on the heterogeneity of anatomy seen in the HLHS, it seems likely that there are multiple pathways to achieve the diagnosis of a nonviable LV. Our definition of HLHS is, to a degree, a convenience and an arbitrary one, derived from the physiological consequences of the anomaly and our management. HLHS, as we define it today, is most likely an umbrella "grab-bag" term for a number of differently originating, but related, disorders.

Prenatal Physiology and Management

The intracardiac pathways of blood flow are different from normal in the fetus with HLHS. Superior and inferior vena caval return is to the right atrium and the ductus venosus drains in the normal fashion into the intrahepatic portion of the inferior vena cava. The eustachian valve, a membrane-like tissue at the orifice of the inferior vena cava that usually guides inferior caval flow toward the atrial septum, can at times be small and poorly formed.[14] Pulmonary venous return is typically to the left atrium. However, as opposed to the normal *right-to-left* flow across the atrial septum, shunting occurs in a *left-to-right* manner across the atrial septum in order to decompress the left atrium when the LV is hypoplastic.

A number of anatomical features of HLHS affect the physiology and are worthy of discussion.

The Atrial Septum and Pulmonary Vasculature

Patency of the atrial septum through either a foramen ovale or an atrial septal defect is a critical factor in the normal development of the fetus with HLHS. A severely restrictive or intact atrial septum is seen in approximately 6% of infants with HLHS. In such cases, egress from the left atrium is obstructed, left atrial pressure is increased, and pulmonary venous return is impaired. Infants born with HLHS and an intact atrial septum are at high risk for mortality after birth.[15] The fetus with an intact atrial septum is clinically asymptomatic because the placenta, and not the lung, is the organ of fetal oxygenation. However, at birth, these infants are extremely cyanosed and hypoxemic owing to the inability for oxygenated

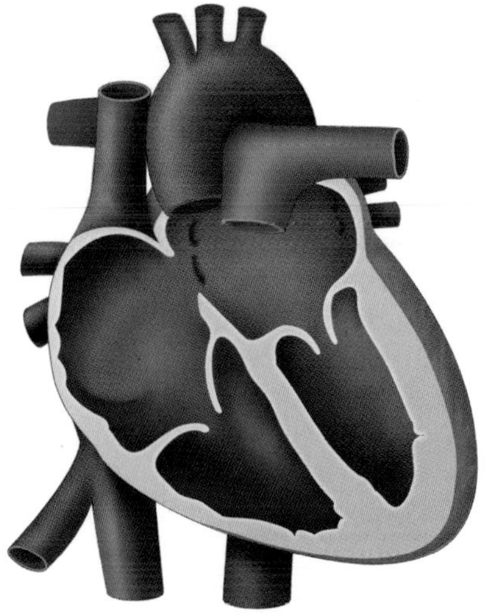

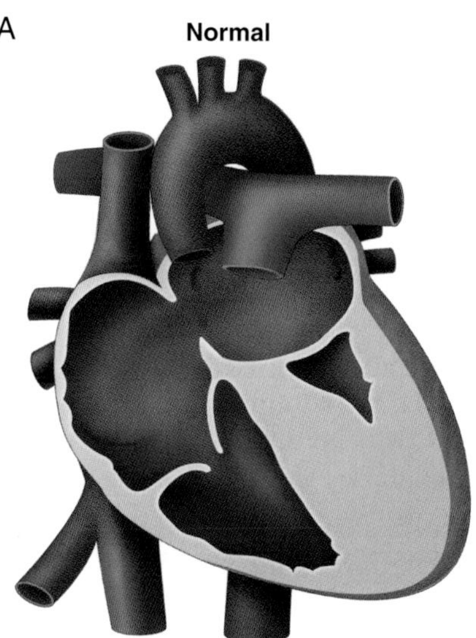

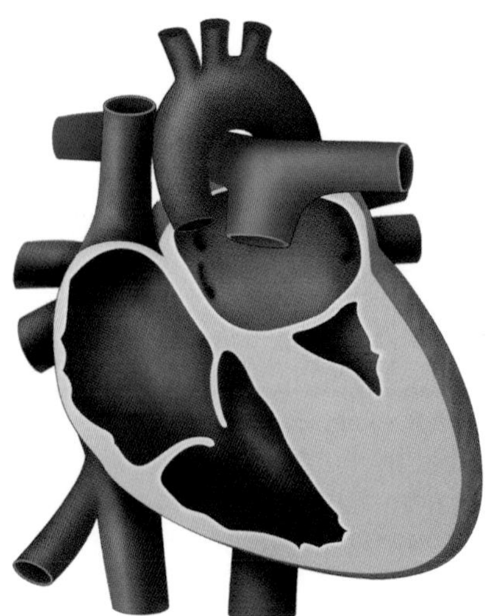

Figure 22-3. Direction of atrial level shunting in the fetus. **(A)** Normal fetal right-to-left shunting at the atrial level with preferential streaming of relatively highly oxygenated venous return from the ductus venosus directed toward the atrial septum and left atrium. **(B)** HLHS with an open atrial septum. There is left-to-right shunting at the atrial septal level. **(C)** Intact atrial septum with no atrial level shunting.

blood returning from the lungs to exit the left atrium and mix with the systemic venous return on the right side of the heart (Figure 22-3). These infants do extremely poorly at birth with marked hypoxemia and early demise, despite prenatal diagnosis.[16] Early postnatal identification and immediate intervention in infants with an intact atrial septum does not appear to substantially improve upon the relatively poor outcome in all, because it is believed that the inability for blood to exit the left atrium causes damage to the developing fetal lung vasculature in some fetuses. Histological analysis of the pulmonary veins in the newborn with HLHS and intact atrial septum reveals dilated vessels with thickened "arterialized" walls and multiple elastic laminae, suggesting a problem with pulmonary vascular development during fetal life (Figure 22-4).[15] Fetal intervention with balloon atrial septoplasty of the atrial septum has been performed and is in the early stages of development as a possible treatment for this disorder.[17] The goal is to relieve left atrial hypertension and promote flow through the pulmonary veins by allowing for unimpeded egress out of the left atrium. The efficacy of the technique and the optimal timing of when in gestation to intervene in hopes of preventing the pulmonary vasculopathy that develops are yet to be determined.[18] Ideally, it would be most helpful if such an intervention could take place before any permanent changes in pulmonary vasculature with vasculopathy takes place.

Identifying the precise nature of the patency of the atrial septum can be difficult. In addition, decompressing vessels such as a levoatrial cardinal vein may drain blood away from the left atrium, but yet not be detectable on fetal echocardiography. Hence, in addition to visualization of the septum, Doppler sampling in the pulmonary veins is of great use in gauging the presence and degree of impediment to left atrial egress. If there is an open, or only mildly restrictive, interatrial communication, there will be a normal pulmonary vein Doppler flow pattern consisting of a predominance of antegrade, biphasic flow into the atrium, with a short interval of low-velocity retrograde waveform concordant with atrial systole.[19] As the degree of restriction at the atrial septum increases, the time interval and velocity of the retrograde atrial waveform will increase (Figure 22-5). Investigators have determined that a velocity-time integral (area under the Doppler waveform) ratio of antegrade flow to retrograde flow of less than 5 suggests the presence of important atrial level restriction that may require attention and urgent atrial opening at birth.[20]

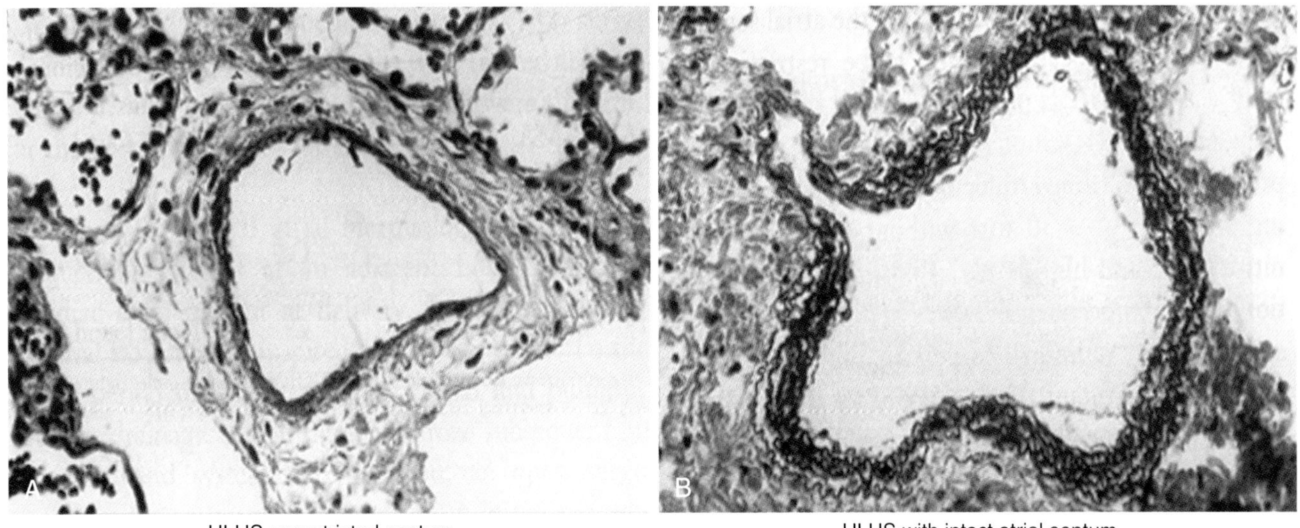

Figure 22-4. Histological assessment of pulmonary vein via endothelial stains. **(A)** A case of HLHS and a wide-open, unrestrictive atrial septum. Pulmonary vein wall is thin and normal in appearance. **(B)** A case of HLHS with intact atrial septum. Note the thick endothelial wall and the presence of multiple elastic laminae, suggestive of the process of "arterialization" of the pulmonary vein.

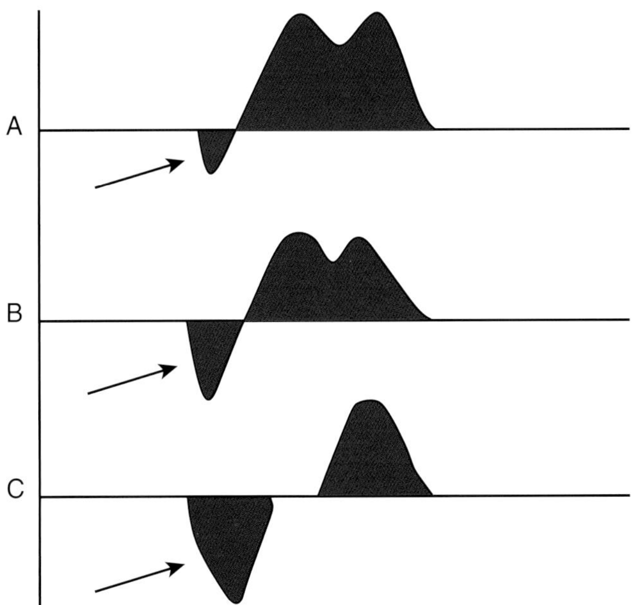

Figure 22-5. Schematic diagrams of Doppler pulmonary venous flow patterns in the HLHS. **(A)** Widely patent atrial septum with no restriction to left atrial egress. There is a predominance of antegrade flow (above baseline) with a very small amount of retrograde flow with atrial contraction (below baseline; *arrow*). **(B)** Moderate degree of restriction at the atrial septum. There is still a predominance of antegrade flow, but also a prominent waveform with atrial reversal *(arrow)*. Such fetuses warrant observation and benefit from serial prenatal surveillance. **(C)** Severe degree of restriction at the atrial septum, as seen in an intact atrial septum. There is equal reversal of flow with atrial contraction *(arrow)* as there is antegrade flow. This suggests significant obstruction to left atrial egress and left atrial hypertension and is a marker for severe cyanosis at birth.

In addition to pulmonary vein flow analysis, we have added another component of direct evaluation of pulmonary vascular health in our fetuses with HLHS. In congenital diaphragmatic hernia, it is known that normal, healthy fetal pulmonary vasculature will vasodilate in response to maternal hyperoxygenation, whereas abnormal pulmonary vasculature will not.[21] We, therefore, applied this principle to our mothers carrying fetuses with HLHS.[22] By offering 100% oxygen through a nonrebreather mask for 15 minutes, adequate levels of oxygen should cross the placenta and result in relaxation of the pulmonary vasculature. We assessed the pulsatility index (PI) as a measure of vascular resistance and sampled at different sites in the pulmonary artery of fetuses with HLHS and varying degrees of atrial level restriction. The Doppler signals obtained from sampling in the pulmonary artery vary slightly from proximal to distal sites. We, therefore, sampled at a proximal pulmonary artery site just at the bifurcation (P1), midportion of the pulmonary artery as it just enters the lung parenchyma (P2), and distal in the lung bed beyond the hilum and into the lung parenchyma (P3). Case 22-1E and F demonstrates the contour change in the pulmonary artery Doppler waveform that takes place from room air sampling to maternal hyperoxygenation. There is a characteristic increase in peak velocity and an overall increase in diastolic flow and decrease in PI with maternal hyperoxygenation if the vasculature is normal. We found that fetuses with HLHS and an open atrial septum had good vasoreactivity, with at least a 10% decrease in PI with hyperoxygenation, whereas those with HLHS and an intact or highly restrictive septum had very little vasoreactivity and little change in PI with hyperoxygenation. The highest resistance measure is seen at site P3, the most distal aspect of the pulmonary artery measured. This is also the site of greatest sensitivity to change and vasodilation when the atrial septum is wide open. Those fetuses with little vasoreactive response to maternal hyperoxygenation were also those who had severe hypoxemia at birth, requiring urgent care and had in general poorer outcome. We advocate the use of maternal hyperoxygenation in all of our fetuses with HLHS and use the data to determine candidacy for either fetal atrial septoplasty intervention or urgent immediate opening of the septum at birth. Maternal hyperoxygenation is safe, with no untoward effects noted in the fetus and no evidence for ductal constriction in close to 100 fetuses thus far evaluated in this manner.

Patterns of Aortic Blood Flow

The pattern of blood flow in the aorta is altered in HLHS. In the absence of an LV or in aortic atresia, perfusion of the ascending aorta and, hence, the coronary circulation is in a retrograde manner originating distally, beyond the isthmus of the aorta, from the ductus arteriosus (Figure 22-6). Often, in the presence of a small LV with aortic stenosis, a small amount of antegrade flow may take place in the ascending aorta; however, the transverse aorta and the cerebral vasculature arising therefrom are perfused retrograde from the ductus arteriosus. Dependency of the cerebral circulation upon retrograde perfusion from the ductus arteriosus into a variably hypoplastic aorta may limit the volume of blood flow and alter the regulatory mechanisms for cerebrovascular resistance. We have found lower cerebrovascular resistance as assessed by lower middle cerebral artery PI in fetuses with HLHS in comparison with normal and other forms of congenital heart disease.[23] One explanation may be that the brain is autoregulating blood flow and attempting to increase perfusion by vasodilation under conditions in which there are structural impediments to flow, such as in HLHS.

Alterations in cerebral blood flow patterns in utero may be one explanation for the relatively high prevalence of neuroanatomical differences in infants with HLHS and may in part explain some of the neurocognitive deficits seen in a growing number of the survivors of surgery.

The Right Ventricle and Cardiac Output

Inadequacy of the LV to support the systemic perfusion has little obvious clinical impact in the fetus because the right ventricle takes over the task of blood flow delivery to the fetal body and placenta through ejection into the ductus arteriosus. In the absence of an adequate-sized LV, the right ventricle receives the full complement of venous return. Owing to the increase in blood volume, the right ventricle dilates, as does the tricuspid valve annulus. Ostensibly, on the surface of it, fetal perfusion looks to be preserved in the absence of right ventricular dysfunction or tricuspid valve insufficiency. However, upon deeper scrutiny, we have identified a decrease in the Doppler-derived measure of cardiac output in fetuses with HLHS with good ventricular function and no valvar dysfunction.[24] Comparison of age-matched fetuses with HLHS and normal (mean gestational age 29 wk) reveals a lower "combined ventricular" cardiac output of 380 ±

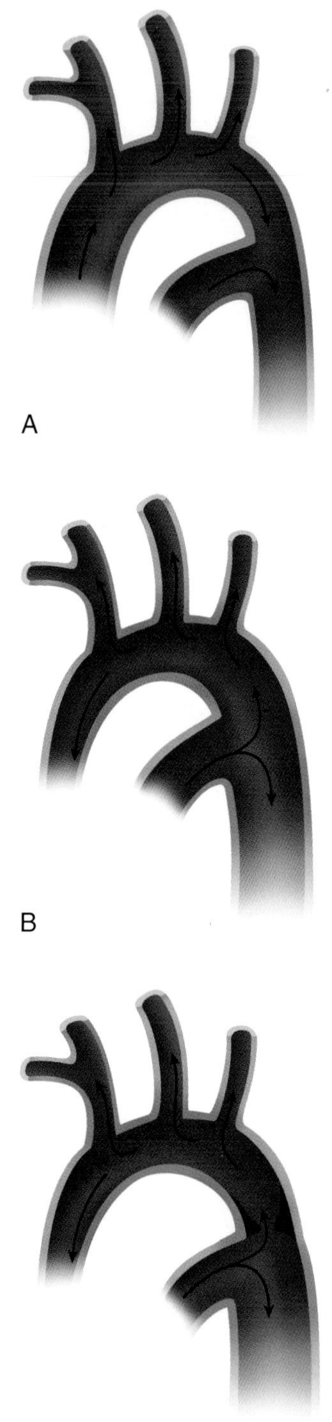

Figure 22-6. Flow patterns in the aorta. **(A)** Normal antegrade flow in the ascending aorta and ductus arteriosus. Note that the ascending aorta is larger in diameter than the transverse or isthmus. **(B)** Abnormal retrograde flow with perfusion of the ascending aorta via the ductus arteriosus. Note that the transverse aorta is larger in size than the ascending aorta, which is typically the case in aortic atresia. **(C)** Abnormal retrograde flow in the aorta with development of juxtaductal narrowing at the insertion of the ductus arteriosus. Hence, there is a discrete coarctation of the aorta as well as ascending aortic hypoplasia.

124 mL/min/kg for the HLHS group versus 461 ± 45 mL/min/kg for the normal heart group ($P < 0.05$). This is nearly a 20% decrease in cardiac output of the fetus with HLHS relative to normal. The overall impact of a diminished cardiac output for the developing fetus with HLHS is unclear. The vast majority of fetuses with HLHS progress to term without any difficulties. Hydrops fetalis of a cardiac etiology does not occur in HLHS unless there are problems with severe tricuspid regurgitation or severe right ventricle dysfunction. However, it is possible that a chronic low cardiac output may influence organogenesis and may contribute to the small weight for gestational age seen in HLHS. It may also have implications for mode of delivery because the fetus with a borderline poor cardiac output may not tolerate a long and strenuous vaginal delivery as well as a normal fetus. This area is ripe for further investigational work.

Prenatal Diagnostic Determination of Left Ventricle Inadequacy: Will the Left Ventricle Be Viable after Birth?

It is relatively straightforward to determine the inadequacy of the left-sided structures in the presence of mitral or aortic atresia with an absent or very small LV. However, cases in which there is ventricular size discrepancy between the LV and the right ventricle with a small borderline-sized LV can present a diagnostic challenge; it can be difficult to predict the viability and adequacy of the LV to provide for postnatal systemic perfusion. A number of abnormalities may result in the appearance of size discrepancy between the two ventricles (Box 22-1).[25] Distal aortic obstruction such as in coarctation of the aorta may present with a borderline small LV as may a number of anomalies in which the filling volume of the LV is altered from the normal. For example, in the presence of an interrupted inferior vena cava with azygos continuation to the superior vena cava, there is a decrease in the normal complement of streaming blood flow across the atrial septum. Filling of the LV is diminished, while an increased amount of flow is channeled to the superior vena cava and directed across the tricuspid valve, resulting in a relative increase in volume load to the right ventricle. Anomalous return of the pulmonary veins, either complete or partial, may limit volume filling of the LV in utero and provide for the appearance of a small cavity size. In congenital diaphragmatic hernia, abdominal contents may be positioned in the chest, potentially compressing the left-sided heart structures, thereby limiting LV filling by impeding right-to-left flow at the atrial level. In addition, lung compression and pulmonary hypoplasia may reduce the amount of pulmonary venous return to the LV, also contributing to a relatively smaller LV cavity volume.

In the fetus with ventricular size discrepancy and a small, but ultimately viable LV, the measurements of LV length and mitral valve annulus are no less than 3 standard deviations from the mean for the expected dimensions for gestational age (no less than −3 Z-score). If the dimensional measurements are less than −3 Z-score for gestational age, the LV is most likely to be inadequate in makeup and size. Other factors may contribute to inadequacy and/or nonviability of the LV such as the presence of endocardial fibroelastosis, severe structural abnormality of the mitral valve, or severe left ventricular outflow tract obstruction. A diagnostic formula for predicting the adequacy of the fetal LV when dimensional Z-scores are greater than −3 is not available; hence, each subject should be considered individually on a case-by-case basis (Box 22-2).

Doppler flow patterns may be helpful in discriminating between those with a prohibitively small LV and those with a borderline small but viable LV.[26] The following are general guidelines:

1. **Direction of flow across the atrial septum.** Left-to-right flow across the atrial septum is a strong indicator of left atrial hypertension and left ventricular inadequacy.
2. **Direction of flow in the ascending aorta.** Retrograde flow in the ascending portion of the aorta reflects an inability for the LV to eject blood forward, suggesting LV inadequacy.

Box 22-1 Anomalies That May Result in Ventricular Size Discrepancy and Variably Small Left Ventricle

- Hypoplastic left heart syndrome
- Unbalanced atrioventricular canal defect
- Coarctation of the aorta
- Interrupted inferior vena cava with azygos continuation to the superior vena cava
- Total anomalous pulmonary venous connection
- Partial anomalous pulmonary venous connection
- Dilated coronary sinus due to left superior vena cava
- Congenital diaphragmatic hernia

Box 22-2 Prenatal Variables That May Predict for Inadequacy of the Left Ventricle

- Mitral valve z score < −3
- Aortic valve z score < −3
- Severe structural abnormality of the mitral valve
- Severe left ventricular outflow tract obstruction
- Endocardial fibroelastosis
- Left-to-right atrial level shunting
- Retrograde blood flow in the ascending aorta

Prenatal Intervention: Can We Prevent the Evolution of Hypoplastic Left Heart Syndrome?

Investigators have reported the phenomenon of relatively late gestational age development of HLHS, this in the fetus with aortic stenosis. A fetus with a normal, or a dilated, LV in the presence of aortic stenosis can theoretically undergo "arrest" of left ventricular development, presumably due to impaired flow through the LV.[27,28] Such patients typically have poor LV function. Techniques have been developed for a maternal percutaneous approach to the developing second-trimester fetus, which would allow for a needle-guided balloon valvuloplasty of the aortic valve. The intention of such an intervention is to create forward flow across the aortic valve in the hopes of promoting continued growth and development of the LV and prevent HLHS.[29] The results of this undertaking are still limited because the experience is currently in its beginning stages. Identifying with certainty which fetus with aortic stenosis will progress to LV hypoplasia and which will continue to have LV growth and be amenable to a simple aortic balloon valvuloplasty at birth is controversial. Left-to-right shunting at the atrial level and reversal of flow in the transverse aortic arch in the face of aortic stenosis and LV dysfunction have been advocated as reliable predictors of evolving HLHS. In addition, the most appropriate gestational timing of the intervention and the most effective technique are still in question.

No doubt that fetal intervention, and the ability to divert development of structural heart disease by altering flow in utero, may potentially revolutionize our thinking about the treatment of congenital heart disease in the coming decades. Unfortunately, this approach is applicable to a very small fraction of all fetuses with HLHS because the vast majority already have marked LV hypoplasia, mitral atresia, or aortic atresia at presentation. Perhaps some have LV inadequacy at early formation in the first trimester and will not be responsive to changes in flow at all but will be amenable to gene therapy in the future.

Postnatal Course and Management

Infants born with HLHS typically exhibit cyanosis and respiratory distress at birth. Often, there may be no cyanosis at all or little symptoms whatsoever as long as the ductus arteriosus remains patent. Commensurate with the natural constriction and closure of the ductus arteriosus, which usually occurs at 24 to 48 hours of life, the infant begins to exhibit signs of systemic hypoperfusion with hypotension and metabolic acidosis. As systemic perfusion decreases, pulmonary perfusion increases with the classic findings of hypotension, cool underperfused extremities, an increase in systemic oxygen levels, and an enlarged heart with increased pulmonary vascular markings on chest radiograph. In the absence of identification of this anomaly, death ensues shortly after natural closure of the ductus arteriosus. Prenatal identification allows for administration of prostaglandin E_1 infusion at birth, with maintenance of ductal patency until the time of surgical intervention.

Although it is one of the most challenging anomalies to treat, HLHS is nonetheless currently amenable to successful management through a variety of different surgical strategies. The medical caretaker counseling the family carrying a fetus with HLHS must be fully aware of the various forms of surgical strategies available as well as the current outcomes for intervention. Whereas non-intervention results in 100% uniform death, surgical intervention through staged surgical reconstruction has been reported to provide as high as 80% to 90% survival.[30,31]

Major strides and dramatic improvement in surgical outcome has been achieved in just the recent past few years; hence, one must avoid quoting old, obsolete data concerning dismal surgical outcomes to families. The goal for this anomaly in particular is to provide objective, nonjudgmental information to expectant parents because the anomaly and its management appear to have been stigmatized by faulty information in the past. In a recent review, we stratified fetuses presenting to our Fetal Heart Program at CHOP based on being "high risk" versus "standard risk."[32] Based on experience and prior observations, a number of categorical risk factors were identified as possibly leading to poor outcome and were analyzed. These categorical risk factors were (1) the presence of any extracardiac, genetic, or chromosomal anomalies, (2) prematurity, defined as birth before 34 weeks' gestation, or fetal echocardiographic identification of additional cardiac risk factors such as (3) an intact or highly restrictive atrial septum, (4) severe degree of tricuspid regurgitation, or (5) ventricular dysfunction. Any fetus with these risk factors was considered "high risk," whereas a fetus without these risk factors was considered "standard risk." Two hundred and forty fetuses were evaluated over a 5-year period from 2004 to 2009 (Figure 22-7). Family decision of either termination of pregnancy or non-intervention at birth was chosen in 16% of cases. Overall, 68% were standard risk and 32% were high risk. Survival to hospital discharge after stage 1 surgical reconstruction was strikingly different between the two groups, with 93% survival for standard risk and 57% survival for high risk. This analysis highlights the importance of karyotype assessment and careful obstetrical ultrasound evaluation for extracardiac anomalies in the proper counseling of the family of a fetus with HLHS.

Heart transplantation is the treatment of choice in a diminishingly small number of centers in the United States today. Transplantation entails morbidity and mortality in relation to awaiting receipt of a donor heart and the lifelong risks related to organ rejection.[33] Most centers today have undertaken a program of staged surgical reconstruction utilizing a three-stage surgical approach

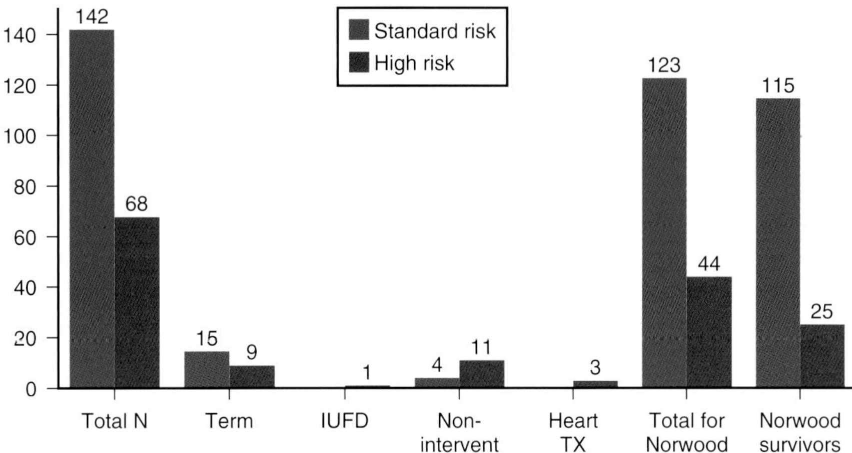

Figure 22-7. Outcomes for prenatal diagnosis of HLHS stratified based on standard or high risk. Of the 210 fetuses, 142 were standard risk and 68 high risk. There were 24 terminations of pregnancy (Term), 15 in the standard-risk and 9 in the high-risk category. There was 1 intrauterine fetal demise (IUFD). Fifteen families chose no intervention at birth: 4 standard risk and 11 high risk. Three fetuses were referred directly for heart transplant (Heart Tx) at birth, primarily due to tricuspid regurgitation. Of the 123 with standard risk presenting for Norwood stage 1 surgery, 115 survived (93%); of the 44 with high risk presenting for surgery, only 25 survived (57%).

resulting in utilization of the right ventricle as the systemic ventricle and connection of the venae cavae directly to the pulmonary arteries. The strategy involves, first, reconstruction of the aorta via a pulmonary artery–to–aorta anastomosis with arch augmentation. By doing so, the task of systemic perfusion is transferred to the right ventricle. An atrial septectomy is performed to allow for unimpaired egress from the left atrium and a source for pulmonary blood flow such as an aortopulmonary shunt is placed. At the second stage, the aortopulmonary shunt is removed and the superior vena cava is connected to the pulmonary artery, as the new source for pulmonary blood flow. At the third stage, the inferior vena cava is connected to the pulmonary artery, such that the full complement of systemic venous return is channeled into the lungs without the use of an interposed pumping chamber (the Fontan principle).

Newer techniques continue to develop and offer promise for reduction in morbidity and mortality. One such technique is the use of a tube graft from the right ventricle to the pulmonary arteries in lieu of an aortopulmonary shunt as part of the initial stage 1 reconstruction.[34] The theoretical benefit in the use of a tube graft lies in the elimination of diastolic flow, or potential "steal," that occurs in the presence of an aortopulmonary shunt and has been implicated as a possible cause of sudden death after initial surgery. A "hybrid" approach utilizing catheter and surgical techniques has been described in which a stent is placed across the ductus arteriosus and across the atrial septum to create patency for systemic perfusion and left atrial decompression, respectively. The branch pulmonary arteries are then "banded" to limit pulmonary blood flow.[35] Cavopulmonary connections are then created at a later point in time.

Outcomes

Survival after reconstruction for HLHS is 85% to 90% following stage 1 and over 95% for stage 2 and stage 3. Risk factors for stage 1 survival in our center are the presence of extracardiac anomalies or genetic or chromosomal abnormalities, an intact or restrictive atrial septum, tricuspid regurgitation, or right ventricle dysfunction. Survival is variably diminished based on the presence of these factors. Studies looking at the intermediate-term outcome for HLHS (>15 yr) demonstrate that the vast majority of these children are thriving, attending school, participating in sports activities (with some limitations), and partaking in a relatively good quality of life, for the most part. Because the oldest survivors are currently in their late teens and early 20s, long-term outcome much beyond the second decade of life is still uncertain. Continued scrutiny of these very special patients is ongoing. Concerns have been raised about the longevity of patients with HLHS because potential long-term complications are many. Ventricular dysfunction, thromboembolism, hepatic dysfunction, and protein-losing enteropathy are serious problems, being recognized with increasing frequency in survivors of single-ventricle surgery.[36] What is the likelihood that the fetus born today with HLHS will have a normal lifespan and a decent quality of life? This is a common question asked during fetal counseling, with an unknown answer. However, one response is that just as the likelihood of neonatal survival was once unimaginable, so it is believed that new and effective solutions will be discovered in the coming years that will provide a long and decent quality of life to these patients.

Imaging Essentials and Key Points

- Smallness of the left side of the heart can be found in a number of anomalies including coarctation of the aorta, aortic stenosis, or HLHS. The degree of "smallness" or hypoplasia obviously differs between these. The extent of the descent of the LV toward the apex is one clue.
- The most important distinguishing feature in the fetus that predicts for adequacy or inadequacy of the LV is the direction of flow across the atrial septum. Normal right-to-left atrial level shunting predicts an adequate left side, whereas left-to-right atrial level shunting predicts LV inadequacy. Bidirectional shunting across the atrial septum can be seen, which certainly bodes for concern but is not helpful in predicting LV adequacy. We have certainly seen cases of left-sided heart disease in which a fetus with bidirectional atrial level shunting has manifested LV adequacy at birth, whereas in other cases it has not.
- Serial evaluation of the fetus with a "borderline" LV is essential. Findings as close to gestational term as possible will yield the most reliable predictive data as to LV viability.
- We have developed the habit of evaluating our fetuses with congenital heart disease every 4 weeks. In HLHS, serial evaluation of the atrial septum is important for a variety of reasons:
  - A fetus with a borderline mildly restrictive atrial septum may develop more severe restriction over time.
  - Abnormalities of the tricuspid valve are common, and the presence or degree of tricuspid regurgitation can change with advancing gestation.
  - Right ventricular function typically remains stable; however, we have seen cases of development of systolic ventricular dysfunction during gestation. Qualitative estimates of right ventricular function are warranted during periods of serial fetal echocardiographic evaluation.
- Those who have an intact atrial septum at initial discovery of HLHS at 18 to 24 weeks will be most likely to exhibit abnormal pulmonary vasoreactivity at maternal hyperoxygenation testing. Conversely, some fetuses who have an open atrial septum early on may acquire restriction or an intact atrial septum at 26 weeks or greater. These fetuses may have abnormal pulmonary venous Doppler flow patterns as left atrial egress is impaired; however, often, there is normal pulmonary vasoreactivity at maternal hyperoxygenation because the restrictive process has not occurred at a critical period of pulmonary vascular development. Such fetuses have a better outcome at birth. This is a situation in which the maternal hyperoxygenation test has provided essential information for management.
- Families who have declined a fetal intervention for intact atrial septum but wish to continue with aggressive care are candidates for what we call the "IMPACT" procedure (immediate postpartum access to cardiac therapy). This is a scheduled cesarean section delivery in a cardiac operating room suite or hybrid surgical catheterization suite, where immediate intervention can be offered to the newborn within minutes of birth. The IMPACT procedure involves the orchestration of multiple teams from various disciplines including perinatology, obstetrics, cardiology, surgery, and anesthesiology as well as an appropriate facility for maternal and neonatal care.
- Karyotype assessment and careful obstetrical ultrasound in search for extracardiac anomalies is key for the accurate counseling of families carrying a fetus with HLHS because outcomes vary widely based on the presence or absence of additional anomalies.

References

1. Rychik J. Hypoplastic left heart syndrome: from in-utero diagnosis to school age. *Semin Fetal Neonatal Med.* 2005;10:553-566.
2. Rychik J. Aortic stenosis or atresia with associated hypoplasia of the left ventricle: imaging before and after reconstructive surgery. *Echocardiography.* 1996;13:325-336.
3. Natowicz M, Chatten J, Clancy R, et al. Genetic disorders and major extracardiac anomalies associated with the hypoplastic left heart syndrome. *Pediatrics.* 1988;82:698-706.
4. Natowicz M, Kelley RI. Association of Turner syndrome with hypoplastic left-heart syndrome. *Am J Dis Child.* 1987;141:218-220.
5. Schultz AH, Wernovsky G. Late outcomes in patients with surgically treated congenital heart disease. *Semin Thorac Cardiovasc Surg Pediatr Card Surg Annu.* 2005:145-156.
6. Hinton RB, Andelfinger G, Sekar P, et al. Prenatal head growth and white matter injury in hypoplastic left heart syndrome. *Pediatr Res.* 2008;64:364-369.
7. Goldberg CS, Schwartz EM, Brunberg JA, et al. Neurodevelopmental outcome of patients after the Fontan operation: a comparison between children with hypoplastic left heart syndrome and other functional single ventricle lesions. *J Pediatr.* 2000;137:646-652.
8. Glauser TA, Rorke LB, Weinberg PM, Clancy RR. Congenital brain anomalies associated with the hypoplastic left heart syndrome. *Pediatrics.* 1990;85:984-990.
9. Shillingford AJ, Ittenbach RF, Marino BS, et al. Aortic morphometry and microcephaly in hypoplastic left heart syndrome. *Cardiol Young.* 2007;17:189-195.
10. Hoffman JI, Kaplan S. The incidence of congenital heart disease. *J Am Coll Cardiol.* 2002;39:1890-1900.

11. Nora JJ, Nora AH. Update on counseling the family with a first-degree relative with a congenital heart defect. *Am J Med Genet.* 1988;29:137-142.
12. Boughman JA, Berg KA, Astemborski JA, et al. Familial risks of congenital heart defect assessed in a population-based epidemiologic study. *Am J Med Genet.* 1987;26:839-849.
13. Hinton RB Jr, Martin LJ, Tabangin ME, Mazwi ML, Cripe LH, Benson DW. Hypoplastic left heart syndrome is heritable. *J Am Coll Cardiol.* 2007;50:1590-1595.
14. Remmell-Dow DR, Bharati S, Davis JT, Lev M, Allen HD. Hypoplasia of the eustachian valve and abnormal orientation of the limbus of the foramen ovale in hypoplastic left heart syndrome. *Am Heart J.* 1995;130:148-152.
15. Rychik J, Rome JJ, Collins MH, DeCampli WM, Spray TL. The hypoplastic left heart syndrome with intact atrial septum: atrial morphology, pulmonary vascular histopathology and outcome. *J Am Coll Cardiol.* 1999;34:554-560.
16. Glatz JA, Tabbutt S, Gaynor JW, et al. Hypoplastic left heart syndrome with atrial level restriction in the era of prenatal diagnosis. *Ann Thorac Surg.* 2007;84:1633-1638.
17. Marshall AC, van der Velde ME, Tworetzky W, et al. Creation of an atrial septal defect in utero for fetuses with hypoplastic left heart syndrome and intact or highly restrictive atrial septum. *Circulation.* 2004;110:253-258.
18. Marshall AC, Levine J, Morash D, et al. Results of in utero atrial septoplasty in fetuses with hypoplastic left heart syndrome. *Prenat Diagn.* 2008;28:1023-1028.
19. Chintala K, Tian Z, Du W, Donaghue D, Rychik J. Fetal pulmonary venous Doppler patterns in hypoplastic left heart syndrome: relationship to atrial septal restriction. *Heart.* 2008;94:1446-1449.
20. Michelfelder E, Gomez C, Border W, Gottliebson W, Franklin C. Predictive value of fetal pulmonary venous flow patterns in identifying the need for atrial septoplasty in the newborn with hypoplastic left ventricle. *Circulation.* 2005;112:2974-2979.
21. Broth RE, Wood DC, Rasanen J, et al. Prenatal prediction of lethal pulmonary hypoplasia: the hyperoxygenation test for pulmonary artery reactivity. *Am J Obstet Gynecol.* 2002;187:940-945.
22. Szwast A, Rychik J. Current concepts in fetal cardiovascular disease. *Clin Perinatol.* 2005;32:857-875, viii.
23. Kaltman JR, Di H, Tian Z, Rychik J. Impact of congenital heart disease on cerebrovascular blood flow dynamics in the fetus. *Ultrasound Obstet Gynecol.* 2005;25:32-36.
24. Szwast A, Tian Z, McCann M, Donaghue D, Rychik J. Right ventricular performance in the fetus with hypoplastic left heart syndrome. *Ann Thorac Surg.* 2009;87:1214-1219.
25. Quartermain MD, Cohen MS, Dominguez TE, Tian Z, Donaghue DD, Rychik J. Left ventricle to right ventricle size discrepancy in the fetus: the presence of critical congenital heart disease can be reliably predicted. *J Am Soc Echocardiogr.* 2009;22:1296-1301.
26. Kovalchin JP, Brook MM, Rosenthal GL, Suda K, Hoffman JI, Silverman NH. Echocardiographic hemodynamic and morphometric predictors of survival after two-ventricle repair in infants with critical aortic stenosis. *J Am Coll Cardiol.* 1998;32:237-244.
27. Allan LD, Sharland G, Tynan MJ. The natural history of the hypoplastic left heart syndrome. *Int J Cardiol.* 1989;25:341-343.
28. Tworetzky W, Wilkins-Haug L, Jennings RW, et al. Balloon dilation of severe aortic stenosis in the fetus: potential for prevention of hypoplastic left heart syndrome: candidate selection, technique, and results of successful intervention. *Circulation.* 2004;110: 2125-2131.
29. McElhinney DB, Marshall AC, Wilkins-Haug LE, et al. Predictors of technical success and postnatal biventricular outcome after in utero aortic valvuloplasty for aortic stenosis with evolving hypoplastic left heart syndrome. *Circulation.* 2009;120:1482-1490.
30. Tabbutt S, Dominguez TE, Ravishankar C, et al. Outcomes after the stage I reconstruction comparing the right ventricular to pulmonary artery conduit with the modified Blalock Taussig shunt. *Ann Thorac Surg.* 2005;80:1582-1590; discussion 1590-1591.
31. Tweddell JS, Hoffman GM, Mussatto KA, et al. Improved survival of patients undergoing palliation of hypoplastic left heart syndrome: lessons learned from 115 consecutive patients. *Circulation.* 2002;106:I82-I89.
32. Rychik J, Szwast A, Natarajan S, et al. Perinatal and early surgical outcome for the fetus with hypoplastic left heart syndrome: a 5 year single institutional experience. *Ultrasound Obstet Gynecol.* 2010;36:465-470.
33. Chrisant MR, Naftel DC, Drummond-Webb J, et al. Fate of infants with hypoplastic left heart syndrome listed for cardiac transplantation: a multicenter study. *J Heart Lung Transplant.* 2005;24: 576-582.
34. Sano S, Ishino K, Kawada M, et al. Right ventricle-pulmonary artery shunt in first-stage palliation of hypoplastic left heart syndrome. *J Thorac Cardiovasc Surg.* 2003;126:504-509; discussion 509-510.
35. Galantowicz M, Cheatham JP, Phillips A, et al. Hybrid approach for hypoplastic left heart syndrome: intermediate results after the learning curve. *Ann Thorac Surg.* 2008;85:2063-2070; discussion 2070-2071.
36. Khairy P, Fernandes SM, Mayer JE Jr, et al. Long-term survival, modes of death, and predictors of mortality in patients with Fontan surgery. *Circulation.* 2008;117:85-92.

CASES

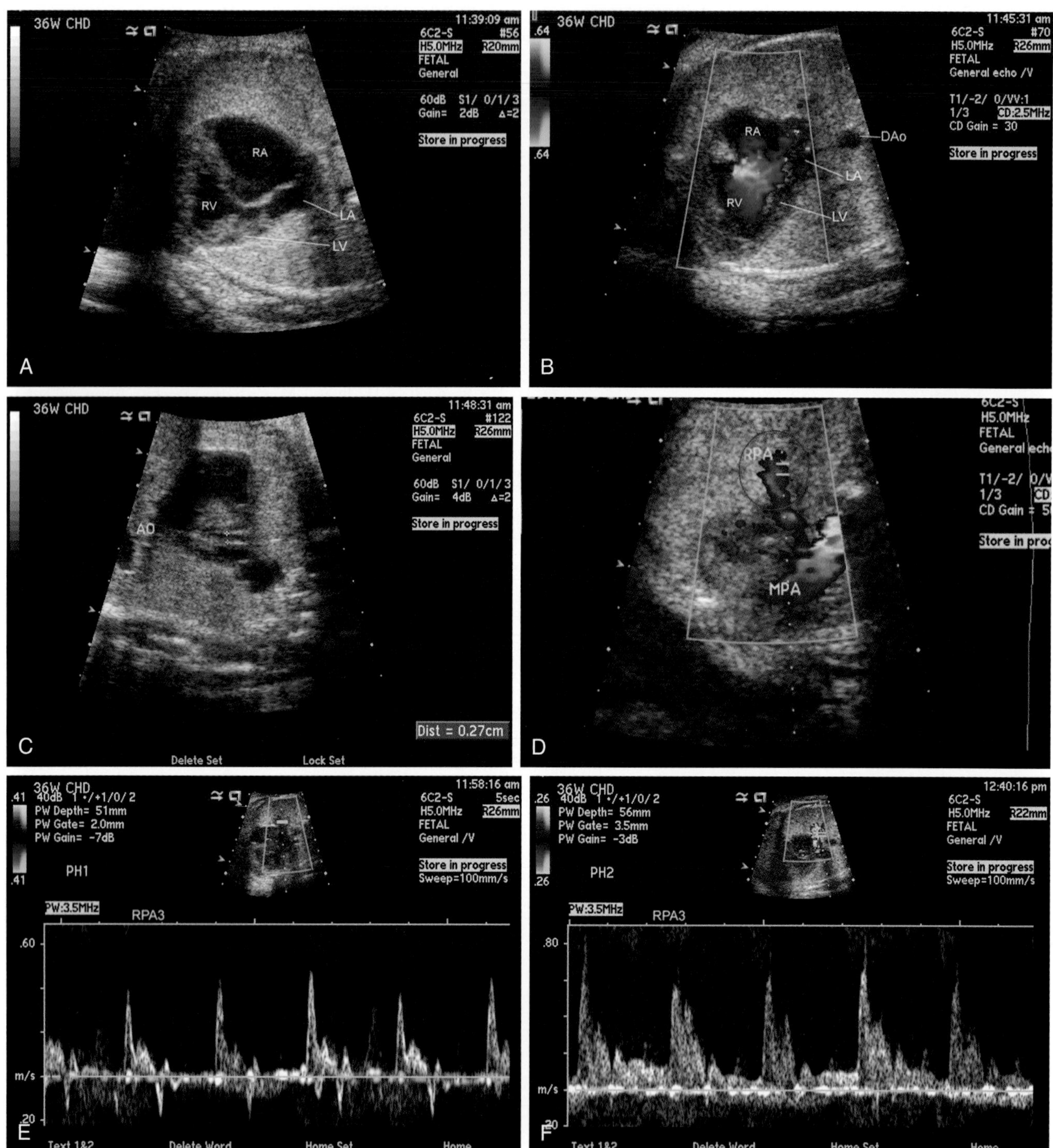

Case 22-1. **(A)** Apical view demonstrates a dilated right atrium (RA) and dilated right ventricle (RV). The left atrium (LA) is small and the left ventricle (LV) is severely hypoplastic and barely visible. **(B)** Color flow in diastole. There is filling of a dilated RV, but no color flow is seen entering any LV. DAo, descending aorta. **(C)** Hypoplasia of the ascending aorta. The aorta (AO) measures less than 3 mm in diameter, which is markedly hypoplastic at 36 weeks' gestation. The walls of the ascending aorta in the hypoplastic left heart syndrome (HLHS) are commonly very echo-bright, as seen in this image. **(D)** Sampling for evaluation of pulmonary vasoreactivity in response to maternal hyperoxygenation. Color flow identifies the right pulmonary artery (RPA) and its course into the right lung parenchyma. A pulmonary intraparenchymal site is chosen for sampling, typically at 1 to 2 cm beyond the origin and branching from the main pulmonary artery (MPA). **(E)** Doppler sample of the branch RPA from a distal intraparenchymal site obtained in room air. Note the very "spiky" initial upstroke, reflecting high pulmonary vascular resistance. There is very little diastolic flow. This is the expected normal pattern seen in room air, which reflects a "constricted," high-resistance state. **(F)** Doppler sample at the same site in the branch RPA after 20 minutes of maternal hyperoxygenation with 60% supplemental oxygen. Note the broadening of the initial upstroke with increased peak velocity (~80 cm/sec) and a substantial increase in diastolic flow. This is the anticipated favorable response indicating pulmonary vasoreactivity with a decrease in resistance and increased flow. This reflects a normal, healthy pulmonary vasculature in the fetus with an open, unrestrictive interatrial communication.

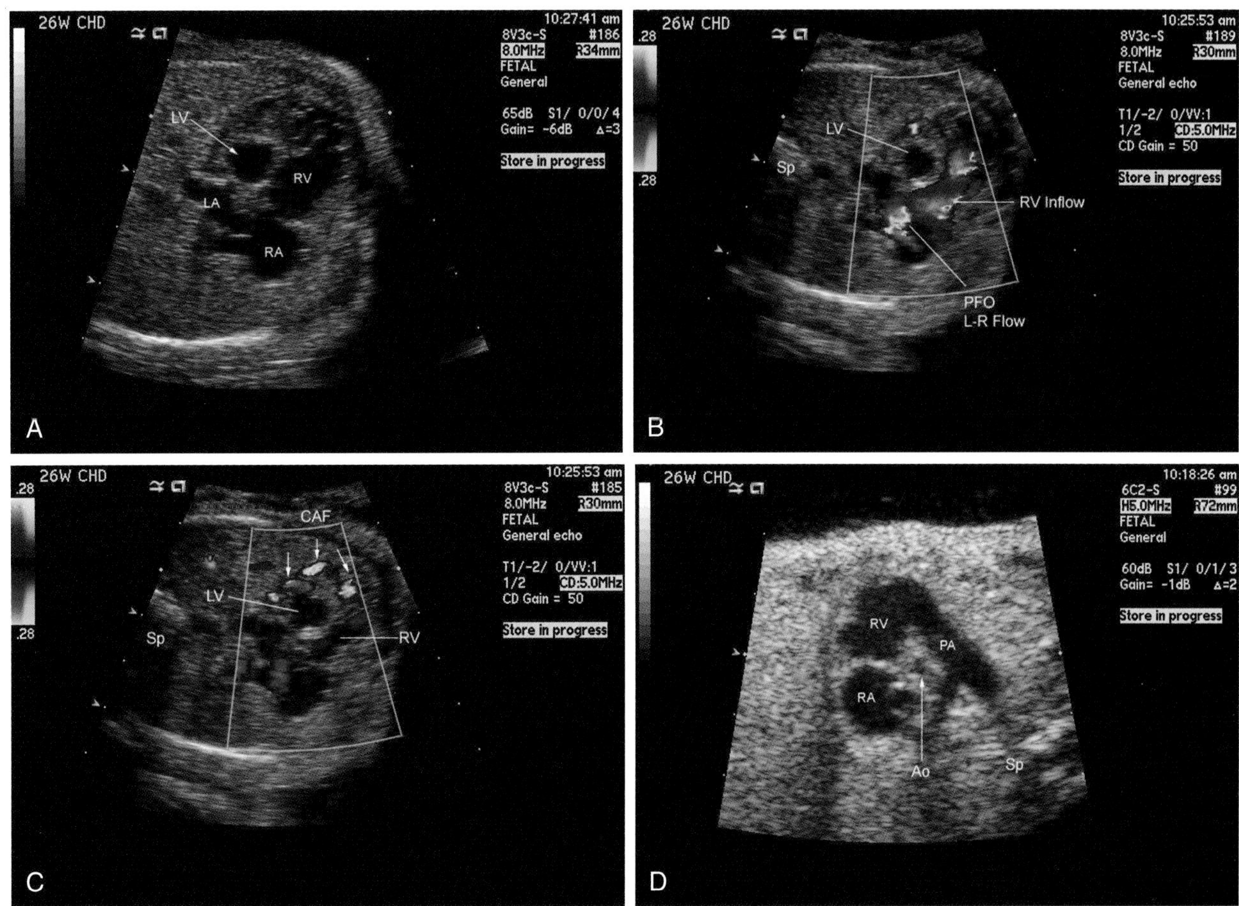

Case 22-2. **(A)** Four-chamber view of a case of mitral stenosis and aortic atresia. There is a small, rounded LV cavity with inflow across a very hypoplastic mitral valve. Note the flap of the atrial septum bows from LA to RA. **(B)** Color flow in diastole demonstrates a broad swath of red color traversing the tricuspid valve into the RV; however, no color is seen entering the left ventricular cavity because the velocity is extremely low. Nevertheless, there is a small high-velocity jet of color near the apex of the LV, which reflects evidence for a coronary-cameral fistula. This suggests that there is entry of blood into this ventricular chamber across the mitral valve and egress via this fistulous connection. There is left-to-right shunting across the patent foramen ovale (PFO) from LA to RA. **(C)** Angling with focus toward the body and apex of the LV reveals multiple color jets, which represent coronary artery–to–ventricular fistulous connections (CAF). **(D)** Short-axis view demonstrates a small aorta (Ao) arising from its normal central location. Note the size discrepancy between the aorta and the pulmonary artery (PA). Sp, spine.

Continued

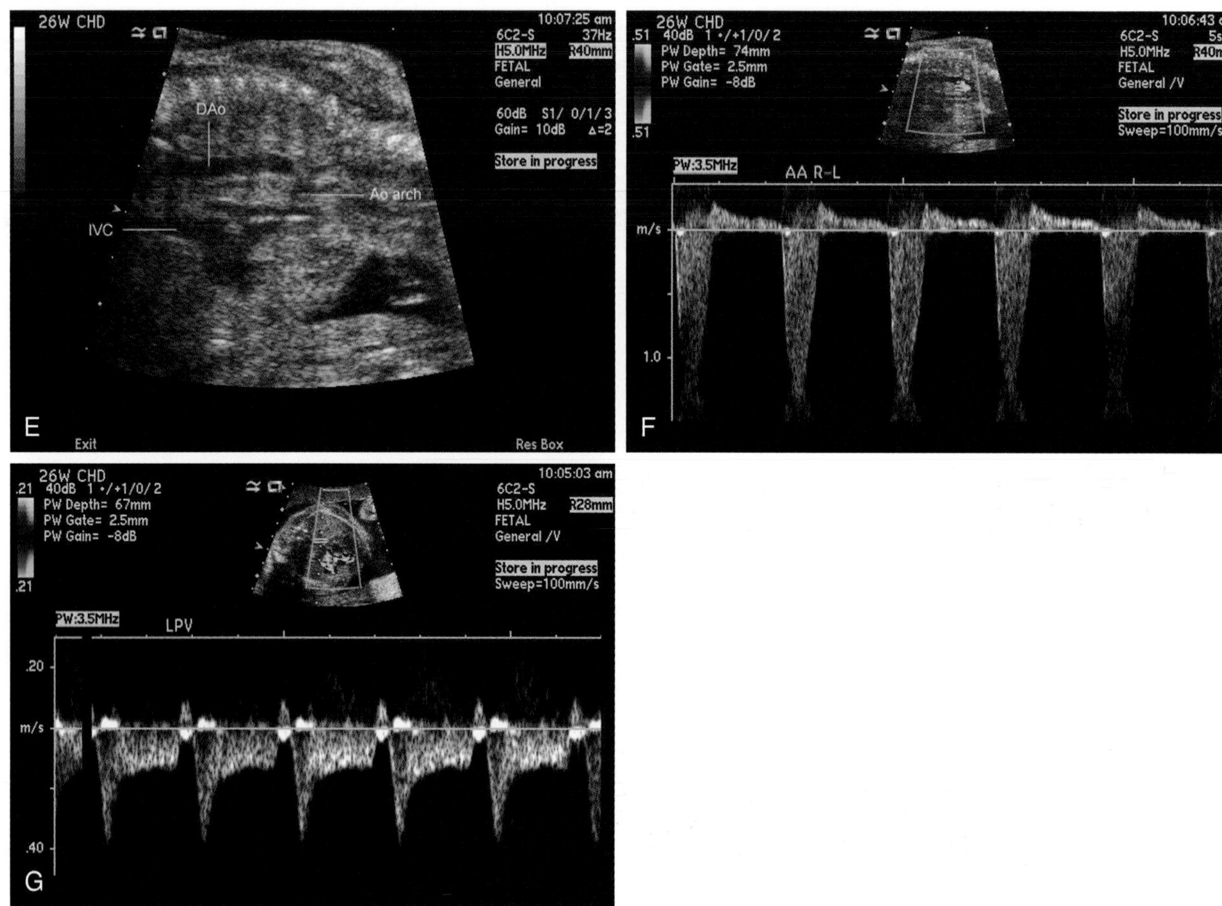

Case 22-2, cont'd **(E)** View of the aortic arch. There is marked size discrepancy between the descending aorta (DAo) and the transverse portion of the aortic (Ao) arch. The transverse arch is identified by its giving rise to the head vessels. Note the acute right angle with which the transverse arch joins with the DAo. IVC, inferior vena cava. **(F)** Doppler sampling at the junction between the DAo and the transverse aortic arch (AA). There is retrograde flow into the transverse aorta in systole (flow below the baseline). Hence, the head vessels are being perfused in a retrograde manner from ductal flow. **(G)** Doppler interrogation of the left pulmonary vein (LPV). This is the typical pulmonary venous flow pattern seen when there is no significant obstruction to egress out of the LA and there is an open, unobstructed atrial septum. There is predominantly antegrade flow (below the baseline from this angle), which is biphasic. There is a small amount of reversal of flow with atrial contraction (above the baseline). A small amount of reversal with atrial contraction is normal because the left atrial compliance is slightly lower than in the normal fetus.

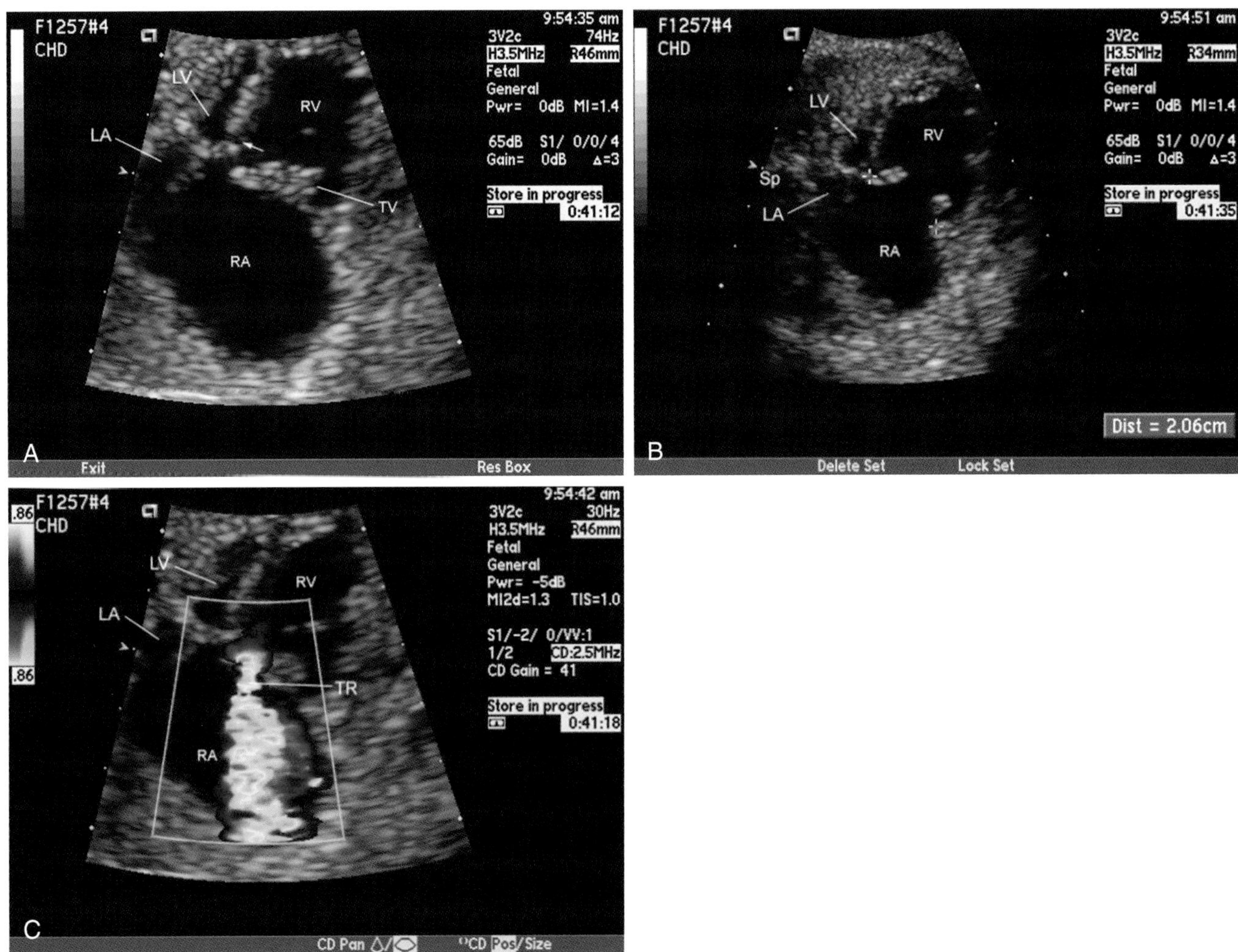

Case 22-3. **(A)** A case of HLHS in which there is mitral atresia, but with a small ventricular septal defect *(arrow)*, and hence, an LV cavity is present. The LA is small and the RA is strikingly enlarged. The tricuspid valve (TV) appears unusually thickened. **(B)** In diastole, the TV is open and again appears quite thick and dysplastic. The RA is markedly dilated. **(C)** Color Doppler imaging during systole. There is severe tricuspid regurgitation (TR). This finding is a significant risk factor for survival after stage 1 Norwood operation.

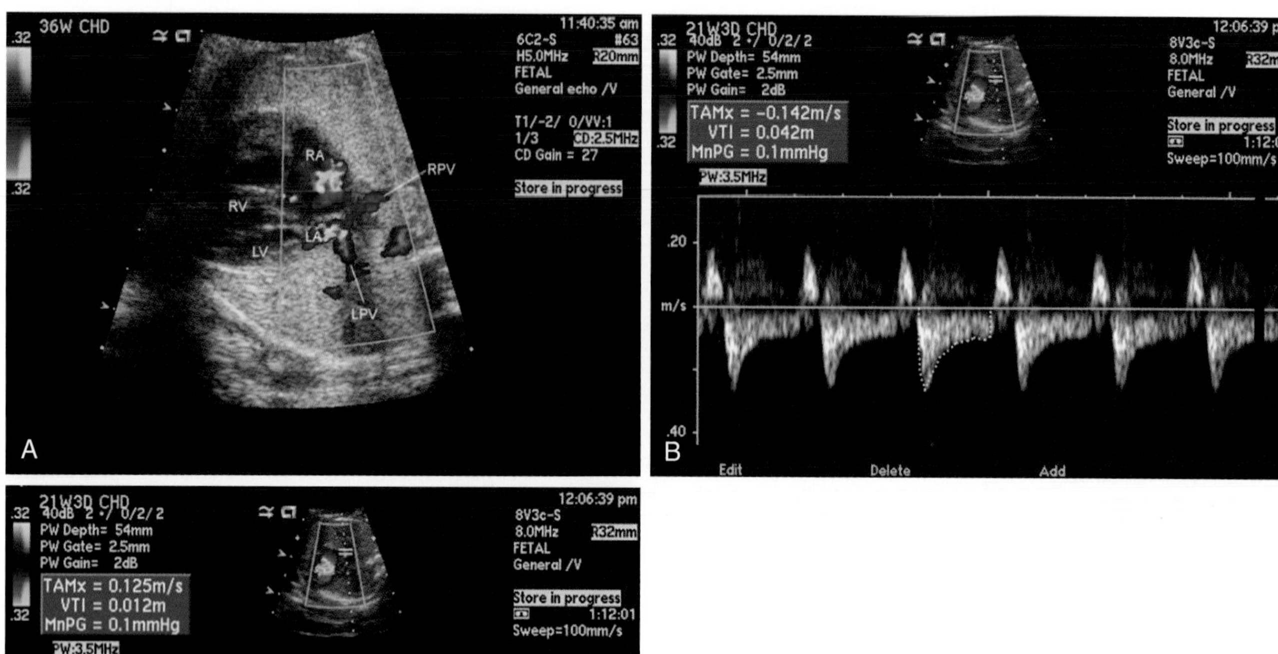

Case 22-4. **(A)** Assessment of Doppler flow patterns of the pulmonary veins is an essential aspect of the evaluation of the fetus with HLHS. In this color Doppler image, the right pulmonary vein (RPV) and LPV are seen returning to the small LA. **(B)** Doppler spectral display of flow in the pulmonary vein. There is predominantly antegrade flow (below the baseline); however, there is also a prominent retrograde waveform with atrial contraction. The antegrade waveform is traced and the velocity-time integral (VTI) is 4.2 cm. **(C)** In the same cardiac cycle, the retrograde waveform (above baseline) is traced and the VTI is 1.2 cm. Hence, the ratio of antegrade to retrograde flow is equal to 3.5; a ratio less than 5 suggests an element of restriction and raises the suspicion for possible left atrial hypertension and the need for postnatal assessment and urgent opening of the atrial septum. In our experience, this ratio reflects only mild atrial level restriction and is still acceptable and would predict good outcome without the need for urgent postnatal intervention, in particular if there is evidence for pulmonary vasoreactivity upon maternal hyperoxygenation. A ratio less than 3 would suggest a more severe form of obstruction. However, because this fetus is still only at 21 weeks' gestation, progression of narrowing at the atrial level is possible and serial evaluation is crucial with repeat sampling of the pulmonary veins and calculation of the antegrade-to-retrograde ratio of VTI flow.

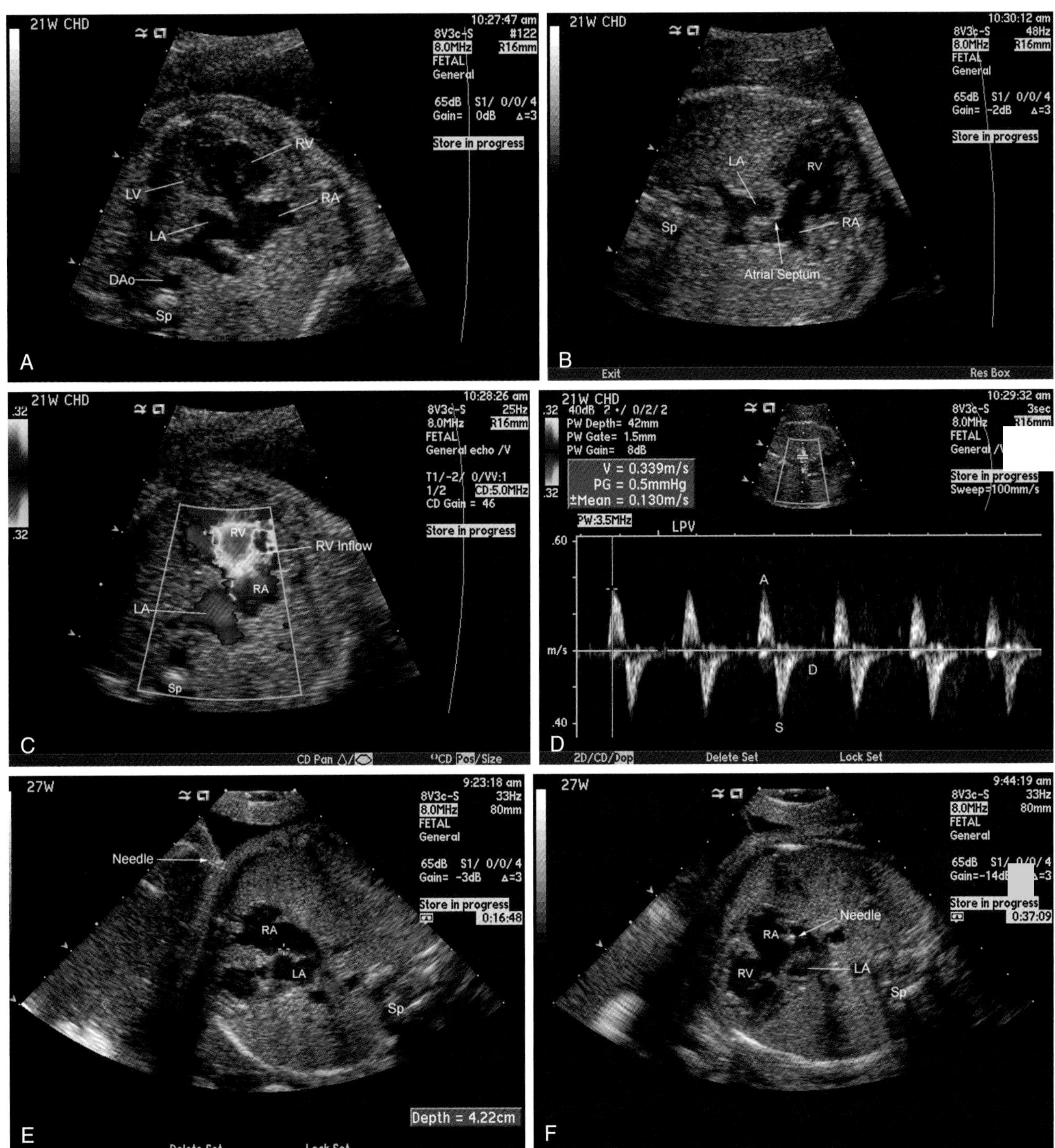

Case 22-5. **(A)** Fetus at 21 weeks' gestation with HLHS and intact atrial septum. Note the "double-chamber" appearance to the LA. The LA is tense and cannot normally empty. The confluence of the pulmonary veins that connects to the back of the LA is dilated, as are the individual RPV and LPV. **(B)** Abnormally thickened atrial septum in this fetus with HLHS and intact atrial septum. **(C)** Color flow imaging demonstrates absence of any left-to-right shunting at the atrial level. **(D)** Doppler interrogation of the pulmonary vein in this fetus with HLHS and intact atrial septum. There is an almost 1 : 1 ratio of antegrade flow (below baseline) to retrograde flow (above baseline), indicating a severe degree of obstruction to left atrial egress. This Doppler pulmonary venous flow pattern is highly predictive of severe hypoxemia at birth and the need for urgent intervention to open the atrial septum. Often, despite immediate postnatal intervention, the pulmonary vasculature is malformed owing to chronic fetal left atrial hypertension and hypoxemia does not improve. This supports the argument for prenatal intervention in such severe cases. **(E)** At 27 weeks' gestation, this fetus with HLHS and intact atrial septum is undergoing fetal intervention to open the atrial septum. A 19-gauge needle is introduced across the maternal uterus and guided toward the fetal chest. The target *(crosshair)* is the atrial septum, with the goal of entering the LA, passing a wire into the pulmonary vein. A 3-mm coronary balloon is threaded across and positioned over the atrial septum and inflated in order to create a communication. **(F)** The needle has entered through the fetal chest into the RA and is aiming at the atrial septum.

Continued

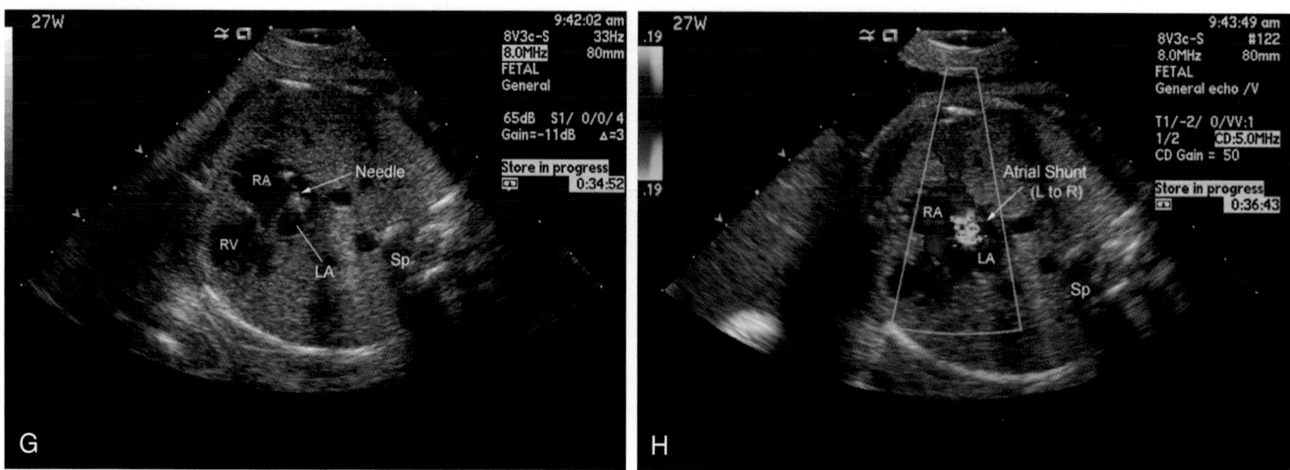

Case 22-5, cont'd **(G)** The balloon is threaded over a wire and is positioned onto the atrial septum and inflated. **(H)** Color flow imaging identifies the creation of an interatrial communication with left-to-right shunting from LA to RA.

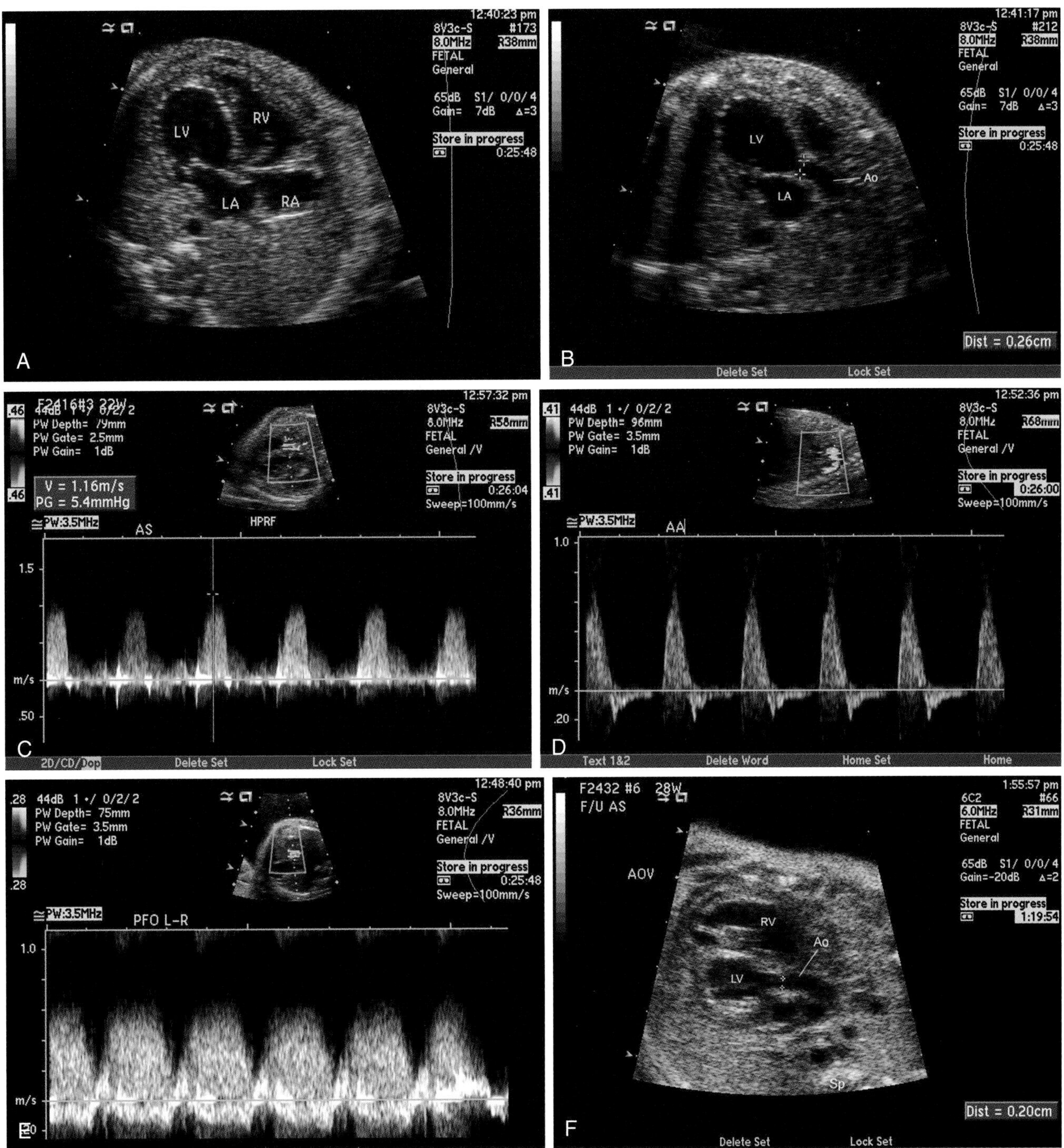

Case 22-6. **(A)** Four-chamber view of a fetal heart at 22 weeks' gestation with a dilated, poorly functioning LV. There is an echo-bright LV endocardium, suggesting the presence of endocardial fibroelastosis. At this stage, the LV does not appear to be hypoplastic, and without further data, it would be hard to say that this is HLHS. **(B)** The aortic (Ao) annulus is slightly small at 2.6 mm and the aortic valve appears slightly thickened. **(C)** Doppler flow interrogation across the aortic valve demonstrates turbulent, nonlaminar flow and a slightly increased peak velocity of greater than 1 m/sec. **(D)** Doppler interrogation across the transverse arch. Flow is retrograde (above the baseline) in systole in the transverse aortic arch (AA). This suggests that the LV is unable to generate adequate forward flow across the stenotic aortic valve to create antegrade, forward flow in the transverse aorta. Flow to the head and neck vessels is dependent upon retrograde perfusion from the ductus arteriosus via the RV. **(E)** Doppler interrogation across the PFO is all left-to-right flow. This fetus fulfills criteria that would predict the "arrest of LV development" and the evolution of HLHS: (1) dilated, poorly functioning LV with evidence for endocardial fibroelastosis in conjunction with aortic stenosis, (2) left-to-right shunting at the atrial level, and (3) retrograde perfusion in the transverse aortic arch. **(F)** This fetus is now at 28 weeks' gestation. There is now easy recognition of size disproportion between the RV and the LV, with the LV appearing smaller. The aorta is essentially unchanged in size from the prior evaluation at 22 weeks; however, the right-sided structures have continued to grow. We now see evidence for left ventricular hypoplasia.

Continued

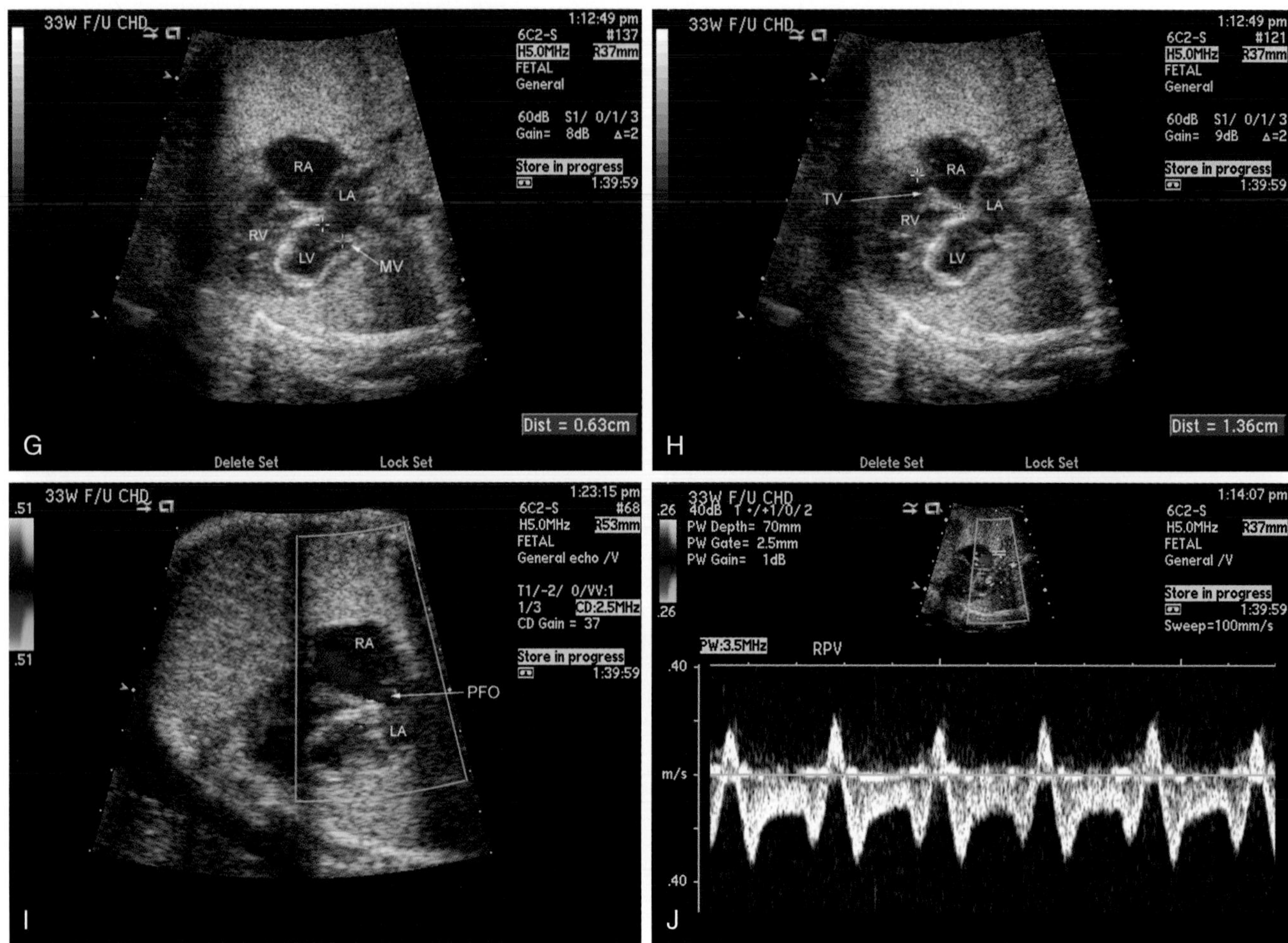

Case 22-6, cont'd (G) This fetus is now at 33 weeks' gestation. There is increasing discrepancy in ventricular size with clear development of LV hypoplasia. The mitral valve (MV) is small for gestational age and the LV continues to exhibit significant endocardial echo-brightness. **(H)** The TV annulus size is more than twice the MV annulus size. Note the bowing of the atrial septum from left to right. **(I)** Color flow imaging demonstrates the presence of a PFO with left-to-right shunting from LA to RA. **(J)** Doppler interrogation of the RPV. There is a normal pulmonary vein flow pattern as the LA empties easily both across an open atrial septum and into a hypoplastic LV, which is ejecting into the ascending aorta. Hence, left atrial egress is unimpeded and is reflected in this pulmonary vein Doppler flow pattern with predominantly antegrade flow.

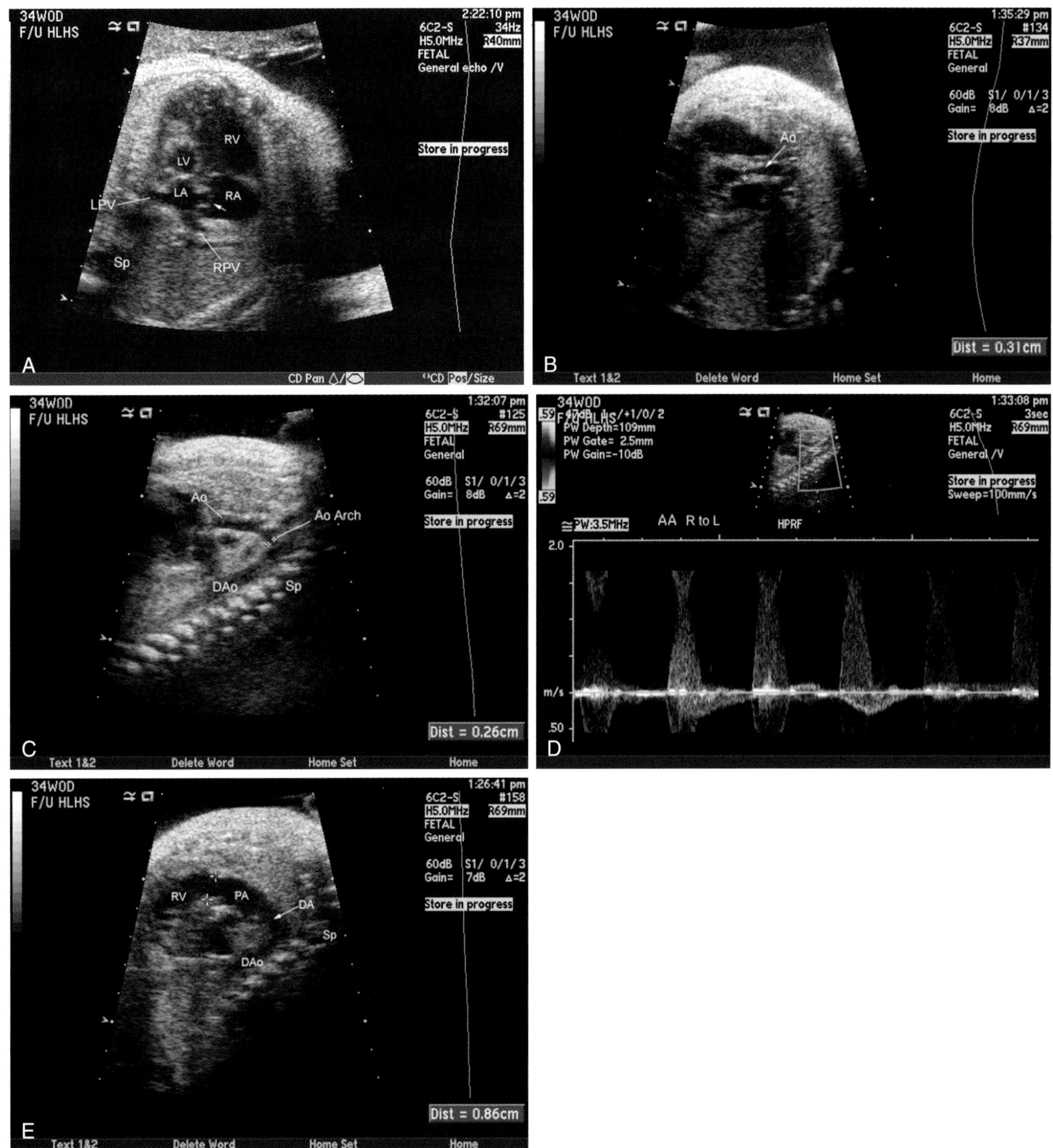

Case 22-7. **(A)** HLHS with mitral hypoplasia. Note the position of the atrial septum *(arrow)*, which is bowing left to right. **(B)** Long-axis view of the hypoplastic LV and aorta (Ao). There is aortic hypoplasia, but the pathway is patent. The aortic annulus measures 3.1 mm at 34 weeks' gestation. **(C)** Image of the aortic arch. The isthmus measures 2.6 mm, which is moderately hypoplastic for gestational age. **(D)** Pulse Doppler flow shows retrograde flow in the aortic arch. **(E)** Demonstration of the ductal arch and its natural-appearing curvature arising from the RV to the PA and ductus arteriosus (DA), connecting to the descending aorta (DAo).

23

Aortic Stenosis and Mitral Valve Dysplasia Syndrome

Lindsay Rogers and Jack Rychik

Key Echocardiographic Features

- Left ventricle dilation with poor contractility.
- Aortic annular hypoplasia, with aortic stenosis or atresia.
- Abnormal mitral valve with small annulus, thickened leaflets, stenosis, and severe regurgitation.
- Markedly dilated left atrium in the presence of severe mitral regurgitation.
- Highly restrictive or intact atrial septum.
- Abnormal Doppler flow pattern may be noted when sampling the pulmonary veins ("double-reversal" pulmonary vein flow pattern).
- Echo-bright left ventricle endocardium, reflecting endocardial fibroelastosis.
- Retrograde flow in the transverse and ascending aorta secondary to perfusion via the ductus arteriosus.
- Right ventricle may be compressed secondary to left-sided dilation.
- Hydrops fetalis possible when the right ventricle is compressed by the left ventricle.

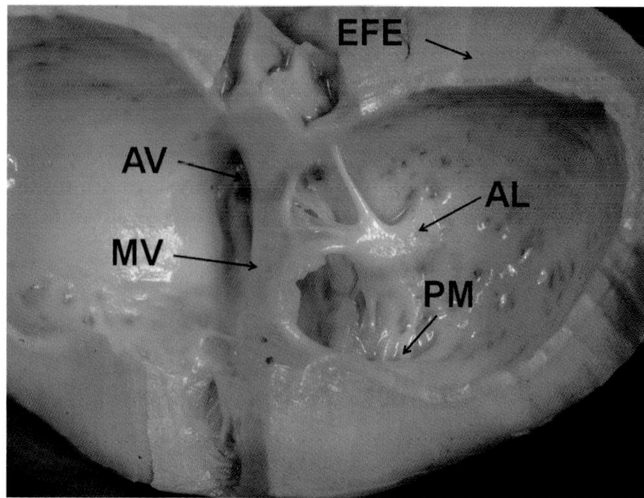

Figure 23-1. Autopsy specimen from a neonate with mitral valve (MV) dysplasia syndrome (MVDS). We are looking from the apex of the left ventricle up toward the outflow tract. Note the glistening white endocardium, which has an "egg-shell" appearance. This is endocardial fibroelastosis (EFE). The EFE covers much of the MV and chordae as well as the inner lining wall of the left ventricle (LV). The chordae are shortened and thickened. AL, anterolateral papillary muscle; AV, aortic valve; PM, posteromedial papillary muscle.

Anatomy and Anatomical Associations

Mitral valve dysplasia syndrome (MVDS) is an uncommon form of congenital heart disease that is often thought to be synonymous with hypoplastic left heart syndrome (HLHS) or critical aortic stenosis. The anomaly is unique with specific characteristics and a constellation of findings that make this disorder deserving of recognition as a separate entity. Patients with MVDS share many anatomical and physiological similarities to those with HLHS, such as mitral stenosis and severe aortic stenosis/atresia leading to left ventricular outflow tract (LVOT) obstruction. In addition, they often have dilated, dysfunctional left ventricles, like patients with critical aortic stenosis. However, unique from those forms of left-sided obstructive heart disease, patients with MVDS have a primary abnormality of the mitral valve (MV). The MV is thick and dysplastic, resulting in significant mitral regurgitation (MR). In utero, these fetuses have marked left atrial dilation and restriction of the atrial septum. In addition, left ventricular *dilation* and *dysfunction*, often compromising right ventricular function, is characteristic of the disease. This combination of aortic outflow obstruction, severe MR, left heart dilation, and restriction of the atrial septum is what defines MVDS as a unique entity.

Pathological review of specimens with MVDS reveals the presence of a thick, dysplastic MV with absent chordae, characteristic of MV arcade (Figure 23-1). In addition, they typically have severe aortic stenosis or atresia, with a monocuspid aortic valve. Left ventricle dilation and the presence of endocardial fibroelastosis (EFE) are common. The left atrium is thick-walled, with evidence of left atrial hypertension, and a restrictive or intact atrial septum is usually present.

MVDS is a rare constellation of cardiac findings, and to our knowledge, there are no other associated anatomic or extracardiac anomalies.

Frequency, Genetics, and Development

MVDS is a rare disorder. Because these patients have historically been categorized as having HLHS, the exact incidence is not known. In our institution, a review of our fetal database from 2002 to 2009 revealed 10 cases of MVDS diagnosed in utero. In addition, a handful of isolated case reports in the literature have described patients with this disease process, but no large case series has been reported.

The developmental progression of MVDS in the fetus may be similar to the development of HLHS. As hypothesized in HLHS, patients with MV dysplasia have aortic stenosis and decreased flow across the LVOT in utero. In addition, aortic stenosis leads to dilation and dysfunction of the left ventricle. Elevated end-diastolic pressures in the LV change flow dynamics such that there is left-to-right flow across the foramen ovale, with less systemic venous return directed into the left heart. In HLHS, this leads to severe mitral stenosis/atresia and poor development of the left ventricle with the consequence of ventricular hypoplasia.[1] However, in patients with significant MR, such as in MVDS, there is an increased volume load on the left heart. The developing fetus with MVDS has both critical impediment to outflow across the aorta and severe MR with volume load. Therefore, there is continued, often progressive, left ventricular dilation and significant dysfunction. Severe incompetence of the dysplastic MV and MR lead to progressive left atrial dilation and left atrial hypertension. Elevated left atrial pressure may alter the geometry of the atrial septum with impetus for apposition of septum primum against septum secundum as left atrial pressure markedly exceeds right atrial pressure. This leads to progressive restriction, or at times complete closure, of the foramen ovale.

There are no identified extracardiac associations seen with MVDS, and no known genetic cause has been identified.

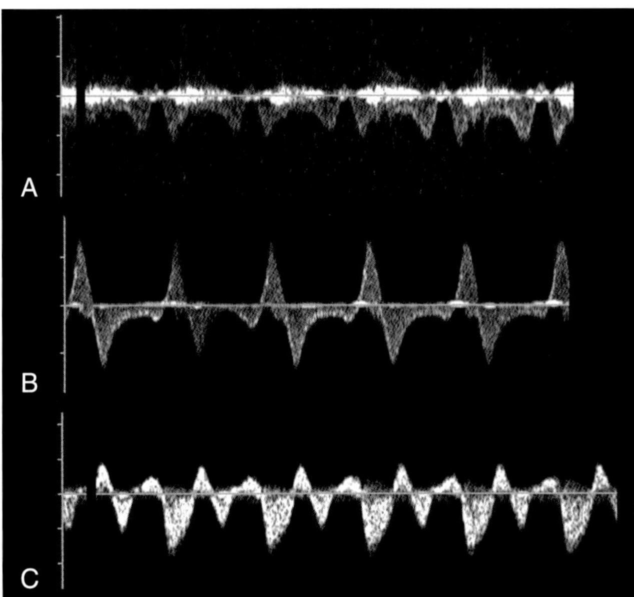

Figure 23-2. Doppler samples obtained from the pulmonary veins. (A) A normal flow pattern. (B) A prominent atrial contraction reversal waveform suggests elevated left atrial pressure. (C) A "double-reversal" flow pattern seen in the fetus with MVDS and severe mitral regurgitation. This Doppler flow pattern predicts poor outcome and reflects the worst end of the spectrum of this disease.

Prenatal Physiology

MVDS has a significant and profound impact on fetal cardiovascular physiology. As described previously, aortic stenosis results in little antegrade flow in the ascending aorta and the coronary arteries are primarily supplied via retrograde flow from the ductus arteriosus and right side of the heart. Aortic stenosis leads to left ventricular hypertrophy, dilation, and dysfunction. EFE limits diastolic relaxation of the ventricle. In addition, significant MR causes left atrial hypertension and severe left atrial dilation, sometimes to more than twice the size of the right atrium. Left heart dilation, left ventricular dysfunction, and significant MR are the key echocardiographic features of this disease in utero.

Key physiological features of MVDS include significant MR, left-to-right flow across the atrial septum, and atrial septal restriction. This restriction likely results from elevated left atrial pressures causing adherence of septum primum to septum secundum.[2] With significant atrial septal restriction, elevated left ventricular filling pressures and significant MR contributing to left atrial hypertension, the pulmonary veins are engorged with limited ability to empty into the left atrium. Pulse wave Doppler sampling of the pulmonary veins often shows flow reversal during atrial systole. In addition, depending on the degree of atrial septal restriction and degree of MR, some patients can have blunting and/or reversal of pulmonary venous flow during ventricular systole. Hence, these fetuses have reversal of pulmonary venous flow with ventricular systole and with atrial contraction, revealing a unique "double-reversal" Doppler flow. This additional wave of retrograde pulmonary venous flow is unique to MVDS (Figure 23-2).

The effects of left-to-right flow across the atrial septum and obstruction to pulmonary venous egress have a significant impact on fetal cardiovascular and lung development. However, given the unique ability of the fetus to redistribute blood flow, it is possible to have significant left atrial hypertension with restricted egress from the left atrium and yet no overt signs of altered cardiac output—hydrops fetalis—so long as the right side of the heart is functioning normally. Left-to-right flow at the level of the foramen ovale means that essentially all of the fetal cardiac output is provided via the right ventricle, with right-to-left flow across the patent ductus arteriosus. In addition, only approximately 10% to 25% of fetal cardiac output traverses to the pulmonary vascular bed and alterations in pulmonary venous return are of little clinical significance from the perspective of cardiac output during fetal life.[3] However, pulmonary venous hypertension and impaired egress of blood from the left atrium can alter pulmonary vascular development creating a pulmonary vasculopathy, which becomes clinically apparent as soon as the fetus must use its own lungs, resulting in profound hypoxemia at umbilical cord separation at birth.

In some cases of MVDS, significant hydrops fetalis can occur. In these fetuses, hydrops likely results from massive left-sided dilation impinging upon filling of the right side with compression of the right ventricle. The inability of the right ventricle to fill raises right atrial pressure, leading to venous hypertension and hydrops. Because no effective perfusion can be achieved from the left side owing to the structural anomalies inherent in the disorder, right-sided function with ejection into the ductus arteriosus is vital for fetal survival. Cardiac output in such a scenario is diminished and fetal demise may occur. Alternatively, significant MR can lead to overall volume overload on the left heart and, if the foramen is patent, onto the right side of the heart as well. Animal studies have shown that the resting fetal heart is at near-maximum ventricular output and any increase in preload can exceed the fetal heart's ability to increase stroke volume, leading to heart failure.[4]

Despite these physiological changes, Doppler patterns of the umbilical artery and vein, ductus venous, and middle cerebral artery remain unchanged from normal in the majority of patients with MVDS, supporting the observation that the fetus can effectively redirect flow from the left to the right side of the heart. If right ventricular compression is present, changes in the ductus venosus consistent with right-sided restriction can be seen, and if cardiac output is limited, middle cerebral artery resistance will drop relative to umbilical artery resistance. In the presence of significant left atrial dilation in utero, arrhythmias may be observed in patients with this disorder. Of 24 prenatally diagnosed patients in two series reported on this disease, 2 patients had fetal arrhythmia, 1 with reentrant supraventricular tachycardia and the other with permanent junctional reciprocating tachycardia.[5,6]

Prenatal Management

Serial fetal echocardiograms are essential to prenatal management and counseling of families who are carrying fetuses with MVDS. Identified fetal echocardiographic characteristics have been described that can predict patients who may need an immediate postnatal intervention to open the atrial septum and those who are at highest risk for poor outcome. In our review, we found that a total left heart area (traced left atrium plus left ventricle) that was 1.5 times the size of the right heart area (traced right atrium plus right ventricle) on the final fetal echocardiogram before birth was 100% predictive of mortality in the neonatal period. In addition, the presence of a "double-reversal" pulmonary venous Doppler flow pattern was 100% predictive of the need for an immediate postnatal intervention to open the atrial septum and overall mortality.[6]

The most appropriate prenatal management of fetuses with MVDS remains unclear. Left unaltered, the natural history carries significant risk for infant mortality; therefore, in utero intervention aimed at altering the disease makes sense and would be an ideal option for patients with MVDS. In our center's experience, prenatal intervention was undertaken in 3 of 10 patients (Table 23-1). Two patients had balloon aortic valvuloplasty in an attempt to relieve aortic outflow obstruction, promote forward flow, and recruit the left ventricle with the hopes of also reducing the degree of MR. This strategy was utilized based on existing data that in utero aortic valvuloplasty may be a successful strategy for some patients in halting the progression of aortic stenosis toward HLHS.[7] In both of these patients, the procedures were technically successful but also resulted a significant increase in aortic valve regurgitation (AR) without any change in the severity of the MR. The AR, in combination with continued MR, was a significant volume load on the left heart resulting in continued left ventricular dilation and severe dysfunction. Both patients underwent heart transplantation shortly after birth. One patient in our series had balloon atrial septostomy as a fetus, in order to compress the left atrium, potentially improve upon pulmonary vascular development, and potentially improve filling of the right heart thereby increasing cardiac output. In our case, there was technical difficulty in opening the atrial septum, which led to a fetal demise during the procedure. Other investigators[5] have argued that opening the aortic valve and promoting forward flow alone or in combination with opening of the aortic valve may be helpful; however, mortality for this undertaking is quite high. Fetal hydrops was treated using maternal digoxin in 1 patient in our series, with some beneficial effect.

Current strategy for prenatal management of MVDS entails close observation of the fetus for signs of hydrops fetalis and preparation of the family for a complicated postnatal course, utilizing echocardiographic predictors noted previously. However, given that this rare disease is known to have poor postnatal outcomes, the opportunity to alter its natural progression likely lies with in utero intervention. In our view, because the primary defect of this disorder lies in the abnormality of the MV, creating forward flow across the aorta may not improve matters. An attempt toward complete recruitment of the left ventricle with ultimate two-ventricle repair may not be feasible in the presence of a profoundly incompetent and stenotic MV. Encouraging a change in the morbid pathophysiology in the hopes of creating a better single-ventricle palliation candidate by opening the atrial septum, thereby reducing left atrial hypertension and improving right ventricular filling, may be the better strategy. Prenatal intervention to open up the restrictive/intact atrial septum may provide a more stable postnatal course, especially in those patients at highest risk for morbidity and mortality at birth. It can provide for more normal lung development by allowing normal pulmonary venous emptying into the left atrium during fetal life. The optimal strategy is yet unclear, and currently, there are no existing data to support the benefit of prenatal intervention in these patients. More research will be needed to provide a clear pathway for management of this rare but difficult disease.

Postnatal Physiology

The transition from fetal to postnatal life in infants with MVDS can sometimes be fatal unless immediate postnatal intervention is undertaken. At birth, the greatest

Table 23-1 Ten Fetuses with Mitral Valve Dysplasia Syndrome, Their Fetal Course, Postnatal Course, and Outcome

	1	2	3	4	5	6	7	8	9	10
GA at initial diagnosis (wk)	27.7	28	21	21	23.3	35.7	32	30.7	24.9	28
GA at last fetal echocardiogram (wk)	39	37	35	36	38	35.7	34	33	24.9	29.3
Hydrops	Yes	No	No	No	No	No	No	Yes	No	Yes
Left/right heart area ratio	0.99	0.77	1.1	1.82	0.54	NA	2.3	2.73	1.52	2.05
PV Doppler flow pattern	Nl	Nl	AR	AR	AR	NA	DR	DR	AR	DR
Fetal intervention	None	None	BAV	BAV, Digoxin	None	None	None	Digoxin	None	BAS
GA at delivery (wk)	39	37.4	38.6	38.1	37.9	36	34.7	33.7	37	Fetal demise
Atrial septal status at birth	Restr	Restr	Restr	Intact	Restr	Restr	Intact	Intact	Unknown	NA
Immediate postnatal intervention	None	None	None	Atrial stent	Atrial stent	Atrial septectomy	Attempted atrial stent	Atrial stent	None	NA
Postnatal operative strategy	Norwood	Norwood	OHT	OHT	Norwood	Norwood	NA	Hybrid procedure	Palliative care (no intervention)	NA
Age at operation (days)	8	2	36	36	3	0	0	7, 16	NA	NA
Survival to hospital discharge	Yes	Yes	No	Yes	Yes	Yes	No	No	NA	NA
Current status	Alive (Fontan)	Alive (BDG)	Dead	Alive (s/p OHT)	Alive (BDG)	Alive (Fontan)	Dead	Dead	Dead	Dead

AR, atrial reversal type of Doppler flow pattern; BAS, balloon atrial septostomy; BAV, balloon aortic valvuloplasty; BDG, bidirectional Glenn; DR, double-reversal; GA, gestational age; Nl, normal; NA, not applicable; OHT, orthotopic heart transplant; PV, pulmonary vein; Restr, restrictive atrial septum.

determinant of cardiovascular instability is the degree of atrial septal restriction that is present. In all infants, transition to extrauterine life means a significant drop in pulmonary vascular resistance and resultant increase in pulmonary blood flow. This change in flow dynamics allows for the left ventricle to provide a substantial portion of the cardiac output almost immediately at birth. In infants with obstruction of flow into the left ventricle (mitral stenosis/atresia) or LVOT obstruction, pulmonary venous return is obligated to cross the atrial septum into the right heart. Therefore, systemic output is dependent upon the right ventricle and right-to-left flow across the patent ductus arteriosus. However, if there is obstruction to flow across the atrial septum, in combination with left heart obstruction, pulmonary venous return has no egress from the left atrium. The left atrium becomes significantly hypertensive leading to profound cyanosis, pulmonary edema, and significant respiratory distress. Without immediate intervention to open the atrial septum, these patients become profoundly hypoxemic, hypercarbic, and acidotic, leading to cardiovascular collapse.

Therefore, it is imperative that all patients with this disease process deliver in a center where access to immediate postnatal intervention is available. In our center, such fetuses are delivered in a cardiac operating room with cardiac anesthesia and an interventional cardiologist present.

In patients without significant restriction of the atrial septum, transition to extrauterine life is made with little difficulty with a physiology very similar to that of HLHS. The physiology in the immediate newborn period is similar to that in fetal life, the only difference being that the amount of pulmonary blood flow is increased and oxygen saturations can range from the mid-80s to low 90s. Systemic output is dependent upon right-to-left flow across the patent ductus arteriosus and, therefore, ductal patency should be maintained with prostaglandin E_1 infusion. The head and neck vessels and coronary arteries are supplied via retrograde flow across the transverse and ascending aorta from the ductus arteriosus. As pulmonary vascular resistance progressively falls, more of the cardiac output is shunted to the lungs at the expense of the systemic circulation. This can lead to hypoperfusion and acidosis; therefore, diligent monitoring for signs of decreased end-organ perfusion is essential.

Clinically, there is no known genetic syndrome that associates with MVDS, so infants generally do not appear dysmorphic. Physical examination is notable for a systolic murmur due to high volume flow across the right ventricular outflow tract and sometimes an MR murmur. Their femoral pulses can be bounding if a large ductus arteriosus is present.

Postnatal Management

Once the adequacy of the atrial septal communication has been assessed and intervention undertaken if necessary, the medical management of these patients relies on maintaining an open ductus arteriosus. Low-dose prostaglandin E infusion is often started in the delivery room. Infants should be closely monitored in an intensive care unit setting for signs of circulatory instability, until surgical correction is undertaken.

Maintaining a well-balanced systemic and pulmonary circulation can be a challenge as pulmonary vascular resistance falls and there is increased pulmonary blood flow. Increasing oxygen saturation and tachypnea are often accompanied by decreased systemic perfusion. However, tachypnea in these infants can also be a sign of pulmonary edema from residual restriction at the atrial septum and reassessment of the foramen ovale by echocardiography may be necessary.

By the time these patients are born, the left ventricle is often dilated and severely dysfunctional, with echobright endocardium signifying EFE. Therefore, such neonates may not be candidates for two-ventricle repair and in our view a stable circulation is ultimately achieved by staged, single-ventricle palliation. The left ventricle may be of normal size or dilated and appear seductively attractive for a two-ventricle repair via either catheter balloon dilation of the aortic valve or aortic valve surgery; however, one must remember that the primary pathology is that of an abnormal MV. Relief of aortic outflow obstruction alone will not address the dysfunction of the MV, its stenosis and profound insufficiency, and in our view, a two-ventricle strategy is a poor one that often results in failure. A single-ventricle palliative strategy is best applied in this anomaly. In some cases, the left ventricular dilation can be so severe that the left ventricle negatively affects right ventricular mechanics, impairing cardiac output after birth. Therefore, with the first-stage Norwood palliation, oversewing of the MV should be considered to help decrease left ventricular size. In patients in whom right ventricular mechanics are severely affected or severe aortic insufficiency occurs from fetal intervention, primary cardiac transplantation may be the best option.

Outcomes

The significant morbidity and mortality of MVDS occurs in early postnatal life. Patients with intact or significantly restrictive atrial septa in utero are at highest risk for mortality in the newborn period. In our institutional experience of 10 patients, there are currently 5 survivors, the oldest of whom is 8 years of age at the time of this publication. One of the survivors underwent primary cardiac transplant as an infant, and the other 4, including our oldest survivor, all had single-ventricle palliation. Of the 5 nonsurvivors, 1 death occurred during fetal balloon atrial septoplasty; 1 secondary to non-intervention at birth; 1 from complications during catheter-based intervention; 1 after hybrid procedure; and 1 after heart transplant.

In a case series from Boston Children's Hospital, 14 fetuses were diagnosed with this syndrome and only 2 survived, the oldest was 45 months of age at the time of publication. One underwent a balloon aortic valvuloplasty (BAV) as a neonate and the other had BAV followed by a neonatal Ross operation and MV repair. All patients diagnosed postnatally with this disease died in the neonatal period.

Besides the two previously discussed case series, review of the literature shows only isolated case reports of patients with the constellation of anomalies associated with MVDS. One such case report describes a patient prenatally diagnosed at 30 weeks, born at 35 weeks by cesarean section secondary to fetal hydrops. The patient underwent an aortic valvotomy immediately after birth and was unable to successfully separate from cardiopulmonary bypass, dying in the operating room.[8]

A second small case series reports three autopsy specimens all with prenatal diagnosis of premature closure of the foramen ovale, aortic valve stenosis, abnormal MV and large, dysfunctional left ventricle. Only one patient had MR and was prematurely stillborn at 24 weeks.[9]

Unfortunately, based on our limited data, the outcomes of patients with this rare disorder is at best 50% survival beyond the neonatal period. Currently, efforts to improve the stabilization shortly after birth will have the largest impact on overall survival in this population. Identifying these fetuses as a distinct group, different from critical aortic stenosis and HLHS, and realizing they are at high risk for perinatal mortality is an important step. Delivery in a location where immediate interventional and/or surgical care is available can significantly alter the disease course. In the future, as more information through experiences becomes available, it may become clear that particular fetal or early postnatal interventions can provide improved outcomes.

Imaging Essentials and Key Points

- MVDS is an anomaly with characteristics that identify it as a unique disorder separate from critical aortic stenosis and HLHS.
- The primary aspect of the disorder that distinguishes it from critical aortic stenosis and HLHS is the presence of an abnormal MV.
- The pathology of the MV in MVDS is typically that of an "arcade" with a small annulus, mitral stenosis limiting inflow into the left ventricle, and thickened leaflets that are incompetent, leading to severe MR.
- On fetal echocardiography, there is a dilated dysfunctional left ventricle with echo-bright endocardium, aortic stenosis or atresia, and severe MR with left atria enlargement.
- The atrial septum bows left to right and may be highly restrictive or intact.
- Doppler sampling of the pulmonary veins is important in order to discern flow patterns that may identify those fetuses at greatest risk.
- A dilated left side may negatively affect the right side, compressing the right ventricle, which can be associated with the development of hydrops.
- Fetal intervention may play a therapeutic role in MVDS and should be considered in this anomaly with very high mortality.

References

1. Trines J, Hornberger LK. Evolution of heart disease in utero. *Pediatr Cardiol.* 2004;25:287-298.
2. Rychik J, Rome JJ, Collins MH, et al. The hypoplastic left heart syndrome with intact atrial septum: atrial morphology, pulmonary vascular histopathology and outcome. *J Am Coll Cardiol.* 1999; 34:554-560.
3. Keane JF, Lock JE, Flyer DC. *Nadas' Pediatric Cardiology.* 2nd ed. Philadelphia: Elsevier; 2006:75-79.
4. Silverman NH, Kleinman CS, Rudolph JA. Fetal atrioventricular valve insufficiency associated with nonimmune hydrops: a two-dimensional echocardiographic and pulsed Doppler ultrasound study. *Circulation.* 1985;72:825-832.
5. Vogel M, McElhinney DB, Wilkins-Haug LE, et al. Aortic stenosis and severe mitral regurgitation in the fetus resulting in giant left atrium and hydrops. *J Am Coll Cardiol.* 2011;57:348-355.
6. Rogers L, Peterson AL, Gaynor JW, Rome JJ, Weinberg PM, Rychik J. Mitral valve dysplasia syndrome: a unique form of left-sided heart disease. *J Thorac Cardiovasc Surg.* 2011. In press.
7. McElhinney DB, Marshall AC, Wilkins-Haug LE, et al. Predictors of technical success and postnatal biventricular outcome after in utero aortic valvuloplasty for aortic stenosis with evolving hypoplastic left heart syndrome. *Circulation.* 2009;120:1482-1490.
8. Bharati S, Patel A, Varga P, et al. In utero echocardiographic diagnosis of premature closure of the formen ovale with mitral regurgitation and large left atrium. *Am Heart J.* 1991;122:597-600.
9. Nowlen TT, Ayres NA, Kearney DL, et al. Premature closure of the foramen ovale associated with aortic stenosis, left ventricular dilation with thrombus and early mortality. *Am J Cardiol.* 2000;85: 1159-1161.

CASES

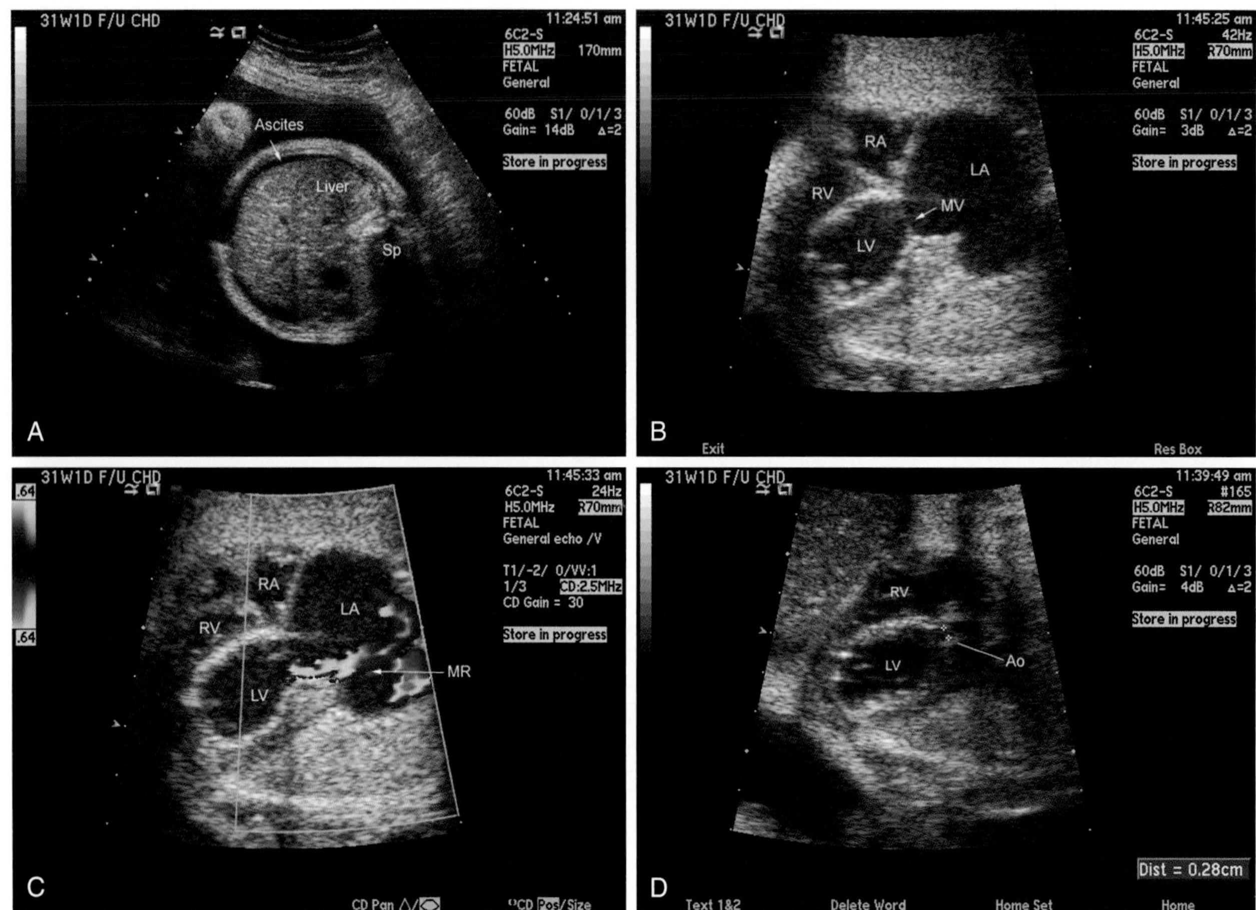

Case 23-1. **(A)** Fetus presented at 31 weeks' gestation with mitral valve dysplasia syndrome (MVDS). There is fetal hydrops with ascites present. Sp, spine. **(B)** Four-chamber view. The left atrium (LA) is gigantic and the left ventricle (LV) is also enlarged. There is an echo-brightness to the endocardium of the LV indicating endocardial fibroelastosis. The combined LA and LV are substantially larger than the right atrium (RA) and right ventricle (RV) combined, indicating a poor prognosis. MV, mitral valve. **(C)** Severe mitral regurgitation (MR) into the gigantic LA. The atrial septum is intact with bowing left to right and no shunting noted across. Blood essentially is ineffectively propelled back and forth between the LV and the LA without exiting to perfuse the fetus. **(D)** The aortic (Ao) valve is stenotic and there is aortic annular hypoplasia. The aortic annulus measures less than 3 mm at 31 weeks' gestation.

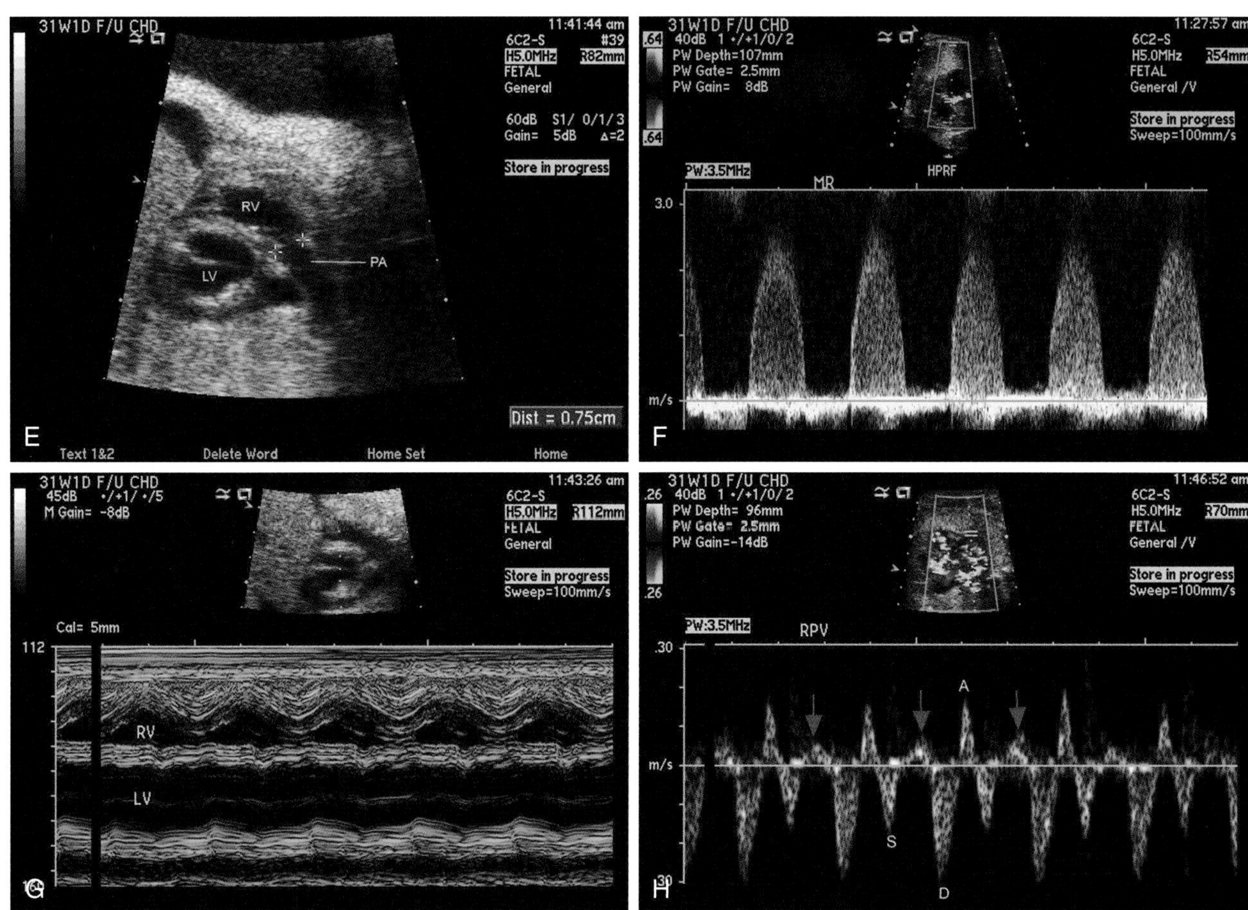

Case 23-1, cont'd **(E)** The pulmonary artery (PA) annulus is more than twice the size of the aortic annulus at 7.5 mm. **(F)** Doppler sample of the peak velocity of the mitral regurgitant jet. The velocity is only approximately 2.5 to 2.8 m/sec, indicating an LV intracavitary pressure of 30 mm Hg greater than the LA pressure. This is a low LV pressure in the face of aortic outflow tract obstruction and confirms the presence of a very poorly contractile LV. **(G)** M-mode tracing through the RV and LV. Note the LV dilation and relatively narrow cavity of the RV. The LV is extremely hypocontractile and is compressing the RV cavity, limiting inflow and cardiac output, which is predominantly dependent upon the RV in this scenario. **(H)** Doppler sample obtained from the right pulmonary vein (RPV). There is evidence of "double-reversal" with the *red arrows* pointing out the reversal of flow within the pulmonary vein coincident with the mitral regurgitant jet. This indicates that the LA is markedly tense and hypertensive and cannot empty properly.

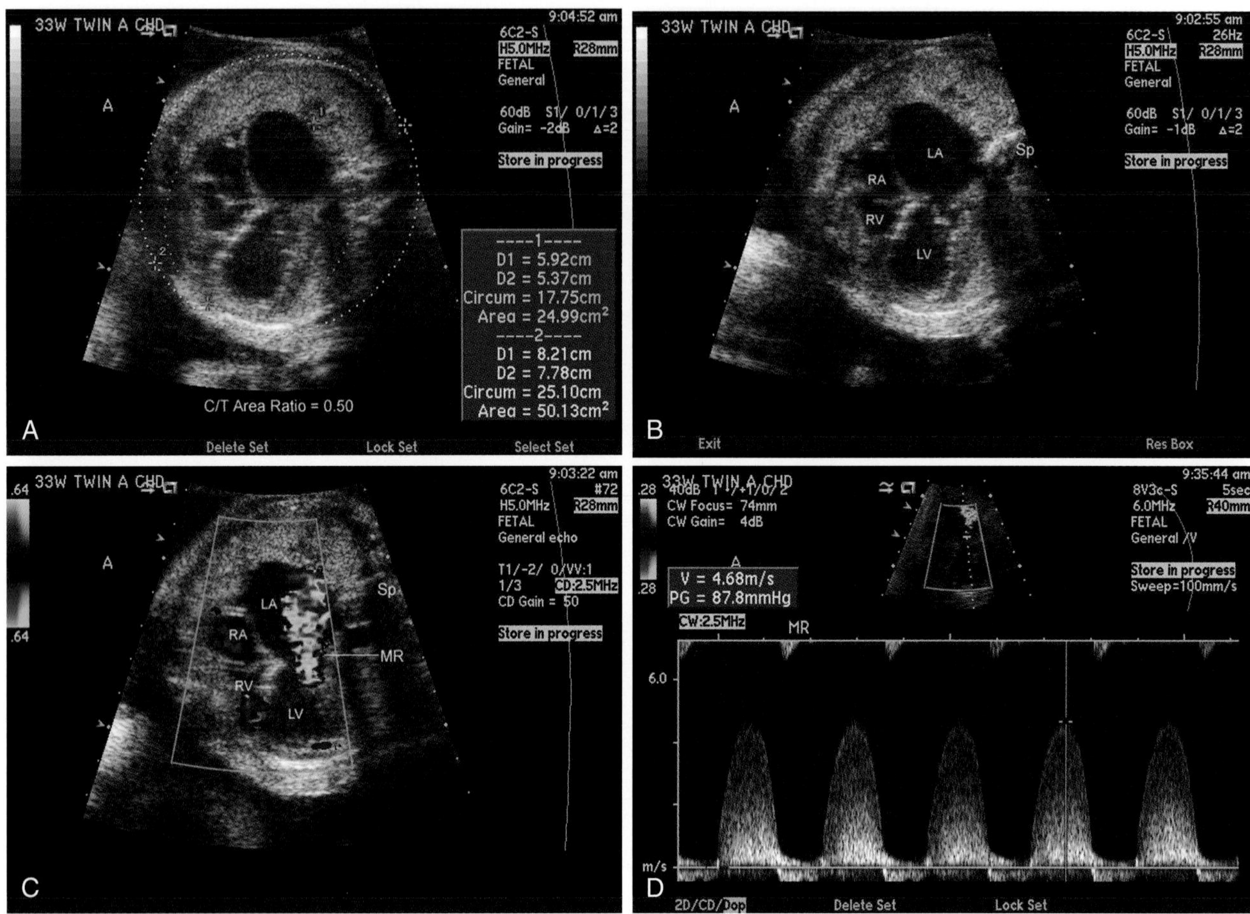

Case 23-2. **(A)** A case of MVDS seen at 33 weeks' gestation. Fetuses with this anomaly often present late because the early 20-week four-chamber view obstetrical screen may appear normal, if LV dysfunction is not identified. At this point, the heart is quite enlarged with cardiothoracic ratio (C/T ratio) = 50%. **(B)** The LA and LV are markedly dilated. There is echo-brightness to the endocardium of the LV. **(C)** There is severe MR, with the color jet filling more than half of the dilated LA area. **(D)** In this case, the peak velocity of the mitral regurgitant jet indicates an intracavitary LV pressure of approximately 90 mm Hg greater than the LA pressure. This suggests that the LV can muster a significant pressure head in the face of aortic outflow obstruction and indicates relatively good LV function.

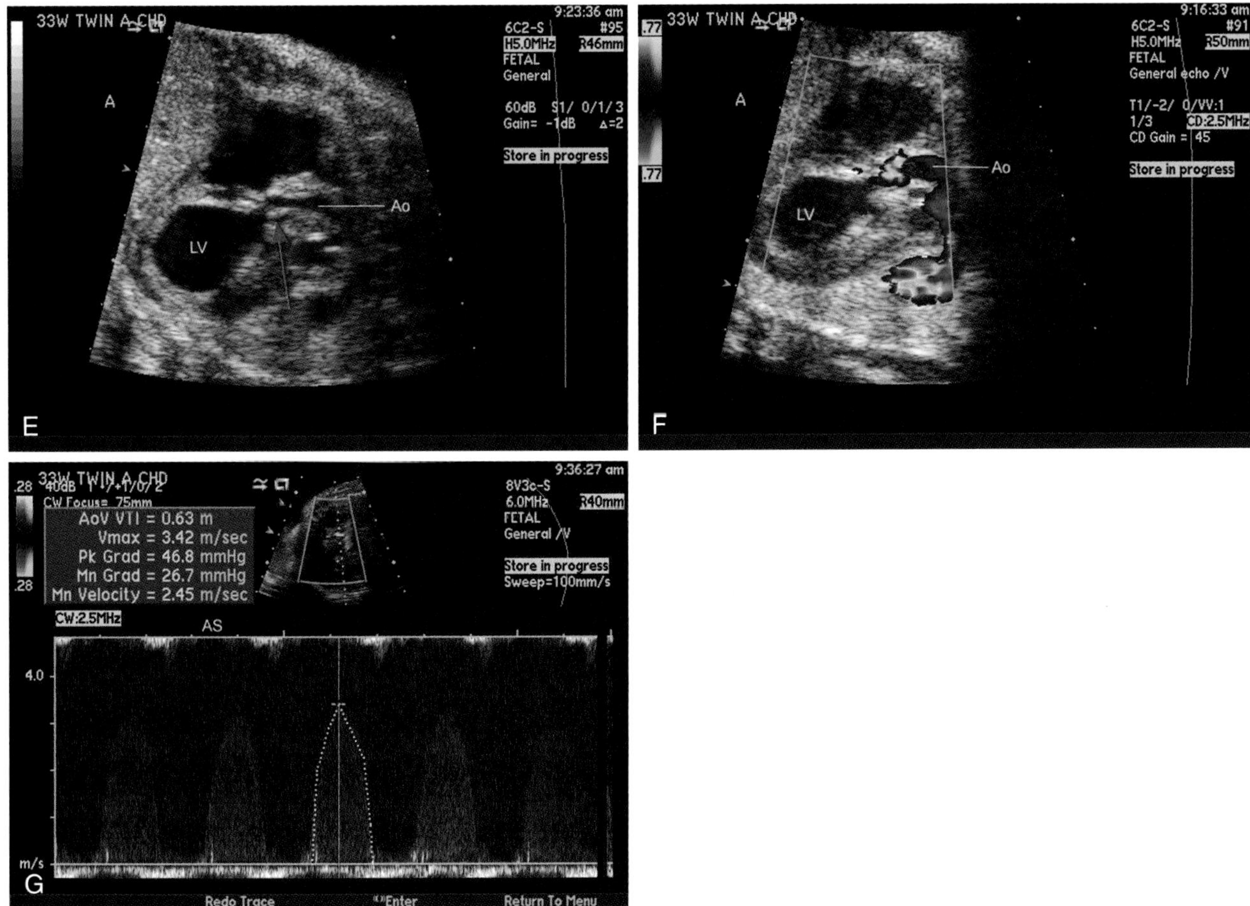

Case 23-2, cont'd **(E)** Long-axis view of the LV. There is aortic stenosis with a thickened aortic valve *(red arrow)*. **(F)** Color flow imaging across the aortic valve. There is a jet of antegrade flow just above the aortic valve *(speckled color)*; however, there is retrograde flow *(blue color)* in the ascending aorta (Ao). **(G)** The peak velocity across the aortic valve suggests a peak instantaneous gradient of approximately 45 to 50 mm Hg, yet the quantity of antegrade aortic flow is limited by the massive degree of MR. AS, aortic stenosis.

V

Congenital Heart Anomalies: Right-Sided Heart Defects

24

Pulmonary Stenosis

Anita Szwast

Key Echocardiographic Features

- Size of the pulmonary annulus in comparison with the aortic annulus.
- Laminar or turbulent flow across pulmonic valve?
- Peak systolic velocity across the pulmonic valve.
- Morphology of the pulmonary valve.
- Size of the tricuspid annulus compared with the mitral annulus.
- Degree of tricuspid regurgitation.
- Right ventricle pressure estimate based on tricuspid regurgitation peak velocity.
- Right atrial size.
- Right ventricle size and function.
- Degree of right ventricular hypertrophy.
- Direction of flow within the ductus arteriosus.
- Size of the branch pulmonary arteries.
- Size and appearance of the foramen ovale.
- Evidence for elevated central venous pressure as marked by reversal of flow with atrial contraction in the ductus venosus.
- Evidence for elevated central venous pressure as marked by pulsations within the inferior vena cava.
- Presence of any ventriculocoronary "sinusoid" connections.

Anatomy and Anatomical Associations

Pulmonary stenosis is a heterogeneous disorder. The obstruction may occur at the subvalvar, valvar, or supravalvar levels (Figure 24-1). In subvalvar stenosis, the obstruction may be caused by either muscle or fibrous tissue. Muscular subvalvar stenosis includes obstruction secondary to malalignment of the conal septum or hypertrophic cardiomyopathy. Fibrous subvalvar stenosis typically occurs in association with conotruncal abnormalities and may be caused by abnormal chordal attachments or abnormal atrioventricular valve leaflet attachments.

Valvar pulmonary stenosis may be classified into six anatomic subtypes: (1) doming (42%), (2) unicommissural (16%), (3) bicuspid (10%), (4) tricuspid (6%), (5) hypoplastic annulus (6%), and (6) dysplastic (19%). In doming pulmonary stenosis, the valve appears dome-shaped or conical with a small central orifice varying in size from a pinhole to several millimeters in diameter. There is no separation into leaflets in doming pulmonary stenosis. In unicommissural pulmonary valve stenosis, there is a single commissure (natural split between the leaflets) and a single thickened leaflet. In bicuspid pulmonary valve stenosis, two commissures and two thickened leaflets are present. In tricuspid pulmonary valve stenosis, there is moderate thickening of all three leaflets

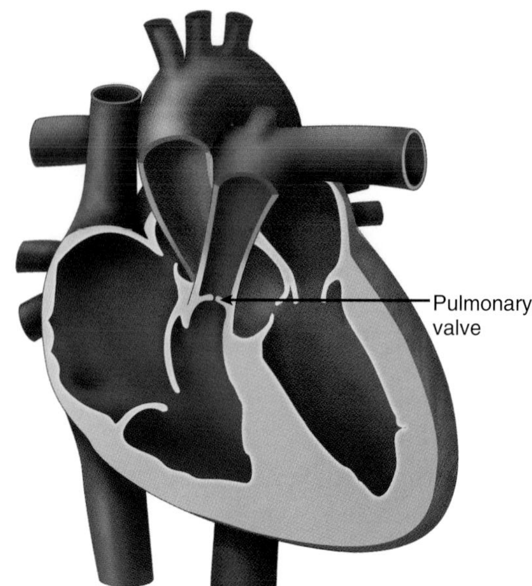

Figure 24-1. Pulmonary stenosis.

and partial fusion of all three commissures. In hypoplastic pulmonary valve stenosis, the annulus is markedly narrowed. Finally, in dysplastic pulmonary valve stenosis, the three leaflets are markedly thickened and redundant, although the commissures are not fused. Dysplastic pulmonary valves are present in the majority of cases of Noonan's syndrome and in some nonfamilial cases of pulmonary stenosis. In supravalvar pulmonary stenosis, the obstruction occurs above the annulus of the pulmonary valve.

Pulmonary stenosis may be seen in association with a number of different types of congenital heart disease, including conotruncal abnormalities such as tetralogy of Fallot, double-outlet right ventricle or transposition of the great arteries, ventricular septal defect, tricuspid atresia or stenosis, Ebstein's anomaly, and congenitally corrected transposition of the great arteries. With more severe degrees of valvar obstruction, the infundibulum (conus) of the right ventricle may become hypertrophied, producing dynamic subvalvar stenosis. Poststenotic dilation of the main pulmonary artery may occur on account of the high-velocity jet of flow being ejected through the stenotic pulmonary orifice. Tricuspid regurgitation may occur secondary to increased right ventricular pressure. The right atrium may dilate secondary to elevated filling pressures within the hypertrophied right ventricle and altered compliance. Smallness or hypoplasia of the right ventricle can be seen in association with isolated, but severe, pulmonic stenosis. Finally, in severe degrees of obstruction seen in the fetus, in the absence of significant tricuspid regurgitation, connections between the hypertensive right ventricle cavity and the developing coronary circulation—coronary sinusoids—may form. Abnormalities within the coronary circulation, including stenoses, interruptions, or even atresia of the origin of the coronary artery, place the fetus at risk for myocardial ischemia and infarction within the subendocardium of the right ventricle. Although these can be seen in severe pulmonic stenosis, they are more common in the presence of pulmonary atresia.

Frequency, Genetics, and Development

Isolated pulmonary valve stenosis occurs in 7% to 12% of patients with congenital heart disease. In contrast, if associated lesions are included, pulmonary stenosis occurs in 25% to 30% of all patients with congenital heart disease. Familial studies suggest a 2.1% incidence of congenital heart disease, usually either tetralogy of Fallot or pulmonary stenosis, in siblings of patients with pulmonary stenosis.[1] If a parent has pulmonary stenosis, the incidence of pulmonary valve stenosis in a child is 2.8%.[2] In twin studies, 8.3% of monozygotic twins and 2.2% of dizygotic twins had pulmonary stenosis.

Genetic syndromes may be associated with pulmonary stenosis. These include neurofibromatosis, multiple lentigines or LEOPARD (lentigines, electrocardiogram abnormalities, ocular hypertelorism, pulmonary stenosis, abnormal genitalia, retardation of growth, and deafness) syndrome, and Noonan's syndrome. Up to 50% of patients with Noonan's syndrome have a congenital heart defect, usually a dysplastic pulmonary valve, and up to 25% of patients with Noonan's syndrome have hypertrophic cardiomyopathy, which may also be associated with pulmonary stenosis.[3,4] In Williams's syndrome, supravalvar pulmonary stenosis can be seen. Systemic diseases such as glycogen storage disease may be associated with infundibular and valvar pulmonary stenosis.

Prenatal Physiology

Fetal physiology depends upon the severity of the pulmonary valve stenosis. Mild forms of pulmonary stenosis are well tolerated in utero and may not even be detected by screening fetal echocardiography. Diagnosis depends upon careful inspection of pulmonary valve morphology and pulse wave Doppler interrogation of the pulmonary valve. A peak velocity greater than 1 m/sec across the pulmonary valve is abnormal and should alert the clinician to the possibility of pulmonary valve stenosis. With moderate to severe pulmonary stenosis, right ventricular hypertrophy, tricuspid regurgitation, and poststenotic dilation of the main pulmonary artery may be seen. Flow within the ductus arteriosus may be reversed (aorta-to-pulmonary artery) in order to augment pulmonary blood flow. With severe degrees of obstruction, right ventricular filling pressures may be high, leading to increased right-to-left shunting across the patent foramen ovale and dilation of the left side of the heart as a consequence. Right ventricular hypoplasia to varying degrees can also be seen in such cases. As blood is diverted away from the right ventricle, growth is impaired. Normally, the tricuspid valve annulus is larger than the mitral valve annulus throughout gestation. In severe pulmonic stenosis, the right ventricular cavity and tricuspid valve annulus may not grow at an expected rate, leading to the finding of a mitral valve annulus that is larger than the tricuspid.

In "critical" pulmonary stenosis in the absence of significant tricuspid regurgitation, the right ventricular pressure may become even higher than that in the left ventricle (suprasystemic pressure). Coronary sinusoids may form from the right ventricular cavity to the coronary circulation. Abnormalities within the coronary circulation, including stenoses, interruptions, or even atresia of the origin of the coronary artery, places the fetus at risk for myocardial ischemia and infarction.

Prenatal Management

Family counseling depends upon the severity of the obstruction. Mild to moderate cases of pulmonary stenosis are well tolerated in utero and typically do not require neonatal intervention. However, pulmonary valve stenosis may progress over the course of gestation from a milder to a more severe form.[5,6] Consequently, serial surveillance over the course of gestation is appropriate. Severe cases of pulmonary stenosis will require neonatal intervention, either in the cardiac catheterization laboratory or in the operating room.

A number of important features are to be imaged and assessed at initial diagnosis and at subsequent prenatal visits when pulmonary stenosis is suspected (see Key Features). Vaginal delivery is generally well tolerated by most fetuses with pulmonary stenosis. However, cesarean section may be recommended for fetuses with critical pulmonary stenosis if impending hydrops fetalis is suspected, if there is evidence for left ventricular dysfunction, or if there is a restrictive patent foramen ovale. Prostaglandin should be recommended at birth if there is inadequate antegrade flow across the pulmonary valve and reversal of flow within the ductus arteriosus.

Most fetuses with pulmonary stenosis have perhaps a somewhat small but adequate size right ventricle and achieve a biventricular repair after birth. Consequently, prenatal intervention is usually not recommended. However, some centers have advocated balloon valvuloplasty in utero in cases of critical pulmonary stenosis in order to prevent the development of hydrops fetalis and to ensure a biventricular circulation postnatally.[7-9] Indications cited for in utero intervention include impending hydrops fetalis, marked by the appearance of ascites, pericardial, or pleural effusions, decreased left ventricular shortening, marked flow reversal with atrial contraction within the ductus venosus, pulsations within the inferior vena cava, and restrictive flow across the patent foramen ovale.[8]

Postnatal Physiology

Postnatal physiology depends upon by the severity of the obstruction. In mild to moderate pulmonary stenosis, neonates are asymptomatic and tolerate natural closure of the ductus arteriosus without any trouble. With more moderate degrees of obstruction, there may be right-to-left shunting at the patent foramen ovale, leading to mild cyanosis in the neonatal period. Neonates with more severe degrees of obstruction or critical pulmonary stenosis may be quite cyanotic in the neonatal period on account of marked right-to-left shunting at the patent foramen ovale and inadequate forward flow across the pulmonary valve. In these neonates, pulmonary blood flow is supplied primarily by reversed flow (aorta to pulmonary artery) across the ductus arteriosus. If the ductus arteriosus were to close, these neonates may develop life-threatening cyanosis. In neonates with severe tricuspid regurgitation or a restrictive patent foramen ovale, symptoms of right heart failure may be seen.

Postnatal Management

Postnatal management depends upon the severity of the obstruction. Newborns with mild to moderate degrees of obstruction are usually discharged from hospital with outpatient follow-up. Cyanotic newborns with critical pulmonary stenosis, however, require intervention in the neonatal period. Supplemental oxygen may be necessary. Prostaglandin should be administered to maintain ductal blood flow if there is inadequate forward flow across the pulmonary valve. Inotropic infusion and anticongestive medications may be required if there is significant right heart failure.

Most neonates with critical pulmonary stenosis should be referred for balloon valvuloplasty as the initial intervention. However, subvalvar stenosis secondary to muscle or fibrous tissue and conditions of marked hypoplasia of the pulmonary annulus are not amenable to balloon dilation of the pulmonary valve in the cardiac catheterization lab. These patients should be referred for surgical intervention. Effective balloon dilation of the pulmonary valve may be safely performed in over 90% of patients. Antegrade flow through the pulmonary valve is improved significantly in most patients such that prostaglandin may be weaned off. Mild to moderate cyanosis secondary to right-to-left shunting across the patent foramen ovale may persist until the compliance of the right ventricle improves. In cases of incomplete relief of pulmonary stenosis with balloon valvuloplasty, surgical intervention may be required if the patient is unable to be weaned from prostaglandin infusion. Although the right ventricle may be mildly hypoplastic and markedly hypertrophied in some cases, cavity growth and reduction in hypertrophy should occur over time if adequate relief of valvar obstruction has been achieved.

Surgery for pulmonary stenosis is uncommon because most are amenable to catheter procedure and balloon valvuloplasty. However, rarely, there may be ineffective relief via balloon technique or the association of severe right ventricular hypoplasia, which leads to the need for surgery. The type of surgical intervention depends upon whether the patient is deemed appropriate for either a biventricular repair or, if there is significant ventricular hypoplasia, a single-ventricle palliation. If deemed a candidate for a biventricular repair, as is the case in most, a pulmonary valvotomy can be performed or a transannular patch, if the annulus is deemed too hypoplastic. If the pulmonary valve is dysplastic, the valve itself may need to be partially or completely excised and a homograft valve possibly inserted. If deemed best a candidate for a single-ventricle palliation, which is quite rare in pulmonary stenosis, a systemic-to-pulmonary shunt would be performed in the neonatal period, followed by a bidirectional Glenn procedure at 4 to 6 months of age and a Fontan operation at 2 to 3 years of age (see Chapter 25).

Long-term Outcomes

Outcomes for isolated pulmonary valve stenosis are excellent. Studies have been performed elucidating the lifelong natural history of pulmonary stenosis. According to the Second Natural History Study, mild cases of pulmonary stenosis with peak velocity less than 25 mm Hg across the pulmonary valve do not require intervention.[10] Exercise tolerance in these patients is normal. Management of moderate pulmonary valve stenosis, defined as a peak gradient between 25 and 50 mm Hg remains controversial. In the Second Natural History Study, 20% of patients with peak gradients between 25 to 49 mm Hg required surgery.[10] Although most patients were asymptomatic, indications for surgical intervention included subnormal cardiac output response during formal exercise testing and abnormal increase in right ventricular end-diastolic pressure. In the current era, many centers recommend elective balloon dilation of the pulmonary valve with a gradient greater than 40 mm Hg. Over time, disproportionate growth of the child compared with the pulmonary valve may lead to worsening of the obstruction. Consequently, infants with even mild to moderate degrees of obstruction should be followed over time to ensure that the gradients do not progress and require intervention at a later date. Moderate to severe pulmonary stenosis with peak velocity greater than 50 mm Hg should definitely undergo either balloon dilation valvuloplasty or surgical valvotomy. None of the natural history studies previously performed to date have included prenatal findings; hence, predicting with accuracy which of these pathways a fetus with pulmonary stenosis will take is difficult.

Excellent results are achieved in patients who undergo initial balloon dilation as a child or as an adult.

Following effective pulmonary valvuloplasty, a long-term outcome study in a group of 134 patients reported a 77% freedom from re-intervention at 15 years.[11] Of the 17 patients who required surgical intervention for persistent obstruction, 11 had the unique finding of dysplastic valves, an association seen in Noonan's syndrome.[11] Clinical status for the entire cohort was excellent at a mean follow-up of 11.9 years.[11] There were no arrhythmias and only 2 patients in New York Heart Association class II.[11]

In neonates undergoing balloon valvuloplasty, 90% have successful reduction in their gradients, although up to 10% of these patients require additional procedures within months after the initial procedure in order to achieve long-term relief of obstruction.[12] In addition, hemodynamically significant pulmonary insufficiency requiring pulmonary valve replacement at some point in life occurs more frequently in neonates who require intervention.[13]

Imaging Essentials and Important Points

- Mild pulmonary stenosis can be missed on fetal echocardiography.
- The pulmonary valve can be imaged in multiple planes. Examples of excellent views include the short axis at the level of the great vessels and long-axis angling anteriorly toward the right ventricular outflow tract. From the four-chamber view, anterior angling just beyond visualization of the left ventricular outflow tract will reveal the right ventricular outflow tract. This view provides an opportunity for optimal Doppler sampling across the pulmonary valve.
- In pulmonary stenosis, Doppler interrogation across the pulmonary valve will reveal "turbulent" flow and loss of laminar flow as well as a peak velocity that is greater than 1 m/sec.
- Both the pulmonary annulus and the tricuspid annulus are larger than the aorta and mitral valve in the normal fetus. In pulmonary stenosis, however, the pulmonary annulus may be smaller than normal and should be measured and plotted as gestation progresses.
- The degree of associated tricuspid valve hypoplasia reflects the degree of right ventricular hypoplasia that is present. In many cases, the tricuspid annulus will be small, but of adequate size, typically at a gestational age Z-score of greater than –3 (no smaller than 3 standard deviations from the expected mean for gestational age).
- A general sense and qualitative impression of the cavity size of the right ventricle should be made in every fetus with pulmonic stenosis. Actual measurement of cavity volume can be extremely challenging because of the geometric nature of the right ventricle and its hypertrophied state in pulmonary stenosis. This does not lend itself to accurate formulaic equations that can be applied. The best indirect gauge of right ventricular capacity is measurement of the tricuspid valve annulus.
- Doppler evaluation of tricuspid valve inflow, ductus venosus, and umbilical vein flow in the fetus can help assess right ventricular compliance and predict who may have significant diastolic dysfunction after birth, with right-to-left shunting at the foramen ovale and consequential cyanosis. Features such as (1) single-peak inflow across the tricuspid valve, (2) absence or reversal of forward flow with atrial contraction in the ductus venosus, or (3) venous pulsations in the umbilical vein reflect altered right ventricular compliance and should be noted.
- Signs of hydrops fetalis in association with pulmonary stenosis are troubling. Abnormal Doppler flow patterns as described previously have not been demonstrated to progress to hydrops in the fetus with pulmonic stenosis and do not predict impending hydrops because diastolic dysfunction may remain stable throughout fetal life without any significant clinical manifestations until birth. However, the combination of a restrictive foramen ovale with the venous Doppler changes described previously may place the fetus at risk for impediment to forward flow and may impair cardiac output. Such a fetus is at substantial risk for hydrops.
- Severity of tricuspid regurgitation, if present, should be monitored carefully. Severe tricuspid regurgitation is a risk factor for development of hydrops.
- The tricuspid valve should be inspected carefully when there is tricuspid regurgitation in the presence of pulmonary stenosis. Abnormalities such as Ebstein's anomaly or dysplasia of the tricuspid valve can be seen. Careful attention should be paid to the septal leaflet of the tricuspid valve as a mild Ebstein anomaly can be missed.

References

1. Campbell M. Factors in the aetiology of pulmonary stenosis. *Br Heart J*. 1962;24:625-632.
2. Driscoll DJ, Michels VV, Gersony WM, et al. Occurrence risk for congenital heart defects in relatives of patients with aortic stenosis, pulmonary stenosis, or ventricular septal defect. *Circulation*. 1993; 87:1114-1120.
3. Burch M, Sharland M, Shinebourne E, et al. Cardiologic abnormalities in Noonan syndrome: phenotypic diagnosis and echocardiographic assessment of 118 patients. *J Am Coll Cardiol*. 1993;22: 1189-1192.

4. Noonan JA. Hypertelorism with Turner phenotype. A new syndrome with associated congenital heart disease. *Am J Dis Child.* 1968;116:373-380.
5. Rice MJ, McDonald RW, Reller MD. Progressive pulmonary stenosis in the fetus: two case reports. *Am J Perinatol.* 1993;10:424-427.
6. Todros T, Presbitero P, Gaglioti P, Demarie D. Pulmonary stenosis with intact ventricular septum: documentation of development of the lesion echocardiographically during fetal life. *Int J Cardiol.* 1988;19:355-362.
7. Galindo A, Gutierrez-Larraya F, Velasco JM, de la Fuente P. Pulmonary balloon valvuloplasty in a fetus with critical pulmonary stenosis/atresia with intact ventricular septum and heart failure. *Fetal Diagn Ther.* 2006;21:100-104.
8. Tulzer G, Arzt W, Franklin RC, et al. Fetal pulmonary valvuloplasty for critical pulmonary stenosis or atresia with intact septum. *Lancet.* 2002;360:1567-1568.
9. Tworetzky W, Marshall AC. Fetal interventions for cardiac defects. *Pediatr Clin North Am.* 2004;51:1503-1513, vii.
10. Hayes CJ, Gersony WM, Driscoll DJ, et al. Second natural history study of congenital heart defects. Results of treatment of patients with pulmonary valvar stenosis. *Circulation.* 1993;87:I28-I37.
11. Garty Y, Veldtman G, Lee K, et al. Late outcomes after pulmonary valve balloon dilatation in neonates, infants, and children. *J Invasive Cardiol.* 2005;17:318-322.
12. Colli AM, Perry SB, Lock JE, et al. Balloon dilation of critical valvar pulmonary stenosis in the first month of life. *Cathet Cardiovasc Diagn,* 1995;34:23-28.
13. Berman W Jr, Fripp RR, Raisher BD, et al. Significant pulmonary valve incompetence following oversize balloon pulmonary valvuloplasty in small infants: A long-term follow-up study. *Cathet Cardiovasc Intervent.* 1999;48:61-65.

CASES

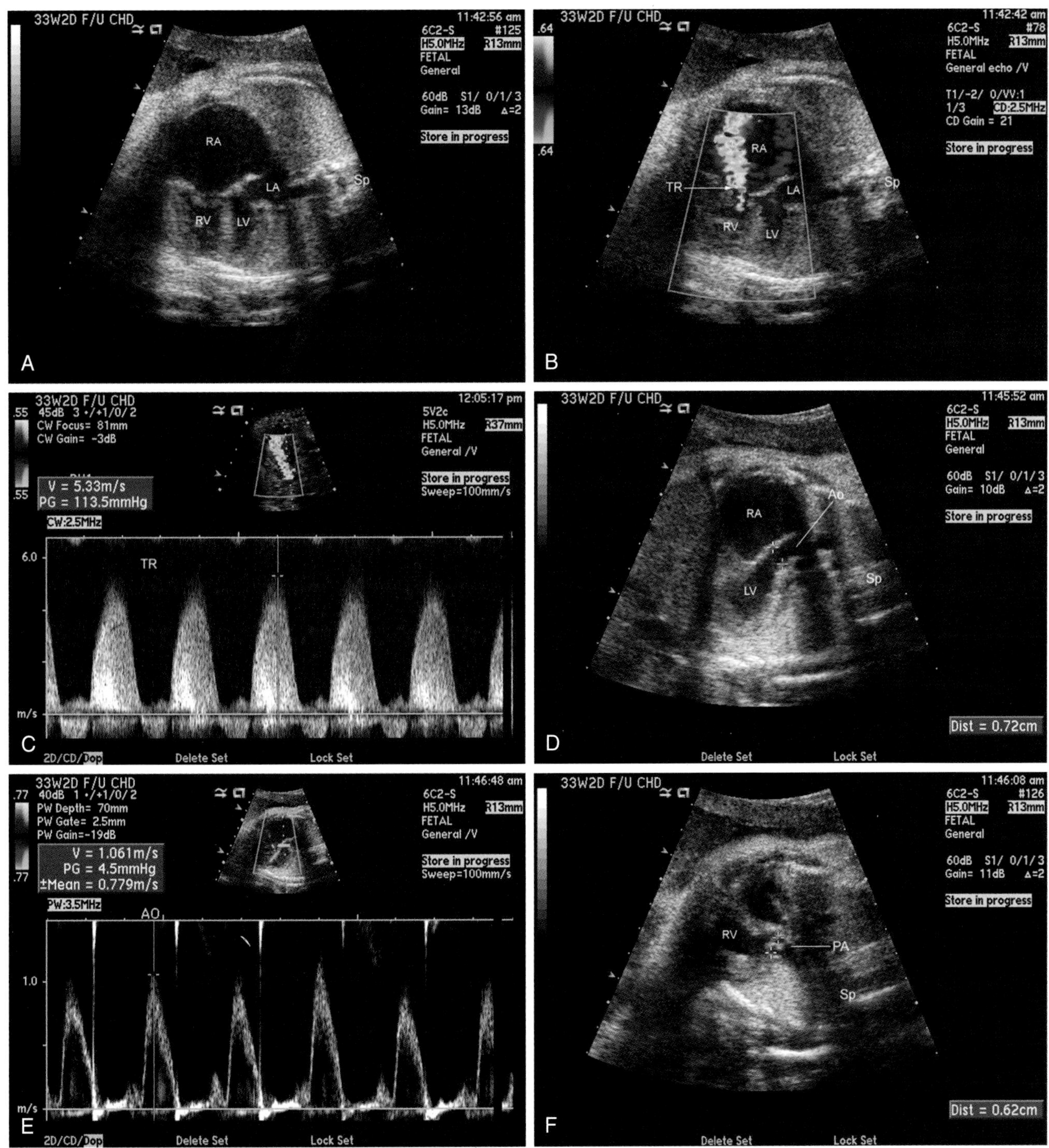

Case 24-1. (**A**) Four-chamber view of the fetal heart at 32 weeks' gestation. The overall heart size is enlarged, but this is mostly related to a markedly dilated right atrium (RA). LA, left atrium; LV, left ventricle; RV, right ventricle; Sp, spine. (**B**) Color Doppler imaging demonstrates severe tricuspid regurgitation (TR). (**C**) Continuous wave Doppler assessment of the peak systolic velocity of the tricuspid regurgitant jet is over 5.3 m/sec. Right ventricular pressure estimate is extremely high and markedly over the LV pressure at 113 mm Hg over the right atrial V wave. This suggests right-sided outflow obstruction. (**D**) The aortic annulus measures 7.2 mm and is unobstructed. Ao, aorta. (**E**) Doppler flow pattern across the aortic valve. The flow is laminar. (**F**) The pulmonary valve is thickened. The pulmonary annulus (PA) measures 6.2 mm and is smaller than the aortic annulus, which is an abnormal finding. Pulmonary annular hypoplasia is associated with valvar pulmonic stenosis.

Continued

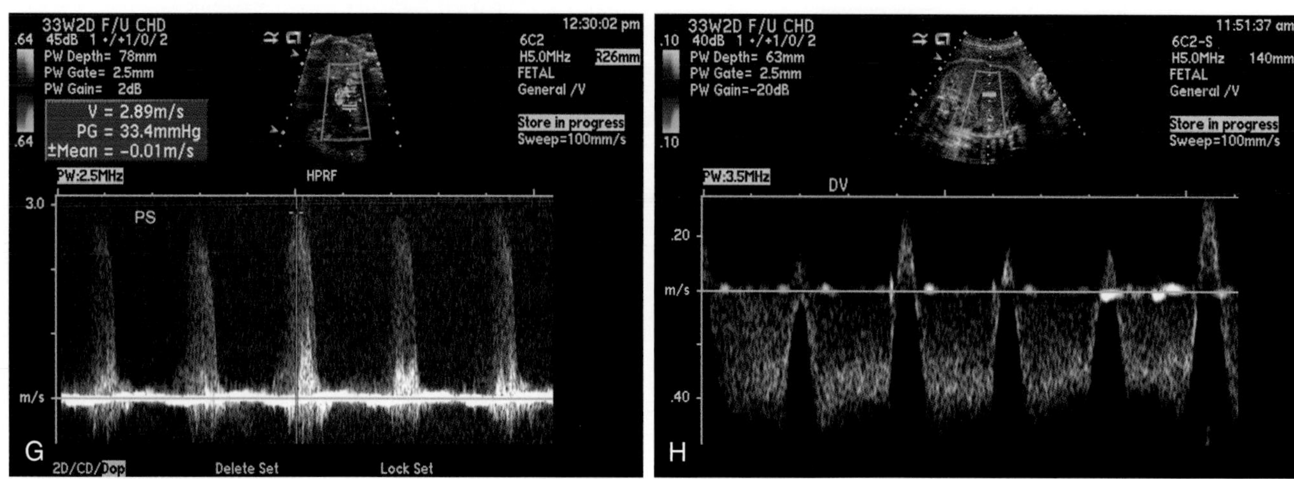

Case 24-1, cont'd (G) Doppler flow pattern across the pulmonic valve. There is turbulent flow and the peak velocity is increased to 2.9 m/sec. (H) Doppler flow pattern in the ductus venosus (DV) demonstrates reversal with atrial contraction. This is caused by increased right atrial pressure as a consequence of the TR and a poorly compliant, hypertrophied RV.

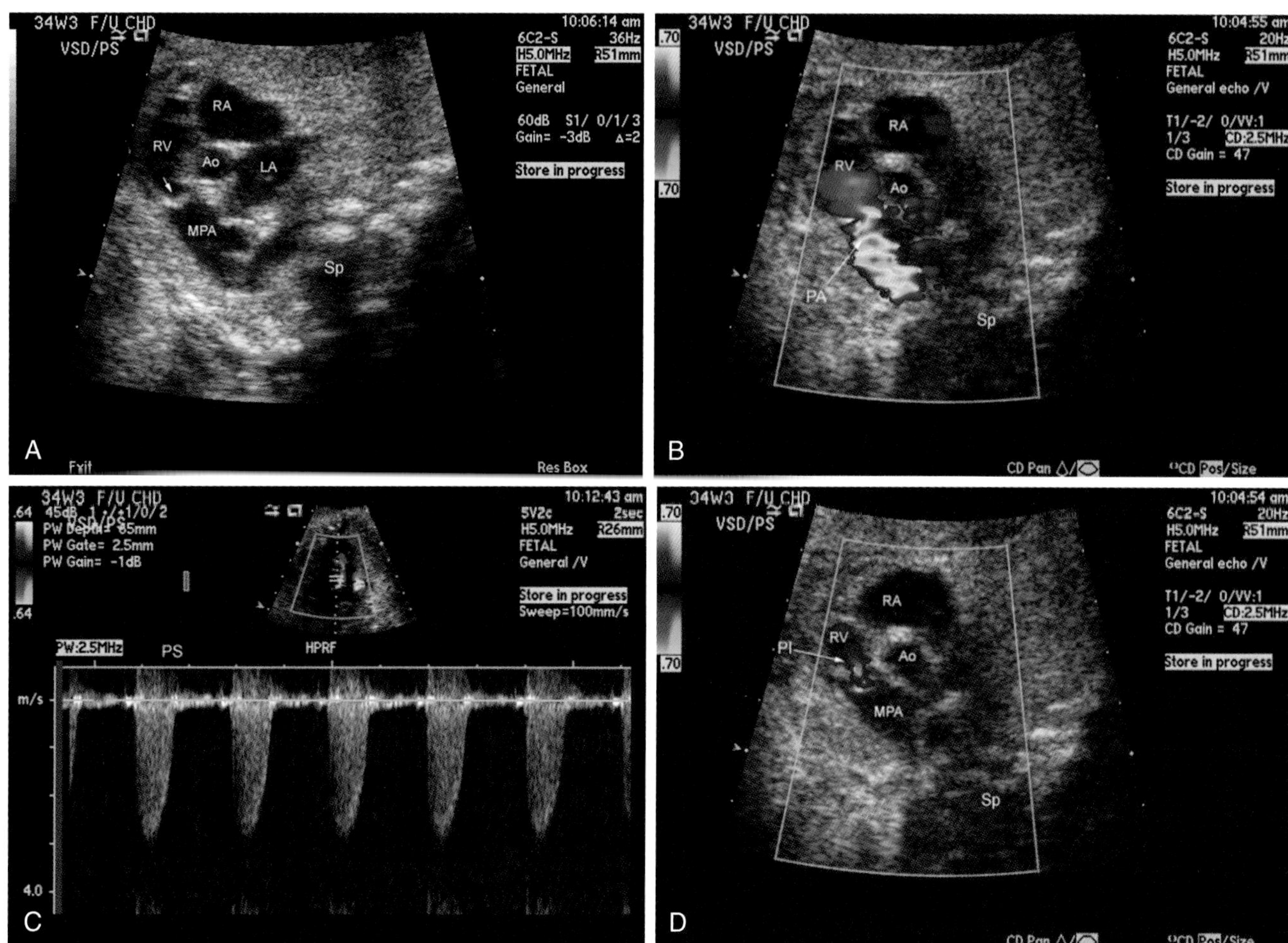

Case 24-2. **(A)** Short-axis view of the heart. The *arrow* points to the stenotic pulmonary valve, which is seen doming in systole. Ao, aorta; LA, left atrium; MPA, main pulmonary artery; RA, right atrium; RV, right ventricle; Sp, spine. **(B)** Color flow across the stenotic pulmonary valve demonstrates turbulence above the valve, with multiple colors seen, suggesting high-velocity nonlaminar flow. PA, pulmonary artery. **(C)** Pulsed-wave Doppler across the stenotic pulmonary valve (PS). The peak velocity across is approximately 3 m/sec, suggesting a peak instantaneous velocity of 36 mm Hg. **(D)** Pulmonary insufficiency (PI) in diastole. The jet originates from the abnormal valve and flows back into the RV.

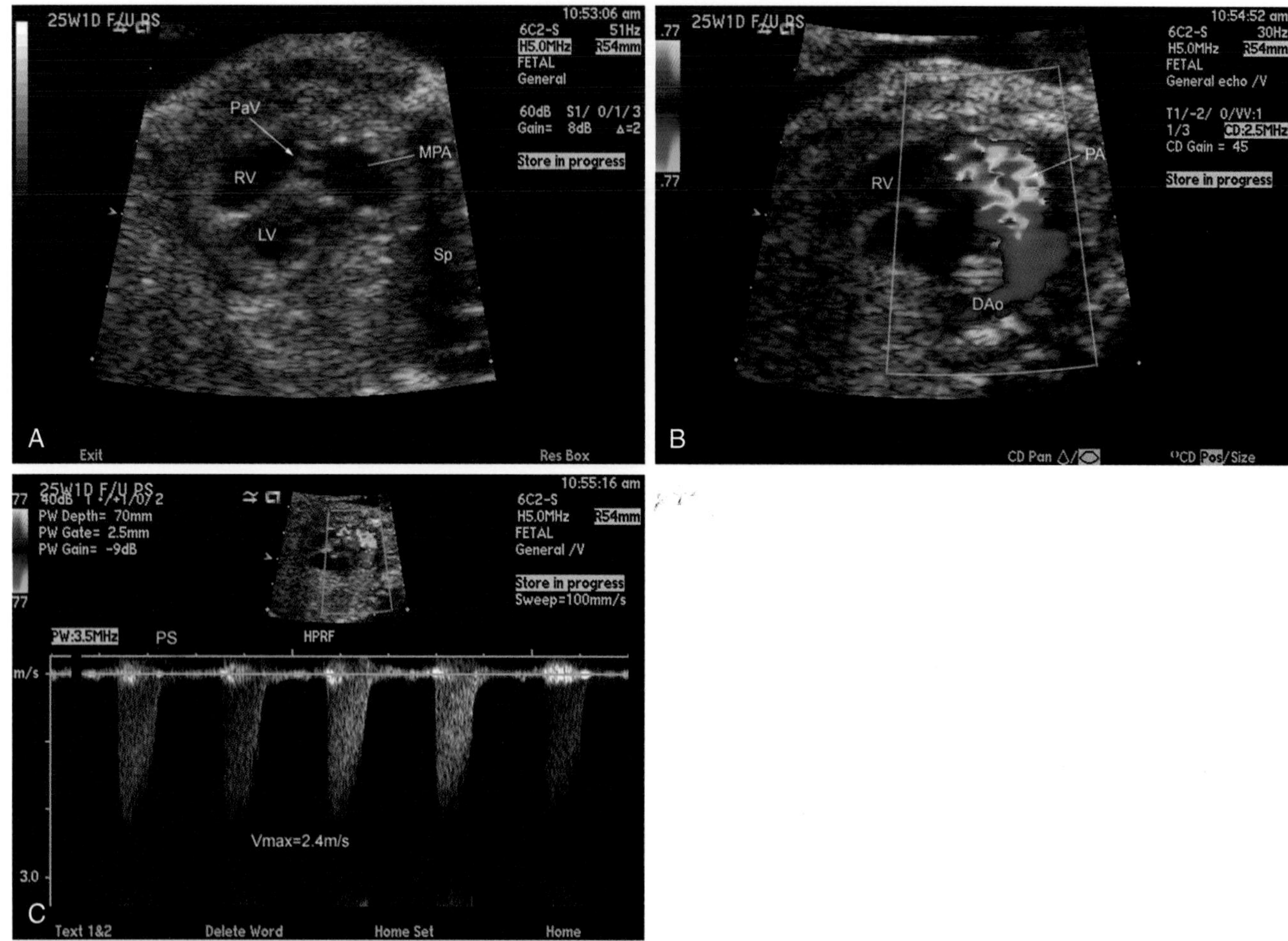

Case 24-3. **(A)** Long-axis view of the right ventricle (RV). The *arrow* points to the stenotic pulmonary valve (PaV). Note there is also a dilated appearance to the main pulmonary artery (PA) indicating poststenotic dilation of the MPA. **(B)** Color flow imaging further highlights the stenosis of the pulmonic valve as seen by turbulent flow above the valve and the poststenotic dilation. There is also some ductal dilation as well in its continuity with the descending aorta (DAo). **(C)** Pulse wave Doppler above the pulmonic valve. There is a peak velocity of 2.4 m/sec, hence, a peak instantaneous gradient of 23 mm Hg across the valve. PS, stenotic pulmonary valve.

25

Pulmonary Atresia with Intact Ventricular Septum

Anita Szwast

Key Echocardiographic Features

- Size and function of the right ventricle in comparison with the left ventricle.
- Morphology of the right ventricle (i.e., tripartite?).
- Morphology of the pulmonary outflow tract.
- Patency of the pulmonary valve.
- Tricuspid valve size and morphology.
- Presence or absence of tricuspid regurgitation.
- If tricuspid regurgitation is present, estimate the intracavitary right ventricular pressure by Doppler estimate of the peak velocity of the regurgitant jet.
- Presence or absence of right ventricle coronary-cameral fistulas.
- Presence or absence of coronary artery dilation along the septum or surface of the heart.
- Presence or absence of left ventricular outflow tract obstruction (i.e., septal bowing).

Anatomy and Anatomical Associations

Pulmonary atresia with intact ventricular septum (PA/IVS) is an anomaly in which the pathway from the right ventricle (RV) to the pulmonary artery is completely sealed off (PA) and there is no ventricular septal defect. PA/IVS is a morphologically heterogeneous disorder. The RV is commonly small or hypoplastic, or it can be markedly dilated, as when associated with Ebstein's anomaly or tricuspid valve (TV) dysplasia and severe tricuspid regurgitation. There may be muscular atresia of the right ventricular infundibulum with no outflow chamber at all or there may be platelike valvar atresia. In addition, PA may be acquired over the course of gestation. Critical pulmonary stenosis may progress to PA.[1] In addition, decreased forward flow through the right ventricular outflow tract in the setting of severe tricuspid regurgitation, as in Ebstein's anomaly[2,3] or the twin-twin transfusion syndrome,[4,5] may lead to "functional" PA in which the valve leaflets do not open based on hemodynamics but, anatomically, do have the potential to open. Such cases of "functional" atresia can progress to true, anatomical PA. At birth, the pulmonary valve leaflets may be fused and appear clinically indistinguishable from congenital forms of PA.

Extracardiac anomalies are unusual in PA/IVS, although many different cardiac anomalies can be seen. Atrial septal defects and abnormalities of the right side of the heart are common. In PA/IVS, the TV leaflets are frequently dysplastic. The chordae of the TV may be thickened and may not adequately coapt, causing severe regurgitation in utero. In addition, in many cases, the TV annulus is small. It may be moderately to severely hypoplastic, causing tricuspid stenosis or, in some cases, fully seal off and manifest tricuspid atresia.

The morphology of the RV may be abnormal and is an important component of the anomaly. The RV is anatomically considered to consist of three parts (tripartite). It can be divided into (1) an inlet or sinus portion, which is the region just beneath the TV, (2) a trabecular or muscular portion, which makes up the apex, and (3) an outlet portion, which consists of the infundibulum. In PA/IVS, there may be severe underdevelopment and distortion of the ventricle so that only an inlet portion is recognized (Figure 25-1). Interestingly, pulmonary arterial abnormalities are rare in PA/IVS. The branch pulmonary arteries are typically of good size and perfused by the ductus arteriosus.

Coronary abnormalities are common in PA/IVS, especially in the setting of a hypertrophied, hypertensive RV with little or no tricuspid regurgitation. There is an inverse relationship between RV size and coronary abnormalities—the smaller the RV and tricuspid annulus, the more likely there will be coronary abnormalities. There may be atresia of the coronary os from the aortic root, hemodynamically significant coronary stenoses, or even coronary interruptions. In these cases, coronary arterial flow depends upon perfusion from the RV through connections into the right ventricular cavity called *right ventricular sinusoids* or *fistulas*. If a portion of the myocardium is solely dependent upon coronary perfusion from the RV alone, there is "RV-dependent coronary circulation."

The prevalence of coronary arterial abnormalities in PA/IVS is as follows. Fistulous communications between the RV and the coronary arteries are noted in 75% of

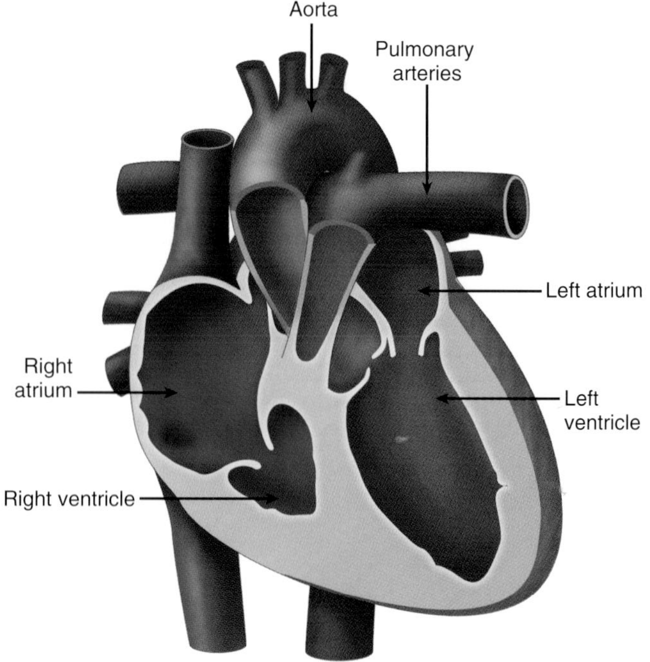

Figure 25-1. Pulmonary atresia/intact ventricular septum.

patients. Of these, 34% have coronary interruptions, 16% have atresia of the aortocoronary os, and 5% have a single coronary orifice.[6] In one study, 40% of patients were deemed to have RV-dependent coronary arterial circulation.[6] Myocardial abnormalities may be seen in conjunction in PA/IVS. These abnormalities include myocardial disarray, spongy myocardium, and ventricular endocardial fibroelastosis. In the setting of coronary abnormalities, ischemia, fibrosis, infarction, and myocardial rupture have been observed in fetuses with PA/IVS.

Finally, left heart abnormalities may be seen in PA/IVS. Left ventricular outflow tract obstruction may occur at the subvalvar and valvar levels. In cases of suprasystemic right ventricular pressure with severe septal hypertrophy, the septum may bow right to left into the left ventricular outflow tract causing subaortic obstruction. In utero infarction of the ventricular septum can cause septal aneurysm and distortion, leading to left ventricular outflow obstruction.

Frequency, Genetics, and Development

PA/IVS is a rare congenital heart defect with no known genetic etiology. The prevalence of PA ranges from 4.1 to 8.3 per 100,000 live births and accounts for approximately 3% of serious congenital heart defects. Males and females are affected equally. Multifactorial inheritance suggests a risk of recurrence of 3% to 5%.

The coronary arteries develop from the epicardial surface of the heart and normally migrate toward the aorta. In PA/IVS, normal coronary development is altered. The hypertensive RV may act as an "attractant," directing coronary migration toward it. Alternatively, very early natural connections between the developing RV and the coronary circulation may persist in order to allow for decompression and a pathway out of the embryonic RV, when the pulmonary valve is atretic. Over time, as the RV develops further hypertension, these primitive RV-to-coronary connections are preserved, and competitive flow between the aorta and the RV lead to narrowing and dilation (stenosis and ectasia) at the connections.

Prenatal Physiology

In the fetus with PA/IVS, there is no antegrade flow across the pulmonary valve. Consequently, all flow across the ductus arteriosus is retrograde (aorta–to–pulmonary artery), supplying the branch pulmonary arteries. Because blood cannot effectively make its way across the right side of the heart, there is increased right-to-left shunting at the atrial communication, leading to relative dilation of the left side of the heart. Restriction at the atrial communication will impair venous return and may lead to development of hydrops fetalis. The size of the TV and the degree of tricuspid regurgitation dictate the course.

In cases of severe tricuspid regurgitation with a normal TV annulus, the right atrium and RV become dilated, placing the fetus at risk for arrhythmia and hydrops fetalis. Marked cardiomegaly with cardiothoracic area ratios greater than 0.60 may compromise pulmonary vascular and lung development.[7]. In these, the prognosis is extremely poor.[7] In cases of severe tricuspid stenosis with little tricuspid regurgitation, the RV is severely hypertrophied and noncompliant. Pressures within the hypoplastic right ventricular cavity may reach suprasystemic and fistulous communications between the RV and the coronary arteries may be present. These coronary sinusoids place the fetus at risk for myocardial ischemia, arrhythmia, and potential fetal demise.

Prenatal Management

At initial encounter of a fetus with PA/IVS, prognosis and counseling hinge on assessment of the anatomy as being most favorable for a two-ventricle (biventricular) repair strategy or a single-ventricle palliative strategy. In essence, the questions to be answered are, (1) Can the RV undertake the task of perfusing the pulmonary circulation? and if so, (2) How best to get there and achieve this goal? If deemed that the RV cannot be recruited to this task based on anatomical features that make it prohibitive, a single-ventricle palliative strategy is to be undertaken.

Many investigators have looked into identifying fetal predictors of the eventual postnatal circulation. Gardiner and coworkers[8] published gestational age–specific criteria for predicting postnatal single-ventricle palliation versus biventricular repair. Predictive variables included the TV/mitral valve annular diameter ratio, Z-scores for the pulmonary valve (indexed to fetal size based upon femoral length), the right atrial "pressure score" (a composite based upon the TV Doppler, foramen ovale, and ductus venosus Doppler flow patterns), and the presence of coronary fistulas.[8] Salvin and colleagues[9] established the importance of the TV Z-score in the mid–gestational age fetus. In their study, all fetuses with a TV Z-score greater than −3 achieved a biventricular repair postnatally. Finally, Roman and associates[10] established a scoring system utilizing four criteria for discriminating fetuses with PA/IVS likely to achieve a biventricular repair from a single-ventricle palliation. In their study, fetuses most likely to require a single-ventricle palliation had (1) TV/mitral valve annular diameter ratio less than 0.7, (2) RV/LV (left ventricle) length ratio less than 0.6, (3) TV inflow duration less than 32% of the cardiac cycle, and (4) fistulous connections to the RV.[10]

Once the diagnosis is established, serial fetal echocardiography should be performed with focus on the features (see Key Features) as well as those in the previously discussed, published criteria in order to survey for findings that may change the prognosis from a two-ventricle to a single-ventricle strategy.

When coronary artery abnormalities are present in PA/IVS, it is important to distinguish between two categories of patients. In the first, there are connections between the RV and the coronaries (sinusoids or coronary-cameral fistulas) but dual supply from both the aorta and the RV, without any impediment to normal aorta-to-coronary perfusion. In the second, there are connections between the RV and the coronaries, but there is also impediment to aortic supply distal to the connection due to stenosis or atresia; hence, the distal coronary circulatory bed is dependent upon perfusion from the RV. This is referred to as an "RV-dependent coronary circulation." In the first category, postnatal rehabilitation of the RV through relief of outflow obstruction and decompression is permissible, because coronary flow will continue via the aorta. However, in the second, such decompression will reduce RV pressure and eliminate the source for coronary perfusion resulting in myocardial ischemia. Distinguishing between these two categories using fetal echocardiography is not possible. Diagnosis of RV-dependent coronary circulation is best made using cardiac catheterization after birth.

Most fetuses with PA/IVS have no significant problems in utero. However, the presence of extensive fistulous communications places the fetus at risk for ischemia, arrhythmia, and sudden death in utero. Fistulous connections between the RV and the coronaries can be seen on fetal echocardiography. Color Doppler imaging scale should be lowered in order to increase the sensitivity of observing low-velocity flow. However, delineating details of coronary anatomy such as stenosis or source of perfusion is a challenge and should be left for postnatal assessment via cardiac catheterization.

Severe dilation of the right heart secondary to severe tricuspid regurgitation and massive cardiomegaly compromises lung development and may lead to hydrops fetalis. Impending hydrops fetalis may be an indication for early delivery via cesarean section. Fetal intervention for PA/IVS remains controversial, although proponents argue that fetal pulmonary valvuloplasty is indicated in cases of impending hydrops.[11,12] In addition, in utero intervention may preserve the possibility for a biventricular repair postnatally.[11,12] It can be said that, once specific features are seen, it is possible to determine which fetuses have an inadequate RV for a two-ventricle repair. However, predicting which fetuses with a current profile suggesting an adequate RV will go on during gestation to develop findings of an inadequate RV is a challenge. Such a path, and the prognostic echocardiographic features that would predict such, has not yet been described in the literature.

Postnatal Physiology

At birth, pulmonary blood flow is entirely dependent upon the patency of the ductus arteriosus. As the ductus arteriosus closes, severe hypoxemia occurs, leading to death. Consequently, all neonates with PA/IVS require an infusion of prostaglandin to maintain ductal patency. Neonates with severe tricuspid regurgitation and marked cardiomegaly may become hypoxemic and acidotic. Symptoms of right heart failure may develop if the atrial communication becomes restrictive. Finally, neonates with coronary-to-RV cameral fistulas and RV-dependent coronary circulation are at risk for ischemia.

Postnatal Management

All neonates with PA/IVS require prostaglandin infusion to maintain ductal patency because there is no other source for pulmonary blood flow. Supplemental oxygen may be required for hypoxemia. Inotropic agents may be needed for symptoms of right heart failure related to severe tricuspid regurgitation. A balloon atrial septostomy may be required for a restrictive patent foramen ovale. A full postnatal echocardiogram should be performed to assess candidacy for a biventricular repair strategy versus a single-ventricle palliation strategy. Many criteria have been established for two-ventricle repair in the neonate with PA/IVS. The presence of a good-sized TV with Z-score greater than −3 and absence of RV-dependent coronary circulation best predicts success.

A diagnostic cardiac catheterization is routinely performed in all neonates with PA/IVS in order to accurately identify the presence and extent of coronary artery abnormalities and determine whether there are sinusoid connections with dual supply or RV-dependent coronary circulation. This cannot be accurately elucidated via echocardiography alone.

A two-ventricle repair strategy involves relief of right ventricular outflow tract obstruction by opening of the atretic pulmonary valve. RV-dependent coronary circulation is an absolute contraindication to lowering right ventricular pressure by opening up the right ventricular outflow tract. In neonates without RV-dependent coronaries who are deemed appropriate candidates for biventricular repair, the right ventricular outflow tract may be opened by radiofrequency perforation of the pulmonary valve followed by balloon dilation of the pulmonary valve plate. As adequate antegrade flow is established and oxygen saturations improve, prostaglandin infusion may be weaned off. If balloon dilation does not result in successful relief of pulmonary outflow obstruction, surgical relief can be achieved via valvotomy or placement of a patch across the pulmonary annulus. Occasionally, the RV is still small or noncompliant and unable to provide adequate pulmonary blood flow. Then an alternative source of pulmonary blood flow can be established—either with a stent placed in the ductus arteriosus or with a surgical aortopulmonary shunt (modified Blalock-Taussig shunt). Either of these alternative sources of pulmonary blood flow may be coiled in the cardiac catheterization laboratory at a later date once oxygen saturations have improved. By opening up the right ventricular outflow tract, the compliance of the RV gradually improves and the degree of tricuspid regurgitation also usually improves. Repeat pulmonary valvuloplasty may be required in infancy or childhood to relieve recurrent obstruction. Finally, the atrial septal defect or patent foramen ovale may be closed in childhood via device closure in the cardiac catheterization laboratory.

Neonates with PA/IVS unsuitable for biventricular repair owing to severe RV hypoplasia, or with RV-dependent coronary circulation will require a surgical shunt in the neonatal period. These children will undergo a single-ventricle palliation strategy consisting of a bidirectional Glenn procedure at 4 to 6 months of age and a Fontan operation at 2 to 3 years of age. Some patients with significant dysplasia of the TV in association with PA/IVS may require a tricuspid valvuloplasty or a TV replacement. Finally, heart transplantation is an option to consider in patients with RV-dependent coronary circulation, particularly if there is already evidence of significant myocardial ischemia or anatomical atresia of the aortocoronary os.[13]

Outcomes

Long-term outcomes for PA/IVS are quite variable depending upon the anatomy and type of repair performed. Daubeney and coworkers[14] published the early and medium-term outcomes for their population in a U.K. and Ireland Collaborative Study of PA/IVS. Between 1991 and 1995, 183 patients with PA/IVS were identified.[14] There were 15 patients who underwent no intervention and died, 67 underwent a right ventricular outflow tract procedure, 18 underwent a right ventricular outflow tract procedure and a shunt, and 81 patients underwent a shunt alone.[14] Survival at 1 and 5 years, respectively, was 71% and 64%.[14] Independent risk factors for death were low birth weight, unipartite (only a single part) right ventricular morphology, and a dilated RV.[14] The presence of coronary-cameral fistulas, RV-dependent coronary circulation, and TV Z-scores were not found to be risk factors for death.[14] This is likely so, because these factors dictated the various surgical strategies, which were individualized based on anatomy. Survival at 9 years of follow-up was 59%; 29% had achieved a biventricular repair, 11% a univentricular repair, and 17% had a mixed circulation.[14]

Odim and colleagues in 2006[15] published a series of 56 patients who underwent either partial or complete repair between 1982 and 2001 at a single institution. Excellent results were reported if the right ventricular outflow tract obstruction was adequately relieved at the time of initial surgery. In their series, 5-year survival was 92% with a median time for reoperation of 6.9 years.[15] In contrast, Guleserian and associates[13] published a series of 32 patients with PA/IVS with RV-dependent coronary circulation managed with a single-ventricle palliation strategy. In their series, the median TV Z-score was −3.62 with a range of −2.42 to −5.15.[13] All patients had moderate or severe right ventricular hypoplasia.[13] Median follow-up was 5.1 years with a range of 9 months to 14.8 years. Actuarial survival by the Kaplan-Meier method at up to 15 years was 81.3% with a mean survival of 12.1 years.[13] All deaths occurred within 3 months of the Blalock-Taussig shunt secondary to presumed myocardial ischemia—and interestingly, there were no late deaths.[13] Atresia of the aortocoronary os was associated with 100% mortality, prompting the recommendation for heart transplantation at birth.[13]

Consequently, in the absence of severe coronary abnormalities, good outcomes may be achieved with a single-ventricle palliation strategy. In contrast, patients with appropriate anatomy and chosen for management with a biventricular repair have excellent survival, although many patients require reoperation on account of recurrent right ventricular outflow tract obstruction.

Imaging Essentials and Important Points

- Document the presence or absence of flow across the pulmonary valve.
- When suspecting PA, one may see no evidence for antegrade flow across and closed pulmonary valve leaflets in systole; however, the valve leaflets appear thin and delicate, and there is pulmonary insufficiency. In such cases, there is "functional" PA, not true anatomical PA, and one should seek an explanation as to why the valve is not opening (usually due to severe tricuspid regurgitation and poor RV function, as in Ebstein's anomaly).
- Identify the nature of the pulmonary atresia—valvar or muscular/infundibular?
- Attempt to identify whether the RV is tripartite with a sinus (inflow) portion, infundibular (outflow) portion, and trabecular (muscular apical) portion.
- RV size follows TV size. Measure the TV annulus and obtain its Z-score based on gestational age. A Z-score less than −3 suggests marked hypoplasia of the TV and RV.
- Measure the TV annulus and compare it with mitral valve annulus. A TV–to–mitral valve annulus ratio of less than 0.7 suggests right ventricular hypoplasia that may be prohibitive for a two-ventricle repair.
- Coronary fistulous connections can be seen on fetal echocardiography; however, distinct coronary

Imaging Essentials and Important Points—cont'd

anatomy cannot be discerned with accuracy. The presence of a small RV with color Doppler evidence of RV-to-coronary connection should raise suspicion of RV-dependent coronary circulation; however, final determination can be made only after birth.

- Assess the foramen ovale for any restriction.
- Assess for presence and degree of tricuspid regurgitation, and estimate the RV pressure.
- Apply pulse Doppler across the TV inflow to assess for blood flow patterns. A single, "monophasic" inflow peak suggests poor compliance.
- Important—documentation of inflow across the TV, but no tricuspid regurgitation, suggests strongly the presence of RV-to-coronary connections. Otherwise, where is the blood entering the RV going?
- Doppler assessment should include analysis of (1) the ductus venosus for reversal with atrial contraction and (2) the umbilical vein for pulsations. These indicate poor RV compliance, but do not necessarily predict reliably for development of hydrops. However, when these are seen (1) in the presence of a restrictive foramen ovale or (2) developing serially over time, it should raise concerns.
- Signs of hydrops should be looked for vigorously. If effusions or early hydrops is present in PA/IVS, features such as (1) restriction at the atrial level, (2) severe tricuspid regurgitation, or (3) ventricular dysfunction related to myocardial ischemia should be considered as possible causes.

References

1. Todros T, Presbitero P, Gaglioti P, Demarie D. Pulmonary stenosis with intact ventricular septum: documentation of development of the lesion echocardiographically during fetal life. *Int J Cardiol.* 1988;19:355-362.
2. Celermajer DS, Bull C, Till JA, et al. Ebstein's anomaly: presentation and outcome from fetus to adult. *J Am Coll Cardiol.* 1994;23:170-176.
3. Hornberger LK, Sahn DJ, Kleinman CS, Copel JA, Reed KL. Tricuspid valve disease with significant tricuspid insufficiency in the fetus: diagnosis and outcome. *J Am Coll Cardiol.* 1991;17:167-173.
4. Barrea C, Hornberger LK, Alkazaleh F, et al. Impact of selective laser ablation of placental anastomoses on the cardiovascular pathology of the recipient twin in severe twin-twin transfusion syndrome. *Am J Obstet Gynecol.* 2006;195:1388-1395.
5. Lougheed J, Sinclair BG, Fung Kee FK, et al. Acquired right ventricular outflow tract obstruction in the recipient twin in twin-twin transfusion syndrome. *J Am Coll Cardiol.* 2001;38:1533-1538.
6. Calder AL, Peebles CR, Occleshaw CJ. The prevalence of coronary arterial abnormalities in pulmonary atresia with intact ventricular septum and their influence on surgical results. *Cardiol Young.* 2007;17:387-396.
7. Chaoui R, Bollmann R, Goldner B, Heling KS, Tennstedt C. Fetal cardiomegaly: echocardiographic findings and outcome in 19 cases. *Fetal Diagn Ther.* 1994;9:92-104.
8. Gardiner HM, Belmar C, Tulzer G, et al. Morphologic and functional predictors of eventual circulation in the fetus with pulmonary atresia or critical pulmonary stenosis with intact septum. *J Am Coll Cardiol.* 2008;51:1299-1308.
9. Salvin JW, McElhinney DB, Colan SD, et al. Fetal tricuspid valve size and growth as predictors of outcome in pulmonary atresia with intact ventricular septum. *Pediatrics.* 2006;118:e415-e420.
10. Roman KS, Fouron JC, Nii M, Smallhorn JF, Chaturvedi R, Jaeggi ET. Determinants of outcome in fetal pulmonary valve stenosis or atresia with intact ventricular septum. *Am J Cardiol.* 2007;99:699-703.
11. Galindo A, Gutierrez-Larraya F, Velasco JM, de la Fuente P. Pulmonary balloon valvuloplasty in a fetus with critical pulmonary stenosis/atresia with intact ventricular septum and heart failure. *Fetal Diagn Ther.* 2006;21:100-104.
12. Tulzer G, Arzt W, Franklin RC, Loughna PV, Mair R, Gardiner HM. Fetal pulmonary valvuloplasty for critical pulmonary stenosis or atresia with intact septum. *Lancet.* 2002;360:1567-1568.
13. Guleserian KJ, Armsby LB, Thiagarajan RR, del Nido PJ, Mayer JE Jr. Natural history of pulmonary atresia with intact ventricular septum and right-ventricle-dependent coronary circulation managed by the single-ventricle approach. *Ann Thorac Surg.* 2006;81:2250-2257.
14. Daubeney PE, Wang D, Delany DJ, et al. Pulmonary atresia with intact ventricular septum: predictors of early and medium-term outcome in a population-based study. *J Thorac Cardiovasc Surg.* 2005;130:1071.
15. Odim J, Laks H, Tung T. Risk factors for early death and reoperation following biventricular repair of pulmonary atresia with intact ventricular septum. *Eur J Cardiothorac Surg.* 2006;29:659-665.

CASES

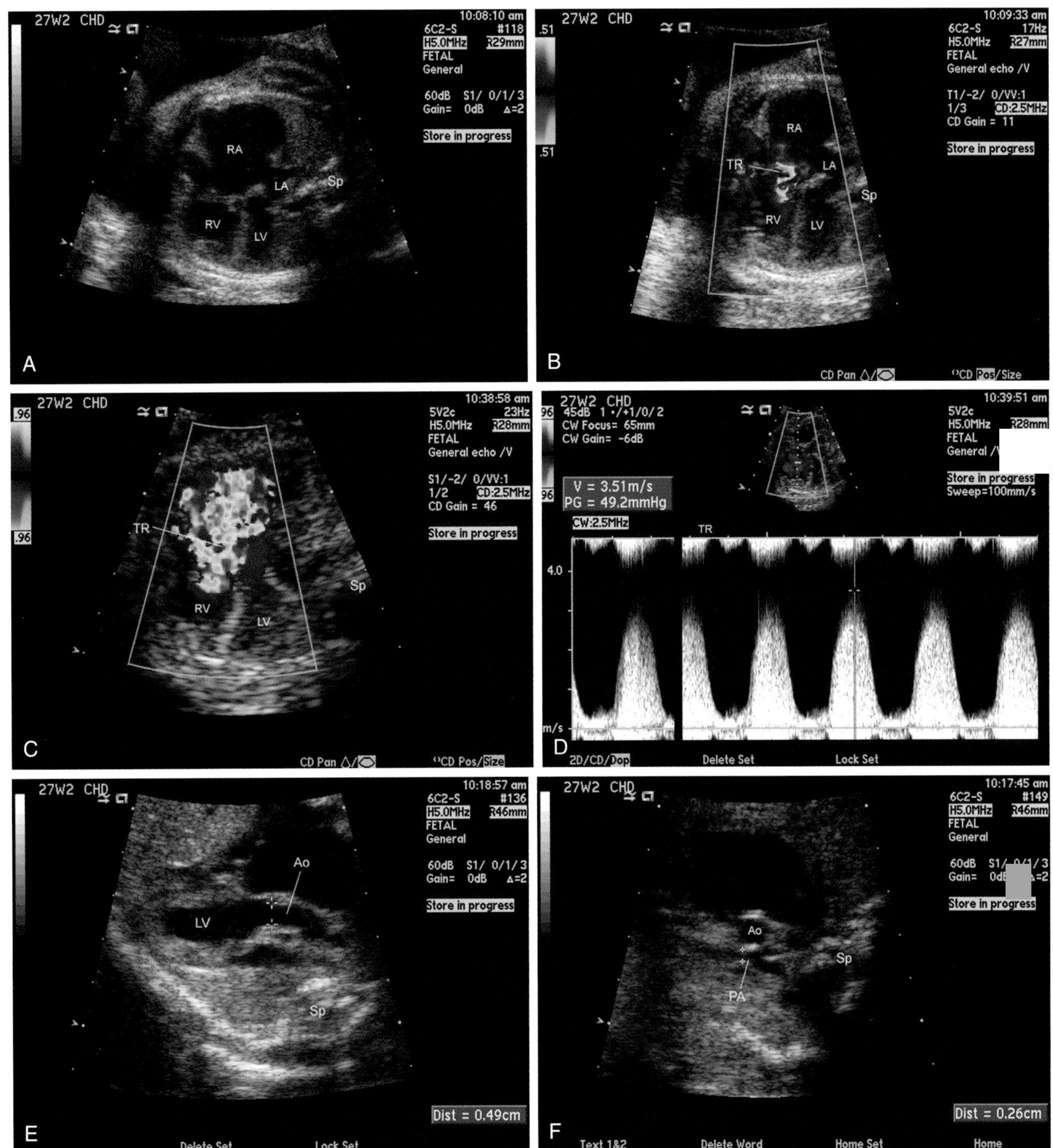

Case 25-1. **(A)** Four-chamber view demonstrates a dilated right atrium (RA) and a well-formed right ventricular cavity. LA, left atrium; LV, left ventricle; RV, right ventricle; Sp, spine. **(B)** Color flow imaging in diastole. There is a good-sized tricuspid (TR) valve annulus present. **(C)** Color flow imaging in systole demonstrates severe tricuspid regurgitation (TR). **(D)** Continuous wave Doppler interrogation demonstrates a peak tricuspid regurgitation velocity of 3.5 m/sec; hence, the right ventricular pressure is approximately 49 mm Hg greater than the right atrial V wave. **(E)** Left ventricular outflow tract. The aortic annulus measures 4.9 mm in diameter. Ao, aorta; LV, left ventricle. **(F)** There is pulmonary atresia. The main pulmonary artery is smaller than the aorta and measures 2.6 mm in diameter.

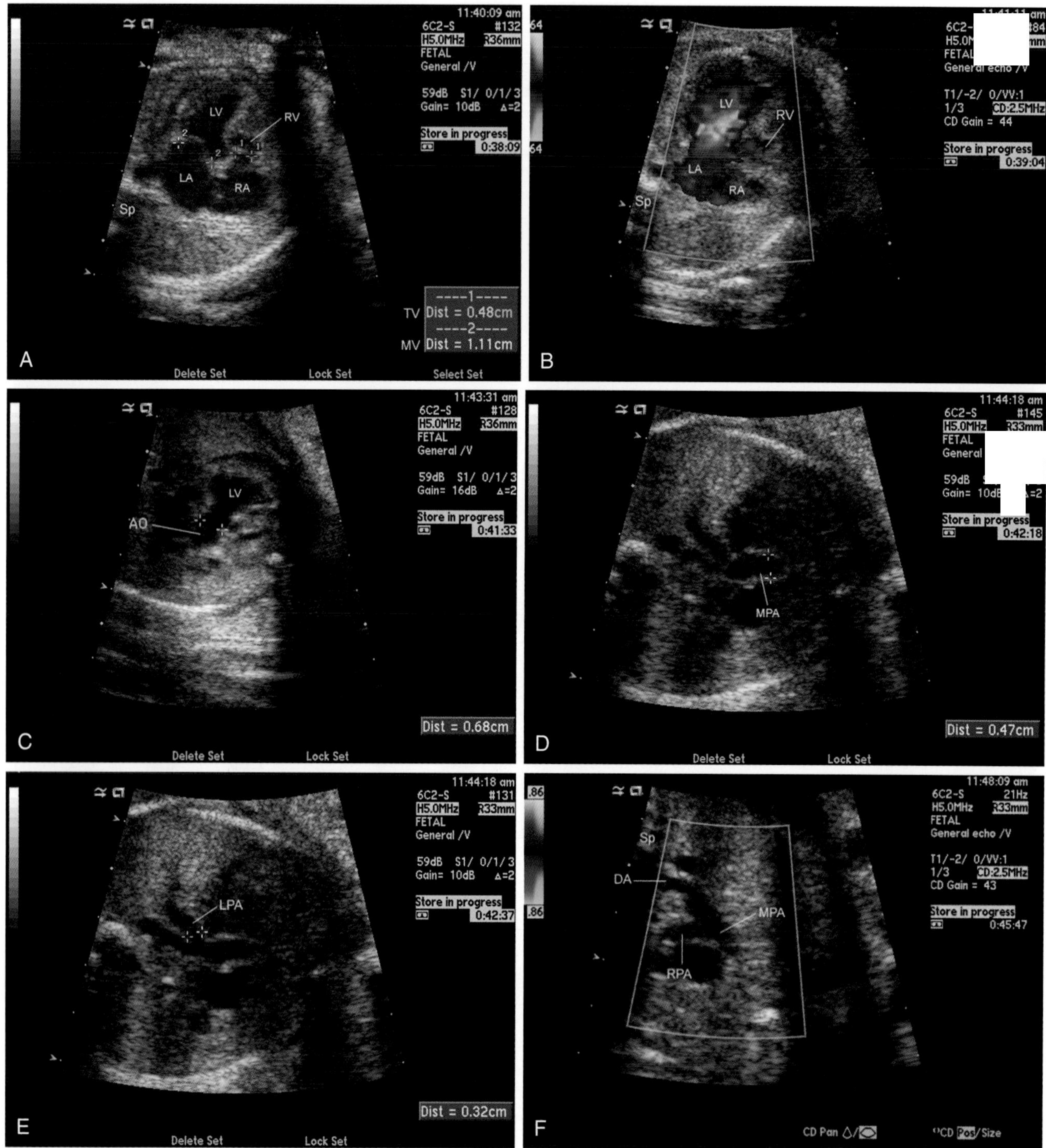

Case 25-2. **(A)** Four-chamber view in a fetus with pulmonary atresia and intact ventricular septum. Note the right ventricle (RV) is small and the trabecular apex is hypertrophied. The tricuspid valve annulus *(crosshairs 1)* measures 4.8 mm and the mitral valve annulus *(crosshairs 2)* measures more than twice as large at 11.1 mm. Normally, the tricuspid valve is larger than the mitral valve, but this is usually not the case in pulmonary atresia with intact ventricular septum. LA, left atrium; LV, left ventricle; RA, right atrium; RV, right ventricle; Sp, spine. **(B)** Color flow imaging reveals filling of the LV in diastole but no such filling is seen on the right side. **(C)** Anterior and superior angling visualizes the aortic outflow tract. The aortic annulus measures 6.8 mm and is unobstructed. AO, aorta. **(D)** The main pulmonary artery (MPA) arises "blindly" from the mass of the heart above the RV. The MPA diameter is 4.7 mm and is smaller than the aortic annulus, an abnormal finding. **(E)** Measurement of the left pulmonary artery (LPA) is 3.2 mm, essentially normal size for this fetus. **(F)** Angulation rightward in the mediastinum visualizes the ductus arteriosus (DA) and the right pulmonary artery (RPA). Both the RPA and the LPA are well formed, and of near-normal size as is commonly the case in pulmonary atresia with intact ventricular septum (PA/IVS).

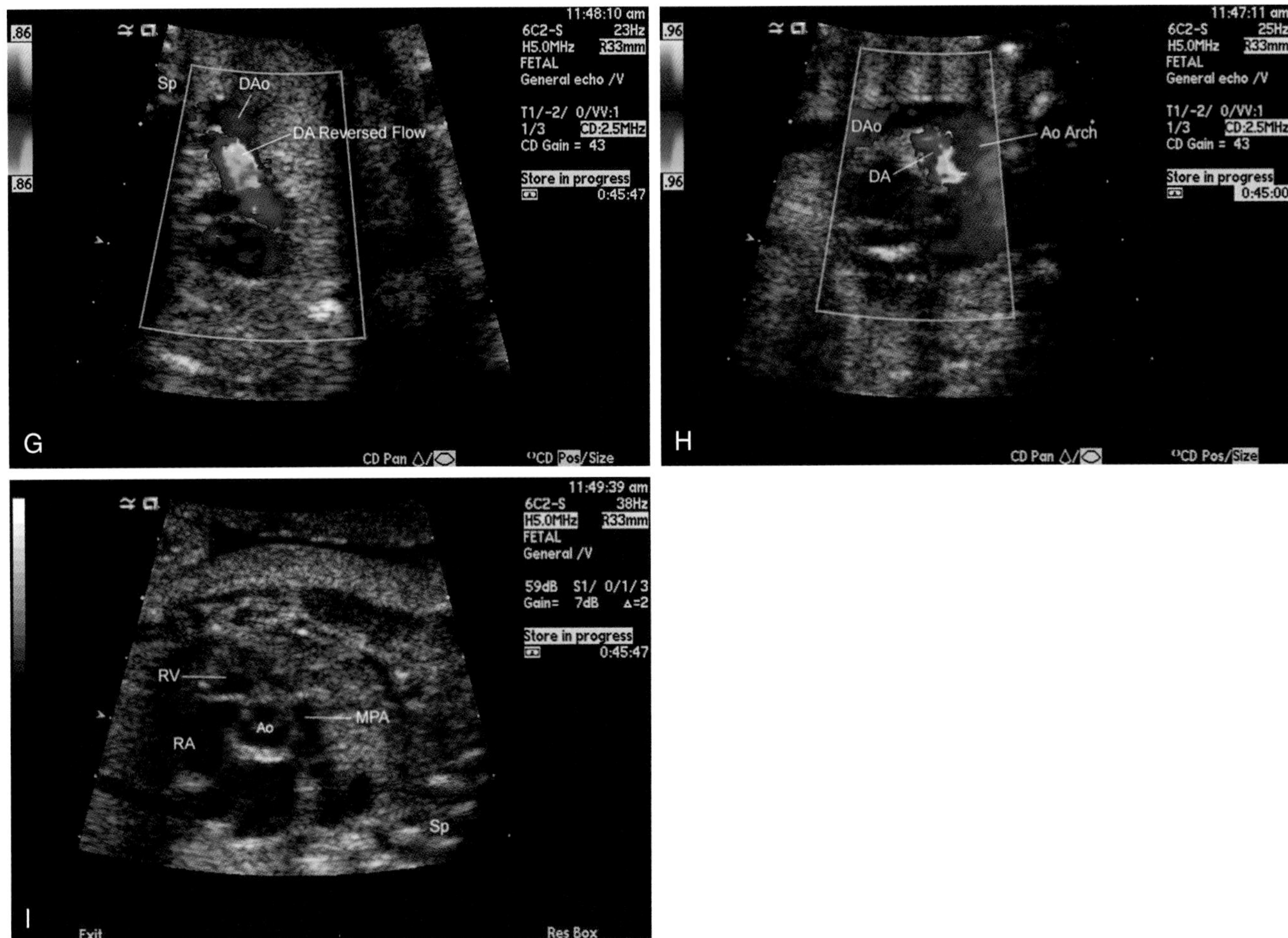

Case 25-2, cont'd (G) Color flow imaging reveals flow in the DA, which is directed retrograde from the descending aorta (DAo) to the MPA. (H) Aortic (Ao) arch view. Flow is antegrade *(red)* into the aortic arch and into the DAo. Retrograde flow *(blue)* is seen in the DA arising from the underside of the arch. (I) Short-axis view at the level of the aortic valve demonstrates the atretic valve plate of the pulmonary artery and the MPA.

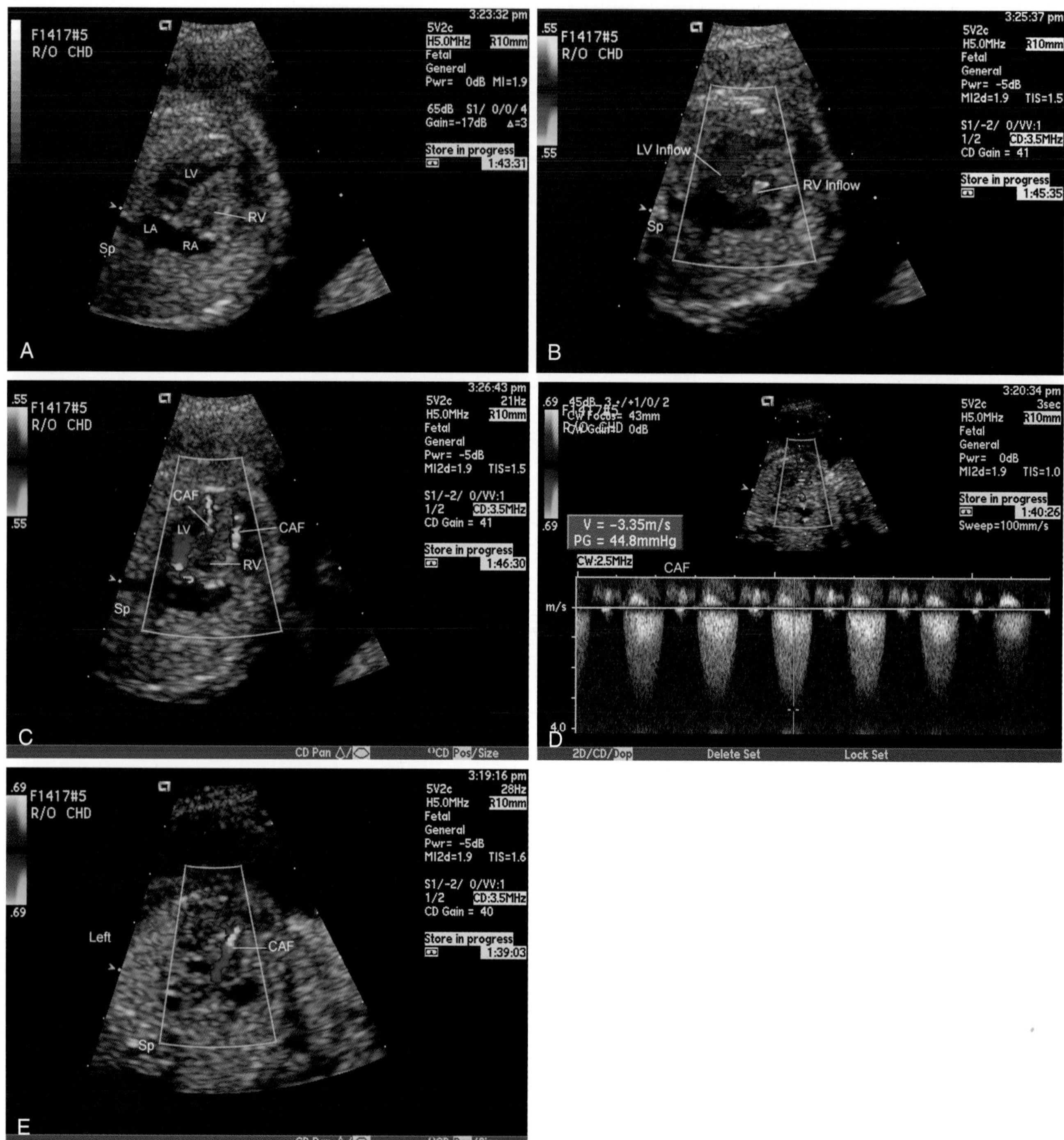

Case 25-3. **(A)** Four-chamber view demonstrates a thickened right ventricle (RV) with a small cavity. The right atrium (RA) is not dilated. LA, left atrium; LV, left ventricle; Sp, spine. **(B)** Color flow imaging during diastole highlights the difference in inflow caliber between the RV and the LV. **(C)** Color flow imaging during systole demonstrates the presence of multiple coronary-cameral fistulas (CAF) between the cavity of the RV and the coronary circulation. **(D)** Pulse Doppler interrogation at one of the sites of connection between the right ventricular cavity and a coronary artery. The high velocity suggests a stenotic connection. **(E)** Color flow imaging identifies a dilated coronary artery, which appears to be filling from the direction of the apex of the RV heading toward the base of the heart *(blue)*. This suggests that the coronary artery is being perfused from the cavity of the RV in a retrograde manner.

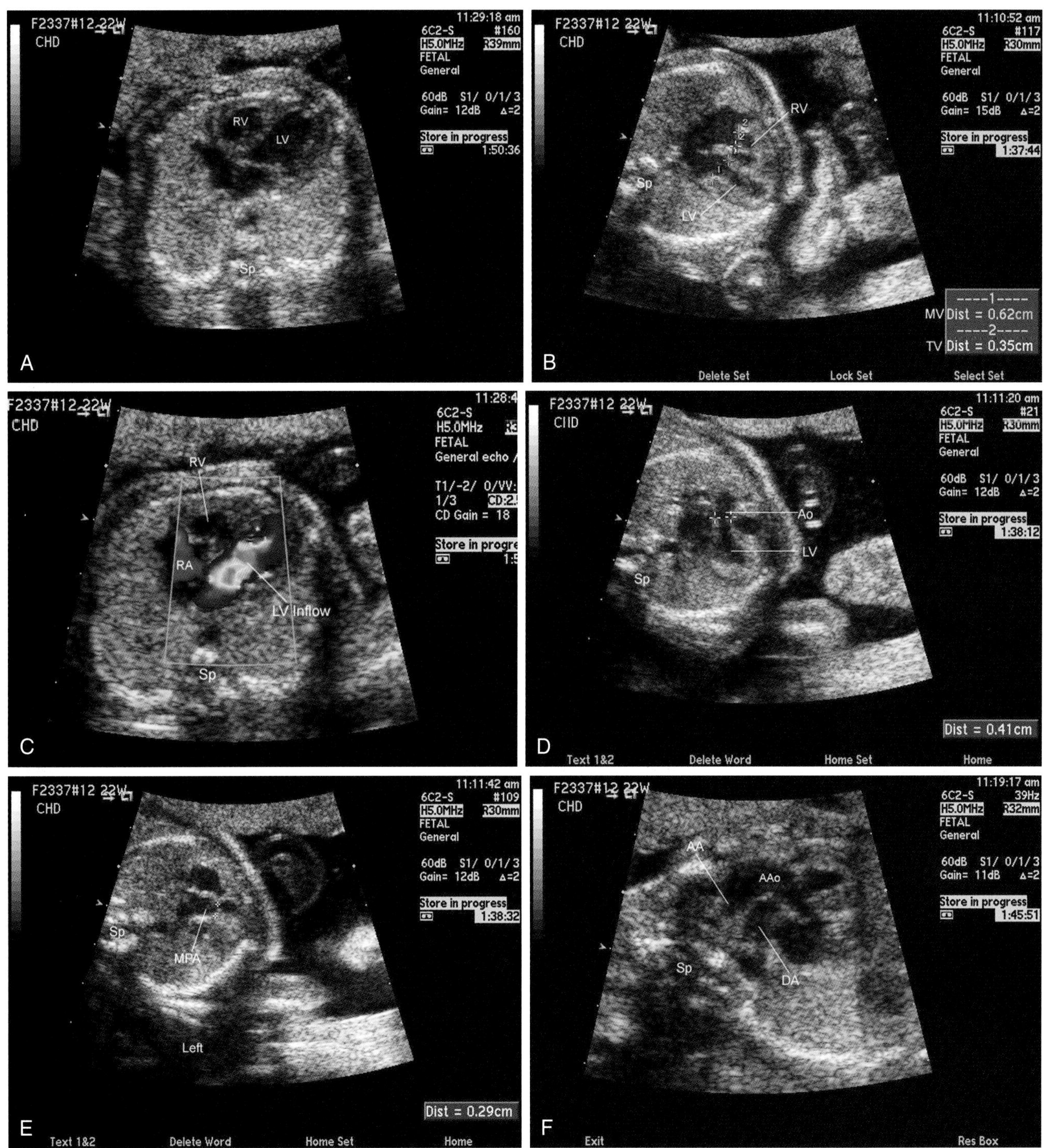

Case 25-4. **(A)** Four-chamber view with size discrepancy between the right (RV) and the left (LV) ventricles with a smaller RV. Sp, spine. **(B)** The RV cavity does not reach the apex of the heart. The tricuspid valve (TV) annulus measures less than the mitral valve (MV) annulus. **(C)** Color flow imaging demonstrates inflow into the LV but not into the RV. **(D)** The left ventricular outflow tract is unobstructed. The aortic annulus measures 4.1 mm. **(E)** The pulmonary valve is atretic and the annulus measures 2.9 mm. MPA, main pulmonary artery. **(F)** Image of the ascending aorta (AAo), proximal aortic arch (AA), and ductus arteriosus (DA) is seen descending to the base of the heart. *Continued*

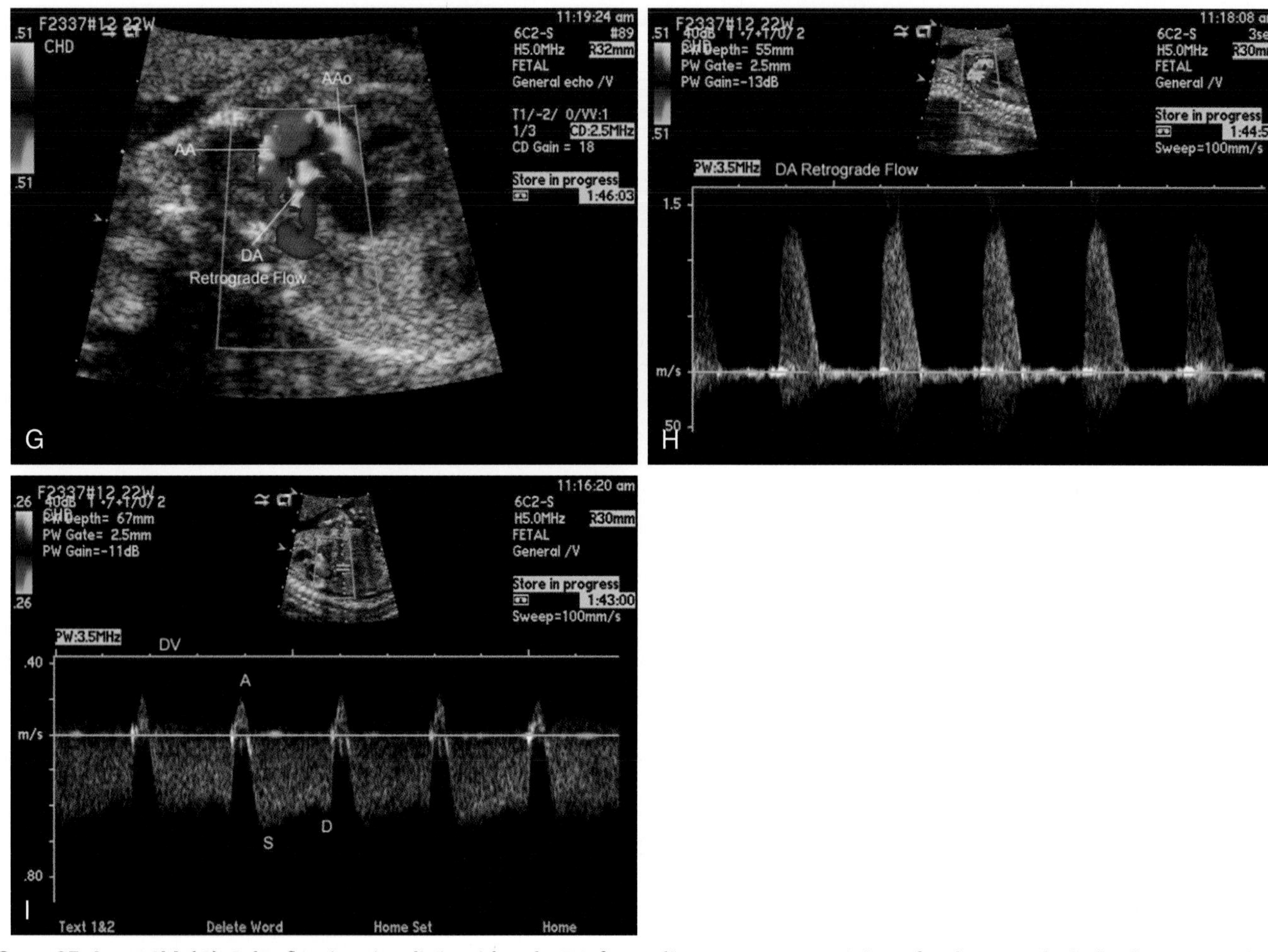

Case 25-4, cont'd **(G)** Color flow imaging distinguishes the DA from adjacent structures as it is perfused retrograde *(red)*. The AAo is *red* as it emerges from the left ventricular outflow tract but then turns *blue* as it curves into the proximal aortic arch (AA). A branch pulmonary artery is seen as *blue flow* adjacent to the DA. **(H)** Pulse Doppler interrogation of the DA demonstrates retrograde flow. **(I)** Doppler flow in the ductus venosus (DV) shows reversal with atrial contraction consistent with the presence of a restrictive, hypertrophied RV and elevated right atrial pressure.

26

Ebstein's Anomaly and Other Abnormalities of the Tricuspid Valve

Anita Szwast

Key Echocardiographic Features

- Heart size, cardiothoracic area ratio
- Heart rhythm
- Degree of displacement of the tricuspid valve
- Effective right atrial and right ventricular size
- Degree of tricuspid regurgitation
- Nature and size of the patent foramen ovale
- Size and patency of the right ventricular outflow tract, with particular attention to the relationship between the displaced tricuspid valve leaflet and the outflow tract
- Appearance of the pulmonary valve, whether it opens in systole or not, and whether there is any pulmonary insufficiency
- Direction of flow within the ductus arteriosus
- Left ventricular outflow tract obstruction
- Branch pulmonary artery size; qualitative assessment of lung volumes
- Ventricular function, left and right ventricle
- Presence or absence of pericardial effusion, pleural effusions, or hydrops

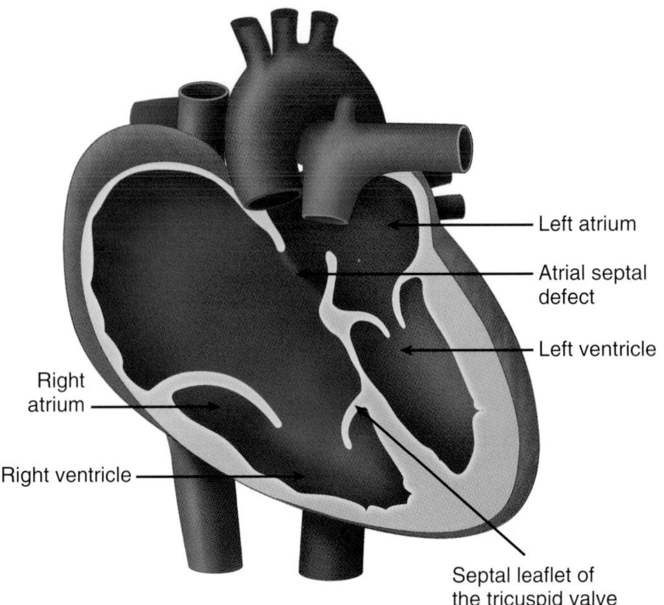

Figure 26-1. Ebstein's anomaly of the tricuspid valve.

Anatomy and Anatomical Associations

Ebstein's anomaly of the tricuspid valve (TV) is an abnormality in which there is inferior displacement of the attachments of the septal leaflet of the TV relative to the annulus. It is to be distinguished from a similar anomaly called *tricuspid valve dysplasia*. In TV dysplasia, the TV attachments are not displaced, although the leaflets are markedly thickened with variable degrees of incompetence. TV dysplasia encompasses a group of diagnoses in which the TV is structurally abnormal, is severely regurgitant, and is not Ebstein's anomaly. There is no "atrialization" of the ventricle, and right ventricular structure is relatively normal. In both TV dysplasia and Ebstein's anomaly, the TV leaflets are often grossly malformed and rudimentary in appearance (Figure 26-1). In both of these anomalies, there can be severe tricuspid regurgitation and massive cardiomegaly.

In Ebstein's anomaly, the septal and inferior leaflet may be tethered to the surface of the right ventricle (RV). The anterior leaflet is normally attached at the TV annulus and appears large and curtain-like, extending to the free wall of the ventricle or to the septum–moderator band complex. Chordae of the anterior leaflet are shortened or absent. With valve closure, the valve leaflets may not adequately coapt, resulting in varying degrees of tricuspid regurgitation. The effective inlet orifice of the TV may be small, leading to varying degrees of functional tricuspid stenosis. The portion of the RV superior to the effective orifice of the TV becomes thin walled and atrialized. With severe tricuspid regurgitation, the atrialized RV and right atrium (RA) dilate massively, leading to severe cardiomegaly, which may compromise lung development.[1] The ventricular septum is frequently abnormal. With marked right ventricular dilation, the ventricular septum may bow into the left ventricular outflow tract, compromising left ventricular function and limiting cardiac output. This ultimately places the fetus at risk for the development of hydrops fetalis.

Atrial septal defects or interatrial communications are present in approximately 90% of patients with Ebstein's anomaly, which leads to right-to-left shunting and variable degrees of cyanosis postnatally. Corrected transposition of the great arteries may be associated with a left-sided Ebstein's anomaly of the TV. Right ventricular outflow tract obstruction is frequent. Fibrous subpulmonary stenosis may be present if the orifice of the TV becomes so displaced that it opens just underneath the pulmonary valve. "Functional" pulmonary atresia can be seen in over 50% of infants. This is a phenomenon in which the pulmonary valve leaflets have the anatomical potential to open but do not do so owing to the inability of the RV to generate an opening force to counter distal, pulmonary resistance. Anatomical "true" pulmonary atresia may be seen in over 20%. In the neonate, cardiomegaly secondary to right atrial dilation may compromise lung development, leading to pulmonary hypoplasia. Left-sided abnormalities can also occur. Mitral valve abnormalities, subaortic stenosis, bicuspid aortic valve, and coarctation have been described in association with Ebstein's anomaly. Ventricular septal defects and tetralogy of Fallot have also been described, but these are extremely rare.

Myocardial abnormalities may be present in Ebstein's anomaly. In Uhl's anomaly, a severe form of Ebstein's anomaly, myocytes fail to develop within the RV. The right ventricular free wall appears thin, translucent, and parchment-like. In the absence of myocytes, the right ventricular free wall fails to contract. Left ventricular dysplasia, resembling noncompaction, has been reported in Ebstein's anomaly. Finally, the presence of muscular bridges behaving as electrophysiological bypass tracts places the fetus at risk for arrhythmia. Approximately one third of patients with Ebstein's anomaly have one or more accessory pathways, predisposing them to supraventricular tachycardia. Ventricular tachycardia is less common, but also reported, in particular in those with myocardial disease. Extracardiac anomalies are rare, but skeletal anomalies and chromosomal abnormalities, especially trisomy 13, have been reported.

Frequency, Genetics, and Development

Ebstein's anomaly of the TV occurs in approximately 5.2 cases per 100,000 live births and accounts for less than 1% of all cases of congenital heart disease.[2] Most cases are sporadic. Familial Ebstein's anomaly is rare, although mutations in the cardiac transcription factor NKX2.5 and deletions in 10p13-p14 and 1p34.3-p36.11 have been reported.[3-5] Maternal lithium exposure can rarely lead to Ebstein's anomaly in the fetus.[6] In the Baltimore-Washington Infant study, additional risk factors for Ebstein's anomaly included twin pregnancies, those with a family history of congenital heart disease, and maternal exposure to benzodiazepines.[2] The presumed embryology of Ebstein's anomaly is incomplete delamination of the TV leaflets from the RV, although the precise mechanism is incompletely understood.

Prenatal Physiology

Fetal physiology is dictated by the severity of the Ebstein's anomaly or the severity of the TV dysplasia. With mild forms of the disease, the fetus is asymptomatic. However, with severe tricuspid regurgitation and marked atrialization of the RV, there can be massive cardiomegaly composed primarily of a dilated RA and RV. Right ventricular systolic function may become compromised with decreased forward flow across the right ventricular outflow tract. With compromised systolic pump function and decreased effective forward flow across the right ventricular outflow tract, the RV may not be able to generate an adequate pressure to open the pulmonary valve, leading to "functional" pulmonary atresia. The pulmonary arteries are then perfused via retrograde (aorta–to–pulmonary artery) flow through the ductus arteriosus. With severe tricuspid insufficiency, right-to-left shunting across the patent foramen ovale increases as RA wall stress increases with RA dilation. Cardiac output is maintained by augmentation of left ventricular stroke volume, up until the left ventricle itself is affected either (1) by compression from the dilated right-sided structures or (2) secondary to ventricular septal dysfunction and altered left-sided myocardial mechanics. A nonrestrictive interatrial communication must be present to maintain cardiac output through to the left side of the heart. Indeed, the presence of a restrictive patent foramen ovale has been associated with hydrops fetalis and fetal demise. With massive dilation of the right side of the heart, lung development may become compromised. The combination of severe tricuspid regurgitation, pulmonary atresia, and lung hypoplasia predicts a particularly poor prognosis for extrauterine life.

Prenatal Management

Prenatal counseling is dictated by the severity of the anomaly. In the past, it was believed that all forms of Ebstein's anomaly diagnosed in the fetus were severe and, hence, boded for a poor outcome. However, in the current era, detection capacity of fetal echocardiography has improved such that the full spectrum of the disease ranging from mild to moderate to severe cases can be seen. Careful prenatal echocardiographic analysis can help distinguish these types.

Quantifying the degree of RA dilation and RV atrialization is one way to assess severity of the Ebstein's anomaly. Celermajer and coworkers[7] developed an index, which is a ratio of the sum of area of the RA and any atrialized portion of the RV to the combined area of the functional RV and left side of the heart. The greater this ratio, the greater is the degree of atrialization of the RV and RA size, and the worse the prognosis. Andrews and colleagues[8] published echocardiographic features associated with increased mortality after birth for TV malformations diagnosed during fetal life. These included increased cardiothoracic area ratio greater than 0.65, Celermajer index greater than 1.5, reduced or absent pulmonary valve flow, retrograde flow in the ductus arteriosus, and a right-to-left ventricular cavity ratio greater than 1.5.[7,8] Fetuses with hydrops fetalis or arrhythmia had particularly poor prognoses, with a high likelihood for intrauterine or neonatal death.[8] In the absence of hydrops fetalis, fetuses with Ebstein's anomaly without cardiac failure tolerate vaginal delivery well. However, premature delivery via cesarean section for the presence of hydrops fetalis is associated with a high risk of neonatal death. In severely affected fetuses with significant right ventricular outflow tract obstruction and reversal of flow in the ductus arteriosus, prostaglandin infusion should be commenced at birth.

Postnatal Physiology

In mild cases of Ebstein's anomaly, neonates are frequently asymptomatic or only mildly cyanotic on account of elevated pulmonary vascular resistance and increased right-to-left shunting across the patent foramen ovale. As pulmonary vascular resistance drops, however, cyanosis decreases over time, with improved compliance of the RV and increased flow across the right ventricular outflow tract. In severe cases of Ebstein's anomaly or TV dysplasia, characterized by cardiomegaly, severe tricuspid regurgitation, and anatomical or functional pulmonary atresia, the neonate faces congestive heart failure and severe hypoxemia secondary to hypoplastic pulmonary arteries and lungs as well as marked right-to-left shunting at the patent foramen ovale. The ductus arteriosus must remain patent in order to supply pulmonary blood flow. Oxygenation and ventilation depend upon the adequacy of the pulmonary vascular bed, which may be abnormal due to massive cardiomegaly in utero. In cases of functional pulmonary atresia, as pulmonary vascular resistance falls, the RV may be able to open the pulmonary valve, leading to improvement in cyanosis and decreased right-to-left shunting at the patent foramen ovale.

Postnatal Management

Postnatal management varies greatly depending upon the severity of the Ebstein's anomaly or TV dysplasia. In mild cases, oxygen therapy may be required for cyanosis. Diuretics and digoxin may be required for treatment of mild congestive heart failure. In severe cases, hypoxemia and severe congestive heart failure predominate, necessitating mechanical ventilation and administration of inotropic agents. Prostaglandin infusion may be necessary to maintain ductal patency. As pulmonary vascular resistance falls, the RV may be able to eject blood into the pulmonary circulation and prostaglandin may ultimately be discontinued.

Surgical intervention may be required if these measures fail to improve symptoms or if there is "true" anatomical pulmonary atresia. In neonates with "true" anatomical pulmonary atresia, a modified Blalock-Taussig (BT) shunt will be performed to provide a stable source of pulmonary blood flow. Placement of the BT shunt allows for right ventricular growth and readjustment of the surgical strategy as necessary at a later date. Some patients will ultimately require a Fontan procedure as the RV is deemed nonviable. In contrast, others may be deemed candidates for a biventricular repair via surgery performed on the abnormal TV (valvuloplasty or valve replacement) at a later date. In severely affected neonates with massive cardiomegaly, severe tricuspid regurgitation, and functional or anatomical pulmonary atresia, one may elect to reduce the RA and oversew the TV in addition to placement of the BT shunt. Less severely affected children and adolescents with adequate right ventricular size may undergo a biventricular repair based upon presentation of clinical symptoms consisting of dyspnea, easy fatigability, cyanosis, or palpitations through a valvuloplasty, which can be performed later in life. Cyanosis at rest or with exercise can be treated with catheter device closure of the foramen ovale in the cardiac catheterization laboratory. In patients with arrhythmias and significant right atrial enlargement, right atrial reduction surgery coupled with surgical cryoablation can be performed and has proved to be effective.

Outcomes

The prognosis varies greatly depending upon the severity of the anomaly. In mild cases, patients may be completely asymptomatic and live 70 years or longer.[9] Women may become pregnant, although miscarriage and fetal loss has been reported in 24%.[10] However, in severe cases presenting either prenatally or in the newborn period, outcomes are much worse. Of all neonates with the diagnosis of *severe* tricuspid dysplasia or *severe* Ebstein's anomaly, 20% to 40% do not survive 1 month and fewer than 50% survive to 5 years of age.[11-13]

Watson[14] published a natural history study in 1974 comprising 505 patients from 61 centers in 28 countries. There were 35 patients younger than 1 year of age, 403 patients between ages 1 and 25, and 67 patients older than 25 years of age. Of the infants, 72% were in congestive heart failure. Of the older patients, 81% were said to have normal growth and development in infancy and childhood. Seventy-one percent of patients ages 1 to 25 and 60% of patients older than 25 years were in New York Heart Association (NYHA) class I or II with little or no functional disability. Mortality was high initially within the first few months of life in infants with congestive heart failure. Between the ages of 1 and 25 years, 12% died of the disease. In patients older than 25 years of age, 16.4% died of the disease.

Celermajer and coworkers[7] reviewed 220 cases of Ebstein's anomaly with 1 to 34 years of follow-up. The median age at time of diagnosis was younger than 1 year of age. Of all live-born patients, actuarial survival was 67% at 1 year and 59% at 10 years.[8] Early mortality was associated with symptoms of congestive heart failure and pulmonary hypoplasia secondary to severe cardiomegaly.[7] Unfortunately, there are as of yet no large-scale studies looking at the outcome of all types of severity of Ebstein's anomaly diagnosed prenatally in the current era of increased sensitivity of fetal diagnosis.

Imaging Essentials and Important Points

- Assessing the degree of septal leaflet displacement is important and is a factor that distinguishes between Ebstein's anomaly and TV dysplasia. Both may exhibit a severely regurgitant TV with RA dilation and cardiomegaly; however, only a true Ebstein's anomaly will have septal displacement of the valve and loss of right ventricular tissue as the atrialization of the RV by septal apical displacement reduces the amount of effective RV present to function as a pulmonary ventricle.
- The TV is normally slightly displaced toward the apex, so how much is normal displacement and at what point is it considered an Ebstein's anomaly? This is a common question in distinguishing a mild case of Ebstein's anomaly and a normal valve, or in distinguishing between Ebstein's and TV dysplasia. Criteria for the normal degree of septal leaflet displacement have been published, based on gestational age. In the four-chamber view, separation between the mitral valve and septal leaflet of the TV progresses with gestation. In general, TV septal leaflet displacement of up to 3 mm away from the crux of the heart is considered normal in the second trimester and up to 5 mm is considered normal in the third trimester up to term. In borderline cases, thinning of the ventricular septum suggesting right ventricular atrialization and elongation or absent delamination of the anterior leaflet should also be looked for as supporting evidence to make the case of a true Ebstein's anomaly.
- Presence of pulmonary insufficiency in the face of what looks to be no antegrade flow across the pulmonary valve suggests "functional" pulmonary atresia, because the valve is anatomically patent if it leaks. Such neonates may benefit from maneuvers to rapidly reduce pulmonary vascular resistance after birth such as hyperventilation or the use of pulmonary vasodilators such as nitric oxide.
- As for many cases of right-sided heart disease in utero, Doppler tracings obtained in the inferior vena cava, ductus venosus, and umbilical vein may be abnormal. Whereas reversal of flow with atrial contraction in the ductus venosus or umbilical venous pulsations may suggest impending hemodynamic collapse and poor prognosis in the fetus with a structurally normal heart, such findings in Ebstein's anomaly may be completely acceptable. Severe tricuspid regurgitation and altered right atrial compliance are typical findings and will certainly influence Doppler signals obtained upstream in the fetal venous system.
- Examination of the foramen ovale is important. Although uncommon, restriction at the level of the atrial septum due to septal tissue redundancy may limit left ventricular filling and thereby reduce cardiac output as well as contribute to the development of hydrops fetalis.
- Left ventricular geometry, form, and function can be negatively affected by the presence of Ebstein's anomaly and should be ascertained and evaluated in a serial manner in all cases.

References

1. Chaoui R, Bollmann R, Goldner B, Heling KS, Tennstedt C. Fetal cardiomegaly: echocardiographic findings and outcome in 19 cases. *Fetal Diagn Ther.* 1994;9:92-104.
2. Correa-Villasenor A, Ferencz C, Neill CA, Wilson PD, Boughman JA. Ebstein's malformation of the tricuspid valve: genetic and environmental factors. The Baltimore-Washington Infant Study Group. *Teratology.* 1994;50:137-147.
3. Benson DW, Silberbach GM, Kavanaugh-McHugh A, et al. Mutations in the cardiac transcription factor NKX2.5 affect diverse cardiac developmental pathways. *J Clin Invest.* 1999;104:1567-1573.
4. Yatsenko SA, Yatsenko AN, Szigeti K, et al. Interstitial deletion of 10p and atrial septal defect in DiGeorge 2 syndrome. *Clin Genet.* 2004;66:128-136.
5. Yang H, Lee CL, Young DC, et al. A rare case of interstitial del(1)(p34.3p36.11) diagnosed prenatally. *Fetal Pediatr Pathol.* 2004;23:251-255.
6. Cohen LS, Friedman JM, Jefferson JW, Johnson EM, Weiner ML. A reevaluation of risk of in utero exposure to lithium. *JAMA.* 1994;271:146-150.
7. Celermajer DS, Bull C, Till JA, et al. Ebstein's anomaly: presentation and outcome from fetus to adult. *J Am Coll Cardiol.* 1994;23:170-176.
8. Andrews RE, Tibby SM, Sharland GK, Simpson JM. Prediction of outcome of tricuspid valve malformations diagnosed during fetal life. *Am J Cardiol.* 2008;101:1046-1050.
9. Giuliani ER, Fuster V, Brandenburg RO, Mair DD. Ebstein's anomaly: the clinical features and natural history of Ebstein's anomaly of the tricuspid valve. *Mayo Clin Proc.* 1979;54:163-173.
10. Connolly HM, Warnes CA. Ebstein's anomaly: outcome of pregnancy. *J Am Coll Cardiol.* 1994;23:1194-1198.
11. Celermajer DS, Cullen S, Sullivan ID, et al. Outcome in neonates with Ebstein's anomaly. *J Am Coll Cardiol.* 1992;19:1041-1046.
12. McElhinney DB, Salvin JW, Colan SD, et al. Improving outcomes in fetuses and neonates with congenital displacement (Ebstein's malformation) or dysplasia of the tricuspid valve. *Am J Cardiol.* 2005;96:582-586.
13. Yetman AT, Freedom RM, McCrindle BW. Outcome in cyanotic neonates with Ebstein's anomaly. *Am J Cardiol.* 1998;81:749-754.
14. Watson H. Natural history of Ebstein's anomaly of tricuspid valve in childhood and adolescence. An international co-operative study of 505 cases. *Br Heart J.* 1974;36:417-427.

CASES

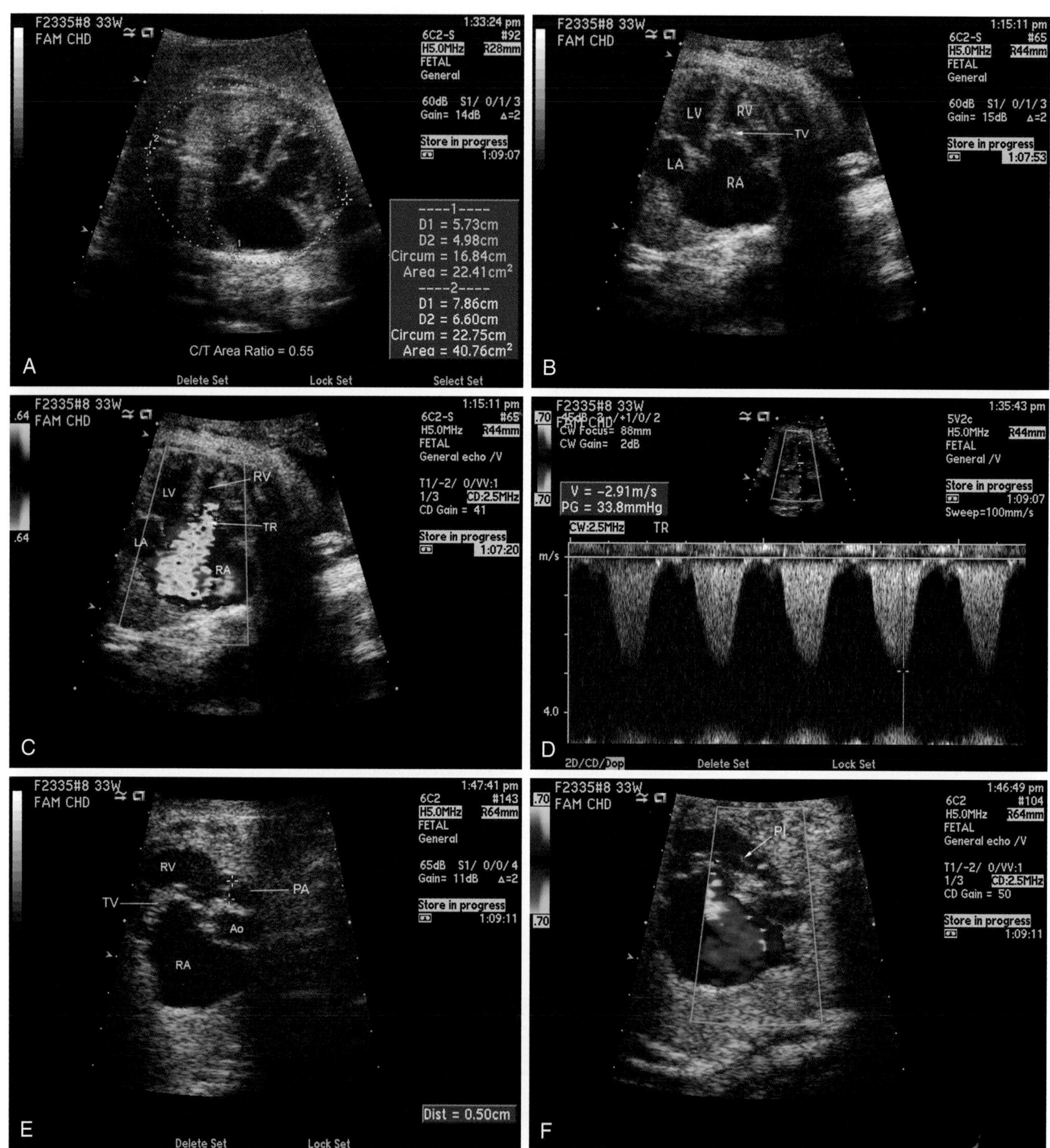

Case 26-1. **(A)** A case of Ebstein's anomaly with marked cardiomegaly. The cardiothoracic area (C/T) ratio is greater than 50%. **(B)** The tricuspid valve (TV) septal leaflet *(arrow)* is displaced apically down into the right ventricle (RV). Note the dilated right atrium (RA) and its large size in proportion to the left atrium (LA). As the valve is displaced apically, it takes away potential cavitary volume from the RV; hence, a portion of the RV is atrialized. LV, left ventricle. **(C)** Color Doppler imaging demonstrates severe tricuspid regurgitation (TR). **(D)** Pulsed wave Doppler spectral display demonstrates a mildly elevated RV intracavitary pressure of 34 mm Hg above the RA V wave. **(E)** Short-axis view demonstrates the dilated RA and displaced tricuspid valve (TV). The pulmonary valve is slightly thickened and did not open in systole. Note the diameter of the pulmonary annulus appears smaller than the aorta, suggesting impaired forward flow and some element of relative pulmonary annular hypoplasia. PA, pulmonary artery. **(F)** Despite the absence of visual confirmation of pulmonary valve opening in systole, color Doppler imaging reveals the presence of pulmonary insufficiency. Hence, the valve is anatomically patent but there is "functional" pulmonary atresia in this case of Ebstein's anomaly.

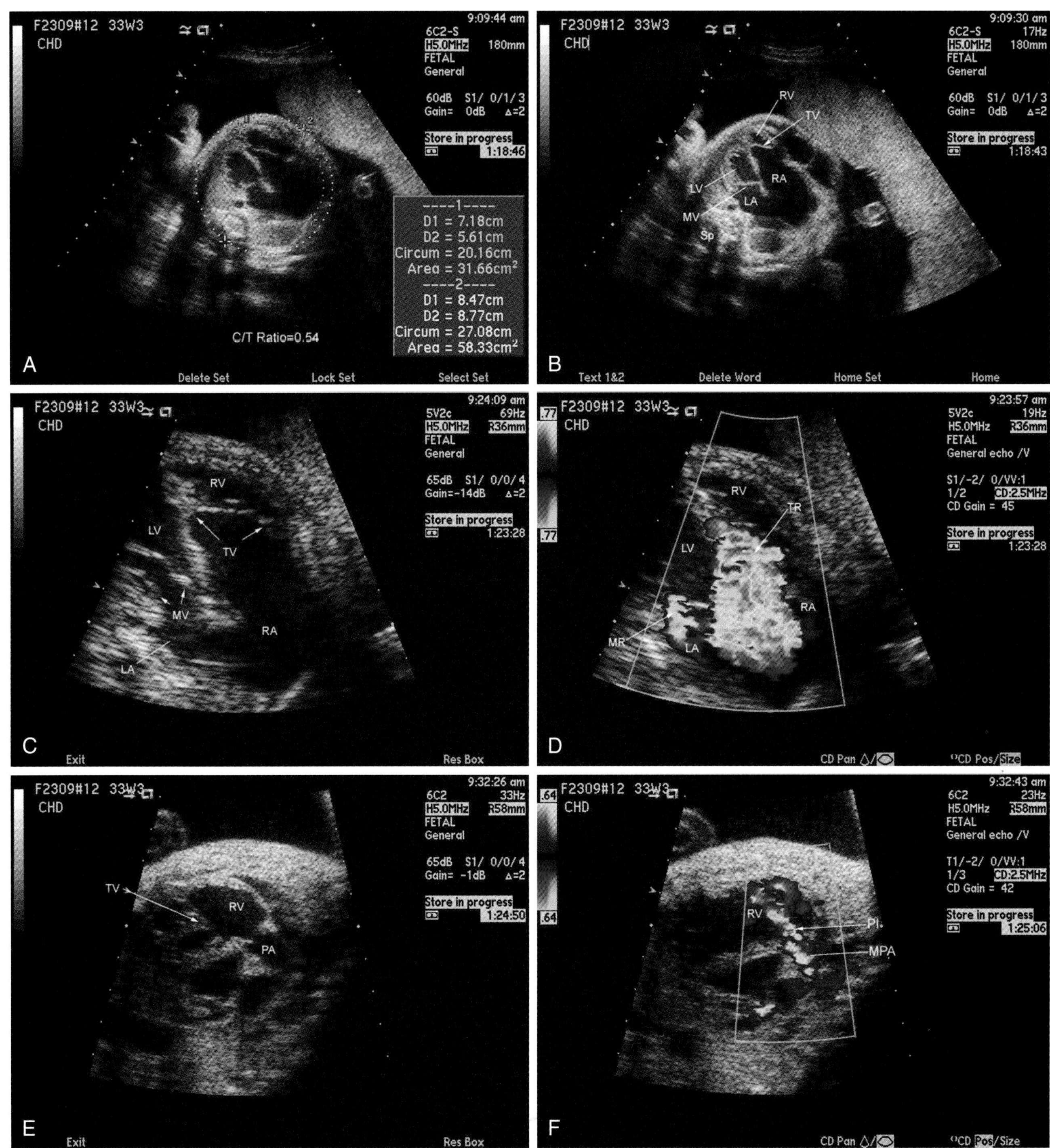

Case 26-2. **(A)** Marked cardiomegaly in this case of severe Ebstein's anomaly. **(B)** Severe displacement of the septal leaflet of the TV. Note that the inlet is essentially at the level of the apex of the RV with marked atrialization and very little effective RV cavity in this plane of view. There is also a pleural effusion on the right side of the chest. So, spine. **(C)** Severe displacement of the septal leaflet of the TV relative to the mitral valve (MV), and poor delamination of the anterior leaflet, which is adherent to the RV free wall for quite a distance apically before separating and coapting with the septal leaflet. **(D)** Severe tricuspid regurgitation (TR). The color jet nearly fills the entire atrialized RV as well as the RA. Owing to alteration of left ventricular geometry and forces on the mitral inlet, mitral regurgitation (MR) is also seen. **(E)** Long-axis view angled toward the pulmonary valve. The TV is displaced and positioned into the right ventricular outflow tract. The pulmonary valve leaflets appear thickened. **(F)** Color flow imaging of the previous view demonstrates severe pulmonary valve insufficiency (PI) originating from the distal main pulmonary artery (MPA) through the pulmonary valve into the body of the RV cavity, demarcated by the displaced TV septal leaflet.

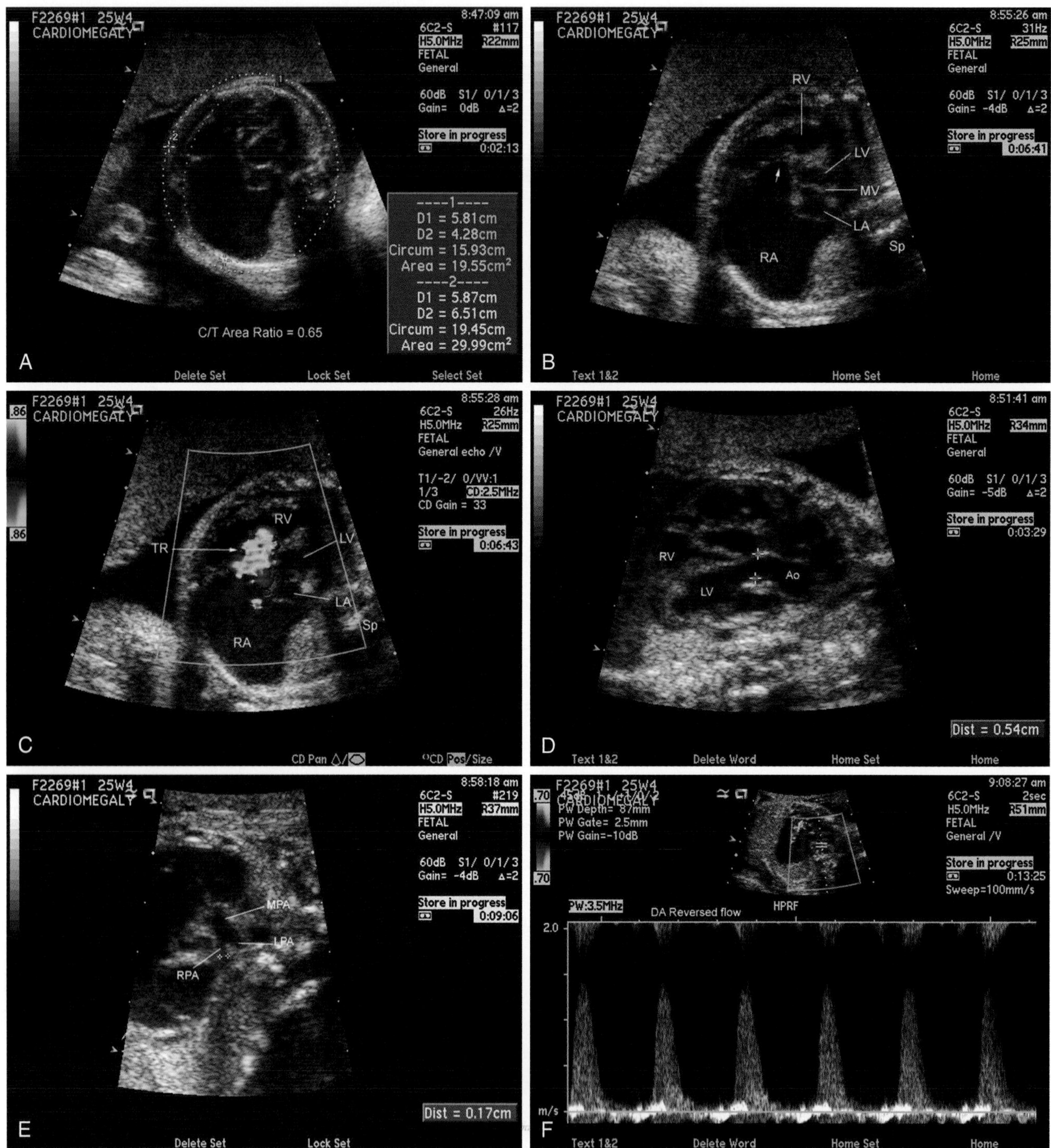

Case 26-3. **(A)** Massive cardiomegaly in this case of Ebstein's anomaly of the TV. **(B)** Apical view demonstrates displacement of the TV *(arrow)* and severe enlargement of the RA. The heart overall is significantly distorted with abnormal morphology and small size of the LA and LV. **(C)** Severe TR originating from the displaced TV leaflets. **(D)** Long-axis view of the heart. The RV cavity is quite small and the myocardium looks thinned and abnormal. The LV is abnormal in shape and with poor function. Ao, aorta. **(E)** There is anatomical pulmonary atresia in this case of severe Ebstein's anomaly. Note the small MPA and tiny branch right pulmonary artery (RPA) measuring less than 2 mm in diameter. Pulmonary artery development typically follows branch pulmonary artery size. This very small size branch pulmonary artery is suggestive of pulmonary hypoplasia. LPA, left pulmonary artery. **(F)** Doppler sampling in the ductus arteriosus (DA) reveals reversed flow from the aorta into the confluence of the small pulmonary arteries.

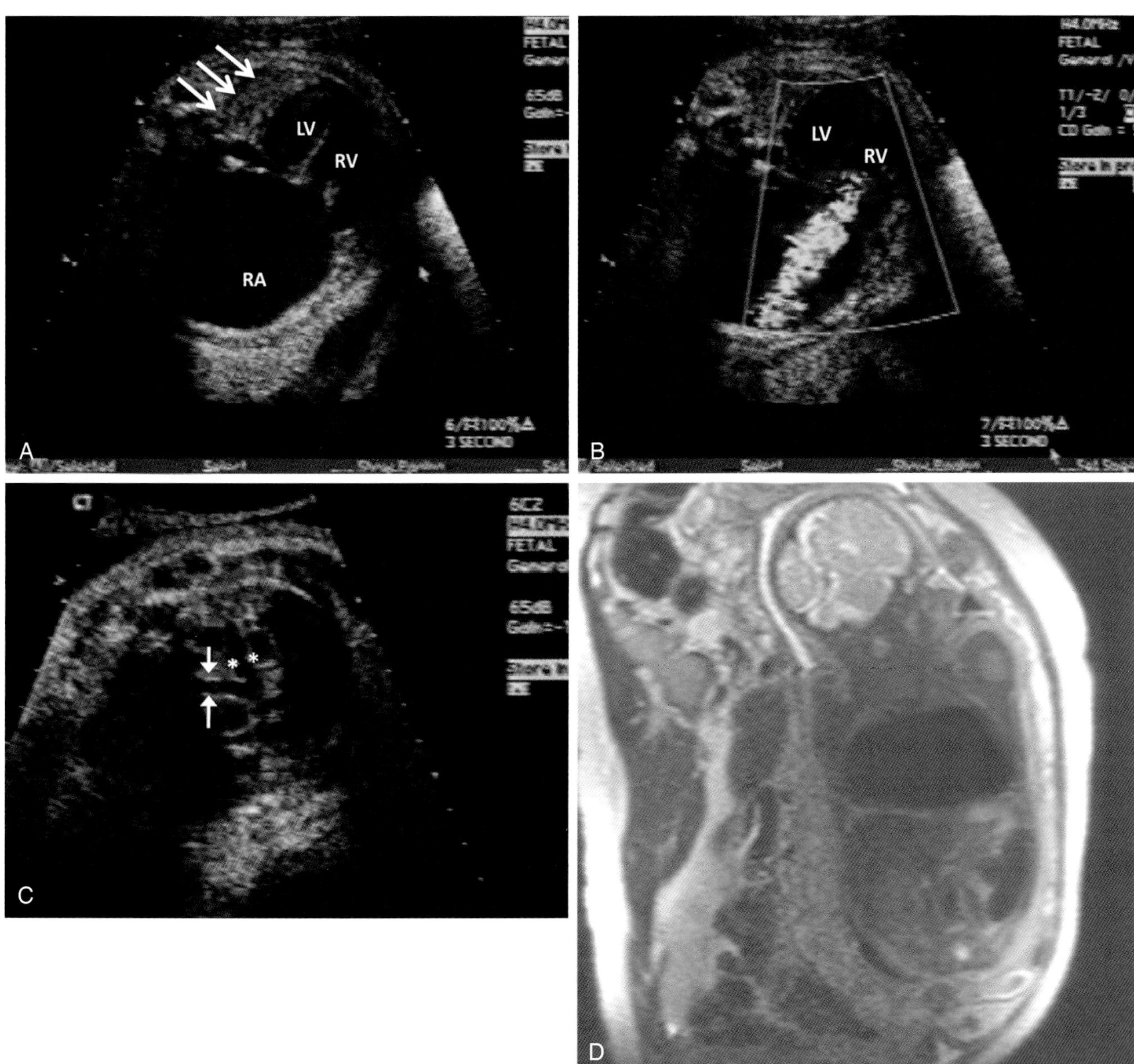

Case 26-4. (A) A case of TV dysplasia, not Ebstein's anomaly. Note there is no displacement of the TV leaflets because they are at the same anatomical level as the MV. There is, however, a massively dilated RA. Owing to the giant heart size, there is compression of the lung tissue, with small lung volume seen on the left side of the chest *(arrows)*. (B) Severe TR in this case of TV dysplasia. (C) Despite the appearance of a very large heart and compressed, small lungs, there was platelike pulmonary atresia with relatively good-sized branch pulmonary arteries. The branch pulmonary artery measure 3 to 4 mm in diameter at 28 weeks' gestation. This nearly normal branch pulmonary artery diameter suggests the presence of well-formed and -developed lung vasculature (and perhaps lung parenchyma) but mechanically compressed lung tissue as a consequence of the heart size. (D) Fetal magnetic resonance imaging (MRI) to assess lung volumes. In this plane, note the giant size heart and the small slivers of lung tissue sitting atop the heart. This fetus manifested conflicting data as to the viability of the lungs because there appeared to be very small lung volumes, but good (near-normal) size branch pulmonary arteries.

Continued

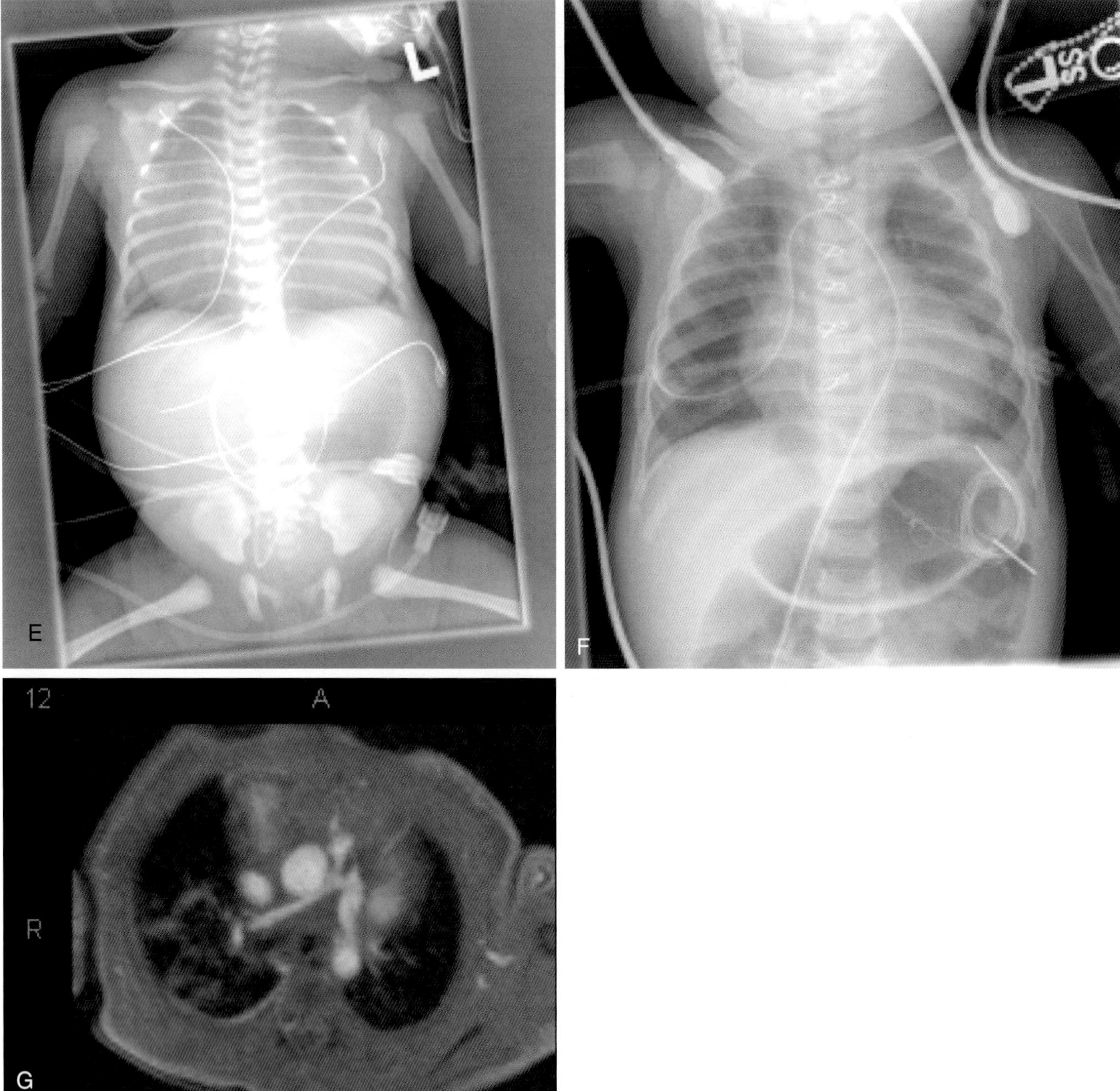

Case 26-4, cont'd **(E)** Chest radiograph of the newborn. There is massive cardiomegaly. Mechanical ventilation supported the notion of viable lung parenchyma. **(F)** The infant underwent surgery consisting of right atrial reduction, plication of the tricuspid annulus, opening of the pulmonary valve, and placement of an aortopulmonary shunt. Note the reduction in heart size and the appearance of adequate-sized lungs. **(G)** Postoperative MRI of the chest demonstrates good-sized lung volumes. This infant went on to successful staged single-ventricle palliation with Fontan operation. Lesson learned—lung viability can be adequately predicted by branch pulmonary artery size in the face of extrinsic lung compression secondary to cardiomegaly.

27

Tricuspid Atresia

Anita Szwast

Key Echocardiographic Features

- Patency of the tricuspid valve
- Size of the right ventricle
- Size and location of the ventricular septal defect, which directs blood into the right ventricle
- Relationship of the great vessels, as normally related or transposed
- Size of the main and branch pulmonary arteries (normally related great vessels)
- Size of the aorta and aortic arch (transposed great vessels)
- Doppler assessment of the presence or absence of antegrade flow across the pulmonary valve
- Doppler assessment of antegrade or retrograde flow across the patent ductus arteriosus
- Left ventricle size, geometry, and function

Anatomy and Anatomical Associations

Tricuspid atresia is an anomaly in which the tricuspid valve is fully sealed off without any flow across. There are four morphologic types of tricuspid atresia: muscular (62%), membranous (29%), Ebstein-like (6%), and valvar (3%). In muscular tricuspid atresia, no valve is present and muscle lines the floor of the atrium. In membranous tricuspid atresia, the membranous atrioventricular septum lines the floor of the atrium. In Ebstein-like tricuspid atresia, the cavity of the right ventricle (RV) is lined with imperforate valve tissue that is displaced apically, with "atrialization" of the RV. Finally, in valvar tricuspid atresia, valve tissue and chordae are visible, although the valve is simply imperforate and sealed. RV hypoplasia is typically seen with tricuspid atresia as well as a ventricular septal defect (VSD). The severity of hypoplasia depends upon the size of the VSD. The inlet portion of the RV is absent because development of the tricuspid valve is related to the inflow (sinus) portion. Thus, in tricuspid atresia, the RV comprises the infundibular and trabecular portions. The branch pulmonary arteries are typically well formed and are perfused by a ductus arteriosus; however, there are cases of associated pulmonary artery hypoplasia.

Tricuspid atresia is classified according to the relationship of the great arteries. In type I tricuspid atresia, which accounts for approximately 70% to 80% of all patients, there are normally related great arteries, Van Praagh segments {S,D,S}. In this type, there is effective pulmonary stenosis because flow is from the left ventricle across the VSD into the RV then into the pulmonary arteries. The size of the VSD dictates the degree of antegrade pulmonary blood flow into the main pulmonary artery (Figures 27-1 and 27-2). In type II tricuspid atresia, which accounts for approximately 12% to 25% of cases, there are transposed great arteries (D-transposition of the great arteries, segments {S,D,D}). With transposed great arteries, the VSD leads to the RV, which gives rise to the aorta and systemic outflow tract, leading to variable degrees of subaortic stenosis and/or coarctation of the aorta (Figure 27-3). Type III is relatively uncommon, accounting for approximately 3% to 6% of patients, and refers to patients with more complex lesions, such as L-transposition or corrected transposition of the great arteries.

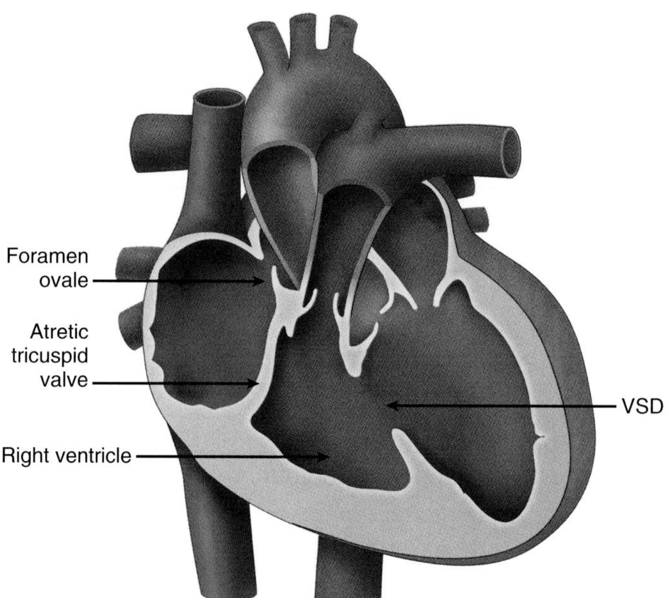

Figure 27-1. Tricuspid atresia, normally related great arteries, large ventricular septal defect (VSD).

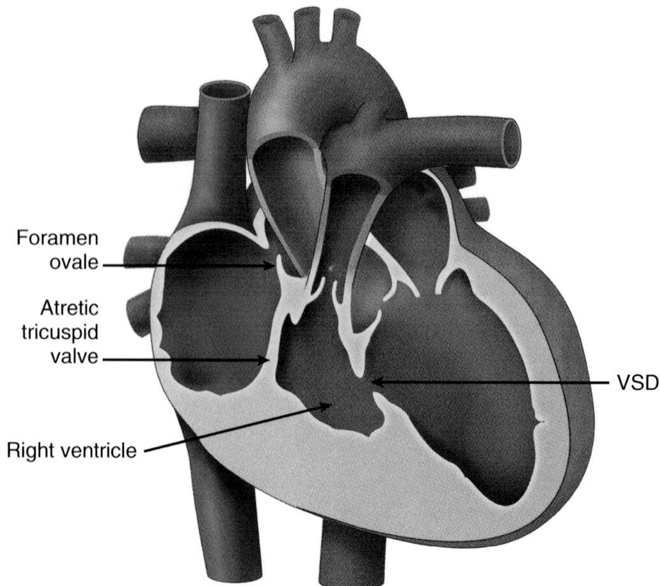

Figure 27-2. Tricuspid atresia, normally related great arteries, small ventricular septal defect (VSD).

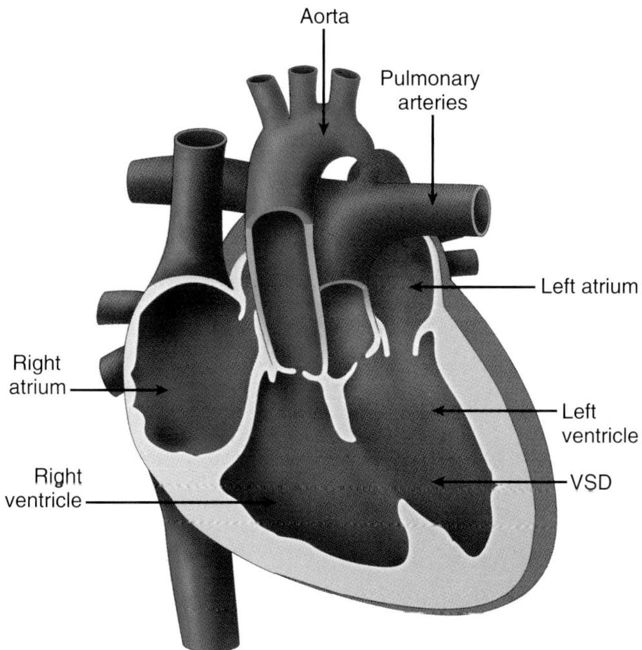

Figure 27-3. Tricuspid atresia, transposition of the great arteries. VSD, ventricular septal defect.

The foramen ovale in tricuspid atresia plays an essential role, because all of the venous return and, hence, cardiac output must travel across it from right to left. In types I and II, the patent foramen ovale is usually large and unrestrictive. In type III patients with L-looped ventricles, the patent foramen ovale may become restrictive over the course of gestation, because the tricuspid valve is then on the left side and guards the chamber receiving pulmonary venous return.

Tricuspid atresia usually occurs as an isolated defect. However, less than 20% of all patients have associated defects. An atrial septal defect is the most commonly seen anomaly. Approximately 8% of patients with tricuspid atresia have coarctation of the aorta, specifically those with transposed great vessels. Other associated cardiac anomalies include left superior vena cava, left juxtaposition of the atrial appendages, and right aortic arch.

Frequency, Genetics, and Development

Tricuspid atresia accounts for 1% to 3% of congenital heart disease. In one study, the prevalence was 0.057 cases/1000 live births.[1] Most cases of tricuspid atresia are sporadic, although families with multiple affected members have been reported.[2] The cause of tricuspid atresia is currently not known, although tricuspid atresia has been reported in mice with Fog-2 or Hey 2 mutations, two transcription factors involved in cardiac morphogenesis.[3,4] Although rare, tricuspid atresia has been reported with 22q11 deletion.[5]

Prenatal Physiology

In the fetus with type I or type II tricuspid atresia, there is obligatory right-to-left shunting across the patent foramen ovale. As a consequence, the patent foramen ovale is typically large and unrestrictive. Increased flow to the left ventricle results in left ventricular dilation and hypertrophy. Restriction at the level of the patent foramen ovale is unusual, although reversal with atrial contraction at the ductus venosus or even venous pulsations may be seen if the patent foramen ovale becomes restrictive. Hydrops fetalis is not typically seen, except in the rare setting of a restrictive patent foramen ovale, which is life-threatening to the fetus.

With normally related great arteries (type I tricuspid atresia), the size of the VSD determines the amount of antegrade pulmonary blood flow. Because the VSD is the proximal controller of blood flow into the RV, hypoplasia of the pulmonary annulus or pulmonary valve stenosis can develop if there is limited flow across the VSD. In its most severe form, with an intact ventricular septum, there is effective pulmonary atresia. Flow in the ductus arteriosus is reversed. With a small or restrictive VSD, antegrade blood flow is limited; there may or may not be flow reversal in the ductus arteriosus. With a large or unrestrictive VSD, there is no reversal of flow in the ductus arteriosus because there is an abundance of antegrade blood flow into the RV. The VSD is typically classified as a perimembranous defect, although muscular VSDs, which may become more restrictive over the course of gestation, may also be seen. Multiple VSDs are also possible.

With transposed great vessels (type II tricuspid atresia), the size of the VSD determines whether or not there is any obstruction to systemic outflow. Consequently, fetuses with tricuspid atresia and transposed great vessels are at risk for subaortic obstruction, aortic hypoplasia, and coarctation of the aorta. With significant aortic arch obstruction, the ductus arteriosus is large and supports the systemic perfusion and there may flow reversal seen in the transverse arch to perfuse the head and neck vessels.

In type III tricuspid atresia with L-looped ventricles, restriction at the level of the patent foramen ovale is more common than in Type I or II. Consequently, with obstruction to pulmonary venous egress, these fetuses are at greater risk for pulmonary hypertension postnatally secondary to maldevelopment of the pulmonary vascular bed.

Prenatal Management

Most fetuses with tricuspid atresia fare well over the course of gestation. In a recent series of 88 fetuses prenatally diagnosed with tricuspid atresia, there were 58 live-born, 4 with in utero demise, 25 terminations of pregnancy, and 1 lost to follow-up.[6] In the absence of hydrops fetalis, fetuses with tricuspid atresia tolerate a vaginal delivery well. Those with restrictive interatrial communications are at risk for development of hydrops fetalis; however, this is a relatively rare phenomenon. In addition, mitral regurgitation and left ventricular dysfunction may progress over the course of gestation, predisposing the fetus to the development of hydrops fetalis.

Diagnosis of tricuspid atresia on fetal imaging is made by assessment of the four-chamber view. On two-dimensional imaging, there is absence of an opening at the site of the tricuspid valve and there is associated right ventricular hypoplasia. Color Doppler imaging will display absence of flow across the region of the tricuspid valve. Assessment of VSD and RV size can be made in multiple planes. The size of VSD and pulmonary annulus, and assessment of the degree of antegrade flow across the pulmonary valve, will dictate whether there will be adequate pulmonary blood flow at birth or the need for prostaglandin E (PGE) infusion to maintain ductal patency as a source of supplemental pulmonary blood flow. If the ductus arteriosus flow in utero is all antegrade, this suggests an adequate size pathway for antegrade pulmonary blood flow. If there is reversal of flow in the ductus arteriosus (aorta to pulmonary artery), it becomes more difficult to judge before birth, and judgment must await postnatal evaluation.

The VSD may become more restrictive over the course of gestation, leading to more severe pulmonary outflow tract obstruction in the case of normally related great arteries or aortic outflow tract obstruction in the case of transposed great arteries. Hence, serial evaluation is called for. In our practice, we evaluate such patients every 4 weeks to reassess the anatomy as well as to continue educational and supportive activities with the family.

There is currently no accepted way to rehabilitate the RV with tricuspid atresia and perform a two-ventricle repair; hence, management involves a single-ventricle palliation. However, not all fetuses with tricuspid atresia require intervention in the neonatal period. In fetuses with pulmonary atresia or severe pulmonary stenosis with flow reversal in the ductus arteriosus, prostaglandin should be initiated at birth to support pulmonary blood flow with plans for a systemic-to-pulmonary artery shunt in the neonatal period. In fetuses with tricuspid atresia, transposed great vessels, and a suspected coarctation of the aorta, prostaglandin is initiated to maintain ductal patency in support of systemic circulation in anticipation of a stage 1 Norwood procedure.

Postnatal Physiology

Fetuses with tricuspid atresia have variable degrees of cyanosis at birth secondary to mixing of the systemic and pulmonary venous return within the left atrium. The degree of cyanosis depends upon the amount of pulmonary blood flow. In tricuspid atresia with normally related great vessels, the size of the VSD determines the degree of cyanosis. In tricuspid atresia with transposed great vessels, there will be adequate mixing and the infant often is relatively pink with just mild cyanosis. In cases of tricuspid atresia with pulmonary atresia, pulmonary blood flow is entirely dependent upon ductal flow. As the ductus arteriosus closes, life-threatening hypoxemia ensues unless prostaglandin is administered to maintain ductal patency. In newborns with tricuspid atresia and a restrictive VSD, pulmonary blood flow ultimately decreases over time. The ductus arteriosus may support pulmonary blood flow in the neonatal period, but ultimately closes, leading to decreased pulmonary blood flow. In addition, the VSD may become smaller over time after birth, leading to worsening cyanosis. Finally, in neonates with large, unrestrictive VSDs, there may be little cyanosis at birth on account of unprotected, unlimited pulmonary blood flow pulmonary overcirculation. As pulmonary vascular resistance drops in these neonates, pulmonary blood flow increases, leading to symptoms of congestive heart failure.

In neonates with tricuspid atresia and transposed great arteries, symptoms of pulmonary overcirculation predominate the clinical presentation because there is little or no pulmonary stenosis. In these patients, as the VSD becomes more restrictive over time, left ventricular pressure rises to maintain systemic output. This, in turn, leads to increased pulmonary blood flow and symptoms of congestive heart failure. Most babies with tricuspid atresia and obstruction to systemic outflow at birth require ductal flow to support systemic perfusion. As the ductus arteriosus closes, perfusion to the lower body becomes compromised, leading to clinical symptoms of shock.

Postnatal Management

Postnatal management in tricuspid atresia is dictated by the degree of obstruction to pulmonary or systemic blood flow at birth. In cases of tricuspid atresia type I (normally related great vessels and obstruction to pulmonary blood flow), prostaglandin infusion should be initiated in the neonatal period, with subsequent evaluation for the need of a Blalock-Taussig shunt. Many neonates with this type of tricuspid atresia have balanced pulmonary and systemic blood flow at birth. Consequently, these infants do not require any intervention in the neonatal period and may proceed directly to a bidirectional Glenn procedure at 4 to 6 months of age. Occasionally, the bidirectional Glenn procedure is performed as early as 2 months of age on account of early, progressive cyanosis. Pulmonary overcirculation typically develops in tricuspid atresia type I, in which the VSD is large, once the pulmonary vascular resistance falls. Anticongestive medications such as digoxin or diuretic medications may be initiated. Pulmonary artery banding to limit pulmonary blood flow can be performed once pulmonary vascular resistance has dropped a bit, between 2 and 4 weeks of age. A bidirectional Glenn procedure is then performed at 4 to 6 months of age.

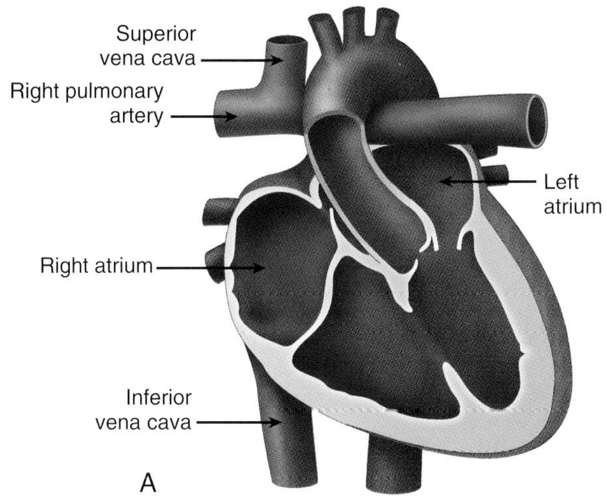

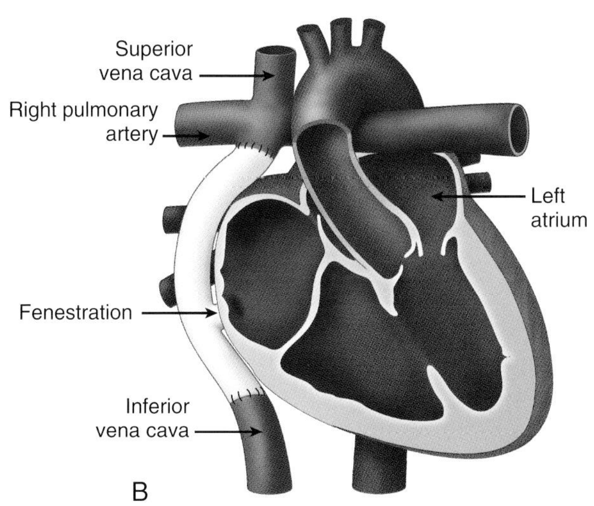

Figure 27-4. Staged Fontan palliation. **(A)** Bidirectional Glenn. **(B)** Fontan completion using an extracardiac conduit.

In cases of tricuspid atresia type II (transposed great vessels with obstruction to systemic outflow) when there is any restriction at the level of the VSD, a modified Norwood stage 1 procedure is typically performed in the neonatal period. A pulmonary artery banding procedure is usually avoided in these patients, because this may promote left ventricular hypertrophy, which may further restrict flow through the VSD to the systemic outflow. Development of subaortic stenosis after a pulmonary artery banding procedure in these patients has been well described in the literature.[7]

All patients with tricuspid atresia ultimately require completion of single-ventricle palliation with a bidirectional Glenn procedure at 4 to 6 months of age and a Fontan completion at 2 to 3 years of age (Figure 27-4).

Outcomes

In the current era, long-term outcomes for tricuspid atresia are favorable. In a recent prenatally diagnosed series, of those infants who were actively managed after birth, survival was 91% at 1 month, 87% at 6 months, 83% at 1 year, and no subsequent deaths for 13 years.[6] In another study of 225 patients who initially presented between 1971 and 1999, 75% had pulmonary outflow obstruction and 11% had aortic outflow obstruction.[8] Palliative procedures were performed in 203 patients (90%). Survival for the entire cohort was 90% at 1 month, 81% at 1 year, 70% at 10 years, and 60% at 20 years.[8] Independent risk factors for mortality included earlier birth date, lower birth weight, aortic arch anomaly, and greater degree of right ventricular hypoplasia.[8]

Management of the Single Ventricle

Tricuspid atresia is the "classic" form of single ventricle for which the initial Fontan operation was first performed and reported in the early 1970s. The concept of the Fontan operation is that one does need to have a ventricle pumping blood into the pulmonary circulation for survival. If pulmonary conditions are appropriate (low pulmonary vascular resistance), connecting the systemic venous return directly to the pulmonary arteries will allow for "passive" flow of blood without the propelling force of a ventricle. This allows for a sufficient degree of pulmonary blood flow and adequate circulation.

In the current era (since 1989), this process of "cavopulmonary connection" has been divided into two parts and is performed in a staged manner. First, the superior vena cava is connected to the branch pulmonary arteries through a procedure called the "bidirectional Glenn" or hemi-Fontan (half of a Fontan) operation. William Glenn is credited with first creating the notion of adequate pulmonary blood flow when he connected the superior vena cava directly to the disconnected right pulmonary artery. The current operation is a "bidirectional Glenn" in that the superior vena cava is connected to the confluent pulmonary arteries and flow reaches both the right and the left pulmonary arteries. The bidirectional Glenn is typically performed at 4 to 6 months of age, when pulmonary vascular resistance has dropped to a relatively low level. This procedure unloads volume from the single-ventricle heart and results in adequate systemic oxygenation with anticipated arterial saturation in the 80% to 85% range. At 2 to 3 years of age, the inferior vena cava is connected to the branch pulmonary arteries by using either a conduit or a baffle to create a tunnel through the right atrium. Occasionally, a small communication or "fenestration" is left between the systemic venous connection, which has been demonstrated to improve early outcome and survival.

This strategy has been demonstrated to be extremely successful in taking a severe form of heart disease and allowing for survival. Many children have now entered their second and third decades of life, with little symptomatic complication. Obviously, the current strategy for single-ventricle care is not a cure, because we cannot replace the missing ventricle. The physiological cost of the Fontan strategy is elevated systemic venous pressure and low cardiac output. Over time, these conditions manifest as a host of complications.[9] Exercise capacity is impaired. Arrhythmias occur as a consequence of the atrial surgery necessary. Ventricular performance changes for the worse over time, because the inherent geometry and functionality of the single ventricle, even the left ventricle as in tricuspid atresia, is not normal. There is a substantial risk for thromboembolism.[10] Elevated systemic venous pressure and impaired cardiac output after the Fontan operation are believed to be the culprits in an odd, but increasingly diagnosed, disorder of protein-losing enteropathy.[11] Hepatic dysfunction with progressive cirrhosis appears to be the destiny of many survivors beyond two decades after surgery.[12]

Early survival and surgical results of all forms of single ventricle continues to improve. However, in counseling families carrying a fetus with single-ventricle type of congenital heart disease, this troubling future should be conveyed. At the same time, it is also important to convey the dynamic aspect of new knowledge in this field of medicine. Twenty years ago, stating with confidence the likelihood of survival with good quality of childhood life for a newborn with single ventricle was not possible, yet such can be done today. Similarly, the expectation is that 20 years henceforth, new knowledge and improved management strategies will be discovered that will allow us to either avoid or overcome some of these late complications, leading to a normal duration and quality of life.

Imaging Essentials and Important Points

- Size of the VSD dictates size of the RV and amount of flow into the RV in tricuspid atresia. The smaller the VSD, the smaller the RV, and hence, the more limited the flow into the pulmonary circulation if there are normally related great vessels (type I), and the more limited the flow into the systemic circulation if there are transposed great vessels (type II).
- More than one VSD can be present; therefore, a careful search of the septum is required, in particular if the size of the RV seems too large and disproportionate to the size of the VSD.
- In tricuspid atresia and normally related great vessels, assess the ductus arteriosus for direction of flow. Forward antegrade flow suggests a good-sized VSD and minimal pulmonary stenosis and predicts an adequate source for pulmonary blood flow after birth.
- A left superior vena cava can be seen in tricuspid atresia. Although of no consequence to the hemodynamics in the fetus or after birth, it is of critical importance to identify before performing the bidirectional Glenn procedure because it needs to be incorporated into the pulmonary arteries.
- The shape of the left ventricle in tricuspid atresia is typically more rounded and globular than normal. This may be related to the fact that it is carrying the entire cardiac output throughout gestation, with a remodeling of chamber architecture.
- Mitral regurgitation in the fetus with tricuspid atresia suggests an inherent anomaly of the mitral valve or an element of ventricular dysfunction.
- Doppler flow assessment should include evaluation of the ductus venosus and umbilical vein. Mild decrease in ductus venosus flow with atrial contraction is *normal* in tricuspid atresia because the right atrium contracts against an atretic valve. It does not suggest restriction at the foramen ovale or predict hydrops. However, venous pulsation in the umbilical vein should warrant closer inspection of the atrial septum for an element of restriction. Most fetuses tolerate mild or moderate restriction at the atrial septum well while in utero. But once cardiac output increases after birth, a moderate degree of restriction may become more severe and should be evaluated urgently in the postnatal period.
- Rarely, a fetus may need to be delivered early for balloon septostomy of the atrial septum, but only if signs of early fetal hydrops are present. No Doppler flow patterns adequately predict which fetus will develop hydrops in the face of atrial level restriction. Close serial follow-up in these unusual cases is indicated.
- In cases of tricuspid atresia and transposed great vessels, careful inspection and measures of the ascending aorta and aortic arch should be performed. Color and pulse wave Doppler evaluation of flow in the aorta can be helpful. Retrograde flow in the aortic arch suggests severe impediment to aortic forward flow and is seen in the most severe cases of VSD restriction and right ventricular hypoplasia. Such patients have a physiology similar to hypoplastic left heart syndrome (HLHS), however, with a systemic ventricle that is a morphologically left ventricle. Management is the same as for HLHS.

References

1. Talner CN. Report of the New England Regional Infant Cardiac Program, by Donald C. Fyler, MD. Pediatrics, 1980;65(suppl):375-461. *Pediatrics*. 1998;102:258-259.
2. Bonnet D, Fermont L, Kachaner J, et al. Tricuspid atresia and conotruncal malformations in five families. *J Med Genet*. 1999;36: 349-350.
3. Donovan J, Kordylewska A, Jan YN, Utset MF. Tetralogy of Fallot and other congenital heart defects in Hey2 mutant mice. *Curr Biol*. 2002;12:1605-1610.
4. Svensson EC, Huggins GS, Lin H, et al. A syndrome of tricuspid atresia in mice with a targeted mutation of the gene encoding Fog-2. *Nat Genet*. 2000;25:353-356.
5. Marino B, Digilio MC, Novelli G, Giannotti A, Dallapiccola B. Tricuspid atresia and 22q11 deletion. *Am J Med Genet*. 1997;72: 40-42.
6. Wald RM, Tham EB, McCrindle BW, et al. Outcome after prenatal diagnosis of tricuspid atresia: a multicenter experience. *Am Heart J*. 2007;153:772 778.
7. Freedom RM, Benson LN, Smallhorn JF, et al. Subaortic stenosis, the univentricular heart, and banding of the pulmonary artery: an analysis of the courses of 43 patients with univentricular heart palliated by pulmonary artery banding. *Circulation*. 1986;73: 758-764.
8. Sittiwangkul R, Azakie A, Van Arsdell GS, Williams WG, McCrindle BW. Outcomes of tricuspid atresia in the Fontan era. *Ann Thorac Surg*. 2004;77:889-894.
9. Rychik J. Long-term outcomes after Fontan surgery. *Nat Clin Pract Cardiovasc Med*. 2008;5:368-369.
10. Coon PD, Rychik J, Novello RT, Ro PS, Gaynor JW, Spray TL. Thrombus formation after the Fontan operation. *Ann Thorac Surg*. 2001;71: 1990-1994.
11. Rychik J. Protein-losing enteropathy after Fontan operation. *Congenit Heart Dis*. 2007;2:288-300.
12. Camposilvan S, Milanesi O, Stellin G, Pettenazzo A, Zancan L, D'Antiga L. Liver and cardiac function in the long term after Fontan operation. *Ann Thorac Surg*. 2008;86:177-182.

CASES

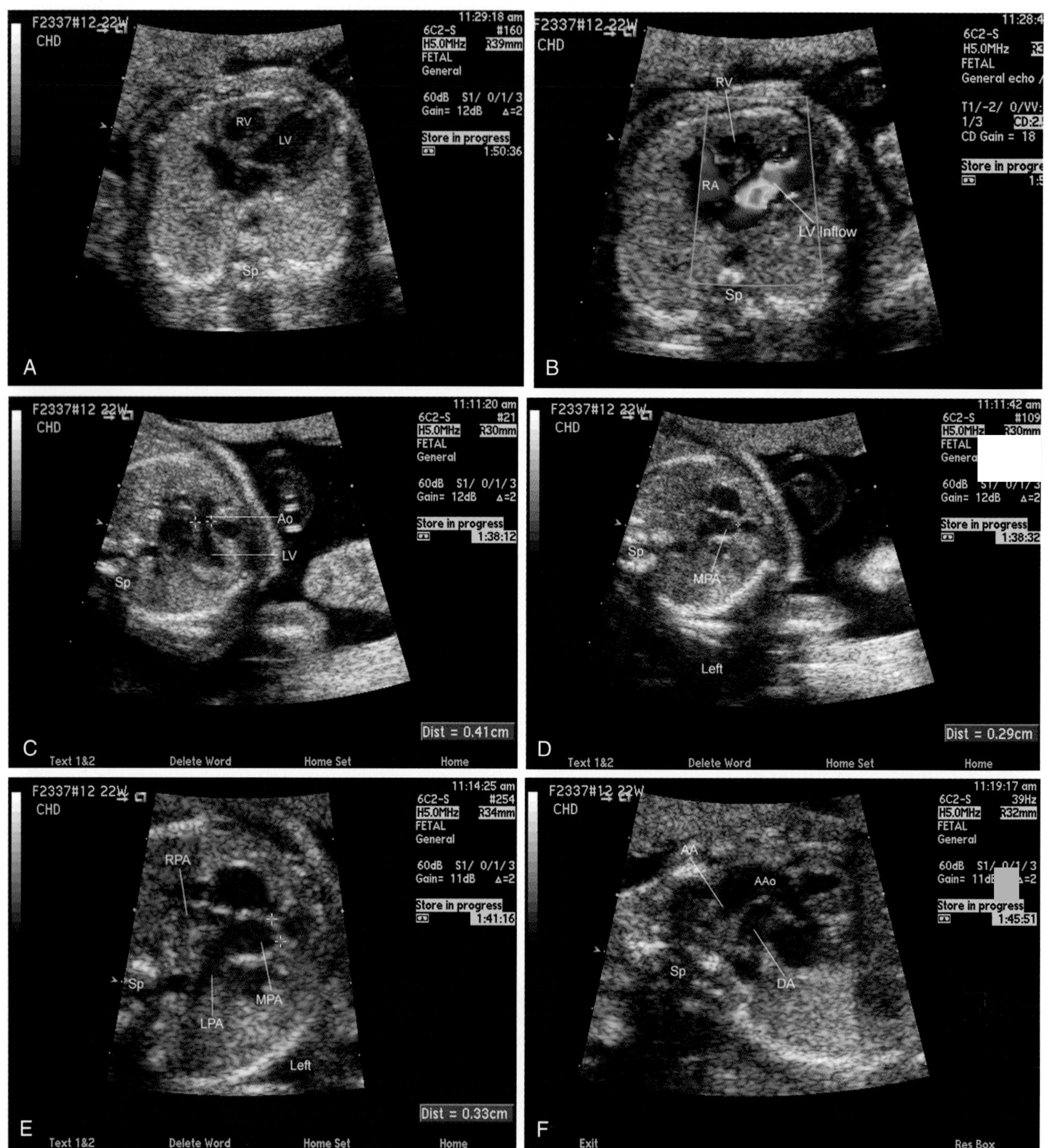

Case 27-1. **(A)** Apical view with size disproportion between the right ventricle (RV) and the left ventricle (LV) with the right smaller than normal. The phase is ventricular systole. Although one cannot yet say this is tricuspid atresia, the valve tissue over the inlet of the RV is thickened. Sp, spine. **(B)** Color flow imaging demonstrates filling of the LV, but no filling of the RV through an atrioventricular inlet, confirming tricuspid atresia. RA, right atrium. **(C)** In this case of tricuspid atresia, there are normally related great vessels. The aorta (Ao) arises from the LV. **(D)** Anterior and leftward angulation demonstrates the main pulmonary artery (MPA) crossing normally with the Ao behind. **(E)** Superior and cephalad angulation reveals a thickened pulmonary valve *(crosshairs)* and the branch pulmonary arteries. Although the MPA is of good size, there is significant pulmonic stenosis. LPA, left pulmonary artery; RPA, right pulmonary artery. **(F)** Imaging of the ascending aorta (AAo) and proximal aortic arch (AA). A large ductus arteriosus is seen (DA).

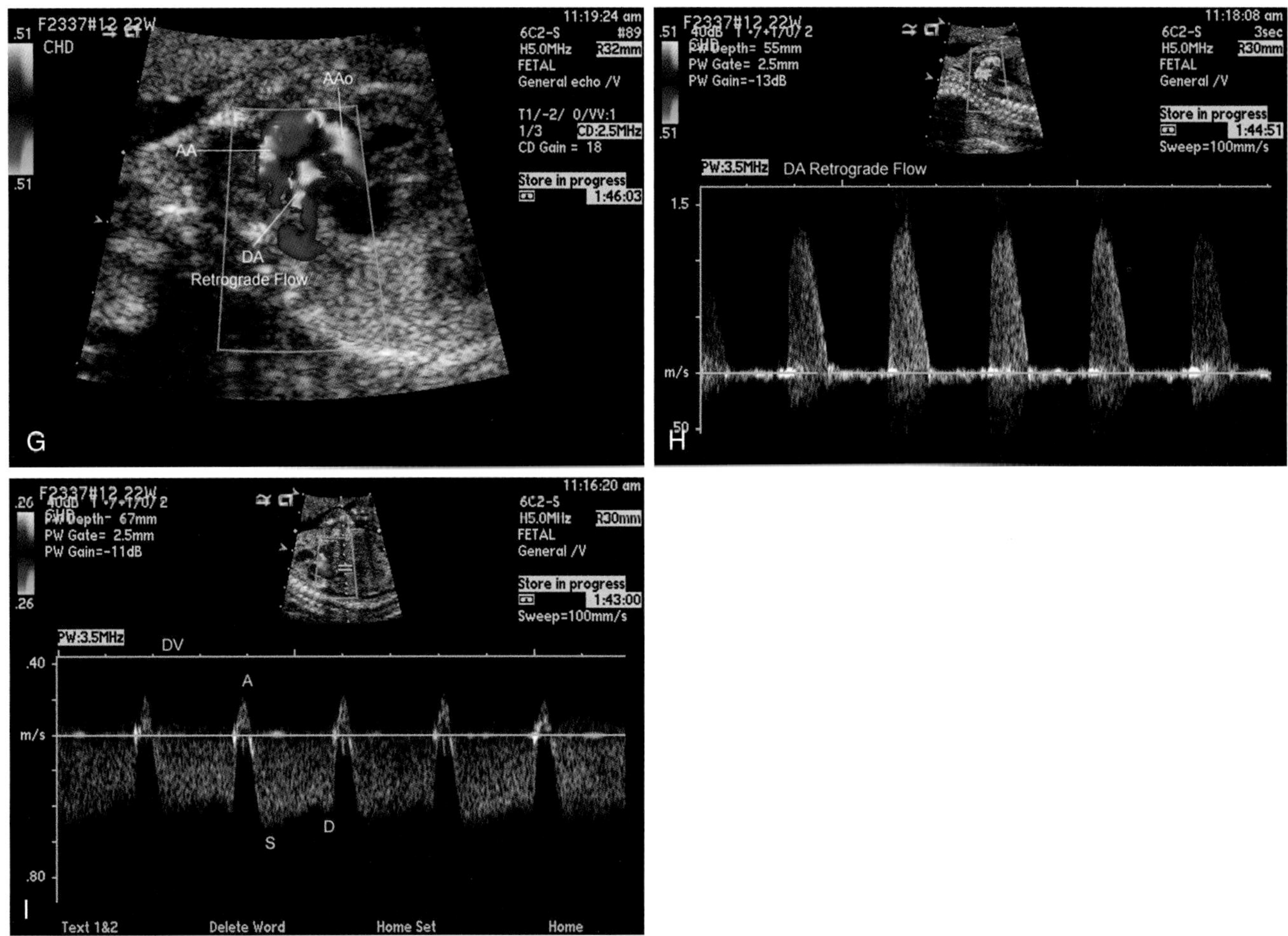

Case 27-1, cont'd (G) Color flow imaging of the arch demonstrates retrograde flow *(red flow)* through the DA. This suggests the presence of significant pulmonic stenosis and the likely need for ductal support of pulmonary blood flow after birth with initiation of prostaglandin infusion. (H) Doppler sampling in the DA demonstrates retrograde (aorta–to–pulmonary artery) flow. (I) Doppler sampling in the ductus venosus (DV). There is retrograde flow with atrial contraction (A wave). Whereas this is considered abnormal in a structurally normal heart, it is completely acceptable in a fetus with tricuspid atresia. The prominent A wave is likely generated by atrial contraction against an atretic tricuspid valve with all of the systemic and umbilical venous blood return propelled across the foramen ovale. A markedly prominent reversal A wave may suggest restriction at the level of the foramen ovale; however, the degree demonstrated here is acceptable.

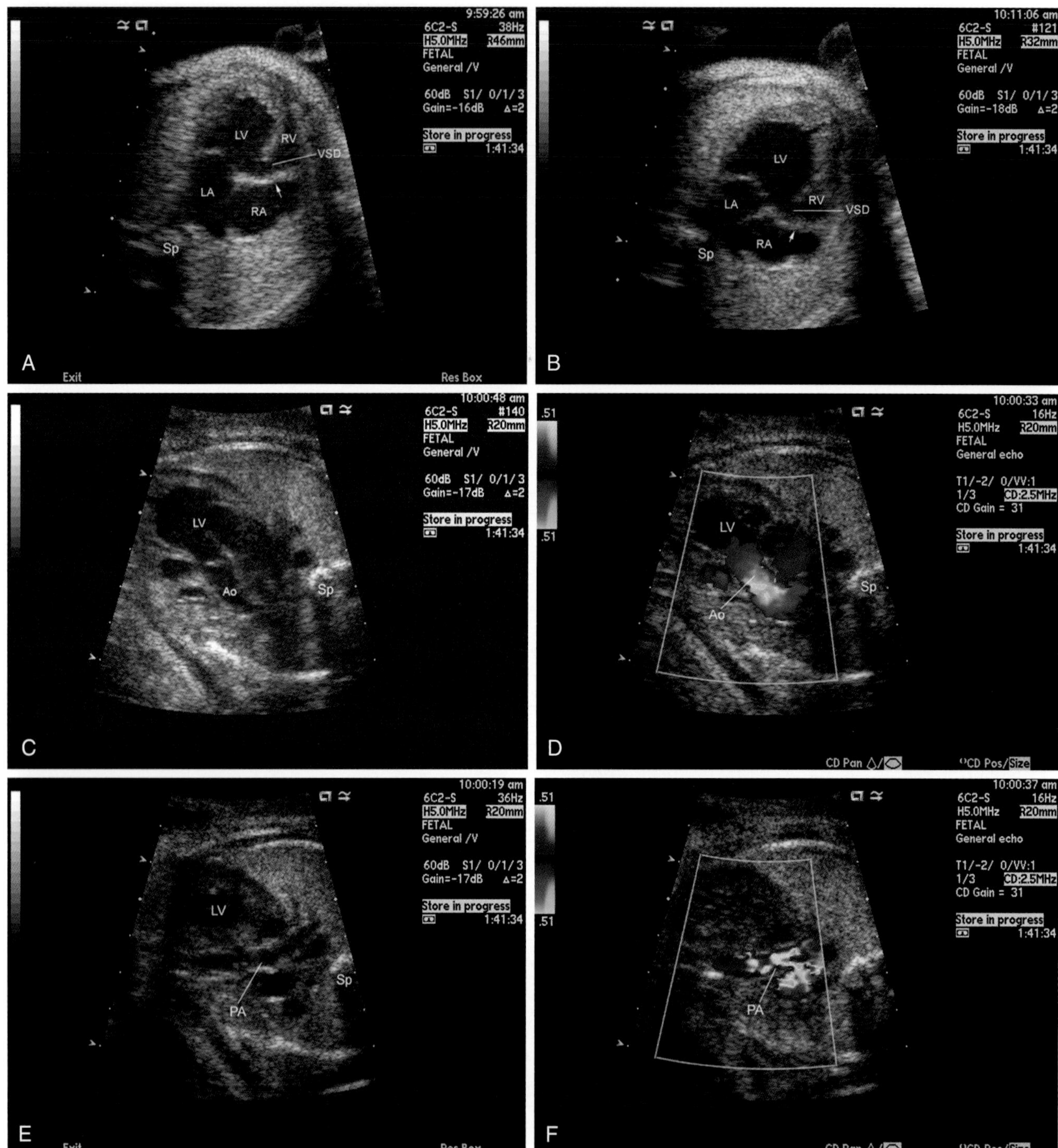

Case 27-2. **(A)** Apical view of tricuspid atresia. There is no right-sided atrioventricular valve. Inlet into the hypoplastic right ventricle (RV) is through a ventricular septal defect (VSD). LA, left atrium; LV, left ventricle; RA, right atrium; Sp, spine. **(B)** More leftward angulation reveals the globular and rounded shape commonly assumed by the LV in cases of tricuspid atresia, as the left takes on the role of the "single ventricle" through which all blood return passes. **(C)** Long-axis view of the aorta arising from the globular-shaped LV. **(D)** Color flow imaging across the large aorta (Ao) arising from the LV in an unobstructed manner. **(E)** The pulmonary artery (PA) arises from the small RV. The PA is smaller than the Ao. **(F)** Color flow imaging demonstrates a very small communication between the LV and the RV. This is the source for pulmonary blood flow and is the anatomical site limiting forward antegrade flow into the PA.

VI

Congenital Heart Anomalies: Single Ventricle

28

Heterotaxy Syndrome and Complex Single Ventricle

Meryl S. Cohen

Anatomy and Anatomical Associations
Frequency, Genetics, and Development
Prenatal Physiology
Prenatal Management
Postnatal Physiology
Postnatal Management
Outcomes

Key Echocardiographic Features

- Identify the location of the abdominal organs (stomach and liver) and determine situs.
- Identify the position of the heart in the chest (levocardia or dextrocardia).
- Identify the systemic venous connections (is there a right superior vena cava? Is there a left superior vena cava? Does the inferior vena cava insert into the heart?).
- Look for the presence of a dilated azygos vein at the level of the diaphragm, which suggests interruption of the inferior vena cava and azygos continuation of inferior systemic venous return.
- Identify the nature of the hepatic venous return and its connections to the atria.
- Identify the presence or absence of the atrial septum (is there a common atrium?).
- Identify the presence or absence of two relatively equal-sized ventricles.
- Look for ventricular septal defects, size, and location.
- Identify the atrioventricular valve connections in relation to the ventricles.
- Identify the presence and degree of atrioventricular valve insufficiency.
- Identify the position and origin of the great vessels.
- Determine the nature of any outflow tract obstruction to the pulmonary artery or aorta.
- Assess the relative size of the pulmonary artery to the aorta.
- Assess aortic arch anatomy and size.
- Assess main and branch pulmonary artery anatomy and size.
- Identify the direction of flow across the ductus arteriosus, as either antegrade from pulmonary artery–to–aorta or retrograde from aorta–to–pulmonary artery.
- Determine the pulmonary venous connection and drainage to the heart.
- Search for any venous structure in the mediastinum or liver in which there is Doppler flow suggesting blood flow away from the heart, because this is highly suggestive of the presence of anomalous pulmonary venous drainage.
- Look for rhythm irregularity that may suggest the presence of heart block.

Anatomy and Anatomical Associations

Heterotaxy is of Greek origin, with *heteros* meaning "other" and *taxis* meaning "arrangement." Heterotaxy syndrome is a disorder of abnormal lateralization of the abdominal viscera, thoracic organs, and cardiac atria. Visceral location falls in a spectrum between situs solitus (normal) and situs inversus (inverted), and cardiac position may vary from levocardia (heart positioned on the left side) to dextrocardia (heart positioned on the right side). In addition to these findings, organs that usually manifest characteristic right-left asymmetry such as the lungs and atrial appendages develop in a mirror-image way. Heterotaxy syndrome can generally be categorized into two subtypes, *polysplenia* (also known as *left atrial isomerism*) and *asplenia* (also known as *right atrial isomerism*), although some patients exhibit features of both. Complex congenital heart disease is a hallmark of both subtypes; in addition, many patients have functional asplenia and malrotation of the intestines. Heterotaxy syndrome results in high morbidity and mortality among children with congenital heart disease despite surgical advances in the current era. The diagnosis is readily made in fetal life when particular cardiac defects are seen in combination or when pathognomonic features of the disease such as organ displacement and organ symmetry are observed.

Heterotaxy syndrome can have a spectrum of congenital heart defects, the hallmarks being systemic and pulmonary venous anomalies, inlet abnormalities, and conotruncal defects.

In *asplenia*, there is bilateral right-sidedness. The atrial appendages both typically have the morphological features of a right atrial appendage (broad-based, triangular shape). There is often absence or unroofing of the coronary sinus and dual sinus nodes.[1,2] Specific characteristics define the right and left lungs. Normally, the right lung has three lobes, and the left two. In the right lung, the bronchi are considered "eparterial," which means the airway sits on top of, or above, the arteries as they run in parallel into the parenchyma, and in the left lung, the bronchi are "hyparterial," which means the airways sit beneath the arteries. In asplenia, regarding the lung anatomy, there are usually two trilobed (right) lungs with bilateral eparterial bronchi.[3] The systemic and pulmonary venous systems are often abnormal with bilateral superior venae cavae and total anomalous pulmonary venous connection (TAPVC, Figure 28-1), frequently to an extracardiac site.[4] The inferior vena cava is often juxtaposed to the descending aorta adjacent to the spine; and hepatic venous drainage may be contralateral to the inferior vena cava because it can enter the atria separately.[3] Complex congenital intracardiac disease is a common feature and typically includes common atrioventricular canal (AVC) in association with a conotruncal abnormality such as transposition of the great arteries or double-outlet right ventricle (DORV). Pulmonary outflow obstruction including pulmonary atresia is usual, whereas systemic outflow obstruction is rare.

In *polysplenia*, bilateral left-sidedness is seen. Both atrial appendages tend to have left appendage anatomy (a long,

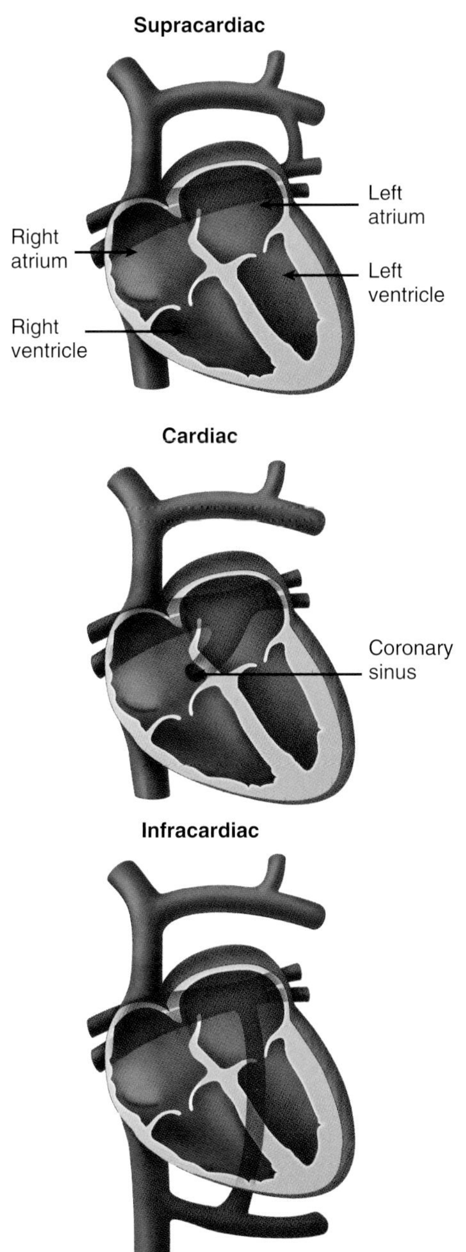

Figure 28-1. Variety of anomalous connections of pulmonary veins.

tubular appearance with a narrow neck). The sinus node may be absent or hypoplastic (because it is typically a right atrial structure).[5] The lungs both have left lung features with two lobes and hyparterial bronchi.[3] The systemic and pulmonary venous connections are also frequently abnormal. Interruption of the hepatic portion of the inferior vena cava with azygos continuation to the superior vena cava is a pathognomonic finding of polysplenia and occurs in approximately 60% to 90% of cases.[6] More than 50% of patients with polysplenia also have bilateral superior venae cavae.[2] With regard to the pulmonary veins, TAPVC to an extracardiac site has been reported in only one case.[6] However, ipsilateral pulmonary veins, in which the right pulmonary veins enter the right atrium and the left pulmonary veins enter the left atrium, is quite common. This occurs in up to 60% of cases, typically in association with a large common atrium with no identifiable atrial septum.[2,6] TAPVC directly to the right atrium can also occur particularly when there is predominantly situs inversus. Intracardiac abnormalities can be less severe than those seen in asplenia. Approximately 15% of those with polysplenia may have normal intracardiac anatomy with interruption of the inferior vena cava as the only feature.[7] When structural heart disease is present, typical cardiac abnormalities include common AVC, common atrium, single ventricle, and pulmonary outflow obstruction.[7,8] In some cases, left-sided obstructive lesions and hypoplastic left heart syndrome can be seen.[9]

In both asplenia and polysplenia, dextrocardia and right aortic arch with mirror image branching occur approximately one third of the time.[9] Up to 20% of both subtypes have absence of the right superior vena cava with isolated left superior vena cava.[2]

Splenic abnormalities including complete absence of the spleen (which can occur in asplenic and polysplenic subtypes) or small, multiple spleens are common in heterotaxy syndrome. In association with the anatomic abnormalities, splenic function may be normal, marginal (polysplenia), or nonexistent (asplenia). Those with splenic dysfunction are vulnerable to particular bacterial infections. The liver is often midline rather than right or left sided. Intestinal malrotation, another common association, affects up to 30% to 40% of children with heterotaxy syndrome and is not readily identified on fetal examination.[10] Biliary atresia has been reported in 3% to 10% of heterotaxy patients and is more common in those with polysplenia.[11] Midline defects such as cleft palate and neurological, musculoskeletal, and genitourinary abnormalities have also been reported.[11] Complete heart block is also unique to patients with polysplenia and carries a very poor prognosis.[12]

Frequency, Genetics, and Development

It is difficult to determine the frequency of heterotaxy syndrome because many different cardiac lesions are seen in association with the syndrome and it is frequently underdiagnosed. It is considered a relatively rare abnormality but accounts for significant morbidity and mortality in most large pediatric cardiac care centers.

Several genes including *ZIC3* and *CRYPTIC* have been associated with heterotaxy syndrome; these genes are likely involved in the regulation of signaling of early embryological left-right patterning.[13] Several mice models including the *inversum viscerum* have abnormalities of left-right asymmetry with mutation of the *Lrd* gene.[14] Many of these mice models also have abnormalities of nodal cilia suggesting features similar to Kartagener's syndrome.

Asymmetrical expression of signaling molecules, including Sonic hedgehog, *cNR1*, *Lefty-2*, and *Pitx2* are involved in the development of heterotaxy syndrome.[15,16] Many of these have had direct mechanistic implications for the development of asymmetrical structures. Nodal cilia in most vertebrates rotate rapidly to produce flow from right to left, a mechanism now identified as the initial event in breaking left-right symmetry.[17] In heterotaxy syndrome, this mechanism appears to be affected very early in development, resulting in either bilateral right- or bilateral left-sidedness.

Prenatal Physiology

The physiology of heterotaxy syndrome as it presents in utero is dependent on the cardiac anatomy. A systematic assessment of the fetal heart and vasculature is necessary in order to diagnose heterotaxy syndrome. This requires knowledge of the segmental approach to anatomical diagnosis of congenital heart disease, as established by Anderson and coworkers[2] and Van Praagh and colleagues.[3,6] In an orderly, sequential manner, this approach addresses cardiac position, systemic and pulmonary venous anatomy, atrioventricular (AV) connections, ventriculoarterial connections, relationship of the great arteries to each other, and aortic arch anatomy. All of these aspects of cardiac anatomy can be abnormal in heterotaxy syndrome.

The diagnosis of heterotaxy syndrome is suggested on fetal echocardiogram when many typical features are seen in combination. Determination of fetal position is essential and should be performed early in the scan so that cardiac position and location of abdominal organs such as the liver and stomach may be correctly identified. Discrepancy between cardiac position and location of visceral structures (i.e., levocardia with stomach on the right or dextrocardia with stomach on the left) should alert the practitioner to the possibility of heterotaxy syndrome. Approximately 20% to 40% of those with heterotaxy syndrome have been reported to have dextrocardia with slightly higher prevalence in those with asplenia.[9,18,19]

Once fetal position and lie are established, the coronal view of the abdomen can identify whether there is interruption of the inferior vena cava (as is seen in polysplenia). If interruption is present, the coronal view will identify two circles side-by-side in the retroperitoneal region just anterior to the spine, one being the aorta and the other the enlarged azygos vein. In the longitudinal view, two vessels can be seen in parallel with flow in opposite directions by color Doppler. The azygos will have a venous flow pattern and be directed toward the heart, and the aorta will be pulsatile and directed away from the heart. No intrahepatic portion of the inferior vena cava can be identified when there is interruption of the inferior vena cava. In asplenia, the inferior vena cava is usually connected to the right atrium (or the left atrium) and can be demonstrated in the longitudinal view, but it is often juxtaposed to the aorta. Other components of the systemic venous anatomy can be identified including presence or absence of the right superior vena cava, assessment for bilateral superior venae cavae, and the connection of the left superior vena cava to the heart (i.e., directly into the roof of the left atrium or to the coronary sinus).

The pulmonary venous anatomy must be determined (Figure 28-2). Functional single ventricle in association with extracardiac TAPVC carries a very poor prognosis.[12,20,21] Therefore, identification of TAPVC is important for family counseling and for postnatal management. In contrast to other congenital heart defects, obstructed TAPVC is a surgical emergency with maintenance of ductal patency providing little to no assistance in stabilizing the postnatal physiology. TAPVC occurs in 60% of patients with asplenia syndrome and should always be highly suspected in this population.[2] Although TAPVC cannot always be identified accurately,[12] the practitioner should look for abnormal venous structures posterior to the heart that may be carrying the pulmonary venous blood flow to an extracardiac site such as the innominate vein, superior vena cava, left superior vena cava, or below the diaphragm into the liver.

In heterotaxy syndrome, particularly in those with asplenia, the AV connection is typically an AVC defect (see Chapter 9). The unbalanced form of AVC occurs frequently in heterotaxy, with one viable ventricle present. In the short-axis view, the common AV valve can often be seen en face. Because the common AV valve can be

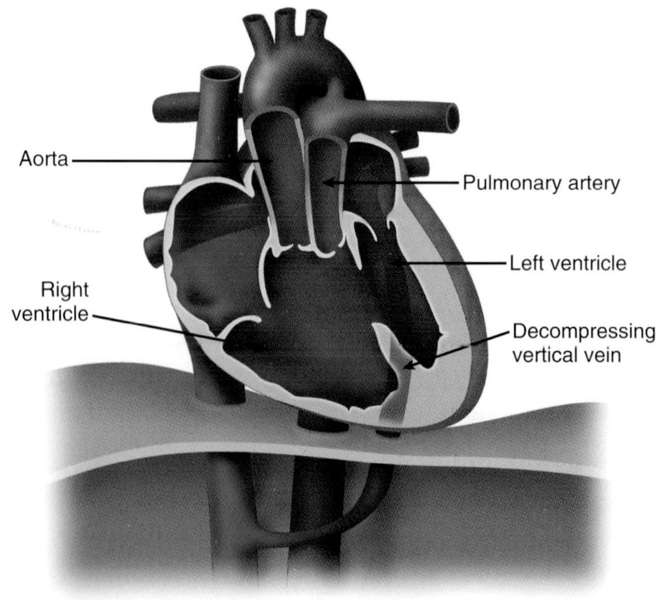

Figure 28-2. Heterotaxy syndrome. Example of unbalanced atrioventricular canal, double-outlet right ventricle, pulmonic stenosis, with infradiaphragmatic total anomalous pulmonary venous connection.

structurally abnormal, in utero regurgitation may occur. Color flow mapping readily identifies fetal AV valve regurgitation and its severity. If the AV valve regurgitation is severe, volume overload develops. Persistence of severe regurgitation often results in fetal compromise with heart failure and the development of hydrops fetalis.

The ventriculoarterial connections can also be abnormal in heterotaxy syndrome. Conotruncal defects typically seen include transposition of the great arteries, DORV, and right ventricle-to-aorta with pulmonary atresia. The prevalence of these lesions ranges from 50% to 96%, with a higher frequency in asplenia than in polysplenia.[2,9,19,21] These conotruncal anomalies are usually seen in association with common AVC defect so that when both are seen together, heterotaxy syndrome should be highly suspected. On fetal echocardiography, both great vessels should be identified (if present) with determination of their connections to the ventricles. In transposition of the great arteries, the great vessels will be in parallel rather than cross each other. In DORV, blood from the left ventricle (if present) must pass through a ventricular septal defect (VSD) to get to the great vessels. In some cases, one great vessel overrides the VSD. In right ventricle-to-aorta, the aorta arises directly from the right ventricle and the pulmonary valve cannot be identified because there is atresia. Typically, the pulmonary arteries receive blood flow retrograde from the ductus arteriosus, which has a tortuous appearance.

Pulmonary outflow obstruction, either pulmonary stenosis or the more severe pulmonary atresia, is also observed in the majority of patients with asplenia[18,20,21] and approximately half the patients with polysplenia.[2,3,9] Retrograde flow in the ductus arteriosus heralds significant right ventricular outflow tract obstruction.[22] Systemic outflow obstruction is more common in polysplenia, with hypoplastic left heart syndrome seen on occasion.

Complete heart block can be seen in association with the polysplenic subtype of heterotaxy syndrome. This finding alerts the obstetrician to refer for cardiac evaluation because the ventricular rate may be significantly less than normal, often in the range of 50 to 70 bpm. When the ventricular rate is very low, hydrops fetalis can occur.

Prenatal Management

Because most patients with heterotaxy syndrome have complex congenital heart disease, close follow-up is required during the course of gestation. Risk factors for poor outcome include a diagnosis of functional single ventricle in association with TAPVC, significant AV valve regurgitation, or complex heart disease with complete heart block.[12,20,21,23] Fetal demise may occur, particularly in those with complete heart block or hydrops fetalis due to valve regurgitation. Families may consider termination of the pregnancy based on severity of the cardiac disease. If the pregnancy is continued, monthly follow-up echocardiographic studies are suggested to follow progression of disease. In those with pulmonary stenosis, serial echocardiography may identify progression to pulmonary atresia.[24] In cases with minimal or no AV valve regurgitation and no complete heart block, the disease may remain quiescent during gestation with no significant physiological impact on the fetus or the mother.

Direction and restriction of flow at the atrial septum (if there is functional single ventricle such as hypoplastic left heart syndrome or tricuspid atresia) and the ductus arteriosus should be performed at each monthly assessment to help to establish the severity of disease.[22] Serial studies also allow for continued consultation with the family and discussion about any changes that may have taken place.

One of the most important aspects of determining prognosis for the fetus with heterotaxy syndrome is knowing the anatomy and drainage of the pulmonary veins. At initial evaluation, for example, at 18 to 22 weeks, visualization of the pulmonary veins can be extremely challenging, because there is normally very little flow in the pulmonary circulation at this gestational age. Compounding the difficulty may be the presence of pulmonary stenosis further limiting pulmonary blood flow or pulmonary venous obstruction due to anomalous connection. Serial evaluation over time, in particular as the fetus approaches later in the third trimester, at a time when pulmonary blood flow is relatively increased in comparison to the second trimester, may help identify pulmonary venous connection not previously seen.

For those fetuses with complete heart block in association with heterotaxy syndrome, the prognosis is quite poor. In a series of 11 such patients who received aggressive treatment after birth including early pacemaker implantation, there were no survivors.[12] Many of these fetuses are noted to have abnormal-appearing myocardium that may affect outcome. Families carrying fetuses with this combination of defects benefit from being counseled accordingly.

From a cardiac standpoint, cesarean section is not necessary unless there is (1) concern about heart block or (2) concern about obstructed TAPVC, both of which may be a surgical emergency at birth. In those cases, urgent delivery with rapid transition to a cardiology and cardiac surgery team may result in the best outcome. If risk factors are not present, normal labor and delivery is optimal for the transition. As with any significant cardiac defect, premature delivery increases the risk of poor outcome because of the additional potential comorbidities such as lung disease, retinopathy, neurological injury, and necrotizing enterocolitis.

Postnatal Physiology

The clinical presentation of newborns with heterotaxy syndrome varies depending on the underlying cardiac anatomy. With prenatal diagnosis, practitioners are prepared for potential hemodynamic instability after birth. Long-term outcome may improve with prenatal diagnosis of many congenital heart lesions[25]; however, in the case of heterotaxy syndrome, the outcome is often dictated by the severity of the disease.[12,21] Prenatal diagnosis allows for determination of whether the infant will be *ductal dependent* (defined as a clinical situation in which the ductus arteriosus must remain open to provide adequate pulmonary or systemic blood flow). In general, accuracy in the prediction of ductal dependency is quite high for heterotaxy syndrome.[12]

Infants with asplenia who have single ventricle with pulmonary stenosis or atresia will be cyanotic at birth. The cyanosis will be severe if obstructed TAPVC is also present because blood will not be able to exit the lungs. For those with normal pulmonary venous connections, initiation of prostaglandin E_1 will provide hemodynamic stability and the mild cyanosis exhibited will be well tolerated. If obstructed TAPVC is present, prostaglandin E_1 may not improve oxygenation because pulmonary venous blood flow is hindered on its return from the heart. Postnatal echocardiography will help in this determination. In this clinical situation, if the partial pressure of oxygen (PO_2) remains less than 30 torr despite aggressive medical management, urgent surgical intervention may be required.

In polysplenia, a broader spectrum of congenital heart disease may be seen. Patients with severe right or left ventricular outflow tract obstruction will require prostaglandin E_1 after birth until surgery is performed. In those with less severe forms of heart disease, surgery may not be required in the neonatal period and there may be no symptoms in early postnatal life. In patients who have a large VSD with no significant pulmonary stenosis, congestive heart failure will develop as the pulmonary vascular resistance drops (generally at 6-8 wk of life).

Those patients with complex congenital heart disease and complete heart block may exhibit signs of low cardiac output, particularly if the ventricular rate is less than 55 bpm.[26] In some cases, inotropic medications may be required to augment perfusion. If these measures fail, pacing is required.

Postnatal Management

Neonates with single ventricle and ductal-dependent circulation will require an operation soon after birth. Prostaglandin E_1 can stabilize the infant until the surgery is performed. In all cases, surgery is palliative; there is no *corrective* repair for these cardiac lesions.

For those with severe pulmonary stenosis or pulmonary atresia, placement of a modified Blalock-Taussig shunt is usually required to provide a reliable source of pulmonary blood flow. Enlargement of the pulmonary arteries may be performed at the same operation when they are considered significantly hypoplastic.

The rare patient with functional single ventricle and no outflow tract obstruction will likely require a banding procedure of the main pulmonary artery to decrease the pulmonary blood flow and prevent pulmonary overcirculation. Increased pulmonary blood flow results in high-output cardiac failure and poor associated constitutional growth. In the long term, high pulmonary blood flow puts the patient at risk for the development of pulmonary vascular disease. Pulmonary artery banding is generally performed within the first 2 to 3 months of life when the pulmonary overcirculation becomes evident. It is the least invasive of all initial procedures; cardiopulmonary bypass and circulatory arrest are not required.

In those patients with TAPVC (asplenia) who have a vertical vein below the diaphragm (infradiaphragmatic TAPVC), pulmonary venous return will most likely be obstructed and urgent surgery may be necessary. In those with supracardiac TAPVC, obstruction can still occur, particularly if the vertical vein becomes obstructed as it travels between the pulmonary artery and the bronchus. During TAPVC repair, the confluence of the pulmonary veins is connected to the back of the left atrium and the vertical vein is ligated. In cases in which there is concern for recurrent obstruction, a "sutureless" technique may be used; this procedure includes use of a patch roofed over the confluence as it connects to the left atrium.[27]

Patients with hypoplastic left heart syndrome or one of its variants will undergo the Norwood procedure as an initial palliative procedure (see Chapter 22). In some cases of right dominant unbalanced AVC, deciding between a Norwood procedure and a two-ventricle repair can pose a significant challenge to the clinician.[28,29] Careful evaluation of features of adequacy of the left side of the heart come into play in the decision making.

There is a rare group of patients who will not require an initial surgical procedure, namely, those with functional single ventricle who have enough pulmonary stenosis to protect their pulmonary vascular bed from overcirculation but not too much to cause severe cyanosis. These patients require close follow-up to ensure adequate pulmonary blood flow.

The eventual goal of surgical palliation for patient with functional single ventricle is separation of the systemic and pulmonary circulations. Therefore, all patients who undergo an initial palliative procedure (or for those who have an appropriate degree of pulmonary stenosis) will require additional palliative surgery. The eventual goal is to divert all of the systemic venous return directly into the pulmonary vascular bed; this is achieved through a "total cavopulmonary anastomosis" but is more commonly referred to as the *Fontan procedure.* The surgery is generally performed in two stages to avoid significant morbidity and mortality.

At 4 to 6 months of age, the first of these stages, called a *superior cavopulmonary anastomosis,* is performed. The pulmonary arteries are connected directly to the superior vena cava. Depending on the method of this connection, the procedure may be called a *bidirectional Glenn shunt* (bidirectional meaning blood flow to both the right and the left pulmonary artery) or a hemi-Fontan operation.

In those patients with interruption of the inferior vena cava, the procedure is called the *Kawashima operation;* in this case, all the systemic venous blood with the exception of hepatic venous blood is directed to the pulmonary arteries. All of these procedures result in a decrease in the volume load to the single ventricle. Cyanosis is still present because the inferior vena cava (or the hepatic veins in the case of interrupted inferior vena cava) still empties into the atrium, resulting in a right-to-left shunt. When hepatic venous drainage does not reach the pulmonary vasculature, over time, pulmonary arteriovenous malformations may develop and cause increased cyanosis. It is suspected that there is an as yet un-identified "factor" in the hepatic blood that appears to prevent these malformations from developing. Lack of delivery of this "factor" to the pulmonary vascular bed leads to development of pulmonary arteriovenous malformations. Surgical incorporation of the hepatic veins can result in resolution of pulmonary arteriovenous malformations.

At 2 to 4 years of age, the inferior vena cava (or the hepatic veins directly) are redirected to the pulmonary arteries. This procedure, known as the Fontan operation, has many technical modifications. After the Fontan procedure, the systemic and pulmonary circulations are separated, absent the presence of a pulmonary ventricle.

In addition to the cardiac intervention that is typically required in patients with heterotaxy syndrome, other organ systems must also be rigorously evaluated. Routine screening for functional asplenia is recommended so that antibiotic prophylaxis and appropriate immunizations can be initiated. All patients should also undergo screening for intestinal malrotation because it occurs in 30% to 40% of both subtypes.[30,31] Once malrotation is diagnosed, a prophylactic Ladd procedure is generally recommended to prevent volvulus of the midgut, a potentially life-threatening complication. Approximately 3% to 10% of children with polysplenia will also have biliary atresia. Therefore, liver enzyme levels should be evaluated in this group with imaging as indicated. Biliary atresia in association with congenital heart disease has an extremely poor outcome.[32,33]

Outcomes

The natural history for heterotaxy syndrome is poor if complex congenital heart disease is present. With surgical palliation, outcome is still worse than for other patients with similar cardiac disease *without* heterotaxy syndrome.[20,23,32] Mortality is as high as 70% in some series, in particular for those with single ventricle and in those with asplenia compared with those with polysplenia.[20,33] For patients with asplenia, risk factors for poor outcome include the presence of TAPVC, recurrent pulmonary venous obstruction, and significant AV valve regurgitation.[12,20,23] For the polysplenia patients, risk factors include complete heart block, significant AV valve regurgitation, recurrent coarctation of the aorta, and biliary atresia.[33]

For the patients who survive to undergo the Fontan operation, outcome appears to be better, because this is a "selected" group. Studies suggest that this group is not significantly different than the single-ventricle population without heterotaxy syndrome.[34,35] Factors that influence outcome after Fontan in patients with heterotaxy syndrome include complex systemic and pulmonary venous anatomy, common AV valve regurgitation, and cardiac rhythm disturbances.

Although morbidity after Fontan may not be worse in this group, patients with heterotaxy syndrome may experience significant complication over time. They are more likely to develop early pulmonary arteriovenous malformations, prolonged perioperative pleural effusions at the time of Fontan operation, and early and late arrhythmias.[32] Despite these concerns, children with heterotaxy syndrome who have had a Fontan operation and survived appear to have good quality of life. A recent study of the Pediatric Heart Network identified that a cohort of Fontan patients with heterotaxy syndrome had no differences in exercise performance or functional health status compared with Fontan patients without heterotaxy syndrome.[36]

The complexity of heterotaxy syndrome requires a multidisciplinary approach to care and appropriate counseling of families regarding potential risk factors and outcomes. Outcome for these patients has improved over the past several decades, but there are particular areas where improvements are still needed. Better techniques to address obstructed TAPVC may avoid significant morbidity and mortality. Treatment of complete heart block in this setting requires reevaluation and is a potential area where fetal intervention may have an impact on prognosis. In some cases, heart transplant in the neonatal period may be an appropriate option to consider.[12]

Imaging Essentials and Important Points

- Imaging of suspected heterotaxy syndrome can be extremely challenging, perhaps the most difficult anomaly to assess in the fetus. Take a deep breath, and set about the investigation in an orderly, segmental manner, accruing data as you go from segment to segment starting with abdominal situs; and position of heart, atrial and venous connections, AV valves, ventricles, outflow tracts,

Imaging Essentials and Important Points—cont'd

and great vessels. The imaging does not need to be performed in this order; however, the mental construction of the anomaly presenting itself will best be diagnosed if processed in this segmental manner. Taking notes as you go along can help.

- As findings are identified, look to see if they are more common in asplenia or polysplenia syndrome (Table 28-1)
- Combination of AVC and conotruncal anomaly raises high suspicions for heterotaxy syndrome. One of the most common configurations seen for asplenia AVC defect, DORV, pulmonary stenosis or atresia, and/or pulmonary vein anomaly will almost always be the asplenia type of heterotaxy syndrome.
- Common marker for polysplenia: interrupted inferior vena cava with azygos continuation.
- Identification of pulmonary venous anatomy is critical in the heterotaxy syndrome because the prognosis changes dramatically if there are anomalous, obstructed pulmonary veins. All venous flow away from the heart is ominous and, in the setting of heterotaxy, suggests for pulmonary venous obstruction (Box 28-1).
- Serial evaluation is key. Later in gestation, owing to a natural, albeit small, normal increase in pulmonary blood flow, it may be easier to visualize pulmonary venous return. If normal, insertion into the left atrium will be better seen. If anomalous connection, greater flow in the decompressing vessel or other abnormal structure to which it connects will be better seen. However, if the pulmonary veins are severely obstructed, there may not be this normal natural tendency toward increased pulmonary blood flow. Oftentimes, such pulmonary veins are small and develop poorly, making it nearly impossible to see. Hence, absence of visualization of the pulmonary veins in the late third trimester, in particular when other structures are relatively easy to see and acoustic windows are good, suggests anomalous, obstructed pulmonary veins.
- The fetus with heterotaxy syndrome, asplenia, functional single ventricle, pulmonary stenosis, and obstructed pulmonary veins has an extremely poor outcome. In addition to management of the complex heart disease, the pulmonary vasculature is often malformed and poorly developed, further compounding the difficulties at birth.

Table 28-1 Anatomical Features Seen in Heterotaxy Syndrome: Asplenia Syndrome (Right Atrial Isomerism) versus Polysplenia Syndrome (Left Atrial Isomerism)

ANATOMICAL FEATURE	ASPLENIA SYNDROME	POLYSPLENIA SYNDROME
Bilateral superior vena cava	45%	45%
Interruption of the inferior vena cava	<2%	80%
Absence of the coronary sinus	–100%	–60%
Juxtaposition of the aorta and inferior vena cava	–90%	Rare
Extracardiac type of total anomalous pulmonary venous connection	50%	Rare
Ipsilateral type of pulmonary venous connection	4%	45%
Atrioventricular canal defect	90%	50%
Common atrium with no remnant of atrial septum	Rare*	80%
Atrioventricular connection	Effectively univentricular in 70%	Effectively biventricular in 75%
Ventriculoarterial connection	Concordant in only 4%	Concordant in 70%
Pulmonary atresia or stenosis	80%	30%
Left-sided obstructive lesion	<5%	30%
Heart block/bradycardia due to sinus node dysfunction	Rare	25-70%

*Functional common atrium due to a large atrial septal defect as in the atrioventricular canal defect is seen quite often; however, complete absence of any atrial septum is unusual.

Box 28-1 Echocardiographic Observations That Help Suspect and Identify Pulmonary Venous Anomalies in the Heterotaxy Syndrome

- Direct insertion seen of pulmonary veins entering into another structure besides the left atrium such as the right atrium or superior vena cava.
- Venous flow directed away from the heart, anywhere—always abnormal!
- Dilated innominate vein.
- Dilated superior vena cava.
- Dilated venous structure behind the heart (distinguish from azygos vein).
- Evaluate the mediastinum—lower color Doppler scale (20-40 cm/sec) and observe for any unusual color speckling to search for a decompressing vertical vein. Sample any suspected venous structure to see if directed away from the heart.*
- Evaluate the liver—look for unusual degree of hepatic venous dilation.
- Evaluate the liver—lower color Doppler scale (20-40 cm/sec) and observe for high-velocity flow, or unusual color speckling.
- Evaluate the liver—lower color Doppler scale (20-40 cm/sec) and observe for venous flow heading *away* from the heart and *caudad* within the body of the liver.
- Within the lung parenchyma—lower color Doppler scale (20-40 cm/sec), identify intraparenchymal pulmonary veins and trace back to the hilum and then to the heart to help identify destination.
- Inability to identify pulmonary veins in the third trimester despite these techniques suggests the presence of anomalous connection and obstruction.

*Aortopulmonary collateral vessels in the case of pulmonary atresia may also be identified in this manner. Pulse wave Doppler should distinguish between the two. Continuous phasic low velocity for a decompressing vertical vein; pulsatile flow for an aortopulmonary collateral vessel.

References

1. Uemura H, Ho SY, Devine WA, Kilpatrick LL, Anderson RH. Atrial appendages and venoatrial connections in hearts from patients with visceral heterotaxy. *Ann Thorac Surg*. 1995;60:561-569.
2. Anderson RH, Webb S, Brown NA. Defective lateralisation in children with congenitally malformed hearts. *Cardiol Young*. 1998; 8:512-531.
3. Van Praagh S, Kakou-Guikahue M, Hae-Seong K, Becker J, Alday L, Van Praagh R. Atrial situs in patients with visceral heterotaxy and congenital heart disease: conclusions based on findings in 104 postmortem cases. *Coeur*. 1988;19:484-502.
4. Rubino M, Van Praagh S, Kadoba K, Pessotto R, Van Praagh R. Systemic and pulmonary venous connections in visceral heterotaxy with asplenia. *J Thorac Cardiovasc Surg*. 1995;110:641-650.
5. Ho SY, Seo JW, Brown NA, Cook AC, Fagg NLK, Anderson RH. Morphology of the sinus node in human and mouse hearts with isomerism of the atrial appendages. *Br Heart J*. 1995;74:437-442.
6. Van Praagh S, Santini F, Sanders SP. Cardiac malpositions with special emphasis on visceral heterotaxy (asplenia and polysplenia syndromes). In Fyler DC, ed. *Nadas' Pediatric Cardiology*. Philadelphia: Hanley & Belfus; 1992:589-608.
7. Gilljam T, McCrindle BW, Smallhorn JF, Williams, WG, Freedom RM. Outcomes of left atrial isomerism over a 28-year period at a single institution. *J Am Coll Cardiol*. 2000;36:908-916.
8. Phoon CK, Villegas MD, Ursell PC, Silverman NH. Left atrial isomerism in fetal life. *Am J Cardiol*. 1996;77:1083-1088.
9. Cohen MS. Clarifying anatomical complexity: diagnosing heterotaxy syndrome in the fetus. *Progr Pediatr Cardiol*. (Rychik J, ed). 2006;22:61-70.
10. Ditchfield MR, Hutson JM. Intestinal rotational abnormalities in polysplenia and asplenia syndromes. *Pediatr Radiol*. 1998;28: 303-306.
11. Ticho BS, Goldstein AM, Van Praagh R. Extracardiac anomalies in the heterotaxy syndromes with focus on anomalies of midline-associated structures. *Am J Cardiol*. 2000;85:729-734.
12. Cohen MS, Schultz AH, Tian ZY, Donaghue DD, Gaynor JW, Rychik J. Hetertotaxy syndrome with functional single ventricle: Does prenatal diagnosis improve survival? *Ann Thorac Surg*. 2006;82: 1629-1636.
13. Belmont J, Mohapatra B, Towbin JA, Ware SM. Molecular genetics of heterotaxy syndromes. *Curr Opin Cardiol*. 2004;19:216-220.
14. Supp DM, Witte DP, Potter SS, Brueckner M. Mutation of an axonemal dynein affects left-right asymmetry in inversus viscerum mice. *Nature*. 1997;389:963-966.
15. Ryan AK, Blumberg B, Rodriguez-Esteban C, et al. Pitx2 determines left-right asymmetry of internal organs in vertebrates. *Nature*. 1998; 394:545-551.
16. Piedra ME, Icardo JM, Albajar M, Rodriguez-Rey JC, Ros MA. Pitx2 participates in the late phase of the pathway controlling left-right asymmetry. *Cell*. 1998;94:319-324.
17. Hirokawa N, Tanaka Y, Okada Y, Takeda S. Nodal flow and the generation of left-right asymmetry. *Cell*. 2006:125:33-45.
18. Atkinson DE, Drant S. Diagnosis of heterotaxy syndrome by fetal echocardiography. *Am J Cardiol*. 1998;82:1147-1149.
19. Berg C, Geipel A, Smrcek J, et al. Prenatal diagnosis of cardiosplenic syndromes: a 10-year experience. *Ultrasound Obstet Gynecol*. 2003; 22:451-459.
20. Hashmi A, Abu-Sulaiman R, McCrindle BW, Smallhorn JF, Williams WG, Freedom RM. Management and outcomes of right atrial isomerism: a 26-year experience. *J Am Coll Cardiol*. 1998;31:1120-1126.
21. Lim JS, McCrindle BW, Smallhorn JF, et al. Clinical features, management, and outcome of children with fetal and postnatal diagnoses of isomerism syndromes. *Circulation*. 2005;112:2454-2461.
22. Berning RA, Silverman NH, Villegas M, et al. Reversed shunting across the ductus arteriosus or atrial septum in utero heralds severe congenital heart disease. *J Am Coll Cardiol*. 1996;27:481-486.
23. Gaynor JW, Collins MH, Rychik J, Gaughan JP, Spray TL. Long-term outcome of infants with single ventricle and total anomalous pulmonary venous connection. *J Thorac Cardiovasc Surg*. 1999; 117:506-513.
24. Hornberger LK, Sanders SP, Sahn DJ, et al. In utero pulmonary artery and aortic growth and potential for progression of pulmonary outflow tract obstruction in tetralogy of Fallot. *J Am Coll Cardiol*. 1995;25:739-745.
25. Tworetzky W, McElhinney DB, Reddy VM, Brook MM, Hanley FL, Silverman NH. Improved surgical outcome after fetal diagnosis of hypoplastic left heart syndrome. *Circulation*. 2001;103:1269-1273.
26. Lopes LM, Tavares GMP, Damiano AP et al. Perinatal outcome of fetal atrioventricular block: one hundred-sixteen cases from a single institution. *Circulation*. 2008;118:1268-1275.
27. Yun TJ, Coles JG, Konstantinov IE, et al. Conventional and sutureless techniques for management of the pulmonary veins: evolution of indications from postrepair pulmonary vein stenosis

to primary pulmonary vein anomalies. *J Thorac Cardiovasc Surg.* 2005;129:167-174.

28. Cohen MS, Jacobs ML, Weinberg PM, Rychik J. Morphometric analysis of unbalanced common atrioventricular canal using two-dimensional echocardiography. *J Am Coll Cardiol.* 1996;28: 1017-1023
29. Szwast AL, Marino BS, Rychik J, Gaynor JW, Spray TL, Cohen MS. The LV inflow index: a novel echocardiographic parameter for predicting successful biventricular repair in unbalanced atrioventricular canal to the right [abstract]. *J Am Soc Echocardiogr.* 2008;21:605.
30. Choi M, Borenstein SH, Hornberger L, Langer JC. Heterotaxia syndrome: the role of screening for intestinal rotation abnormalities. *Arch Dis Child.* 2005;90:813-815.
31. Ferdman B, States L, Gaynor JW, Hedrick HL, Rychik J. Abnormalities of intestinal rotation in patients with congenital heart disease and the heterotaxy syndrome. *Congenit Heart Dis.* 2007;2:12-18.
32. Cohen MS, Anderson RH, Atz AM, et al. Controversies, Genetics, diagnostic assessment, and outcomes relating to the heterotaxy syndrome. *Cardiol Young.* 2007;17(suppl 2):29-43.
33. Gilljam T, McCrindle BW, Smallhorn JF, William WG, Freedom RM. Outcomes of left atrial isomerism over a 28-year period at a single institution. *J Am Coll Cardiol.* 2000;36:908-916.
34. Morales DL, Braud BE, Booth JH, et al. Heterotaxy patients with total anomalous pulmonary venous return: improving surgical results. *Ann Thorac Surg.* 2006;82:1621-1627.
35. Azakie A, Merklinger SL, Williams WG, Van Arsdell GS, Coles JG, Adatia I. Improving outcomes of the Fontan operation in children with atrial isomerism and heterotaxy syndromes. *Ann Thorac Surg.* 2001;72:1636-1640.
36. Atz AM, Cohen MS, Sleeper LA, et al. Functional state of patients with heterotaxy syndrome following the Fontan operation. *Cardiol Young.* 2007;17:44-53.

CASES

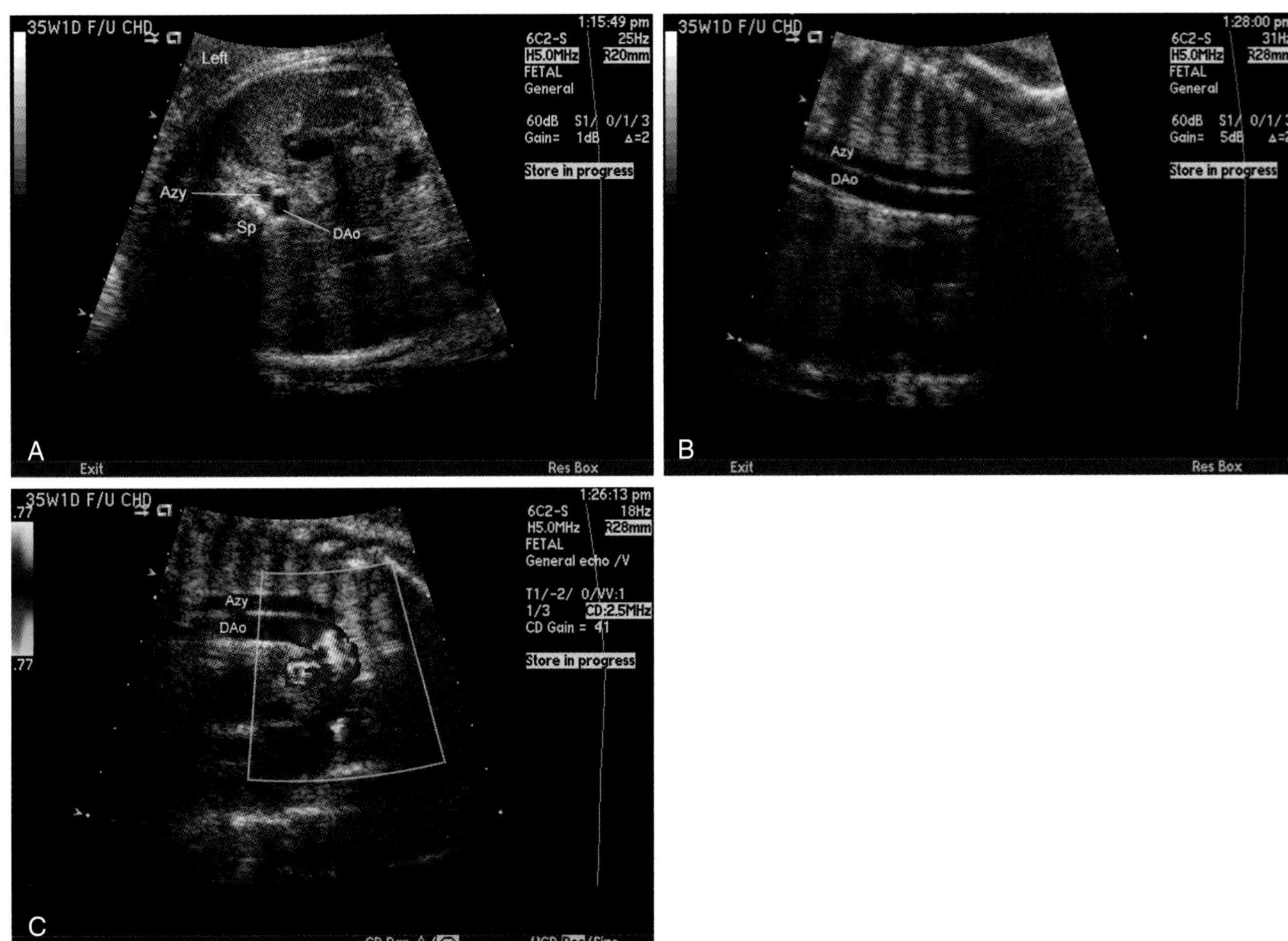

Case 28-1. (A) Fetus at 35 weeks' gestation with interrupted inferior vena cava and azygos continuation. Transverse image at the level of the abdomen with focus on the retroperitoneal space adjacent to the spine (Sp). The descending aorta (DAo) is seen and adjacent to it to the left is another circular structure, which is a dilated azygos vein (Azy). Visualization of the Azy at this level suggests the presence of an interrupted inferior vena cava with azygos continuation. (B) Long-axis view, with transducer turned 90 degrees from the image obtained in **A.** Both the Azy and the DAo are seen in their full length within the abdomen and upper chest. (C) Color flow imaging in the upper mediastinum. A common error is to confuse the insertion of the azygos into the superior vena as being the aortic arch. Color flow imaging can aid with this distinction. In this image, the descending aorta has flow toward the transducer *(red)* and the azygos vein has flow away from the transducer *(blue)* as blood flows into the superior vena cava.

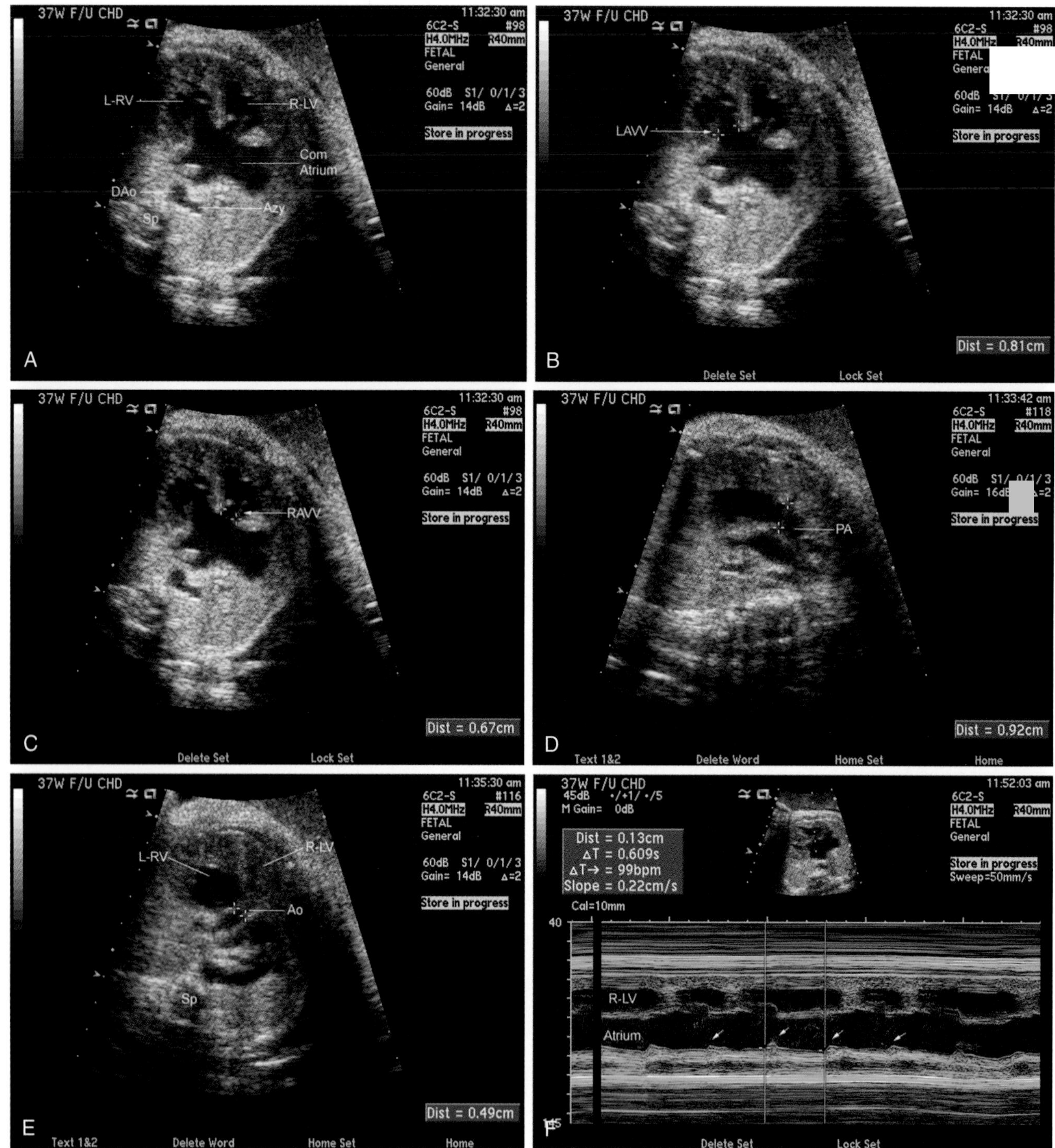

Case 28-2. **(A)** A case of heterotaxy syndrome, polysplenia type, common atrioventricular canal defect and heart block. There is ventricular inversion. The right-sided ventricle is of left ventricle morphology (smooth-walled septal surface, R-LV) and the left-sided ventricle is of right-sided morphology (heavily trabeculated, L-RV). There is a common atrium (Com Atrium). There is a dilated azygos vein (Azy) seen adjacent to the descending aorta (DAo). The DAo is anterior and slightly to the left of the spine (Sp). **(B)** The common atrioventricular valve is mildly unbalanced to the left-sided right ventricle. The left atrioventricular valve (LAVV) component of the common valve measures 8.1 mm at its inlet into the left-sided right ventricle. **(C)** The right atrioventricular valve (RAVV) component of the common atrioventricular valve is smaller than the left and measures 6.7 mm. **(D)** The pulmonary artery (PA) arises from the left-sided right ventricle, is larger in diameter than the aorta (normal), and measures 9.2 mm. **(E)** The aorta (Ao) arises from the right-sided left ventricle, is smaller than the aorta (normal), and measures 4.9 mm. The Ao and pulmonary artery cross as they arise from the heart, in the normal manner. **(F)** M-mode tracing across the right-sided left ventricle (R-LV) and the common atrium. The atrial rate is slow at 99 bpm but is regular without any skipped, or dropped, beats. The *arrows* point to atrial wall activity.

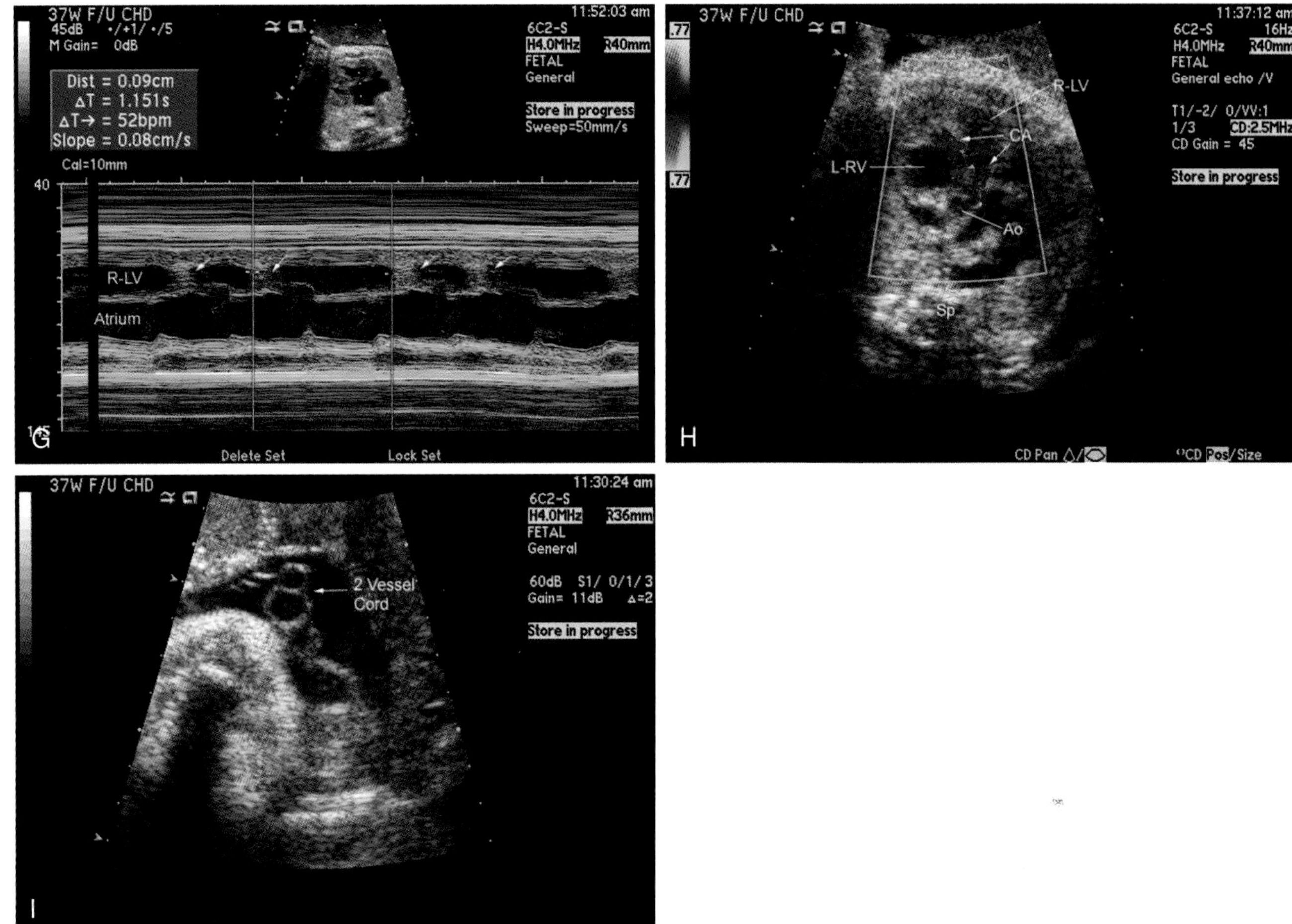

Case 28-2, cont'd **(G)** Same M-mode tracing with the time cursor placed at the onset of ventricular wall movement *(arrows)*. There are dropped beats, and groupings of two ventricular beats are seen, reflecting second-degree heart block. **(H)** Color flow imaging reveals easy visibility of the coronary arteries (CA) in their course within the ventricular myocardium. This reflects coronary vasodilation, perhaps related to a mismatch in myocardial oxygen demand and delivery. Such a mismatch is possible in the setting of increased work of the heart secondary to increased ventricular stroke volume and ventricular dilation in light of the heart block. The slow heart rate also leads to a long diastolic filling time, with a prolonged time for coronary filling. **(I)** A two-vessel cord.

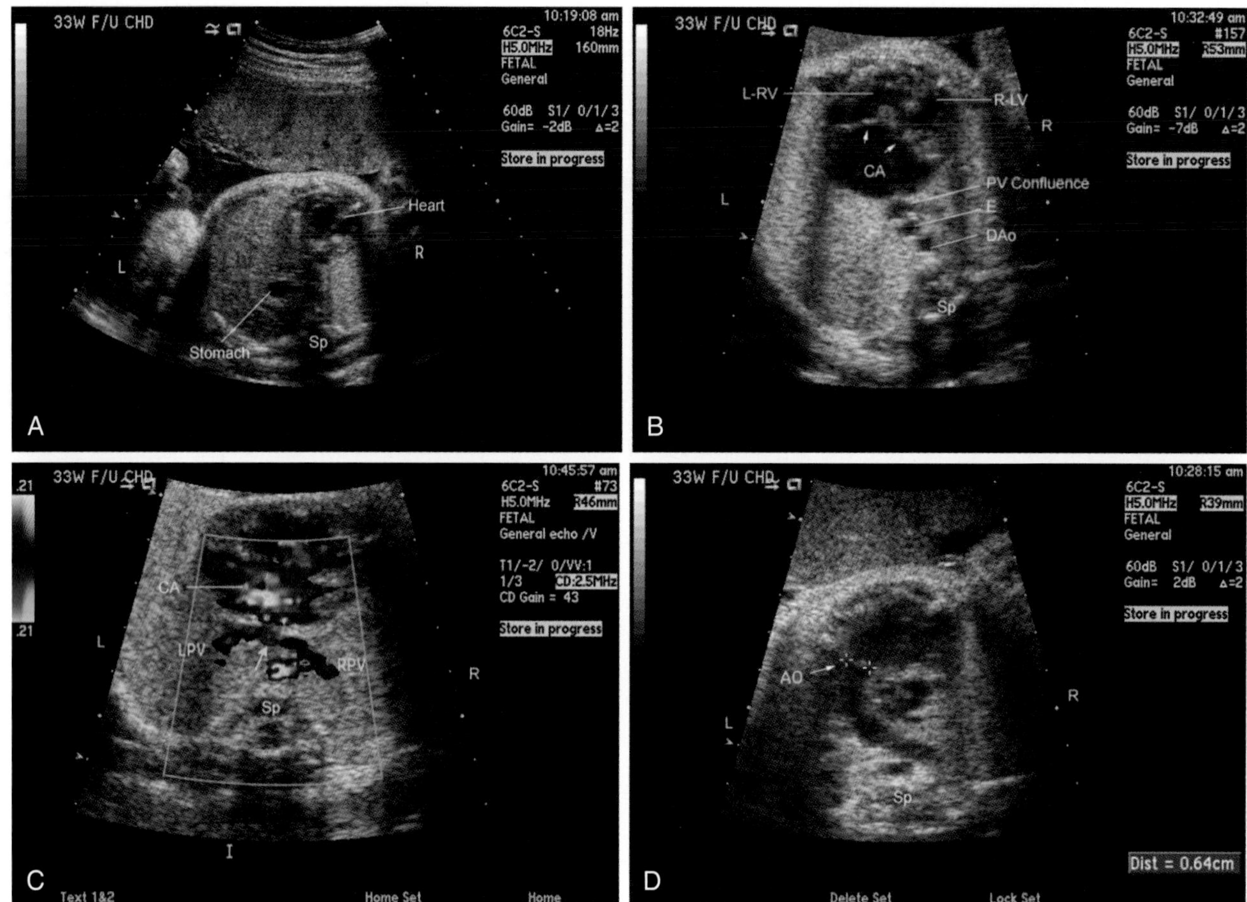

Case 28-3. **(A)** In this case of heterotaxy syndrome, the stomach is to the left of the spine (Sp) as is the liver (Liv). The heart is in the right chest (dextrocardia). **(B)** There is a common atrioventricular canal defect. The morphological left ventricle is on the right (R-LV) and the morphological right ventricle is on the left (L-RV); hence, the ventricles are "L-looped." There is total anomalous pulmonary venous return. Behind the heart in an anterior to posterior manner, one can see a pulmonary venous (PV) confluence, the esophagus (E) in cross-section, and the descending aorta (DAo) in cross-section. **(C)** Color flow imaging demonstrates the confluence of the pulmonary veins behind the common atrium (CA) with entry of one right (RPV) and one left (LPV) pulmonary vein. The veins do not enter into the atrium. **(D)** Double-outlet right ventricle. The aorta (AO) is seen arising from the left-sided right ventricle. The segments of this heart are {A,L,L}: ambiguous situs, L-looped ventricles, and L–great vessel relationship with the aorta arising to the left of the pulmonary artery from the right ventricle.

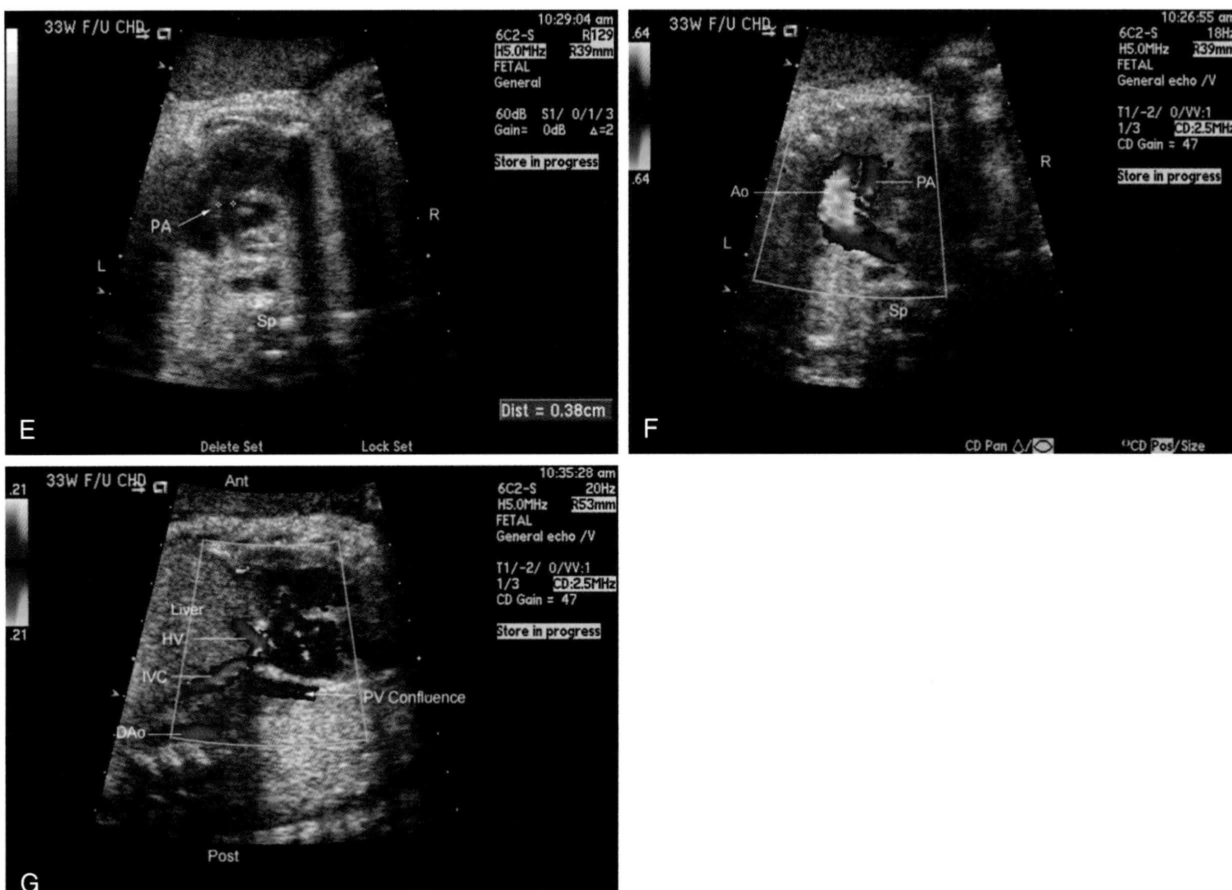

Case 28-3, cont'd **(E)** The pulmonary artery (PA) is to the right of the aorta and is smaller in size. **(F)** Color flow imaging demonstrates the relationship between the aorta (Ao) and the PA. The Ao is to the left of the PA, and the PA is smaller than the Ao. **(G)** View at the level of the diaphragm with color flow imaging. There is a vertical vein draining the pulmonary venous (PV) confluence down toward the liver. Hence, in summary, this fetus has a common constellation of findings seen in the asplenia type of heterotaxy syndrome: double-outlet right ventricle, pulmonic stenosis, complete common atrioventricular canal defect, and total anomalous pulmonary venous return, which is infradiaphragmatic. DAo, descending aorta; HV, hepatic vein; IVC, inferior vena cava.

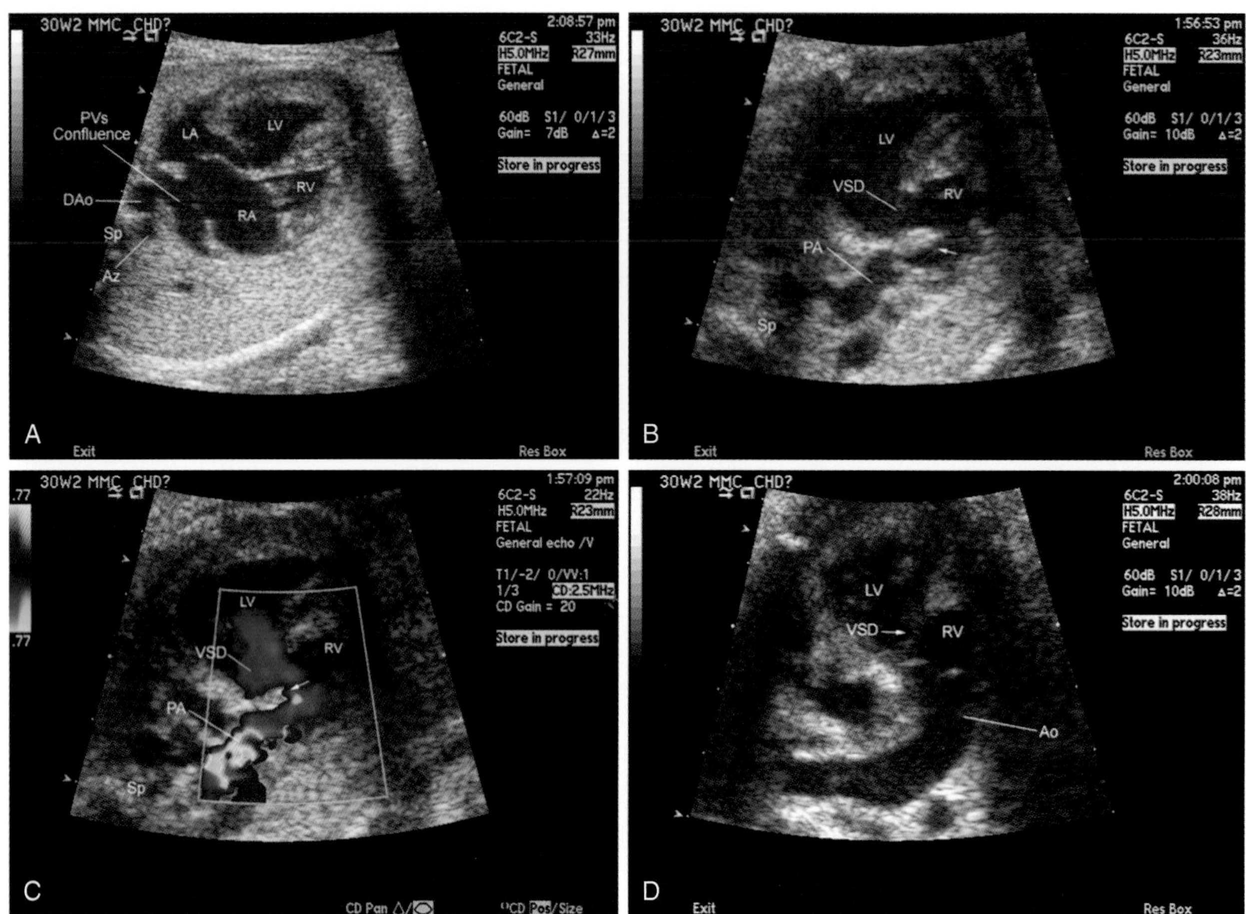

Case 28-4. **(A)** A case of heterotaxy syndrome. Four-chamber view demonstrates a confluence of the pulmonary veins (PVs) to the back of the right atrium (RA). The connection looks to be large and unobstructed. The atrial septum is seen bowing normally toward the left atrium (LA). There is a dilated azygos vein (Az) seen adjacent to the descending aorta (DAo). LV, left ventricle; RV, right ventricle; Sp, spine. **(B)** Angulation toward the outflow tract. There is double-outlet right ventricle with a large ventricular septal defect (VSD). The pulmonary artery (PA) is seen. There is deviation of the infundibular (conal) septum beneath the PA *(arrow)* causing subpulmonic stenosis. **(C)** Color flow imaging demonstrates flow across the VSD from LV to RV. There is infundibular (conal) septal deviation beneath the pulmonary valve causing subpulmonic stenosis. **(D)** Rightward angulation demonstrates the origin of the Ao from the RV. The Ao is of good size and unobstructed.

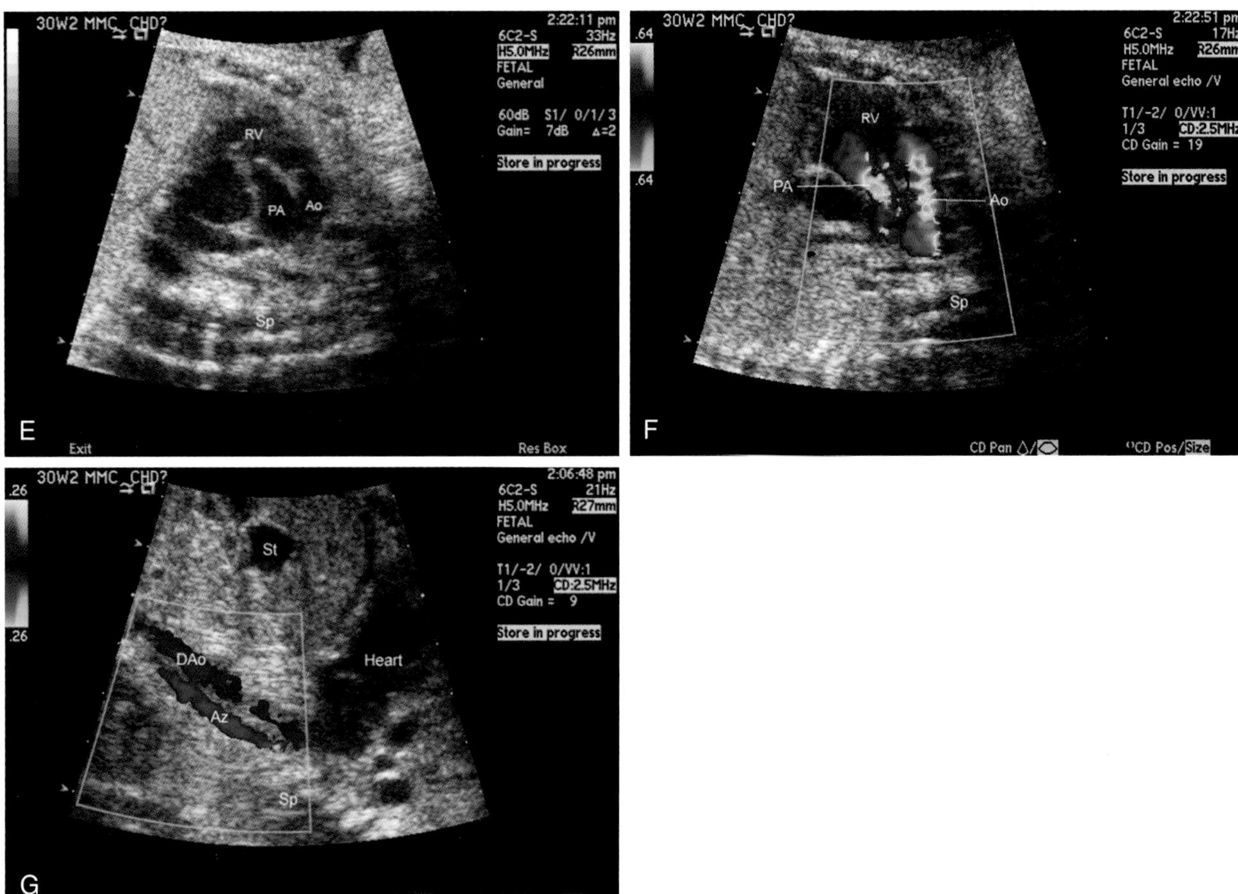

Case 28-4, cont'd **(E)** Both great vessels are seen side-by-side with the Ao to the right of the pulmonary artery (PA). **(F)** Color flow imaging of both great vessels originating from the RV. **(G)** Long-axis color flow imaging at the level just beneath the diaphragm demonstrates a dilated azygos vein (Az) reflecting interruption of the inferior vena cava (IVC). Note the opposite colors of *red flow* in the descending aorta (DAo) headed toward the transducer and *blue flow* in the Az directed cephalad away from the transducer and toward the heart.

29

Double-Inlet Left Ventricle

Jennifer Glatz

Key Echocardiographic Features

- Assess for the morphology of the larger ventricle (left ventricle).
- Identify the atrioventricular valve connections to the left ventricle, and assess size and degree of insufficiency, if present.
- Identify the atrial septum and direction of shunting across.
- If the left atrioventricular valve is small, assess left-to-right gradient across the atrial septum and interrogate the pulmonary veins for Doppler flow pattern in order to determine whether there is obstruction to left atrial egress.
- Identify the position of the small right ventricle as either anterior and rightward, anterior and leftward, or superior.
- Locate and identify the size of the ventricular septal defect communication between the large left ventricle and the smaller right ventricle.
- Identify the great arterial position and origins as either from large left or from small right ventricle.
- Determine the nature of the pathway patency from the large left ventricle to the pulmonary artery and to the aorta.
- Assess direction of flow in the ductus arteriosus, antegrade from pulmonary artery to aorta or retrograde from aorta to pulmonary artery.
- Assess the size of the ascending aorta and aortic arch when the aorta arises from a small hypoplastic right ventricle and the ventricular septal defect is restrictive.
- Identify the direction of flow in the transverse aorta when there is aortic outflow obstruction.
- Assess the size of the branch pulmonary arteries when there is pulmonic outflow obstruction.
- Look for irregularity in heart rhythm, which may reflect heart block.

Anatomy and Anatomical Associations

Double-inlet left ventricle (DILV) is a term used to describe the cardiac malformation in which there are two atrioventricular (AV) valves that drain into a single, large dominant ventricle of left ventricular morphology, which is associated with a diminutive opposing rudimentary outflow chamber. Controversy surrounds the nomenclature of this malformation, and other terms used to describe this anomaly have included *single ventricle* and a *univentricular heart of the left ventricular type.* The main ventricular chamber is of left ventricular morphology with characteristic fine trabeculations. The rudimentary outflow chamber of right ventricle (RV) origin consists only of trabecular and outlet portions and is often in communication with the single left ventricle (LV) through a ventricular septal defect (VSD). The VSD is also often referred to as a *bulboventricular,* or *outlet, foramen.* In this anomaly, the interventricular septum is displaced and malformed, but not absent.[1] The rudimentary right ventricular chamber is located anterior to the main ventricle, either rightward (D-loop) or leftward (L-loop), and is separated by an anterior trabecular septum. Both AV valves are posterior to the trabecular septum and there is no intervening inlet septum between the two.

Diagnosis of DILV excludes those patients with an unbalanced common AV valve. Both AV valves in DILV are in fibrous continuity with the posterior great artery.[2] The RV is variable in size ranging from slitlike to near 80% of the size of a normal RV. There may be either concordance (normal) or discordance (transposition) of the ventriculoarterial relations.

DILV is one of the most common forms of single ventricle and is regarded as the "classic form" because both AV valves communicate into a common chamber. Van Praagh and coworkers[1] distinguished three primary subtypes of DILV based on the relationship of the great arteries: (1) type I DILV has normally related great arteries, (2) type II has a rightward and anterior aorta and rightward outlet chamber, and (3) type III has a leftward anterior aorta. DILV with a hypoplastic subpulmonary, rightward RV and normally related great arteries (type I) is classically referred to as the "Holmes heart" and is relatively rare in our current experience. Type II was observed in 21% of cases of DILV in Van Praagh and coworkers' series. In this form, the outlet chamber is anterior and rightward, consistent with D-looped ventricles, and there is D-transposition of the great arteries, segments {S,D,D}. This type is associated with obstruction of the bulboventricular foramen and, therefore, subaortic stenosis, because the aorta arises from the small chamber. Arch anomalies are reported in approximately 50% of cases.

Type III is the most common form of DILV, accounting for 54% of the cases reviewed by Van Praagh and coworkers.[1] Type III consists of DILV with a left-sided, subaortic, hypoplastic right ventricle (L-loop ventricles) and L-transposition of the great arteries, segments {S,L,L}. Subaortic stenosis is present in approximately 67% of patients with this morphology due to a small bulboventricular foramen or obstruction by left AV valve tissue (Figure 29-1).

Other arterial relations with DILV have included double-outlet arterial connections, with both great arteries arising from the rudimentary right ventricular chamber. Single-outlet connection, most frequently pulmonary atresia, and rare cases of truncus arteriosus have been reported.[3] Bevilacqua and colleagues[4] described a similar spectrum of variety in which out of 57 patients with DILV, 14% had D-looped ventricles with normally related great

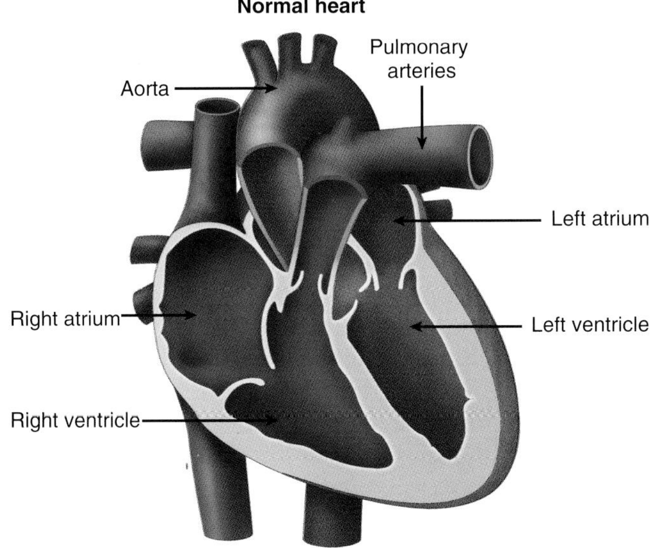

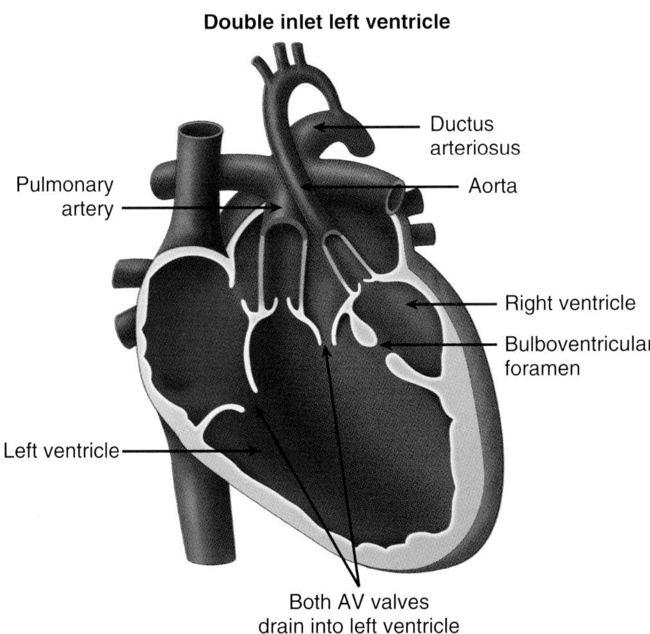

Figure 29-1. DILV segments {S,L,L} with restrictive bulboventricular foramen and coarctation of the aorta.

arteries, 23% had D-looped ventricles with D-transposition of the great arteries, and 63% had L-looped ventricles with L-transposition of the great arteries.[4]

Varying degrees of straddling of the AV valves have been noted in patients with DILV. When straddling occurs, the AV valve that straddles is almost always on the same side as the rudimentary right ventricular chamber.[3] Atresia, stenosis, hypoplasia, and thickening of either AV valve may occur. A parachute-like deformity of the AV valves has also been reported. Shiraishi and associates[5] found a stenotic AV valve in 30% of patients with double-inlet ventricle, most commonly occurring in the left (pulmonary venous) AV valve. When one AV valve is atretic, DILV can be diagnosed if the atretic valve plate overrides the ventricular septum and is committed more than 50% to the LV. Abnormal valves may also lead to AV valve regurgitation.

Pulmonary outflow tract obstruction in DILV occurs with either concordant or discordant ventriculoarterial relations (pulmonary artery from RV or pulmonary artery from LV, respectively). When subpulmonary obstruction occurs within the left ventricular chamber in discordant ventriculoarterial relationship type DILV, it is most frequently due to posterior deviation of the infundibular septum, anomalous attachments of the right AV valve, or herniation of valvular tissue into the pulmonary outflow tracts.[3] When there is concordant ventriculoarterial relation and the pulmonary artery arises from the small RV, subpulmonary obstruction has been reported in 50% of patients with a Holmes heart and can result in hypoxia at birth.[6] Severe pulmonary stenosis and annular hypoplasia can also occur. The pulmonary valve can be thickened and is often bicuspid.[3]

Subaortic obstruction occurs with ventriculoarterial discordance and is located primarily at the level of the interventricular communication. Restriction at this level primarily occurs with a muscular type defect.[4] An interventricular communication, which is smaller in dimension than the aortic root, can be at risk for obstruction over time.[7] Restriction can be severe and may lead to ductal-dependent circulation. Such patients often have coexisting anomalies of the aortic arch including coarctation or interruption. Subaortic obstruction can also be acquired secondary to severe ventricular hypertrophy from muscle bundles within the hypoplastic right ventricular chamber. This occurs more often in patients with associated right AV valve atresia and in patients with DILV and transposed great arteries who are status post-pulmonary artery banding. Pulmonary artery banding in such patients has been associated with progressive ventricular hypertrophy and restriction of the interventricular communication.[7]

Conduction abnormalities have also been associated with DILV due to the abnormal course of the conduction tissue. These abnormalities are found most frequently in patients with discordant arterioventricular relations (L-looped ventricles). Patients with this anatomy are at risk for development of complete heart block.

Frequency, Genetics, and Development

Single-ventricle anatomy accounts for 1.33% to 2.4% of congenital heart disease with a prevalence of 0.054 to 0.08 per 1000 live births.[8,9] Approximately 60% to 70% of all univentricular hearts are characterized by dominant left ventricular morphology.

The developmental origins of DILV are not fully understood. It is speculated that arrest or incomplete movement of the AV septum or the conotruncus results in the malalignment of the inflow and outflow tracts. When the AV septum fails to shift to the right, the right and left AV canals communicate with the LV, forming a DILV. In addition, an abnormality of cardiac looping is often associated with DILV.[3] In a Holmes heart, the interventricular communication represents the primitive bulboventricular foramen.

There are no known specific extracardiac findings or genetic syndromes common to patients with DILV.[10] There is currently no known genetic etiology for DILV.

Prenatal Physiology

The impact of this anomaly on fetal physiology depends primarily on the presence, type, and degree of outflow tract obstruction. Owing to the presence of the ductus arteriosus in fetal circulation and the fact that maternal oxygenation is provided by placental flow, there is minimal hemodynamic compromise to the fetus. If severe aortic outflow tract or aortic arch obstruction is present, as is possible in the case of a rudimentary chamber with ventriculoarterial discordance, systemic perfusion is provided by the right-to-left flow through the ductus arteriosus with retrograde perfusion to the cerebral circulation. When pulmonary outflow is severely obstructed, there is reversal of ductal flow with left-to-right (aorta–to–pulmonary artery) perfusion of the pulmonary vasculature. DILV is not usually associated with significant AV valve regurgitation, ventricular dysfunction, or tachyarrhythmias and, therefore, is not typically associated with hydrops.[11]

Prenatal Management

Prenatal management of this anomaly focuses primarily on accuracy of the diagnosis in order to provide counseling for the family regarding the various options for management. A significant challenge on echocardiography is to distinguish which great vessel is arising from the small outflow chamber—the pulmonary artery or the aorta. In conditions of a very small aorta, the head vessels may falsely appear as if they arise form the large ductal arch, confusing it for the aorta. Identifying which great vessel is small in DILV has ramifications for counseling. If the aorta is small, a modified Norwood operation may be necessary, which carries relatively high risk. If the pulmonary artery is small, a lower-risk initial operation, a Blalock-Taussig shunt, is undertaken.

Fetal echocardiography in DILV should focus on the outflow tract and great vessels relationship as well as delineation of all systemic and pulmonary venous connections, atrial and ventricular anatomy, and structure and function of the AV valves.[11] The fetus is to be followed with serial fetal echocardiography on a regular basis, primarily to monitor for progression of outflow tract obstruction and AV valve regurgitation. Our practice is to see such patients every 4 weeks until term.

Postnatal Physiology

The impact of the transition from fetal to postnatal life depends heavily on the balance of flow to systemic and pulmonary circulations. Because both AV valves drain into the LV, both systemic and pulmonary venous return combine in the left ventricular chamber with mixing of oxygenated and deoxygenated blood. This can lead to a variable degree of cyanosis. Clinical signs of outflow tract obstruction become apparent with closure of the ductus arteriosus, which occurs naturally shortly after birth. In the case of an obstructed pulmonary outflow, cyanosis can be quite pronounced. If pulmonary flow is unobstructed, the normal postnatal decrease in pulmonary vascular resistance will eventually lead to pulmonary overcirculation similar to that seen in a large VSD. If the aortic outflow is severely obstructed, decreased systemic perfusion and signs of shock can develop soon after birth. Prostaglandin therapy is essential for stabilization of infants with ductal-dependent circulation, as in cases of severe subaortic obstruction and arch obstruction or severe pulmonary obstruction.

The clinical features of DILV depend on the presence or absence of aortic and pulmonary outflow tract obstruction. If there is unobstructed pulmonary flow, patients can develop signs and symptoms of congestive heart failure including tachypnea, tachycardia, diaphoresis, hepatomegaly, and failure to thrive within the first 3 months of life.[3] Cyanosis may not be evident due to increased pulmonary blood flow. Infants with unobstructed pulmonary flow who develop symptoms sooner often do so as a result of associated anomalies such as AV valve abnormalities, aortic outflow obstruction, and coarctation of the aorta. Patients with severely obstructed pulmonary blood flow become cyanotic and hypoxemic within the first few hours of life. Those with aortic outflow obstruction and arch anomalies often present with poor perfusion and signs of shock. Streaming of the venous return can also impact symptoms. Infants with DILV and a left-sided subaortic RV, segments {S,L,L}, will have systemic venous streaming preferentially directed to the pulmonary arteries and pulmonary venous return directed to the aorta. Those with a right-sided subaortic RV may have varying degrees of AV valve straddling and may have unfavorable streaming with "transposition-like" blood flow patterns resulting in significant hypoxemia and cyanosis.

On cardiac examination, a soft systolic ejection murmur is occasionally appreciated as a result of flow-related pulmonary outflow obstruction or flow across the interventricular septum to the hypoplastic RV. In the presence of excessive pulmonary blood flow, a diastolic rumble may be heard. A diastolic murmur may also be present in patients with AV valve stenosis. A systolic ejection murmur and thrill may be present with pulmonary or subaortic outflow obstruction. The second heart sound may be single as well. With severe pulmonary stenosis or atresia, a continuous murmur of the patent ductus arteriosus may be heard. In older patients with long-standing pulmonary hypertension, the second heart sound may be single and accentuated.

Postnatal Management

Management of patients with DILV depends on the cardiac anatomy and, in particular, on the presence or absence of outflow tract obstruction. Infants should be delivered in a tertiary care center and postnatal cardiac evaluation should be performed soon after birth. Intravenous prostaglandin therapy should be initiated for those patients with ductal-dependent circulation. A neonatal intervention is often required and may include a systemic-to-pulmonary shunt for obstructed pulmonary blood flow. If severe subaortic obstruction is present, a more complex procedure such as a modified Damus-Kaye-Stansel operation or modified Norwood operation may be required to ensure adequate systemic perfusion.[12] Repair of coarctation of the aorta and other arch anomalies, in conjunction with a pulmonary artery band, although previously used, has fallen out of favor as a reparative strategy. Such patients can develop progressive diminution in VSD size and, hence, progressive subaortic stenosis, which subsequently can be extremely difficult to treat.[13]

Following initial neonatal palliation, the strategy is one of a single-ventricle palliation with ultimate Fontan operation. At approximately 4 to 6 months of life, a bidirectional Glenn (superior cavopulmonary shunt) is typically performed, which provides effective pulmonary blood flow by directing desaturated blood from the superior vena cava directly into the pulmonary arteries. The procedure also reduces ventricular volume loading. The Fontan operation in which inferior vena caval blood flow is channeled to the branch pulmonary arteries is performed at 2 to 3 years of age. The goal of patient management leading up to this procedure is to minimize all possible preoperative risk factors of morbidity and mortality of the Fontan in order to present the best possible candidate for surgery and maximize the chance for success. Current results for this procedure are reassuring and demonstrate low operative and early mortality rates.[14,15]

Outcomes

Rarely, patients with DILV and perfectly balanced circulation can survive into the sixth decade without intervention.[16] Franklin and coworkers published a series of three articles reporting the survival of patients with a single ventricle. There were 191 patients with a double-inlet ventricle, 71% of whom had a dominant ventricle of left ventricular morphology.[16] For patients with DILV, discordant ventriculoarterial connections, and either balanced or restrictive pulmonary blood flow, survival was 96% and 90% at 1 year and 91% and 79% at 10 years, respectively. For those with discordant connections and unobstructed pulmonary blood flow, the 1- and 10-year survival rates were 79% and 60%, respectively.[17]

Studies reporting the outcome for patients who underwent pulmonary band placement demonstrated poor long-term survival if no further interventions were performed. In the second report by Franklin and colleagues,[17] out of 121 patients who underwent pulmonary artery banding, survival was 77% at 1 year and 45% at 5 years. This increased mortality has been associated with subaortic stenosis after pulmonary artery banding, which is a risk factor for those patients with DILV and transposed great arteries. In addition, many of these patients are at risk of myocardial hypertrophy, which is a risk factor for poor outcome after Fontan palliation. In a study by Freedom and associates,[18] functional subaortic obstruction developed in 84% of patients with such anatomy. In addition, a study by Mair and coworkers[14] reviewed 155 patients with DILV and found that 17 patients required subaortic resection at the time of the Fontan, 14 of whom had a prior pulmonary artery band, and an additional 7 required a later operation to relieve the subaortic stenosis.

For those patients with obstructed pulmonary outflow, most commonly, a systemic–to–pulmonary artery shunt is placed early in the neonatal period, which is then followed by a bidirectional cavopulmonary anastamosis and a Fontan completion. Progressive pulmonary stenosis can occur, especially in those patients with a Holmes heart, depending on the initial size of the interventricular communication, the nature of the pulmonary valve, and the infundibulum. Results are similar to other patients with single-ventricle anatomy who undergo this three-stage approach to palliation. Long-term complications of the Fontan operation include ventricular dysfunction, arrhythmias, AV valve regurgitation, development of aortopulmonary collateral blood flow, and protein-losing enteropathy. Progressive left atrial hypertension can also occur if the left AV valve is absent, imperforate, or severely obstructed with a restrictive interatrial communication. Management in infancy should be aimed at optimizing the chances of a successful Fontan procedure because unfavorable outcomes are directly related to the number of preoperative risk factors.

Outcomes for the Fontan operation have improved considerably. Mair and colleagues[14] reported 155 patients with DILV who underwent Fontan palliation. The mortality rate between 1974 and1980 was 21%, but decreased to 9% between 1981 and 1989. Seventeen deaths occurred because of need for reoperation, progressive myocardial failure, sudden arrhythmia, and bleeding varices. At a mean follow-up of 4.9 years, 88% of the patients reported being in good or excellent condition. Seven patients required permanent pacemaker placement for complete heart block, which developed late and was unrelated to prior VSD enlargement or subaortic stenosis resection.

Imaging Essentials and Important Points

- The apical four-chamber view is helpful to determine AV relations and the commitment of the AV valves to the ventricular chambers. DILV is diagnosed if there is drainage of both AV valves either completely or predominantly (>50%) into a dominant chamber of left ventricular morphology. This view also aids in evaluating the misalignment of the atrial and ventricular septa, because the ventricular septum separates the large, well-formed LV from the smaller, abnormally positioned right ventricular outflow chamber.
- Short-axis imaging can help demonstrate ventricular chamber dimensions and ventricular wall thickness and provide a visual estimate of global ventricular contractility.
- Assess AV valve morphology. Short-axis imaging can aid in detailing the valve morphology, straddling of the valve, and the location of the papillary muscles.
- A helpful hint for determining ventricular looping: Both AV valves will drain into the single, large LV. If the AV valve on the right has the morphology of a tricuspid valve with three leaflets and a single papillary muscle, the looping is a "D-looped" ventricle. If the AV valve on the right has the morphology of a mitral valve with two leaflets and two papillary muscles, the looping is one of an "L-looped" ventricle.
- Apical imaging is useful to determine the presence of valve regurgitation and orifice sizes and evaluate for the presence of stenosis.
- Short- and long-axis imaging helps to delineate the VSD and the location of the hypoplastic outlet or rudimentary chamber. Measurement of this communication in comparison with the size of the aortic root can help to determine the risk for subaortic stenosis.
- Apical and parasternal long-/short-axis views are useful for evaluating the anatomy, commitment, and relations of the semilunar valves as well as evaluating for the presence of outflow tract obstruction. If significant subaortic obstruction is seen, it is essential to further image the ascending aorta and the aortic arch to rule out arch obstruction.
- Determination of the direction of ductal flow is useful, especially in the presence of severe pulmonary stenosis in which flow through the ductus arteriosus may be retrograde (aorta to pulmonary artery).
- Assess systemic and pulmonary venous connections to ensure normal venous return.

References

1. Van Praagh R, Van Praagh S, Vlad P, et al. Diagnosis of the anatomic types of single or common ventricle. *Am J Cardiol.* 1965;15:345-366.
2. Snyder AR, Serwer GA, Ritter SB. Ventricular Hypoplasia. In *Echocardiography in Pediatric Heart Disease.* 2nd ed. St. Louis: Mosby-Year Book; 1997:343-363.
3. Srivastava D, Baldwin HS. Molecular determinants of cardiac development. In Allen HD, Gutgesell HP, Clark EB, Driscoll DJ, eds. *Moss and Adams' Heart Disease in Infants, Children, and Adolescents.* Philadelphia: Lippincott Williams & Wilkins; 2001:8-9.
4. Bevilacqua M, Sanders SP, Van Praagh S, Colan SD, Parness I. Double inlet single left ventricle: echocardiographic anatomy with emphasis on the morphology of the atrioventricular valves and ventricular septal defect. *J Am Coll Cardiol.* 1991;18:559-568.
5. Shiraishi H, Silverman NH. Echocardiographic spectrum of double inlet ventricle: evaluation of the interventricular communication. *J Am Coll Cardiol.* 1990;15:1401-1408.
6. Marin-Garcia J, Tandon R, Moller JH, Edwards JE. Common (single) ventricle with normally related great vessels. *Circulation.* 1974;49:565-573.
7. Freedom RM, Benson LN, Smallhorn JF, et al. Subaortic stenosis, the univentricular heart, and banding of the pulmonary artery: an analysis of the courses of 43 patients with univentricular heart palliated by pulmonary artery banding. *Circulation.* 1986;73:758-764.
8. Samanek M, Voriskova M. Congenital heart disease among 815,569 children born between 1980 and 1990 and their 15 year survival: a prospective Bohemia survival study. *Pediatr Cardiol.* 1999;20:411-417.
9. Fyler DC. Report of the New England Regional Infant Cardiac Program. *Pediatrics.* 1980;65(suppl):376-461.
10. Tennstedt C, Chaoui R, Korner H, Dietel M. Spectrum of congenital heart defects and extracardiac malformations associated with chromosomal abnormalities: results of a seven year necropsy study. *Heart.* 1999;82:34-39.
11. Williams RG. Echocardiography in the Management of single ventricle: fetal through adult life. *Echocardiography.* 1993;10:331-342.
12. Jacobs ML, Rychik J, Murphy JD, Nicolson SC, Steven JM, Norwood WI. Results of Norwood's operation for lesions other than hypoplastic left heart syndrome. *J Thorac Cardiovasc Surg.* 1995;110:1555-1561; discussion 1561-1562.
13. Donofrio MT, Jacobs ML, Norwood WI, Rychik J. Early changes in ventricular septal defect size and ventricular geometry in the single left ventricle after volume-unloading surgery. *J Am Coll Cardiol.* 1995;26:1008-1015.
14. Mair DD, Hagler DJ, Julsrud PR, Puga FJ, Schaff HV, Danielson GK. Early and late results of the modified Fontan procedure for double inlet left ventricle: the Mayo Clinic experience. *J Am Coll Cardiol.* 1991;7:1727-1732.
15. Earing MG, Cetta F, Driscoll DJ, et al. Long-term results of the Fontan operation for double-inlet left ventricle. *Am J Cardiol.* 2005;96:291-298.
16. Franklin RC, Spiegelhalter DJ, Anderson RH, et al. Double inlet left ventricle presenting in infancy. I. Survival without definitive repair. *J Thorac Cardiovasc Surg.* 1991;101:767-776.
17. Franklin RC, Spiegelhalter DJ, Anderson RH, et al. Double inlet left ventricle presenting in infancy. II. Results of palliative operations. *J Thorac Cardiovasc Surg.* 1991;101:917-923.
18. Freedom RM, Yoo S. Double inlet ventricle. In Freedom R, Yoo S, Mikailian H, Williams W, eds. *The Natural and Modified History of Congenital Heart Disease.* 1st ed. Boston: Blackwell Publishing; 2004:408-422.

CASES

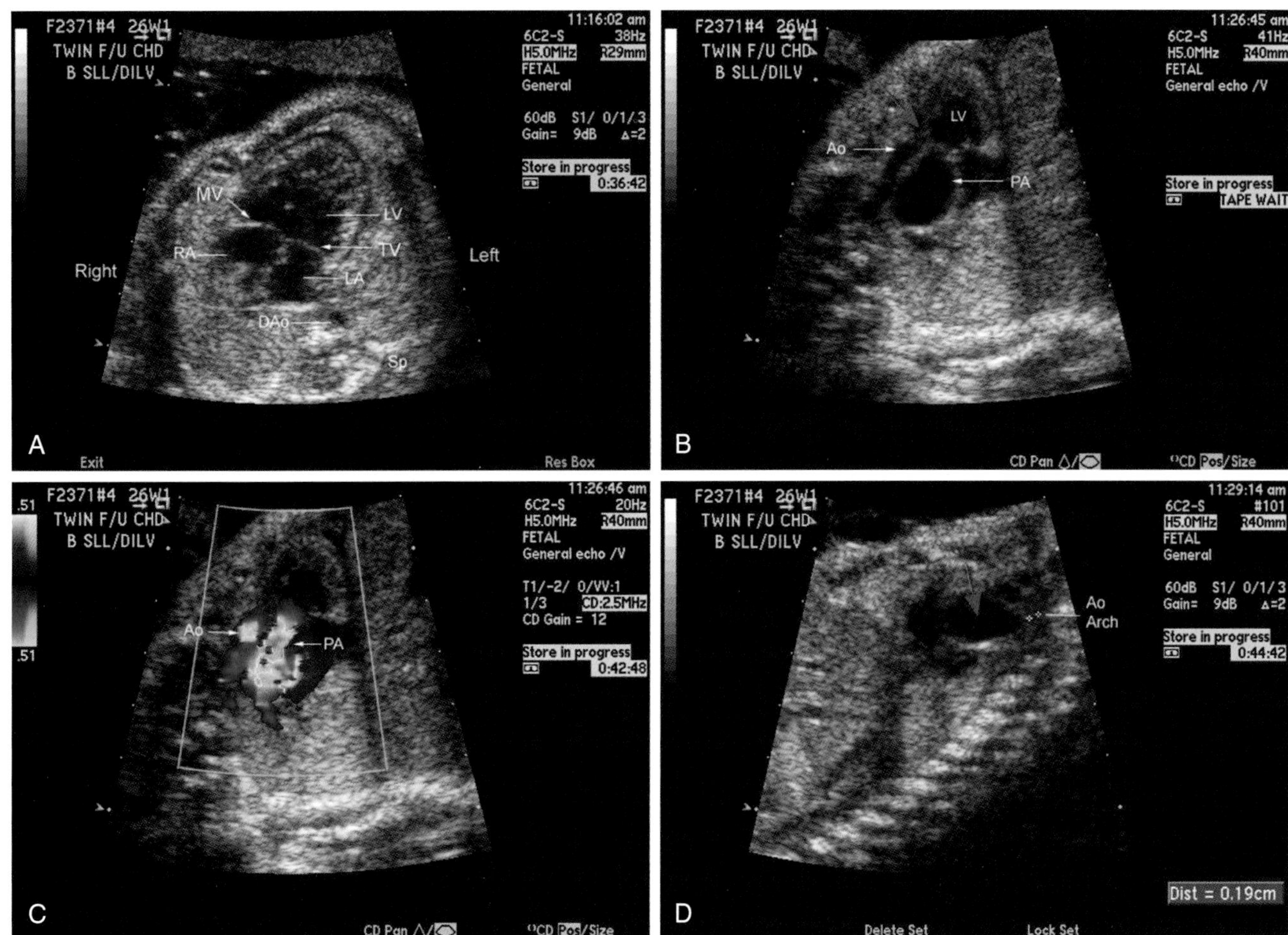

Case 29-1. **(A)** Fetus at 26 weeks' gestation with double-inlet left ventricle {S,L,L}. There are two well-formed atrioventricular valves, with tricuspid valve (TV) on the left side draining the left atrium (LA) into the left ventricle (LV) and a mitral valve (MV) on the right side draining the right atrium (RA). DAo, descending aorta; Sp, spine. **(B)** Long-axis view of the great vessels arising from the heart. The pulmonary artery (PA) arises from the LV and is aneurysmally dilated as the pulmonary valve is thickened and there is mild pulmonic stenosis. The aorta (Ao) is to the left of the PA and is hypoplastic. The Ao arises from a miniscule, very small right ventricle *(red arrow)*. **(C)** Color flow imaging of the great vessels. Both the Ao and the pulmonary artery (PA) arise from the heart in parallel, with the Ao to the left. **(D)** The transverse portion of the aortic arch (Ao Arch) is very small. The main pulmonary artery is dilated *(red arrow)*.

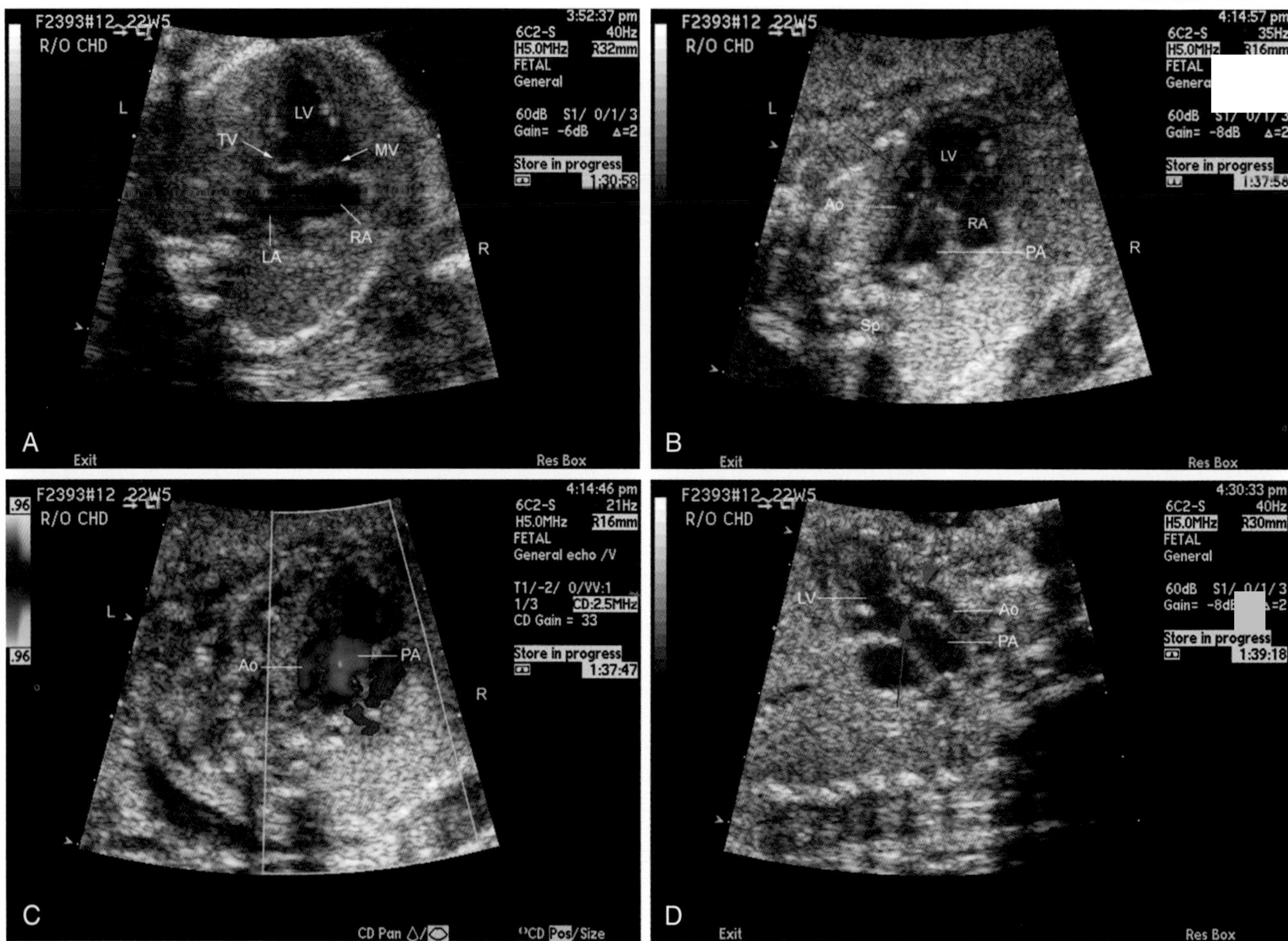

Case 29-2. **(A)** Fetus at 22 weeks and 5 days' gestation with double-inlet left ventricle (LV). The apex is up in this image. Note the "bullet" shape to the LV, typical for a morphological LV. The ventricular configuration is "L-looped"; hence, the mitral valve (MV) drains the right atrium (RA) on the right and the tricuspid valve (TV) drains the left atrium (LA) on the left. The TV is hypoplastic and is smaller in diameter than the MV. **(B)** Imaging of the origins of the great vessels. Both the aorta (Ao) and the pulmonary artery (PA) arise in parallel with the Ao to the left of the PA. Note the small hypoplastic right ventricle *(red arrow)* beneath the Ao, which communicates with the left ventricle (LV) via a small, restrictive ventricular septal defect. Sp, spine. **(C)** Color flow imaging of the Ao and the PA side-by-side with Ao to the left. **(D)** Long-axis view demonstrates the Ao anterior to the PA and arising from a small anteriorly positioned right ventricle *(blue arrow)*. Note the small restrictive ventricular septal defect *(red arrow)*, which is much smaller in diameter than the aortic annulus.

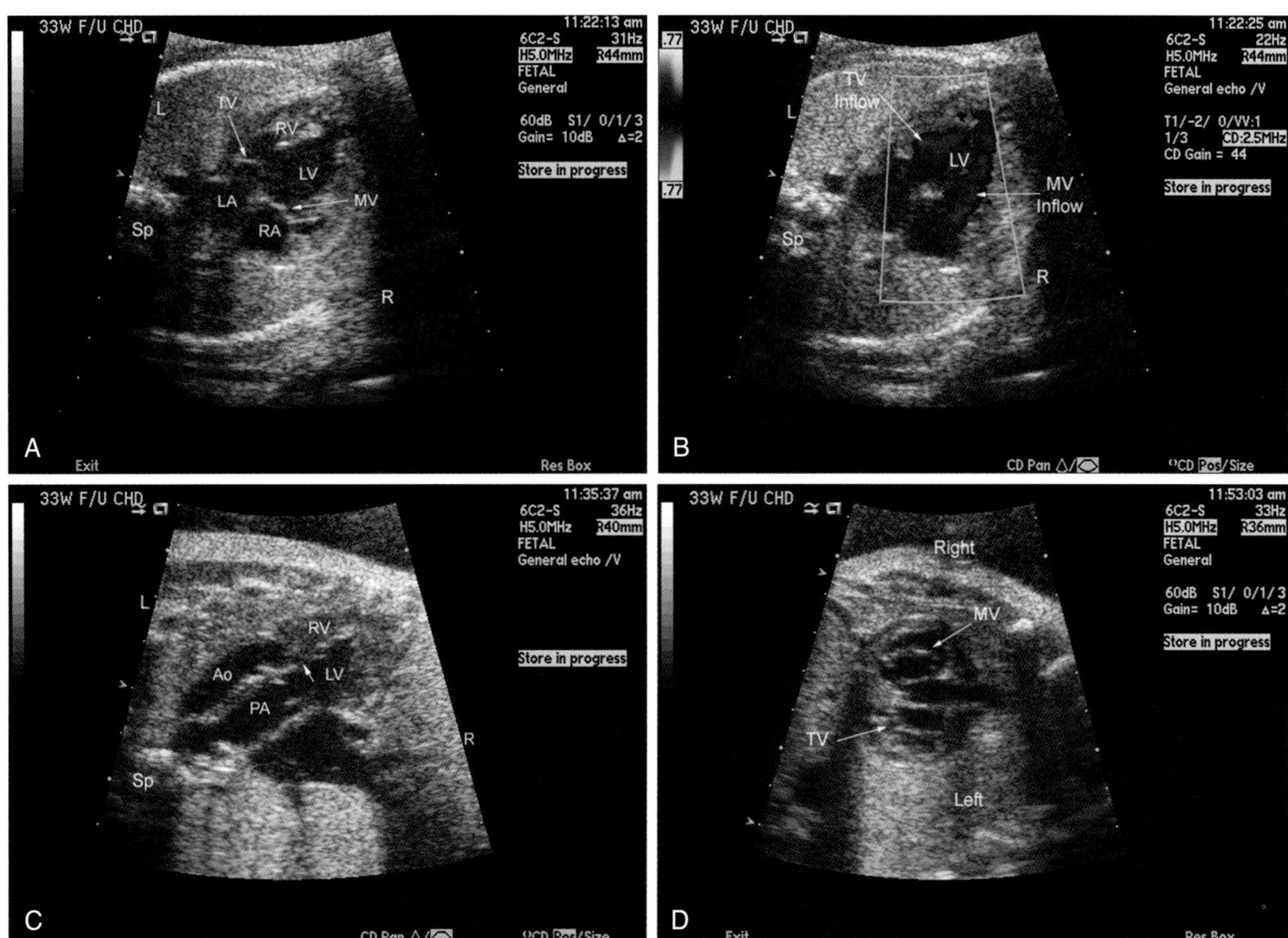

Case 29-3. (**A**) Fetus at 33 weeks' gestation with double-inlet left ventricle (LV). There is a dominant LV and a smaller right ventricle (RV). LA, left atrium; MV, mitral valve; RA, right atrium; TV, tricuspid valve; Sp, spine. (**B**) Color flow imaging demonstrates inflow into the dominant LV from both the left-sided TV and the right-sided MV. (**C**) The pulmonary artery (PA) arises from the LV and the aorta (Ao) from the RV. The RV communicates with the LV through a small restrictive ventricular septal defect *(arrow)*. (**D**) Short-axis of the double-inlet LV at the level of the atrioventricular valves. Note both atrioventricular valves drain into a single large LV. The valve seen superiorly on the right is morphologically of MV appearance in that there is a "fish-mouth" with two leaflets. The inferior leftward valve is morphologically of tricuspid appearance in that it is anchored by a single papillary muscle and has attachment to the ventricular septum between the LV and the smaller RV.

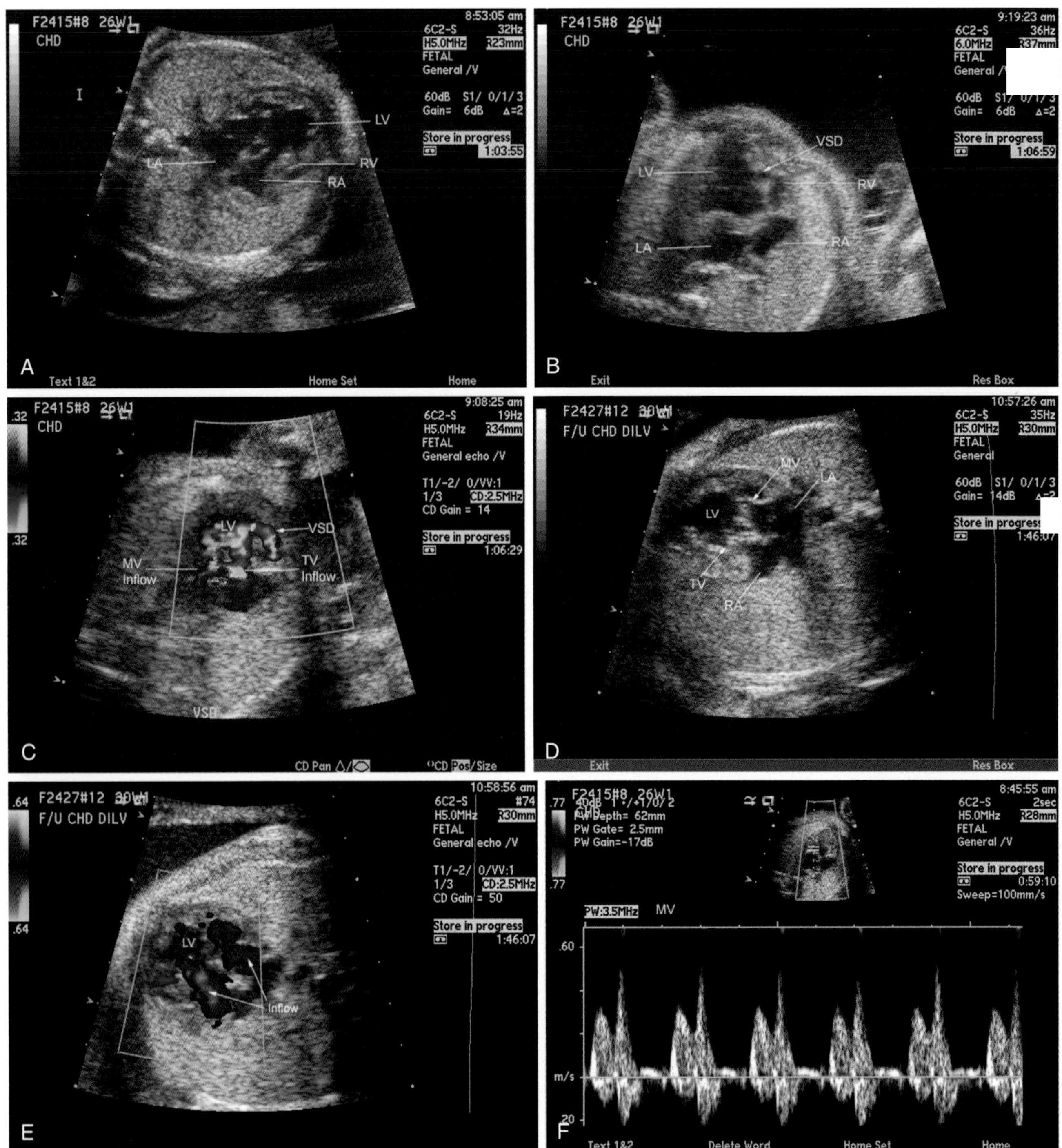

Case 29-4. **(A)** Fetus at 26 weeks' gestation with double-inlet left ventricle (LV), but normally related great vessels with segments {S,D,S} otherwise known as the "Holmes heart." Both atrioventricular valves drain into the dominant large LV. There is a small right ventricle (RV) positioned rightward, which gives rise to the pulmonary artery. Only a small part of the RV and the communicating ventricular septal defect can be seen in this image. LA, left atrium; RA, right atrium. **(B)** With the apex of the heart up, the shape and morphology of the LV is well appreciated as is the small RV and the communicating ventricular septal defect (VSD). **(C)** Color flow imaging demonstrates double-inlet into the large LV and a restrictive VSD communicating with the RV. MV, mitral valve; TV, tricuspid valve. **(D)** Long-axis view demonstrates both the TV and the MV drain into the large LV. The MV drains the LA and the TV drains the RA. **(E)** Color flow imaging demonstrates that both atrioventricular valves drain into the large LV. **(F)** Doppler inflow across the left-sided MV draining into the LV. Normal flow pattern.

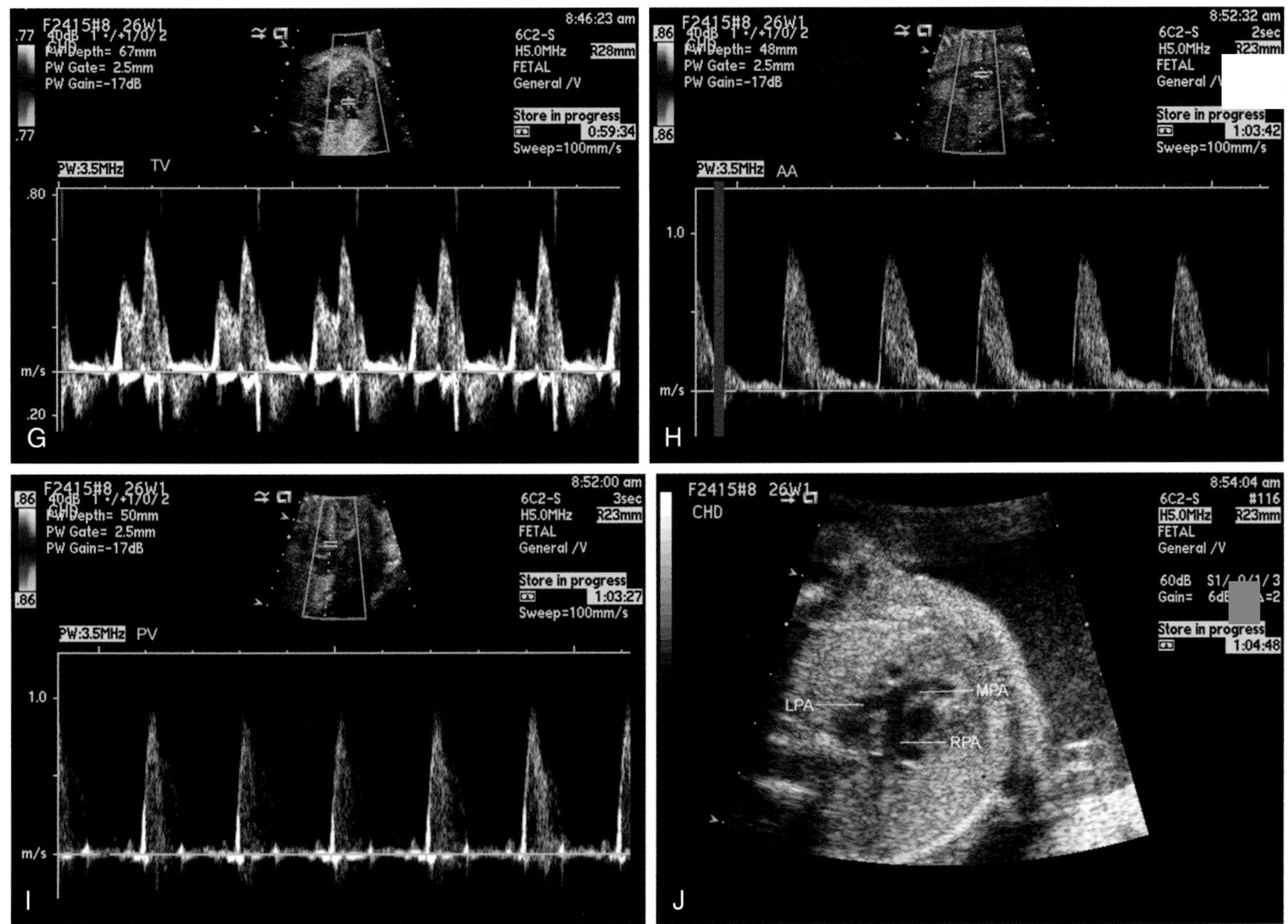

Case 29-4, cont'd **(G)** Doppler inflow across the right-sided TV draining into the LV. Normal flow pattern. **(H)** Doppler flow interrogation within the ascending aorta (AA), which arises from the LV in an unobstructed manner, demonstrates normal laminar flow. **(I)** Doppler flow interrogation across the pulmonary valve (PV) demonstrates mild turbulence of flow and slight increased velocity, as the pulmonary artery arises from the smaller RV. **(J)** Cross-sectional view above the heart at the level of the great vessels shows a relatively normal relationship in this case of double-inlet LV, but normally related great vessels {S,D,S}. LPA, left pulmonary artery; MPA, main pulmonary artery; RPA, right pulmonary artery.

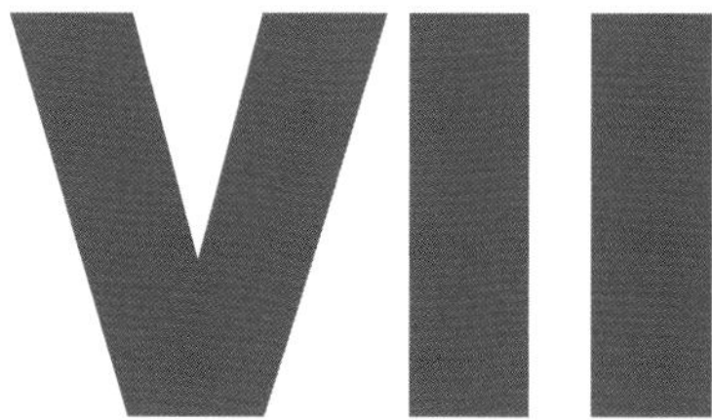

Primary Anomalies and Disorders Affecting the Cardiovascular System in the Fetus

30

Cardiac Masses and Tumors

Donna A. Goff

Key Echocardiographic Features

- Locate the position of the mass within the heart.
- Search for multiple masses and identify the number of masses seen.
- Determine whether the mass is obstructing either right or left ventricular outflow.
- Determine whether the mass is obstructing right or left ventricular inflow across the tricuspid or mitral valves.
- Identify whether there is any distortion of the atrioventricular valve apparatus and presence/degree of atrioventricular valve regurgitation.
- Determine whether the mass is occupying ventricular cavity space and to what degree there may be limitation of ventricular filling.
- Look for heart rate irregularity that may reflect arrhythmia related to the mass.

Cardiac tumors are a relatively rare pathology seen in the fetus. Owing to the timing of ultrasound screening, the true incidence of tumors in utero is difficult to ascertain. Some tumors only increase in size over the course of the latter half of pregnancy, limiting detection in the second trimester when screening ultrasounds are typically performed. Most referrals for fetal echocardiograms are a result of detection of a mass, a pericardial effusion on screening ultrasound, arrhythmias, or family history of tuberous sclerosis.[1,2] Unless the fetus has significant hemodynamic derangements or arrhythmias, they may not present for a fetal echocardiographic evaluation and may go undiagnosed until the neonatal period.[1,3,4] Two cases of symptomatic neonates with cardiac tumors at birth were reported to have normal fetal echocardiograms at 26 and 38 weeks, respectively, demonstrating this point.[3] One patient presented with fetal hydrops at term and was found to have a large left ventricular tumor infiltrating the right ventricle (RV) and atria; diagnosis of a fibroma was made after neonatal demise. The other neonate presented with supraventricular tachyarrhythmia (SVT), was electively delivered, and did well clinically after antiarrhythmic therapy. Postnatal echocardiography demonstrated a small right ventricular mass that was presumed to be a rhabdomyoma.

In a large multicenter study, cardiac tumors were diagnosed in 19 (0.14%) out of 14,000 fetal echocardiograms performed over an 8-year period.[5] The gestational age at diagnosis ranged from 21 to 38 weeks, with rhabdomyoma occurring in the majority of fetuses along with a few cases of fibromas and hemangiomas. In a review of 10,000 fetal echocardiograms from a 12-year period, 11 cardiac tumors (0.1 %) (10 rhabdomyomas, 1 intrapericardial teratoma) were diagnosed in fetuses with gestational ages ranging from 20 to 34 weeks.[1] In a summary of 91 fetal and newborn cases from the literature, rhabdomyoma was the most common tumor accounting for 50% of the cases, followed by teratoma (21%), fibroma (12%), myxoma (8%), and hemangioma (4%) along with the rare occurrence of the malignant tumors rhabdomyosarcoma (3%) and fibrolipoma (1%).[6]

At the Fetal Heart Program at the Children's Hospital of Philadelphia during an 8-year period between 2000 and 2008, there were 17 fetal diagnoses of cardiac tumors. Most of the tumors were solitary (13/17) and were either rhabdomyomas, fibromas, or pericardial teratoma based on the echocardiographic features. Multiple tumors were found in 4 cases consistent with the diagnosis of rhabdomyoma.

In some cases, cardiac neoplasms in the fetus may be the first indication of a genetic disorder including tuberous sclerosis, neurofibromatosis, Gorlin's syndrome (nevoid basal cell carcinoma syndrome), familial myxomas, and Beckwith-Wiedemann syndrome. Although the majority of tumors in the fetus and neonate are histologically benign, their size and location can cause pericardial effusions, compromised blood flow, arrhythmias, myocardial dysfunction, or hydrops fetalis ultimately leading to in utero demise.[7]

Conservative management is the usual approach for fetuses without arrhythmias or hemodynamic compromise. Depending on the gestational age, fetuses with recalcitrant arrhythmias, increasing pericardial effusions, or significant hemodynamic compromise are delivered with anticipation for cardiac surgery to resect the tumor or tumors if technically feasible.[8] Although fetal intervention has been reported for pericardial teratomas, currently, there are no options for prenatal therapy for fetuses with rhabdomyomas and fibromas. Fetal pericardiocentesis was performed in a 28-week fetus with an intrapericardial teratoma after the tumor was noted to be increasing in size with development of pericardial effusion along with concern for progression to hydrops.[9] Although the effusion reaccumulated and hydrops developed at 33 weeks, lung maturity was documented and the patient was delivered at 34 weeks. The patient was immediately taken to surgery for resection of the tumor and did well clinically.

The natural history of cardiac tumors varies depending on their histological composition and anatomical location. Anatomy, pathophysiology, intervention, and clinical outcome are described in the following sections for each individual type of tumor.

Rhabdomyoma

Anatomy and Anatomical Associations

Rhabdomyomas are found most often within the ventricular wall and septum, subepicardial region, and atria and can be single or multiple in nature. Typically, these tumors are not associated with congenital heart lesions, although sporadic cases of rhabdomyoma associated with endocardial fibroelastosis, tetralogy of Fallot, and hypoplastic left heart syndrome have been reported.[5,6,10]

Frequency, Genetics, and Development

Rhabdomyomas are the most common cardiac tumor seen in fetuses, infants, and children.[8] In multiple fetal studies, rhabdomyomas were the predominant lesion ranging from 50% to 91% of the cases.[1-3,5] A summary of 91 fetal cardiac tumor cases reported in the literature found 50% of these cases to be rhabdomyomas.[6]

Rhabdomyomas or hamartomas are considered to be overgrowths of cardiac muscle with only mildly abnormal changes and without true neoplasia. Grossly, these single or multiple tumors are composed of white to yellow-tan circumscribed nodules in the myocardium, primarily in the ventricular wall or septum or subepicardial region of the atria.

Cardiac rhabdomyomas, particularly when there are multiple tumors, have been shown to be the earliest marker of tuberous sclerosis in utero.[7] Tuberous sclerosis is an autosomal dominant disorder with variable expression and penetrance.[11] It effects multiple organs and can result in neurological manifestations including developmental delay and seizures in early childhood. Hamartomas can occur in the skin, eyes, kidney, heart, and brain with the most clinically significant morbidity being the neurological manifestations that may not be present until early childhood. Several small studies have reported the diagnosis of tuberous sclerosis in fetuses or neonates with cardiac rhabdomyomas.[12-15] In one study, 9/11 (81.1%) cases of rhabdomyoma were diagnosed with tuberous sclerosis.[12] In follow-up of patients diagnosed with fetal rhabdomyoma, 15/19 (79%) were diagnosed with tuberous sclerosis. Of these cases with documented tuberous sclerosis, 5 had a fetal brain magnetic resonance imaging (MRI) study suggestive of the disease.[13] In a meta-analysis of 138 cases of prenatal diagnosis of cardiac rhabdomyoma, tuberous sclerosis was present in 85/133 (64%) cases, with multiple tumors being predictive of the disease. Although some studies have shown that multiple rhabdomyomas are predictive of tuberous sclerosis,[14,15] it is unclear whether the same is true for single tumors.[12,13] Because of the significant neurological manifestations that present later in childhood and the limited data available at this time regarding the association of the disease with single rhabdomyomas, fetal diagnosis of a cardiac rhabdomyoma typically leads to further evaluation for tuberous sclerosis. We typically perform fetal MRIs looking for hamartomas in the brain and/or kidneys that contribute to confirmation of the diagnosis. However, it is also known that many of these brain lesions develop after birth, so a clean MRI with no findings, unfortunately, does not rule out the possibility of tuberous sclerosis. In familial cases, molecular testing for mutations in tumor suppressor genes *TSC1* or *TSC2* may be useful because these genes have been implicated in tuberous sclerosis.[7,11] Genetic testing is less helpful in confirmation of tuberous sclerosis in cases without a family history because there is a high likelihood of de novo mutation reportedly as high as 60% to -80%.[11,13] Although sporadic mutations occur with high frequency, fetal diagnosis of a rhabdomyoma with an unknown family history should lead to further evaluation for the disease in parents and siblings.

Prenatal Physiology

Cardiac rhabdomyomas have been detected as early as 18 weeks by fetal echocardiograms.[15] These tumors have distinct echocardiographic features: highly echogenic, well circumscribed, intramural, or intracavitary nodules that sometimes are pedunculated with a homogenous, echobright, finely speckled pattern.[8] Dystrophic calcification of the fetal myocardium can have similar appearances by ultrasound.[16] In half of the cases, these tumors are asymptomatic and discovered only on routine ultrasonography, whereas the other half present secondary to arrhythmias or outflow tract obstruction.[7]

Fetal arrhythmias, either tachyarrhythmias or bradycardias, have been reported in fetuses with rhabdomyomas.[5,17] Left uncontrolled, these can lead to myocardial dysfunction and hydrops. Depending on the location and size of the tumor, there may also be a spectrum of hemodynamic effects ranging from being asymptomatic to poor cardiac output or elevation of venous pressures leading to hydrops.[15,17]

Prenatal Management

Prenatally, limited interventions are available for the fetus with a rhabdomyoma. If the patient develops an arrhythmia such as SVT, drug therapies such as digoxin and sotalol potentially can help control the rapid rate by treating the mother with medication. If the patient develops hemodynamic compromise such as low cardiac output or hydrops as a result of obstruction, the only option, depending on gestational age, is early delivery. Close follow-up is essential because these tumors may remain stable or increase in size during the course of pregnancy.[12,17] Therefore, it is important to perform sequential echocardiograms to monitor the tumor size and hemodynamic changes that may develop.

Postnatal Physiology

Just as described in the fetus, the impact of cardiac tumors on hemodynamics during the neonatal period depends on the location and size of the tumor. Large tumors can cause significant hemodynamic instability leading to the neonate who is critically ill with respiratory distress, congestive heart failure, and low cardiac output. Large rhabdomyomas that are located on the left side of the heart can cause inflow and left ventricular outflow tract obstruction and, if large enough, act as a space-occupying lesion essentially mimicking anomalies such as hypoplastic left heart syndrome. Those on the right side of the heart can cause inflow or right ventricular outflow tract obstruction, resulting in signs and symptoms of right-sided failure and cyanosis, and can mimic lesions such as tricuspid atresia or critical valvar pulmonic stenosis. Neonates may also present with rhythm issues: sinus bradycardia, atrial and ventricular tachyarrhythmias, or first- to third-degree heart block.[8]

Postnatal Management

If the neonate is completely asymptomatic, the approach is to follow conservatively because most rhabdomyomas regress over time.[1,8,18] In contrast, surgical intervention may be necessary if there is compromise of the cardiac output secondary to inflow or outflow obstruction. If there is significant right ventricular or left ventricular outflow tract obstruction, the patient should be started on prostaglandin E1 (PGE_1) infusion. Medical management for heart failure with dopamine and milrinone may need to be initiated to stabilize those who have low cardiac output and poor perfusion. If arrhythmias are contributing to cardiac instability, antiarrhythmic therapy should be added to the treatment regimen.

Outcomes

Rhabdomyomas generally have a favorable outcome with survival for fetuses ranging from 94% to 100%. In a meta-analysis of 138 rhabdomyoma cases summarized from the literature, large cardiac tumor size, fetal dysrhythmias, and hydrops were found to be predictors of a poor prenatal outcome.[15] In another prenatal series, 6/9 fetuses had increase tumor growth up until 30 to 32 weeks' gestation without hemodynamic compromise. In the neonatal period, no patient required medical therapy for arrhythmias or cardiac surgery. Median follow-up was 4.2 years and there was at least partial regression of the tumor. Tuberous sclerosis was diagnosed in 6/9 (67%) cases, with some patients requiring neurosurgery whereas others had neurological symptoms.[12]

In another series of 19 fetuses diagnosed with rhabdomyomas, there was one spontaneous in utero demise at 28 weeks.[13] There was no hemodynamic compromise in the others during the course of the pregnancy. During the neonatal period, 7/19 had cardiac symptoms requiring medical therapy or surgical intervention. Tuberous sclerosis was diagnosed in 15/19 (79%) patients. Beyond the neonatal period in patients for whom clinical information was available, 10/16 were asymptomatic from a cardiovascular standpoint, and in 10/16, tumors spontaneously regressed. In 1 patient, there was substantial tumor growth in utero requiring surgical intervention in the neonatal period.[13]

Teratoma

Anatomy and Anatomical Associations

Teratomas develop primarily from the pericardium and attach to roots of the pulmonary and aortic arteries. Depending upon their size, they can compress adjacent atria or ventricles. A large number of these tumors are located anteriorly and to the right of the heart, causing compression of the cardiac chambers, great vessels, or even the trachea.[19] Occasionally, they occur within the atrium or ventricle. Of the 19 cases summarized from reports in the literature, 17 were intrapericardial with only 2 occurring within the heart, 1 in the right ventricle and the other in the interatrial and interventricular septum.[6,7] There are no reported associations with other congenital heart lesions with this tumor.

Frequency, Genetics, and Development

Intrapericardial teratomas are rare cardiac tumors but are the second most common tumor diagnosed in fetuses and newborns. Grossly, these tumors have a smooth, lobulated surface comprising numerous loculated cysts lined with a variety of epithelia. There are typically intervening solid areas composed of mature or immature neuroglial tissue with thyroid, pancreas, smooth and skeletal muscle, and foci of cartilage and bone. Histologically, these tumors contain all three germ layers: endoderm, mesoderm, and ectoderm.[6,7] To date, there have been no reports of associations with genetic syndromes and no etiology has been identified.

Prenatal Physiology

Teratomas are heterogeneous with cystic components and pericardial calcification, along with the common finding of pericardial effusions and sometimes pleural effusions.[1] They have distinct findings on echocardiogram with cystic areas appearing echolucent and calcifications as echogenic foci.[8] Review of 31 cases reported in the literature reveals that most present with pericardial effusions in the second and third trimesters with 77% of fetuses developing hydrops without intervention.[19] At least in two reported cases, both with pericardial effusions, systolic function was maintained. In both cases, Doppler hemodynamics were normal upon initial evaluation, but in one of the cases a week later, there was an abnormal single peak inflow suggesting compromised filling of the ventricle along with a wave reversal in the ductus venosus and umbilical venous pulsations. These findings are consistent with elevated venous pressures secondary to obstruction from the mass and can come on quite rapidly.[19] Although limited data are available, it appears that Doppler assessment may be useful in determining hemodynamic compromise with this potentially rapid-growing tumor.

Prenatal Management

Intrapericardial teratoma is the only tumor that is amenable to fetal intervention when hydrops and a large pericardial effusion are present. There are numerous reports of successful fetal pericardiocentesis.[9,13,20] It has been suggested by one group that fetal pericardiocentesis is warranted when there is early hydrops with a large pericardial effusion and a small mass. If there is a large mass associated with a large effusion, fetal surgery with resection is likely more efficacious, because there is a low likelihood of having a substantial effect on improving cardiovascular hemodynamics with simple drainage of the pericardial fluid alone.[9] If no hydrops is present, the patient can be followed closely.

Postnatal Physiology

As with all mass lesions, physiology will be variable depending on the location and size of the lesion. If there is a large pericardial effusion, this may need to be drained urgently at birth, if it is found to be causing tamponade symptoms. If the mass is causing significant cardiac compression, there may be cyanosis or low cardiac output necessitating urgent surgical intervention to remove the mass.

Postnatal Management

Some have suggested that a cesarean delivery should be planned because of the risk of cardiac compression during vaginal delivery and the high likelihood of early neonatal distress because the mass may impair the normal transitional physiology. Delivery at a tertiary care center with a neonatal intensive care unit, pediatric surgery, or pediatric cardiac team is important because most patients will require surgery at some point during the neonatal period.[20]

Outcomes

Analysis of 31 fetal cases of intrapericardial teratoma in the literature revealed a survival rate of 58% after all underwent successful surgical intervention in the neonatal period.[19] Long term, once the tumor is removed, these patients typically do well.[8,18]

Fibroma

Anatomy and Anatomical Associations

Cardiac fibromas carry a variety of different names and are included in the terms *fibromatosis, myofibromatosis, fibrous hamartoma,* and *congenital mesoblastic tumor.* These tumors are usually solitary and most commonly arise from the myocardium of the interventricular septum or left ventricular free wall and, less commonly, from right ventricular free wall or cavity. Other congenital heart lesions have not been found in association with this tumor.

Frequency, Genetics, and Development

Cardiac fibromas are very rare tumors and in multiple studies are the third most frequent tumor of the fetal heart.[6] Cardiac fibromas are the second most common reported in infancy and childhood.[21] These tumors have a connective tissue origin. Grossly, they have a firm, white myxoid or trabeculated appearance and may be circumscribed and distinct from, or unencapsulated and blending in with, the myocardium. Histologically, they are composed of spindle-shaped fibroblast cells surrounded by a collagenous matrix. The central aspect of the tumor may have calcification, hematopoesis, elastic fibers, and sometimes microcystic changes.[7] Calcification and cystic changes help differentiate this tumor from a single rhabdomyoma.

Although extracardiac malformations are rare, there have been reports of associations with cleft lip and palate, Beckwith-Wiedemann, and most often with Gorlin's syndrome (nevoid basal cell carcinoma syndrome).[7] The heart may also become involved in congenital generalized fibromatosis, which is associated with a very poor prognosis.[6]

Prenatal Physiology

As previously described for other tumors, the location of the tumor influences the impact on the fetal cardiac physiology. If the tumor develops from the interventricular septum, it may involve the conduction system, predisposing to heart block and arrhythmias such as ventricular tachycardia and ventricular fibrillation. Left or right ventricular inflow or outflow obstruction may develop as a result of tumors located in the free wall or even the interventricular septum.[7] Cardiomegaly and congestive heart failure may develop. In addition, sudden cardiac death may occur as a result of ventricular fibrillation.

Prenatal Management

For fetuses with fibromas that have hemodynamic compromise as a result of the mass or arrhythmia, there are no current options for prenatal therapy. The only option at this time is premature delivery if the fetus is at a gestational age at which the fetal lungs are mature.

Postnatal Physiology

As noted for other tumors, the impact of cardiac tumors on hemodynamics during the neonatal period depends on the location and size of the tumor. Large tumors can cause significant hemodynamic instability, leading to the neonate who is critically ill with respiratory distress, congestive heart failure, and low cardiac output. Large intramural fibromas can obstruct the intracavitary space, causing subaortic stenosis and subpulmonic stenosis. Similar to rhabdomyomas, if the tumor is located on the right side of the heart, it can cause inflow or right ventricular outflow tract obstruction causing signs and symptoms of right-sided failure and cyanosis. Right-sided tumors may mimic lesions such as critical valvar pulmonic stenosis or pulmonary atresia. Neonates may also present with rhythm issues: sinus bradycardia, atrial and ventricular tachyarrhythmias, or first- to third-degree heart block.[8]

Postnatal Management

Urgent surgical intervention may be necessary if there is compromise of cardiac output secondary to inflow or outflow obstruction. If the patient has significant right ventricular or left ventricular outflow tract obstruction, the patient should be started on PGE_1 infusion. Medical management for heart failure with dopamine and milrinone may need to be initiated to stabilize patients who have low cardiac output and poor perfusion. If arrhythmias are contributing to cardiac instability, antiarrhythmic therapy should be added to the treatment regimen.[8] Depending on the location of the tumor, partial or complete resection of the tumor may be feasible. In some cases, transplant may be the only option when complete resection is not technically possible as a result of the size or location of the tumor.[21]

Outcomes

Outcomes are dependent on multiple factors including size, location of tumor, effect on hemodynamics, and whether the tumor is partially or completely resectable. In the majority of cases, surgical resection is necessary because these tumors tend not to regress over time and, if located in the ventricular septum, can predispose to ventricular arrhythmias leading to sudden cardiac death.[21]

Myxomas

Anatomy and Anatomical Associations

Myxomas are quite rare in infants and children. Of the seven neonatal cases compiled from the literature, the most common site is in the right atrium (4/7) followed by the left ventricle and pulmonary valve. This is in stark contrast to the location in the left atrium that is most commonly seen in adults. In the one fetal case reported in the literature, the mass was found attached to the right atrium and to the right atrial wall by a long peduncle and increased in size during the pregnancy without causing any hemodynamic compromise.[22]

Frequency, Genetics, and Development

To date, there has been only one documented case report of fetal echocardiographic diagnosis of a cardiac myxoma at 23 weeks' gestation.[22] Myxomas are thought to arise from the subendocardial multipotential mesenchymal cells with potential for differentiation into myofibroblast, fibroblasts, smooth muscle cells, or endothelial cells. Grossly, they tend to be masses that are polypoid, soft, gelatinous, friable, grayish/white, and mucoid with foci of hemorrhage or thrombus formation. The genetic etiology of this lesion has not been described.

Prenatal Physiology

In the one fetal case, the mass had moderate echogenicity and was pedunculated. Throughout pregnancy, there was no hemodynamic compromise. The mass was noted to pass through the foramen ovale into the right atrium and ventricle.

Prenatal Management

Because there is only one reported case and there was no hemodynamic compromise, the prenatal management was conservative. Elective surgery can be planned.

Postnatal Physiology

Clinical signs and symptoms reported in neonates are cardiomegaly, congestive heart failure, and cyanosis. Some infants, depending on the location of the tumor, also present with a murmur.

Postnatal Management

Postnatal management usually involves surgical resection because embolism of the tumor is a possibility.

Outcomes

Despite intervention, the outcome of neonatal diagnosis was quite poor with only one of seven neonates surviving with this neoplasm.[7]

Cardiac and Pericardial Hemangiomas

Anatomy and Anatomical Associations

Cardiac hemangiomas are incredibly rare tumors in infants and children. In children, these tumors may be intracavitary, on the epicardial surface of the heart or pericardium. In contrast, in the fetus, these tumors are typically found in the lateral wall of the right atrium. Histologically, there are *cavernous* hemangiomas composed of many dilated thin-walled vessel and *capillary* hemangiomas consisting of lobules of smaller vessels resembling capillaries that are found on the endocardium. Intramyocardial hemangiomas have histological features that are similar to intramuscular hemangiomas. In neonates with multiple cutaneous hemangiomas, there should be a high suspicion for such a tumor.[6]

Frequency, Genetics, and Development

Because these tumors are quite rare, there have been only a few case reports of diagnosis in the fetus.[23,24] Of the 91 fetal and newborn cardiac tumor cases summarized from the literature, only 4 were hemangiomas.[6]

Prenatal Physiology

The cardiac manifestations are dependent on the size and location of the mass within the right atrium. If the mass causes inflow obstruction, there can be low cardiac output with development of hydrops and pericardial effusions, which is the more common finding.

Prenatal Management

Because this is quite a rare tumor and the most common presenting symptom is a pericardial effusion, the outcome is dependent on whether there is significant hydrops leading to preterm delivery. Because of the potential development of pericardial effusions and potential tamponade in utero,[23] regular serial fetal echocardiograms should be performed.

Postnatal Physiology

The cardiac manifestations are dependent on the size and location of the mass within the right atrium. If the mass causes inflow obstruction, there can be low cardiac output, with right-to-left atrial level shunting and cyanosis. Pericardial effusions are a common finding and may lead to tamponade symptoms of tachycardia, hypotension, and pulsus paradoxus requiring urgent pericardiocentesis.

Postnatal Management

As noted for other tumors, the impact of cardiac tumors on hemodynamics during the neonatal period depends on the location and size of the tumor. Typically, these tumors cause development of pericardial effusions that can potentially lead to tamponade symptoms requiring urgent pericardiocentesis.

Outcomes

Because this is quite a rare tumor and the most common presenting symptom is a pericardial effusion, the outcome is dependent on whether there is significant hydrops leading to preterm delivery. In general, these vascular tumors tend to regress over time.

Imaging Essentials and Important Points

- For all fetal tumors, the location, number, and size have bearing on prognosis.
- Use different imaging frequencies and switch between harmonic and fundamental imaging frequencies in order to characterize as best as possible the echo "texture" of the tumor. For example, the finding of a capsule around a fetal tumor suggests for the presence of a fibroma. Look to see whether the tumor is homogeneous, cystic, with calcifications, or whether there is vascular flow identified within.
- The impact of other imaging modalities such as cardiac MRI have not yet been established but are worth exploring in these rare circumstances, in order to best attempt to determine prognosis.
- Look for secondary effects of the tumor on overall wellness of the fetal cardiovascular system. The following features aid in providing an overall measure of stability, or lack thereof when there is a fetal cardiac tumor:
  - Presence of pericardial effusion.
  - Presence of pleural effusion.
  - Hydrops.
  - Tricuspid or mitral regurgitation.
  - Degree of distortion of the position and axis of the heart within the chest.
  - Tricuspid or mitral inflow obstruction.
  - Right or left ventricular outflow obstruction.
  - Irregularity of rhythm.
  - Relative ratio of the middle cerebral artery (MCA) and umbilical artery (UA) pulsatility indices as a measure of the ratio of vascular resistances. In a healthy fetus, the MCA pulsatility index (vascular resistance) should be higher than the UA pulsatility index. A MCA/UA pulsatility index ratio less than 1 reflects low cardiac output and is a compensatory attempt to increase cerebral blood flow.
  - Doppler-derived measurement of individual ventricle, or combined cardiac output, can help gauge the impact of a tumor on perfusion.

References

1. Groves AM, Fagg NL, Cook AC, et al. Cardiac tumours in intrauterine life. *Arch Dis Child*. 1992;67:1189-1192.
2. Zhou QC, Fan P, Peng QH, et al. Prenatal echocardiographic differential diagnosis of fetal cardiac tumors. *Ultrasound Obstet Gynecol*. 2004;23:165-171.
3. Geipel A, Krapp M, Germer U, et al. Perinatal diagnosis of cardiac tumors. *Ultrasound Obstet Gynecol*. 2001;17:17-21.
4. Yagel S, Weissman A, Rotstein Z, et al. Congenital heart defects: natural course and in utero development. *Circulation*. 1997;96:550-555.

5. Holley DG, Martin GR, Brenner JI, et al. Diagnosis and management of fetal cardiac tumors: a multicenter experience and review of published reports. *J Am Coll Cardiol.* 1995;26:516-520.
6. Isaacs H Jr. *Tumors of the Fetus and Newborn. Major Problems in Pathology;* vol 35. Philadelphia: WB Saunders; 1997:330-343.
7. Isaacs H Jr. Fetal and neonatal cardiac tumors. *Pediatr Cardiol.* 2004; 25:252-273.
8. Marx G, Moran A. Cardiac tumors. In Allen H, Driscoll DJ, Shaddy RE, Feltes TF, eds. *Moss and Adams' Heart Disease in Infants, Children and Adolescents.* Philadelphia: Wolters Kluwer/Lippincott Williams & Wilkins; 2008:1479-1494.
9. Bruch SW, Adzick NS, Reiss R, et al. Prenatal therapy for pericardial teratomas. *J Pediatr Surg.* 1997;32:1113-1115.
10. Watanabe T, Hojo Y, Kozaki T, et al. Hypoplastic left heart syndrome with rhabdomyoma of the left ventricle. *Pediatr Cardiol.* 1991;12: 121-122.
11. Napolioni V, Curatolo P. Genetics and molecular biology of tuberous sclerosis complex. *Curr Genomics.* 2008;9:475-487.
12. Fesslova V, Villa L, Rizzuti T, et al. Natural history and long-term outcome of cardiac rhabdomyomas detected prenatally. *Prenat Diagn.* 2004;24:241-248.
13. Bader RS, Chitayat D, Kelly E, et al. Fetal rhabdomyoma: prenatal diagnosis, clinical outcome, and incidence of associated tuberous sclerosis complex. *J Pediatr.* 2003;143:620-624.
14. Tworetzky W, McElhinney DB, Margossian R, et al. Association between cardiac tumors and tuberous sclerosis in the fetus and neonate. *Am J Cardiol.* 2003;92:487-489.
15. Chao AS, Chao A, Wang TH, et al. Outcome of antenatally diagnosed cardiac rhabdomyoma: case series and a meta-analysis. *Ultrasound Obstet Gynecol.* 2008;31:289-295.
16. Veldtman GR, Blackburn ME, Wharton GA, et al. Dystrophic calcification of the fetal myocardium. *Heart.* 1999;81:92-93.
17. Lacey SR, Donofrio MT. Fetal cardiac tumors: prenatal diagnosis and outcome. *Pediatr Cardiol.* 2007;28:61-67.
18. Beghetti M, Gow RM, Haney I, et al. Pediatric primary benign cardiac tumors: a 15-year review. *Am Heart J.* 1997;134:1107-1114.
19. Bader R, Hornberger LK, Nijmeh LJ, et al. Fetal pericardial teratoma: presentation of two cases and review of literature. *Am J Perinatol.* 2006;23:53-58.
20. Pachy F, Raiffort C, Mechler C, et al. Intrapericardial teratoma with hydrops leading to in utero demise. *Prenat Diagn.* 2007;27: 970-972.
21. Freedom RM, Lee KJ, MacDonald C, et al. Selected aspects of cardiac tumors in infancy and childhood. *Pediatr Cardiol.* 2000;21:299-316.
22. Paladini D, Tartaglione A, Vassallo M, et al. Prenatal ultrasonographic findings of a cardiac myxoma. *Obstet Gynecol.* 2003;102: 1174-1176.
23. Laga S, Gewillig MH, Van Schoubroeck D, et al. Imminent fetal cardiac tamponade by right atrial hemangioma. *Pediatr Cardiol.* 2006;27:633-635.
24. Tseng JJ, Chou MM, Lee YH, et al. In utero diagnosis of cardiac hemangioma. *Ultrasound Obstet Gynecol.* 1999;13:363-365.

CASES

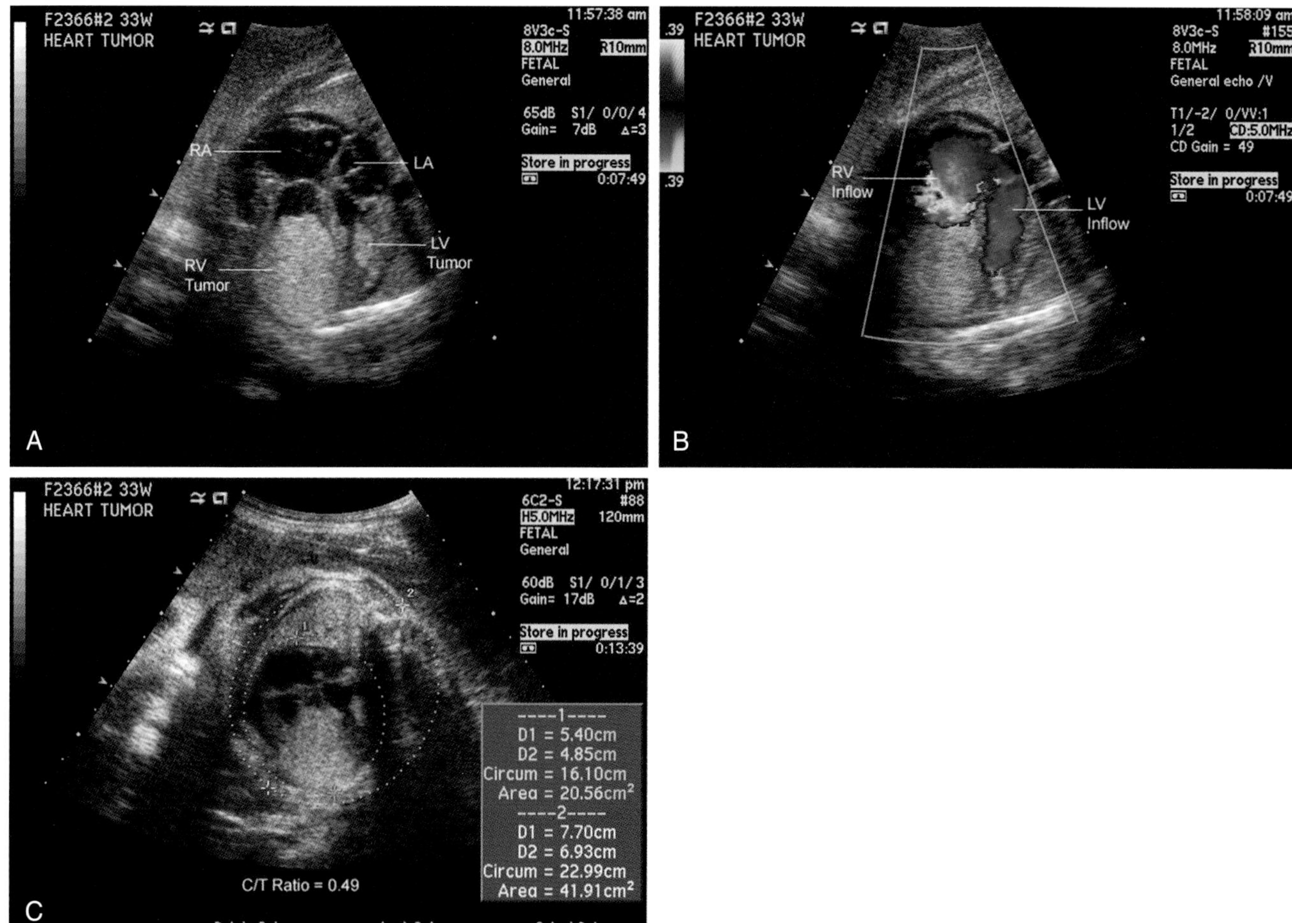

Case 30-1. **(A)** Four-chamber view of a fetus with multiple rhabdomyoma and likely tuberous sclerosis. There is at least one large tumor in the right ventricle (RV) and one in the left ventricle (LV). LA, left atrium; RA, right atrium. **(B)** Color-flow imaging across the inflow of each ventricle. Flow into the RV is limited compared with that of the LV due to tumor impingement. **(C)** Overall, cardiomegaly is a consequence of increased mass due to tumor size. The cardiothoracic (C/T) ratio is nearly 50%.

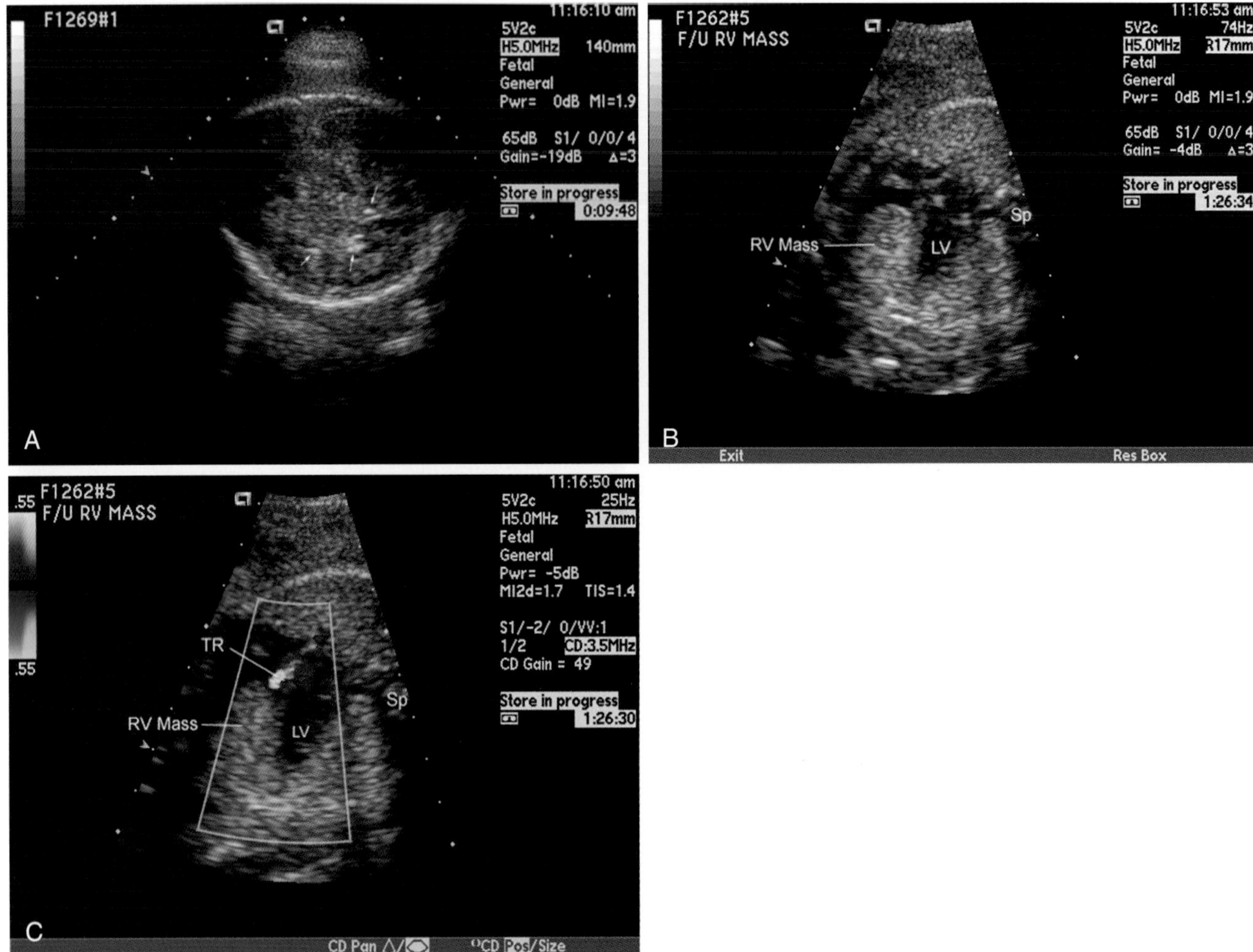

Case 30-2. **(A)** Imaging of the head demonstrates suspicious appearing echo-bright nodules *(arrows)*, which may represent "tubers" consistent with tuberous sclerosis. The presence of these densities may be helpful in making the diagnosis in the fetus; however, their absence does not eliminate the possibility. **(B)** Four-chamber view demonstrates a large right ventricular mass, likely a rhabdomyoma. Sp, spine. **(C)** The mass is altering the function of the papillary muscle of the RV, resulting in tricuspid regurgitation (TR).

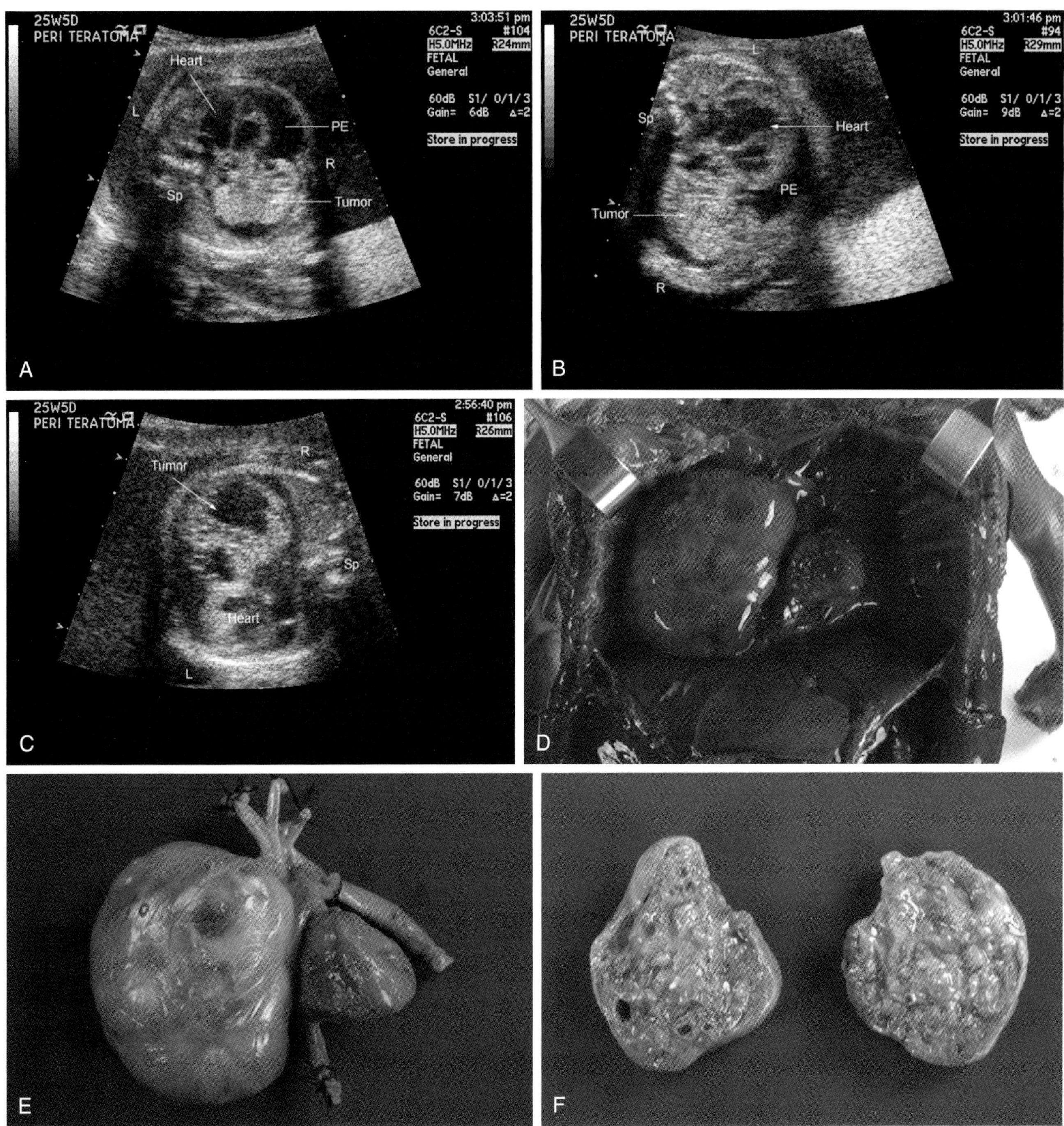

Case 30-3. (**A**) A 31-year-old woman weighing 210 kg presented at 25 weeks' and 5 days' gestation for fetal evaluation as part of screening for gestational diabetes. Imaging was technically challenging. A large heterogeneously echoic mass was seen arising from the pericardial surface of the heart at the right atrioventricular groove region, in addition to a large pericardial effusion (PE) consistent with a diagnosis of a large pericardial teratoma. This is a large pericardial teratoma. Sp, spine. (**B**) Imaging with the left side of the fetus up demonstrates the extent of the tumor and the pericardial effusion. The tumor partially obstructed inflow into the right atrium. (**C**) Imaging with the right side of the fetus up demonstrates a cystic component to the pericardial teratoma. One of the hallmarks of a teratoma is the heterogeneous makeup of the tumor, which may include solid or cystic structures of various densities. Note the large size of the tumor in comparison to the heart. (**D**) The tumor grew rapidly and tamponade physiology ensued with progressive compression of the heart. Attempt was made to tap the cystic component of the tumor but was unsuccessful due to technical issues in relation to maternal body habitus. There was fetal demise at 28 weeks' gestation. The tumor had grown to more than three times the size of the heart. (**E**) The giant pericardial teratoma excised as a block with the heart. The mass originates from the region of the pericardium adjacent to the right atrium and aortic sulcus. (**F**) A slice through the body of the pericardial teratoma reveals a coarse and heterogeneous texture reflecting varying tissues, typical of a teratoma.

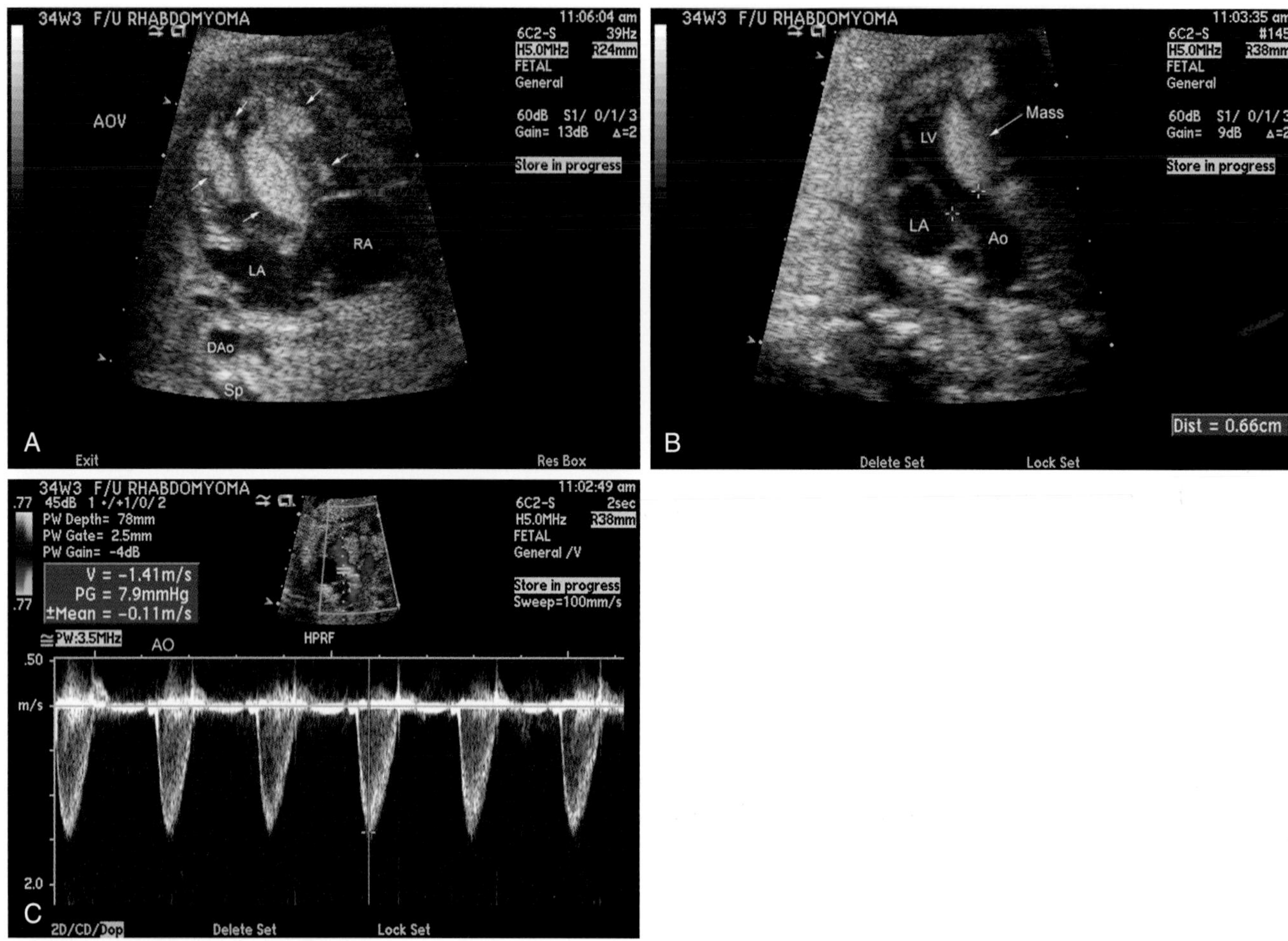

Case 30-4. **(A)** Multiple echo-bright masses seen within the myocardium *(arrows)*, likely a case of multiple rhabdomyoma and tuberous sclerosis. AOV, aortic valve; DAo, descending aorta; LA, left atrium; RA, right atrium. **(B)** Despite the finding of multiple large masses, inflow and outflow pathways are often surprisingly unaffected and without obstruction in some cases of multiple rhabdomyoma due to tuberous sclerosis. Note the large mass in the ventricular septum; however, the left ventricular outflow tract appears unobstructed. Ao, aorta. **(C)** Pulse wave Doppler across the left ventricular outflow tract reveals laminar flow without obstruction. AO, aorta.

31

Echo "Bright" Spot in the Heart

Jack Rychik

Key Echocardiographic Features

- Locate the position of the "echo bright spot" as being solely on the tips of the papillary muscles within the heart.
- Search for any additional "echo bright" regions that may suggest an abnormal pathology such as endocardial fibroelastosis (none should be present in the benign form of echogenic foci).
- Assess for any atrioventricular valve insufficiency (none should be present in the benign form of echogenic foci).
- Assess for ventricular function (should be normal in the presence of the benign form of echogenic foci).
- Identify whether there are any structural abnormalities of the heart (none should be present in the benign form of echogenic foci).

Anatomy and Anatomical Associations

Echogenic foci within the fetal heart, or "echo bright spots," are findings of localized regions of increased ultrasound reflectivity appearing as bright spots within the myocardium. The myocardium itself does not appear distorted by the spot, as might be expected in a tumor or mass, rather the normal myocardium simply appears brighter than its surrounding region. These echogenic foci most commonly appear at the tips of the papillary muscles of the left ventricle. However, they can appear, in order of frequency, within the myocardium of the left ventricle, within the right ventricle, or in both ventricles.[1] They are not associated with any type of structural heart disease and are thought to occur in the normal fetal heart.

The precise pathological origin of this unusual echobrightness is unclear. Histological analysis of myocardial tissue from high-risk pregnancies in which echogenic foci were noted and termination took place has demonstrated these regions to consist of "mineralization" or regions of calcification with surrounding fibrous tissue.[2,3] The fetuses analyzed for these studies all had additional anomalies or aneuploidy; hence, it is unclear whether the same histopathology explains the echogenic foci seen in the normal fetus without anomaly or aneuploidy. One alternative hypothesis is that certain myocardial sarcomere genetic allele subtypes, of which there are a number, may phenotypically reflect ultrasound energy to variable degrees. Hence, visualization of an echogenic focus, although not present in all cases, is simply a reflection of a particular normal variant of myocardium that may have these distinctive properties.

Frequency, Genetics, and Development

The precise etiology of these foci is unknown. Studies have demonstrated the presence of echogenic foci within the heart in obstetrical ultrasound of low-risk, midtrimester pregnancy to be at a prevalence of 1.6% to 6.9% of the population.[1,4-7] They are typically seen around the middle of the second trimester at approximately 20 weeks' gestation. Oftentimes, foci disappear upon follow-up evaluation in later gestation.

When first identified in the 1980s, great concern was raised about the possible association of echogenic bright spots within the fetal heart and aneuploidy such as trisomy 21 or association with other genetic syndromes. Multiple large studies have since dispelled this notion. Numerous investigators have concluded that the finding of an echogenic focus is a variant of normal. When there are no other risk factors such advanced maternal age, biochemical abnormalities on screening, or other abnormalities seen on obstetrical ultrasound, no further testing or follow-up is indicated (e.g., amniocentesis is not indicated).[4-6,8] The presence of multiple bright spots in both the right and the left ventricles, however, may raise suspicion of aneuploidy and may warrant further analysis.[9] Increased nuchal translucency and bilateral echogenic foci have been reported in a case of 22q11 deletion.[10]

Prenatal Physiology

Although quite common, and not associated with structural heart disease or aneuploidy, do these echogenic foci affect myocardial function in any way? Systolic performance has not been noted to be any different than normal; however, diastolic filling patterns have been reported to be different. In one study, investigators found a decrease in the early diastolic–to–late diastolic phase peak velocity ratio (E:A wave) suggesting greater dependence upon atrial contraction for filling and altered ventricular compliance, although to no clinical significance.[11] A more recent study using sophisticated analysis of myocardial deformation found no differences in systolic or diastolic function in fetuses with echogenic foci in comparison with normal.[12] The issue of whether there might be slight differences in diastolic performance in fetuses with echogenic foci is unsettled; however, if present, these differences do not amount to any clinical significance or clinical manifestations because fetal growth, development, and labor are tolerated as perfectly well as in the normal population.

Prenatal Management

The site and number of foci should be evaluated. Isolated echogenic foci in the papillary muscles of the left ventricle require no further evaluation and are considered normal. Isolated foci to the papillary muscle of the right ventricle are similarly normal. Foci found in both ventricles may require attention. We advocate a high-level obstetrical scan if echogenic foci are found in both ventricles, with consideration of an amniocentesis, in particular, if there are any additional risk factors such as advanced maternal age, a small-for-gestational age fetus, Doppler flow abnormalities in the umbilical artery or ductus venosus, evidence of ventricular size discrepancy, or atrioventricular valve regurgitation.

The presence of echogenic foci may be related to technical considerations related to performance of the ultrasound study. One study reported a much higher read of the presence of echogenic foci when using the apical four-chamber view as opposed to the "lateral" view, or long-axis view, of the heart.[13] Axial resolution is maximized in the apical four-chamber view with the beam of ultrasound running parallel to the papillary muscles, which may explain why the yield was better. Another study highlighted the role of the ultrasonic settings and the operator in the ability to visualize the echogenic foci.[14] These studies suggest that perhaps this particular finding is much more pervasive than it seems, further supporting the notion that this is a common phenomenon seen in the general population, and is visualized depending upon by whom and how the study is performed.

Postnatal Physiology

Many echogenic foci "disappear" or are no longer visualized late into the third trimester of pregnancy; however, some may persist into infancy and early childhood.[1] Clinical evaluation and pediatric echocardiography follow-up on fetuses with echogenic foci reveal normal findings.[4,15,16] In fetuses with echogenic foci, left ventricular function as assessed by shortening fraction and myocardial performance index as far out as to 7 years of age are no different than normal.

Postnatal Management

No specific management is necessary for these benign prenatal findings.

Outcomes

Outcome is excellent and is the same as normal, because no study has shown any differences in postnatal heart function or clinical outcome between fetuses with echogenic foci and those without.

Imaging Essentials and Important Points

- Current understanding is that echogenic foci are a variant of normal and do not require any further evaluation, so long as no other associated risk factors are present.
- A benign echogenic focus is typically located at the tips of the papillary muscles of the left ventricle. Deformation of heart tissue or any mass effect related suggests that it is a tumor and not a benign echogenic focus.
- Multiple foci within the myocardium in both ventricles should raise suspicions of tumors, most commonly rhabdomyomas as seen in tuberous sclerosis.

References

1. Petrikovsky BM, Challenger M, Wyse LJ. Natural history of echogenic foci within ventricles of the fetal heart. *Ultrasound Obstet Gynecol.* 1995;5:92-94.
2. Brown DL, Roberts DJ, Miller WA. Left ventricular echogenic focus in the fetal heart: pathologic correlation. *J Ultrasound Med.* 1994; 13:613-616.
3. Tennstedt C, Chaoui R, Vogel M, Goldner B, Dietel M. Pathologic correlation of sonographic echogenic foci in the fetal heart. *Prenat Diagn.* 2000;20:287-292.
4. Dildy GA, Judd VE, Clark SL. Prospective evaluation of the antenatal incidence and postnatal significance of the fetal echogenic cardiac focus: a case-control study. *Am J Obstet Gynecol.* 1996;175: 1008-1012.
5. Barsoom MJ, Feldman DM, Borgida AF, Esters D, Diana D, Egan JF. Is an isolated fetal cardiac echogenic focus an indication for fetal echocardiography? *J Ultrasound Med.* 2001;20:1043-1046.
6. Lamont RF, Havutcu E, Salgia S, Adinkra P, Nicholl R. The association between isolated fetal echogenic cardiac foci on second-trimester ultrasound scan and trisomy 21 in low-risk unselected women. *Ultrasound Obstet Gynecol.* 2004;23:346-351.
7. Simpson JM, Cook A, Sharland G. The significance of echogenic foci in the fetal heart: a prospective study of 228 cases. *Ultrasound Obstet Gynecol.* 1996;8:225-228.
8. Bradley KE, Santulli TS, Gregory KD, Herbert W, Carlson DE, Platt LD. An isolated intracardiac echogenic focus as a marker for aneuploidy. *Am J Obstet Gynecol.* 2005;192:2021-2026; discussion 2026-2028.
9. Wax JR, Philput C. Fetal intracardiac echogenic foci: does it matter which ventricle? *J Ultrasound Med.* 1998;17:141-144; quiz 145-146.
10. Machlitt A, Tennstedt C, Korner H, Bommer C, Chaoui R. Prenatal diagnosis of 22q11 microdeletion in an early second-trimester fetus with conotruncal anomaly presenting with increased nuchal translucency and bilateral intracardiac echogenic foci. *Ultrasound Obstet Gynecol.* 2002;19:510-513.
11. Degani S, Leibovitz Z, Shapiro I, Gonen R, Ohel G. Cardiac function in fetuses with intracardiac echogenic foci. *Ultrasound Obstet Gynecol.* 2001;18:131-134.
12. Perles Z, Nir A, Gavri S, Golender J, Rein AJ. Intracardiac echogenic foci have no hemodynamic significance in the fetus. *Pediatr Cardiol.* 2010;31:7-10.
13. Ranzini AC, McLean DA, Sharma S, Vintzileos AM. Fetal intracardiac echogenic foci: visualization depends on the orientation of the 4-chamber view. *J Ultrasound Med.* 2001;20:763-766.
14. Levine D, Mehta TS, Min KK, Hulka CA, McArdle CR. Technical factors influencing sonographic visualization of fetal echogenic intracardiac foci. *J Clin Ultrasound.* 2000;28:479-484.
15. Wax JR, Donnelly J, Carpenter M, et al. Childhood cardiac function after prenatal diagnosis of intracardiac echogenic foci. *J Ultrasound Med.* 2003;22:783-787.
16. Vettraino IM, Hoprasart NJ, Bronsteen RA, Comstock CH. Clinical implications of the prenatal sonographic finding of fetal myocardial echogenic foci. *J Ultrasound Med.* 2005;24:195-199.

CASES

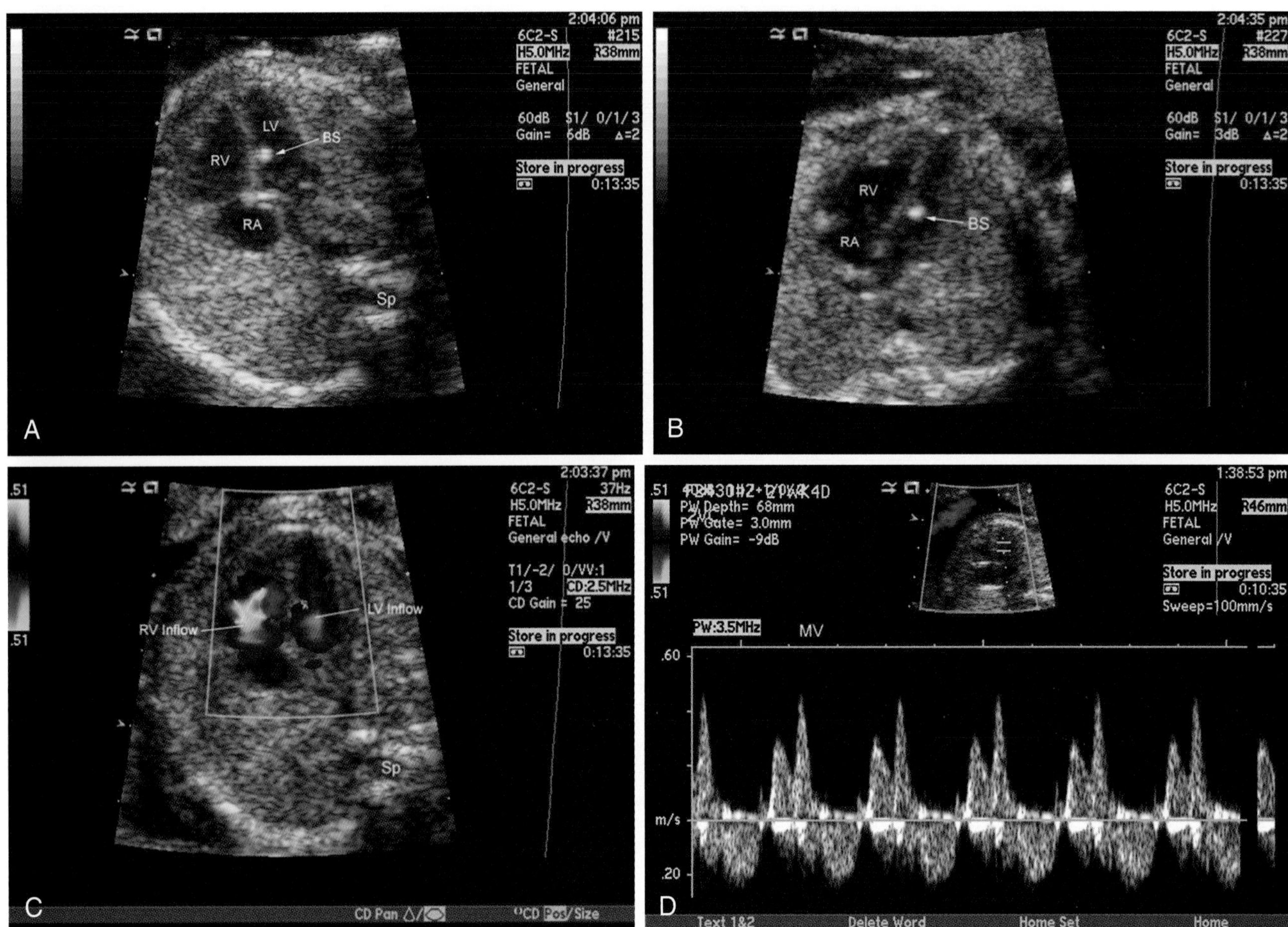

Case 31-1. **(A)** Echo bright spot (BS) in the left ventricle (LV). The lesion is oval and located in the midcavitary portion of the ventricle, at the level of the tip of the papillary muscle as it connects to the chordae of the mitral valve. RA, right atrium; RV, right ventricle; Sp, spine. **(B)** Orthogonal view to **A** demonstrates the position of the BS at the level within the LV, just beneath the mitral valve apparatus. **(C)** Color flow imaging reveals unimpeded inflow into the LV. **(D)** Pulse-wave Doppler across the mitral valve (MV). A completely normal inflow pattern suggests no evidence of any dysfunction of the mitral valve, despite the presence of this echo BS.

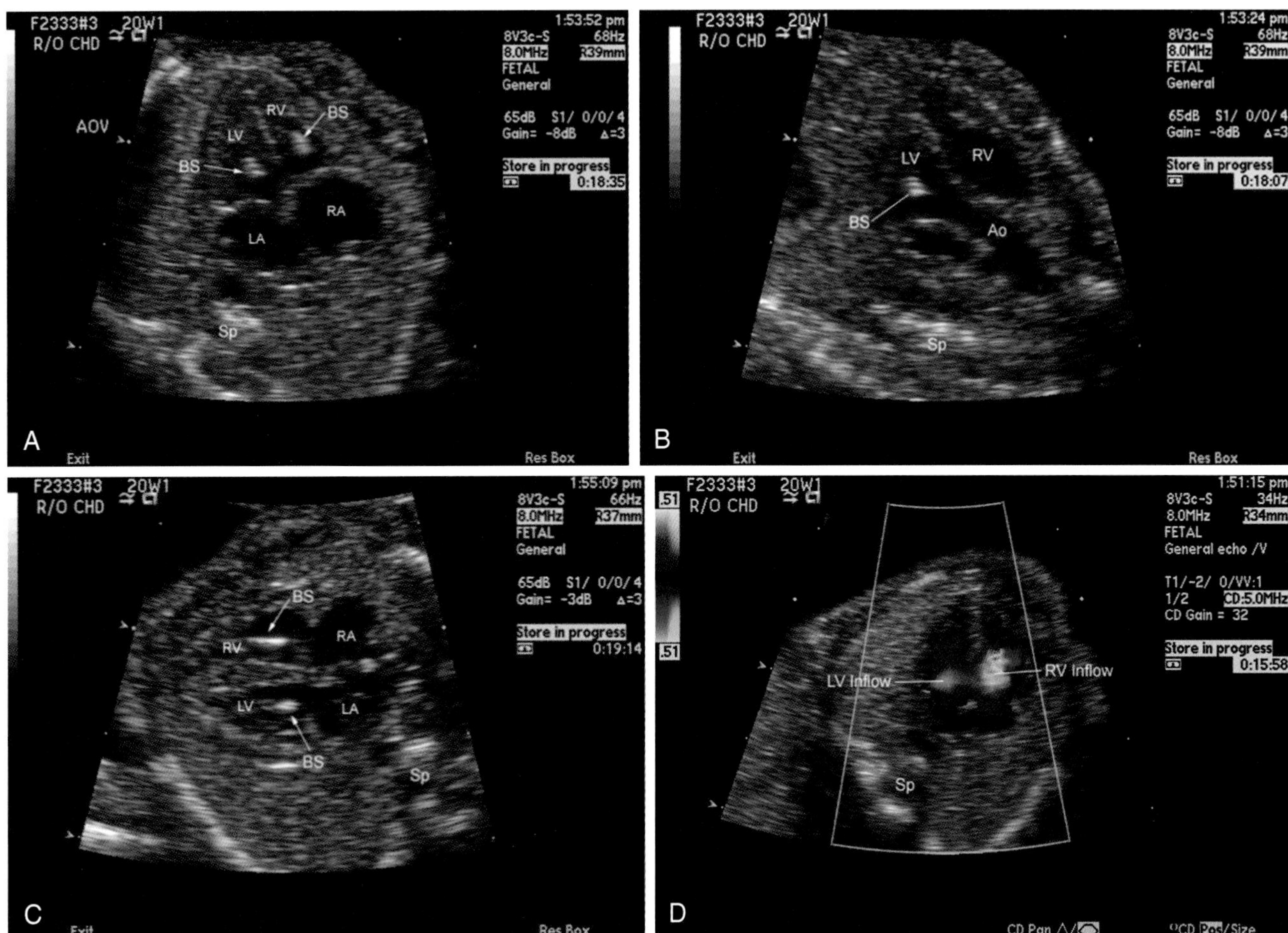

Case 31-2. **(A)** Apical view of a fetal heart at 20 weeks' gestation referred for family history of congenital heart disease. Echo bright spots (BS) are noted in both the right (RV) and the left (LV) ventricles. Both spots are positioned at an equivalent level within the ventricle and are located within the chordal attachments to the tips of the papillary muscles for both the RV and the LV. LA, left atrium; RA, right atrium; Sp, spine. **(B)** Long-axis view with focus on the left ventricular outflow tract and ascending aorta (Ao). Note the location of the BS within the cavity of the LV. **(C)** Long-axis view of both the LV and the RV. The BS are nicely seen precisely located at the junction between the atrioventricular valve and the tips of the papillary muscles. These are the chordae tendinae of the mitral and tricuspid valves. **(D)** Color Doppler imaging demonstrates no impediment to filling across the mitral or tricuspid valves. No regurgitation was seen either. The echo bright spots do not result in any valvar dysfunction.

32
Ectopia Cordis

Jack Rychik

Anatomy and Anatomical Associations

Ectopia cordis is a rare but very dramatic congenital malformation in which the heart is located outside of the confines of the chest cavity.[1-3] The condition can be classified into four types, depending upon the position of the heart: cervical, thoracic, thoracoabdominal, or abdominal. The most common type is thoracic ectopia in which the heart lies partially or completely outside the chest wall with the ventricular apex pointing cephalad.

Ectopia cordis is commonly associated with other anomalies including intracardiac defects and other "midline" body wall defects. In 1958, Cantrell and coworkers[4] described a "pentalogy" of five associated findings including a midline supraumbilical abdominal wall defect, a defect of the lower part of the sternum, a deficiency of the anterior diaphragm, a pericardial defect at the diaphragmatic surface, and a congenital heart malformation. In this syndrome, the heart disease is often a ventricular septal defect or a conotruncal anomaly such as tetralogy of Fallot or double-outlet right ventricle. Diverticulum of the left ventricle apex is also associated, seen in approximately 20% of cases.

Although Cantrell and coworkers described their particular findings as a constellation, in fact patients may have any one of these alone or a wide spectrum of additional anomalies in association with ectopia cordis. These include abdominal wall defects such as omphalocele, diastasis recti, or gastroschisis as well as craniofacial defects such as cleft lip/palate or neural tube defects. Cases of so-called partial pentalogy of Cantrell have been described, in which there is no sternal defect, but rather a large omphalocele with the heart protruding in a thoracoabdominal manner.[5] Hence, two mechanisms for evisceration of the heart outside of the chest wall have been proposed. One is a defect in the sternum with direct protrusion through, referred to as *thoracoschisis.* The other is a *reverse diaphragmatic hernia* in which there is a defect in the diaphragm with the heart protruding into the abdomen in association with an omphalocele within which the abdominal contents including the heart is outside of the body.[6] The embryological mechanisms for these two may be different.

Frequency, Genetics, and Development

Ectopia cordis makes up less than 0.1% of all congenital heart defects. Failure of fusion of the paired cartilage bars of the embryonic sternum leads to a sternal cleft (thoracoschisis), which allows for the potential for the heart to be positioned outside the boundaries of the chest wall. The incidence ranges from 5.5 to 7.9 per 1 million live births. Two thirds of patients are male; one third are born premature or stillborn. Ectopia cordis is part of a developmental field complex defect, which involves deficiency in formation of the sternum, diaphragm, and anterior body wall. A familial pattern has been reported.[7] Ectopia cordis can be associated with a number of genetic and chromosomal anomalies including trisomy 18[8] and can be experimentally induced in animals through a variety of teratogens.[9,10]

Prenatal Physiology

The overall physiology and prognosis depend upon the associated anomalies and their severity. Ectopia cordis is commonly part of a pervasive and fundamental abnormality of body wall development. The fetal cardiovascular physiology will be altered based on the type of heart disease seen. One very important manifestation of thoracic and abdominal content evisceration is the development of a small chest and subsequent pulmonary hypoplasia. Although of no physiological consequence in utero during placental support, postnatal survival is limited if pulmonary hypoplasia is present.

Prenatal Management

Careful evaluation of the cardiac position, the amount of heart sitting outside of the chest, the precise type of congenital heart disease, and other associated anomalies is important. Karyotype evaluation is indicated. Oftentimes, suspicion is first raised by the presence of abnormal elevation in first-trimester serum markers, which then leads to early detailed imaging. Ectopia cordis can be diagnosed in the first trimester of pregnancy, as early as 10 weeks' gestation.[11,12] Partial protrusion of the heart outside of the chest wall as an isolated finding is unusual, and there are commonly many other associated anomalies. Figuring out the anatomy at the junction of the chest, abdomen, and diaphragm can be a challenge. Fetal echocardiography can be complemented by the use of fetal magnetic resonance imaging to obtain a more precise sense of the anatomy with particular focus on the relationship of the heart to the sternum, diaphragm, and abdominal wall defect.[13,14] Considering the poor prognosis in most cases, detailed evaluation and counseling are important as early as possible.

Postnatal Management and Outcomes

Overall prognosis for ectopia cordis is extremely poor with less than 5% survival beyond the neonatal period.[1] There are case reports of neonatal surgery, with survival very much dependent upon additional associated anomalies.[2] The presence of pulmonary hypoplasia is uniformly fatal. Cervical ectopia cordis has extremely poor prognosis, because kinking of vessels and constriction of the heart occur with attempts at repositioning of the heart at surgery.

For thoracic ectopia cordis with associated congenital heart disease, but no other significant extracardiac anomalies, surgical repair can be attempted with some success.[3] The principles of surgical treatment for this disease are to (1) provide soft tissue cover of the heart, (2) reduce the heart into the thoracic cavity, (3) palliate or repair any intracardiac defect, and (4) reconstruct the chest wall. These goals can be achieved in a thoughtful staged manner, in some instances.[15] Single-ventricle palliation has been successfully undertaken in patients with well-formed lungs and no other major anomalies.[16,17] Long-term outcome beyond a few years of age has not been reported.

Imaging Essentials and Important Points

- Overall prognosis is poor. Conditions that may be favorable for consideration of postnatal intervention and, therefore, require careful prenatal evaluation include:
  - Thoracic location.
  - Partial ectopia and not complete.
  - Well-formed lungs with no hypoplasia.
  - No significant extracardiac anomalies.
- Common forms of congenital heart disease include ventricular septal defect or tetralogy of Fallot.

References

1. Amato JJ, Douglas WI, Desai U, Burke S. Ectopia cordis. *Chest Surg Clin North Am*. 2000;10:297-316, vii.
2. Morales JM, Patel SG, Duff JA, Villareal RL, Simpson JW. Ectopia cordis and other midline defects. *Ann Thorac Surg*. 2000;70:111-114.
3. Hornberger LK, Colan SD, Lock JE, Wessel DL, Mayer JE Jr. Outcome of patients with ectopia cordis and significant intracardiac defects. *Circulation*. 1996;94:II32-II37.
4. Cantrell JR, Haller JA, Ravitch MM. A syndrome of congenital defects involving the abdominal wall, sternum, diaphragm, pericardium, and heart. *Surg Gynecol Obstet*. 1958;107:602-614.
5. van Hoorn JH, Moonen RM, Huysentruyt CJ, van Heurn LW, Offermans JP, Mulder AL. Pentalogy of Cantrell: two patients and a review to determine prognostic factors for optimal approach. *Eur J Pediatr*. 2008;167:29-35.
6. Davies BR, Duran M. The confused identity of Cantrell's pentad: ectopia cordis is related either to thoracoschisis or to a diaphragmatic hernia with an omphalocele. *Pediatr Pathol Mol Med*. 2003;22:383-390.
7. Martin RA, Cunniff C, Erickson L, Jones KL. Pentalogy of Cantrell and ectopia cordis, a familial developmental field complex. *Am J Med Genet*. 1992;42:839-841.
8. Shaw SW, Cheng PJ, Chueh HY, Chang SD, Soong YK. Ectopia cordis in a fetus with trisomy 18. *J Clin Ultrasound*. 2006;34:95-98.
9. Ejaz S, Ejaz A, Sohail A, Ahmed M, Nasir A, Lim CW. Exposure of smoke solutions from CNG-powered four-stroke auto-rickshaws induces distressed embryonic movements, embryonic hemorrhaging and ectopia cordis. *Food Chem Toxicol*. 2009;47:1442-1452.
10. Ejaz S, Ashraf M, Nawaz M, Lim CW, Kim B. Anti-angiogenic and teratological activities associated with exposure to total particulate matter from commercial cigarettes. *Food Chem Toxicol*. 2009;47:368-376.
11. Liang RI, Huang SE, Chang FM. Prenatal diagnosis of ectopia cordis at 10 weeks of gestation using two-dimensional and three-dimensional ultrasonography. *Ultrasound Obstet Gynecol*. 1997;10:137-139.
12. Barbee K, Wax JR, Pinette MG, Cartin A, Blackstone J. First-trimester prenatal sonographic diagnosis of ectopia cordis in a twin gestation. *J Clin Ultrasound*. 2009;37:539-540.
13. McMahon CJ, Taylor MD, Cassady CI, Olutoye OO, Bezold LI. Diagnosis of pentalogy of cantrell in the fetus using magnetic resonance imaging and ultrasound. *Pediatr Cardiol*. 2007;28:172-175.
14. Moniotte S, Powell AJ, Barnewolt CE, Annese D, Geva T. Prenatal diagnosis of thoracic ectopia cordis by real-time fetal cardiac magnetic resonance imaging and by echocardiography. *Congenit Heart Dis*. 2008;3:128-131.
15. Alphonso N, Venugopal PS, Deshpande R, Anderson D. Complete thoracic ectopia cordis. *Eur J Cardiothorac Surg*. 2003;23:426-428.
16. Tokunaga S, Kado H, Imoto Y, Shiokawa Y, Yasui H. Successful staged-Fontan operation in a patient with ectopia cordis. *Ann Thorac Surg*. 2001;71:715-717.
17. Okamoto Y, Harada Y, Uchita S. Fontan operation through a right lateral thoracotomy to treat Cantrell syndrome with severe ectopia cordis. *Interact Cardiovasc Thorac Surg*. 2008;7:278-279.

CASE

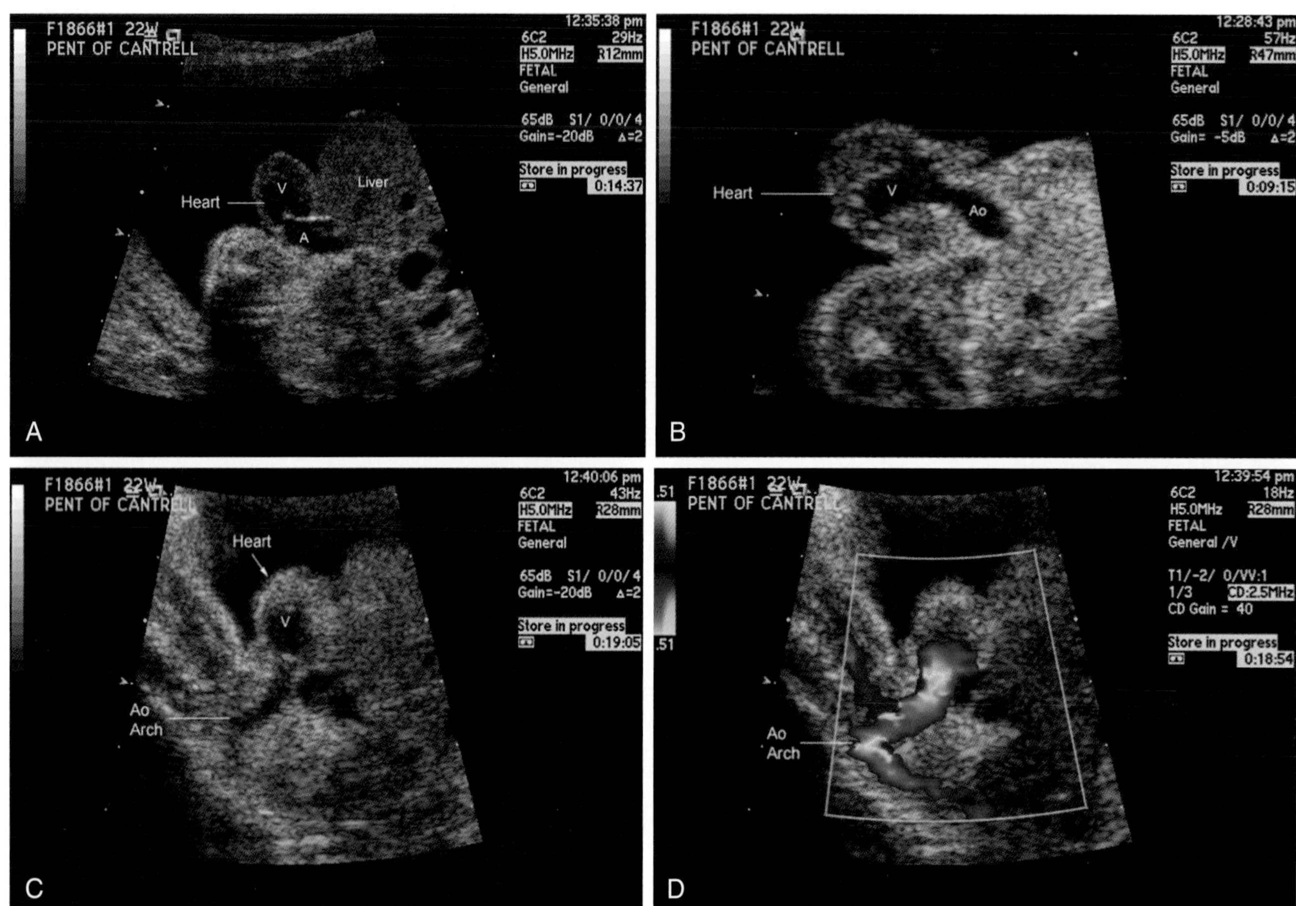

Case 32-1. **(A)** Ectopia cordis in a 22-week fetus with pentalogy of Cantrell. Note both the liver and a substantial portion of the heart are outside of the fetal body. A, atrium; V, ventricle. **(B)** Focused view of the heart demonstrates a dominant single-ventricle type of congenital heart disease, with just one vessel—the aorta (Ao)—arising. **(C)** The single vessel arising from the heart does not bifurcate, suggesting it is the Ao. **(D)** Color flow imaging demonstrates the aortic arch (Ao arch) and a limb vessel coming off.

33

Diverticulum or Aneurysm of the Ventricle

Jack Rychik

Key Echocardiographic Features

- Locate the position of the diverticulum as either at the apex (most common) or originating from the wall of the ventricle.
- Determine the presence or absence of a pericardial effusion.
- Determine whether there is any ventricular dysfunction or regional wall abnormalities near the site of the "outpouching" because none should be present in a true diverticulum.
- Doppler color flow imaging may demonstrate flow between the cavity of the ventricle and the diverticulum.

Anatomy and Anatomical Associations

Outpouchings of the ventricular cavity are referred to as either a "diverticulum" or an "aneurysm" of the ventricle. The terms are frequently used interchangeably; however, some distinctions can be made. A *diverticulum* is described as having all layers of myocardium within the wall and contracts either normally or near normally, whereas an *aneurysm* contains components of fibrotic tissue and does not contract normally. A diverticulum is also described as having a narrow neck and is relatively small; aneurysms are more broad-based and can be quite large.[1-3]

There is an interesting association between a thin-walled ventricular diverticulum and pericardial effusion in the fetus.[4] The pericardial effusion is not related to cardiac dysfunction or hemodynamic abnormality because the diverticulum is often quite small, with no evidence of myocardial compromise. One theory is that the diverticulum acts as a semipermeable membrane allowing for extravasation of fluid into the pericardial space. Intraventricular pressure promotes flux of fluid across and creates a transudate in the pericardial space. These pericardial effusions can become quite large, leading to either cardiac tamponade or pulmonary hypoplasia as it compresses the lungs.

Most commonly, diverticula are seen in isolation. However, they can also be seen in conotruncal anomalies or in association with isolated ventricular septal defects.[5] Diverticulum of the left ventricle can be part of the pentalogy of Cantrell an anomaly consisting of defects in the abdominal wall, sternum, diaphragm, pericardium, and heart. Omphalocele and ventricular diverticulum suggest the presence of this syndrome.[6]

In a review of 35 fetuses with diverticula/aneurysms diagnosed prenatally, 21 were defects in the left ventricle and 14 in the right ventricle. They were located in the apex of the heart in 26, below the atrioventricular valve in 7, and on the lateral free wall in 2.[7]

Frequency, Genetics, and Development

The true incidence of diverticula or aneurysms is not known, because many cases likely are asymptomatic and go unnoticed.

The anatomical features of these outpouchings or "bulges" hint at possible etiologies, although the definitive cause is unknown. Narrow-necked, thin-walled, saccular diverticula are thought to derive from congenital abnormalities of ventricular wall formation and represent a localized, embryogenic defect. Aneurysms appear as broad-based bulges with noncontractile, or dyskinetic, walls and are thought to relate to regional myocardial ischemia or tissue scarring and are perhaps an acquired phenomenon due to disrupted myocardium. These localized areas of ischemia may be due to abnormalities of coronary development in the region affected. Another distinguishing factor is that diverticula typically remain stable in size, whereas ventricular aneurysms can grow, further supporting the notion than the former are discrete congenital abnormalities and the latter relate to ischemic myocardium and respond to intraventricular pressures by potentially changing shape and progressing in size.

Right ventricular aneurysm has been described in the recipient of twin-twin transfusion after fetoscopic laser photocoagulation procedure.[7] The donor died after the procedure and the recipient developed an echogenic focus on the right ventricle free wall with pericardial effusion. Three weeks later, the area developed myocardial disruption with a thin-walled aneurysm and subsequent rupture. The absence of aneurysm before the procedure with identification of an echogenic focus immediately after suggests strongly for an acquired ischemic event, with subsequent myocardial wall scarring and rupture. This case portrays the role of ischemia in the development of fetal ventricular aneurysms, although unlike in this case, most inciting events in other fetuses occur surreptitiously and are of unknown etiology.

Prenatal Physiology

A ventricular diverticulum in the fetus should not cause any hemodynamic compromise on its own; however, when associated with a pericardial effusion, tamponade can occur.[1,2,4] The heart can become compressed with impediment to filling, reducing stroke volume. Tachycardia can be seen as the fetal heart attempts to maintain cardiac output. Furthermore, a large pericardial effusion can compress the lungs as well. When long-standing, such compression can impair pulmonary development.

A ventricular aneurysm in the fetus may cause hemodynamic instability, depending upon the size and degree of myocardium affected.[8] If relatively large, contraction mechanics can be negatively affected with overall reduction in cardiac function, poor cardiac output, and development of fetal hydrops. Regions of the myocardium that support valve function can be affected, and these can present with significant tricuspid or mitral regurgitation. Ischemic regions can also be a source for arrhythmia, and ventricular arrhythmias are possible.[9] Thin-walled scarred tissue may also rupture, leading to fetal demise.

Prenatal Management

Echocardiography will demonstrate the architecture of an aneurysm; however, small ventricular diverticula can be difficult to image. A pericardial effusion should prompt a careful search for a diverticulum.

If a large pericardial effusion is present, pericardiocentesis may be indicated. This has been successfully performed relatively early in gestation, even as early as 14 weeks' gestation. The decision to drain a pericardial effusion will depend upon its impact on hemodynamics or whether there is compression of the lung. Factors that suggest the presence of a hemodynamically significant pericardial effusion include (1) small heart size and general appearance of poorly filled ventricles, (2) single peak filling pattern across the ventricular inflow, (3) Doppler evaluation of the ductus venosus demonstrating reversal with atrial contraction, (4) Doppler evaluation of the umbilical vein demonstrating pulsations, or (5) fetal tachycardia.

Pericardial effusions associated with a ventricular diverticulum can progress and worsen or spontaneously resolve over time.[10] Therefore, if there is a large pericardial effusion but hemodynamics are stable, frequent serial surveillance is important. If a large pericardial effusion is present and the lungs appear compressed, without evidence for any regression of effusion, pericardiocentesis should be considered to relieve intrathoracic pressure and allow for lung expansion.

A ventricular aneurysm should prompt the investigator to look at ventricular function as well as atrioventricular valve regurgitation. Supraventricular arrhythmia, if present, can be treated with maternal administration of digoxin. Ventricular arrhythmias are much more difficult to treat and suggest the presence of "distressed" myocardium, which is an ominous sign.

The fetus with a large ventricular aneurysm and heart failure may benefit from an expectant delivery via cesarean section with an appropriate caretaker team on stand-by, because transitional physiology can add undue load to a sensitive heart, leading to sudden decompensation.

Postnatal Physiology and Management

Ventricular diverticula seen in the fetus frequently disappear at postnatal evaluation. The natural history are for these to remain relatively stable in size while the heart grows. It is rare for these to require surgical intervention. At birth, if a pericardial effusion is present, it may need to be drained, if of significance. However, most will declare themselves before birth, and if not of significance prenatally, it can typically be followed without concern after birth. Newborn echocardiogram and careful assessment for ventricular septal defects are indicated.

Postnatal management of a ventricular aneurysm depends upon the size, location, and impact the defect is exerting on heart or valvular function. Large aneurysms can lead to ventricular dysfunction, atrioventricular valve regurgitation, and heart failure.[5] Inotropic support, heart failure management, surgical resection, or heart transplantation may be required.

Outcomes

Outcome for isolated ventricular diverticulum is excellent. The defects remain small and often disappear after birth. There appear to be no long-term effects into childhood. When indicated, pericardiocentesis is relatively safe and straightforward in experienced hands with excellent results. Once drained, a pericardial effusion in association with ventricular diverticulum rarely returns. This suggests that the transudative phenomenon in this anomaly may be related to gestational age and occurs early only during an immature period of the myocardium.

Outcome for ventricular aneurysm depends upon the size of the defect and its impact on heart function. Reports of sudden rupture of an aneurysm leading to death have also been recorded.[7,11]

Imaging Essentials and Important Points

- When identifying an outpouching, protrusion, or bulge emerging from the right or left ventricle, try to identify the characteristics that distinguish between an aneurysm and a diverticulum.
- Serial evaluation with surveillance for pericardial effusion (diverticulum) or ventricular dysfunction (aneurysm) is indicated.
- Small saccular diverticula originating from the apex are relatively benign so long as there is no significant pericardial effusion.
- In general, diverticula or aneurysms originating from the free wall have a poorer prognosis than those originating from the apex.
- Indications for drainage of a pericardial effusion in association with a diverticulum include cardiac tamponade or lung compression.

References

1. Prefumo F, Bhide A, Thilaganathan B, Carvalho JS. Fetal congenital cardiac diverticulum with pericardial effusion: two cases with different presentations in the first trimester of pregnancy. *Ultrasound Obstet Gynecol.* 2005;25:405-408.

2. McAuliffe FM, Hornberger LK, Johnson J, Chitayat D, Ryan G. Cardiac diverticulum with pericardial effusion: report of two new cases treated by in-utero pericardiocentesis and a review of the literature. *Ultrasound Obstet Gynecol.* 2005;25:401-404.
3. Wax JR, Moran A, Pinette MG, Reyes A, Cartin A, Blackstone J. Prenatal sonographic diagnosis of fetal right ventricular diverticulum. *J Ultrasound Med.* 2007;26:267-270.
4. Johnson JA, Ryan G, Toi A, Smallhorn J. Prenatal diagnosis of a fetal ventricular diverticulum associated with pericardial effusion: successful outcome following pericardiocentesis. *Prenat Diagn.* 1996; 16:954-957.
5. Di Sessa TG, Howard SC, Salim MA. Congenital right ventricular diverticulum associated with a ventricular septal defect: a rare echocardiographic finding. *Echocardiography.* 2006;23:787-789.
6. Halbertsma FJ, van Oort A, van der Staak F. Cardiac diverticulum and omphalocele: Cantrell's pentalogy or syndrome. *Cardiol Young.* 2002;12:71-74.
7. Koshiishi T, Osada H, Hata A, Furugen Y, Murakoshi T, Mitsuhashi N. Prenatal rupture of right ventricular diverticulum: a case report and review of the literature. *Prenat Diagn.* 2007;27:1154-1157.
8. Cavalle-Garrido T, Cloutier A, Harder J, Boutin C, Smallhorn JF. Evolution of fetal ventricular aneurysms and diverticula of the heart: an echocardiographic study. *Am J Perinatol.* 1997;14: 393-400.
9. Tsujimoto H, Takeshita S, Kawamura Y, Nakatani K, Sato M. Isolated congenital left ventricular diverticulum with perinatal dysrhythmia: a case report and review of the literature. *Pediatr Cardiol.* 2000;21:175-179.
10. Del Rio M, Martinez JM, Bennasar M, et al. Prenatal diagnosis of a right ventricular diverticulum complicated by pericardial effusion in the first trimester. *Ultrasound Obstet Gynecol.* 2005;25:409-411.
11. Bernasconi A, Delezoide AL, Menez F, Vuillard E, Oury JF, Azancot A. Prenatal rupture of a left ventricular diverticulum: a case report and review of the literature. *Prenat Diagn.* 2004;24:504-507.

CASES

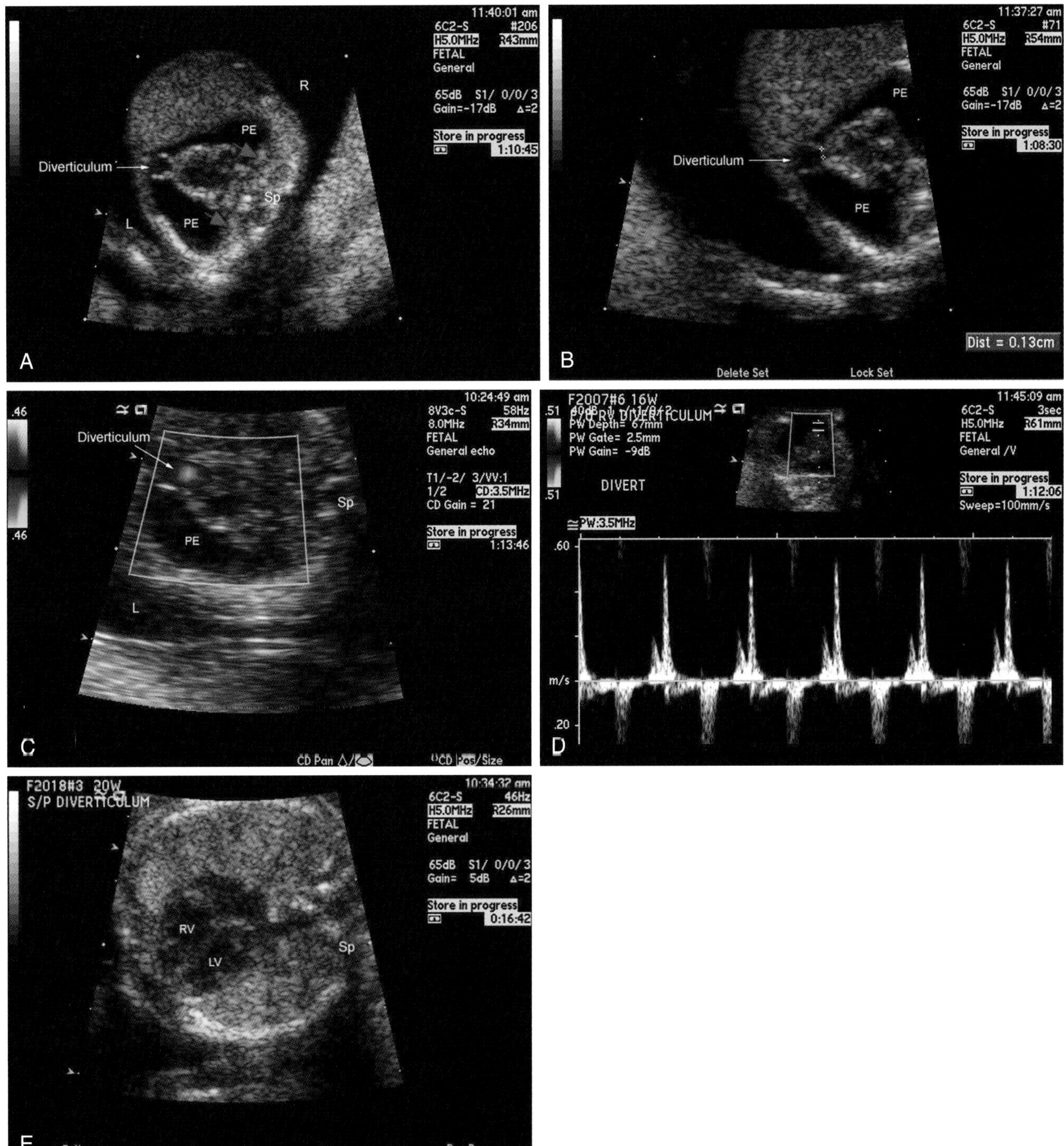

Case 33-1. **(A)** Diverticulum originating from the apex of the heart. There is a large pericardial effusion (PE) and posterior compression of the lungs bilaterally *(red arrows)*. Sp, spine. **(B)** The diverticulum has a neck *(marks)* that originates from the right ventricular cavity. **(C)** Blood flow can be seen entering the diverticulum, with to-and-fro flow between the diverticulum and the ventricle. No blood flow is seen entering the pericardial space. The thinned diverticulum tissue acts as a semipermeable membrane resulting in a transudate of fluid out into the pericardial sac; however, the blood elements remain within the body of the cavity. **(D)** Pulse wave Doppler of flow patterns within the diverticulum demonstrates a typical double-peaked ventricular inflow pattern in diastole and then ejection of blood out of the diverticulum in systole. This suggests that the diverticulum wall tissue, although markedly thinned, is in fact made up of contractile elements and functions in a manner similar to that of the ventricular myocardium. **(E)** Owing to concern about lung compression and impaired lung growth, the PE was tapped with a single needle stick at 18 weeks' gestation. Four milliliters of serous fluid was removed. Follow-up evaluation at 20 weeks reveals no reaccumulation of effusion and the diverticulum was no longer visualized. The fetus was born full term, with no further complications, and postnatal echocardiogram revealed a completely normal heart. LV, left ventricle; RV, right ventricle.

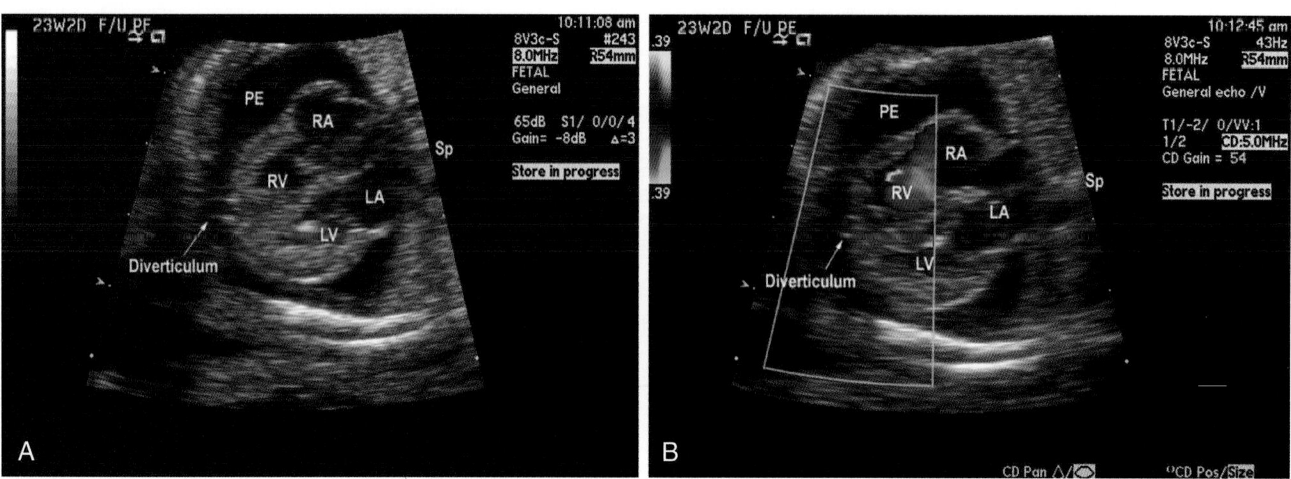

Case 33-2. **(A)** Patient referred at 23 weeks' gestation with fetal pericardial effusion (PE). Initial referring diagnosis was thought to be virally mediated PE. Upon careful inspection, a small diverticulum was identified arising from the apex of the heart. LA, left atrium; LV, left ventricle; RA, right atrium; RV, right ventricle; Sp, spine. **(B)** Color flow imaging reveals a somewhat contracted and underfilled RV secondary to the presence of a PE. Follow-up evaluation at 25 weeks revealed diminishing size of effusion. Without any intervention, spontaneous resolution of the PE occurred.

34

Conjoined Twins

Jack Rychik

Key Echocardiographic Features

- Determine the nature of the heart relationship as being either two separate beating hearts or a single cardiac amalgam.
- If two separate hearts, identify the relative size, function, and anatomy of each individual heart.
- If a single cardiac amalgam, determine the position and degree of apportionment between the two fetal bodies.
- If a single cardiac amalgam identify the number of ventricles, the nature of the communications between the ventricles and the atrioventricular valve connections to the ventricles
- If a single cardiac amalgam, identify the venous connections with particular attention to the presence or absence of the inferior vena cava and its position and insertion in the heart.
- If a single cardiac amalgam, identify the pulmonic and aortic outflow tracts to each twin and the nature of any obstruction.

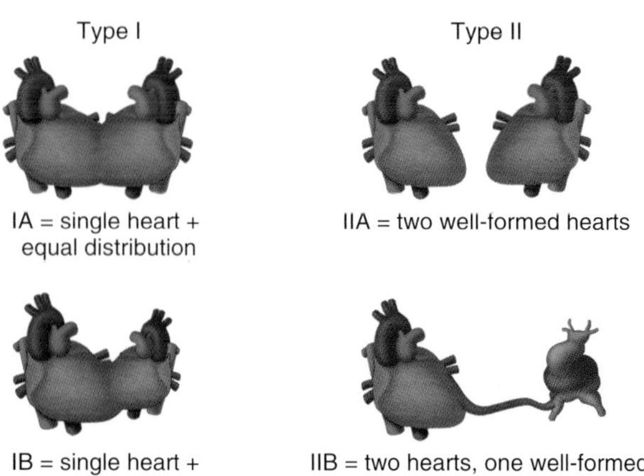

Figure 34-1. Simplified classification system for characterizing cardiac anomalies in conjoined (thoracopagus) twins.

Anatomy and Anatomical Associations

Malformations of the heart are common in conjoined twins. Such twins are classified based on the location of connection, with the term *-pagus* as the suffix, which means "fixed."[1] *Thoracopagus* (joined at the thoracic level) are the most common, accounting for 40% of all cases of conjoined twins, followed by *omphalopagus* (joined at the abdomen predominantly, but may also include the lower thorax) making up 32%. Other forms include *pyopagus* (joined at the sacrum), *ischiopagus* (joined at the hip), or *craniopagus* (joined at the skull). *Parapagus* is a term used to describe twins fused extensively side to side and can also be known as *dicephalus*. Cardiac malformations can be seen in any type of twin fusion; however, it is most common in thoracopagus in which there is a 90% incidence of shared pericardium and a 75% incidence of major myocardial connections. The degree of cardiac fusion and the nature of the associated intracardiac malformation determine the potential for surgical separation as well as long-term survival.

The cardiac anatomy of conjoined twins can be quite varied and complex, ranging from two separate hearts and pericardia to hearts that are fused at the atrial or ventricular levels to what is in essence a single cardiac "amalgam" shared by both twins.[1,2] Coronary arteries and coronary venous drainage may be intertwined and shared.[3] In such fused compound hearts, four is the maximum number of atria and four is the maximum number of ventricles; however, commonly there are fewer of each. One may find a ventricle that is hypoplastic with or without atrioventricular communications leading into it. There can also be multiple communications between the ventricles via ventricular septal defects. The great vessels arising from such a single-heart amalgam to each twin can be abnormally related with conotruncal type anomalies and vessel size discrepancy seen commonly.

In order to simplify the approach to anatomical evaluation of the heart in conjoined twins, we developed a classification system based on the number of hearts present (type) and the location of the cardiac mass (subclass) (Figure 34-1). This classification system allows for a framework of understanding from which the details of the anatomy can be built upon. In type I, a joined single-heart mass with great vessels arising from opposite poles of the heart perfuse the individual twins. In type II, two distinct heart masses for each twin are present. In subclass A, there is an *equal* distribution of cardiac mass for each twin; in subclass B, there is an *unequal* distribution of cardiac mass between the twins. Hence, a thoracopagus with classification IA has a single large heart amalgam compound that is positioned equally between the two twin chests; IIB has a single-heart amalgam compound predominantly positioned within the chest of one twin, but this heart gives rise to vessels that perfuse both twins. In class IIA, each twin has its own separate, relatively equal-sized heart. In addition, each heart may be normal or have an intracardiac abnormality such as a conotruncal anomaly or single-ventricle type congenital heart disease. In class IIB, there are also two separate hearts; however, one is well formed and functions to perfuse the body, whereas the other is primitive and poorly developed. Vascular connections from the twin with the well-formed heart cross over and perfuse its partner.

Although type I with a single-heart amalgam can appear to be a confusing random array of chambers, we have noticed recurring patterns of anatomy. In thoracopagus, the fused twins are typically facing each other. It is best to think of the large heart amalgam in their shared chest as an open book, with the two pages facing you representing the two hearts fused at the center. Often, one can determine a central axis point that distinguishes where the hearts have fused. Typically, there is fusion between the morphologically left ventricles centrally and medially, with the morphologically right ventricles positioned laterally. When there are four ventricles, the two medial left ventricles may share a wall. When there are three or fewer ventricles, the single large central ventricle is typically a fused left ventricle with right ventricles of varying size located on each side. The great vessels can arise from the medial or lateral ventricles but always travel from the ventral conjoined surface of the twins toward the dorsal aspects of each. Pulmonary obstruction or aortic obstruction can be present. Interestingly, when there is vessel obstruction in one twin, the other may have the same type of vessel obstructed or no obstruction. We have not seen any cases in which there was pulmonary obstruction to one twin but aortic obstruction to the other in our fused class I type conjoined heart.

We reviewed a series of 25 conjoined twins evaluated at the Fetal Heart Program at CHOP (unpublished data). Of these, 12 were type IA, 8 type IB, 4 type IIA, and 1 type IIB. Of the type I (single-heart amalgam, $n = 20$), pulmonary obstruction to both twins was present in 10 (50%), pulmonary obstruction to one twin in 7 (35%), aortic obstruction to both twins in 2 (10%), and no obstruction to either great vessel in 1 twin set (5%). Of the type II (two cardiac masses, $n = 5$), the hearts were normal in both twins in 2; in 1 set there was transposition of the great vessels in both twins; in 1 set, there was a normal heart in one twin and double-outlet right ventricle in the other; and in 1 set, there was a normal heart in one twin and a rudimentary, primitive single-ventricle heart with complete heart block in the other twin.

Extracardiac abnormalities in conjoined twins are common including congenital diaphragmatic hernia, abdominal wall defects, and imperforate anus. In omphalopagus, a shared liver can be seen, with either one or two bile drainage systems.

Frequency, Genetics, and Development

Conjoined twins occur in the range of 1 in 50,000 to 100,000 pregnancies. Because 60% are stillborn or die shortly after birth, the true incidence is approximately 1 in 200,00 live births. The female to male ratio is 3 : 1.

In the case of conjoined twins, a woman produces only a single egg, which does not fully separate after fertilization. The developing embryo starts to split into identical twins during the first few weeks after conception, but stops before the process is complete. The partially separated egg develops into a conjoined fetus. The twins are, therefore, "identical" with similar genetic makeup. Since in thoracopagus twins, the single heart is multiventricular; it suggests very early union with fusion of the cardiac amalgam before significant differentiation has taken place.[4]

In general, as a consequence of assisted reproductive technologies, the number of twins are increasing, and in combination with improved accuracy of early imaging, conjoined twins are being more readily diagnosed early in pregnancy. Intracytoplasmic sperm injection (ICSI) type of in vitro fertilization has been reported in association with conjoined twinning[5]; however, the overall numbers of such are too small to declare a cause-and-effect relationship.

Prenatal Physiology

Conjoined twins that present at the tail end of the first or beginning of the second trimester have already self-selected as demonstrating a stable cardiovascular system. Nonviable cardiovascular systems will undergo demise in the first trimester. Physiological disturbances of the cardiovascular system in first-trimester survivors depend upon the classification type and the intracardiac anatomy. Most single amalgam fused hearts (type I) function well with normal myocardial contractility and normal perfusion of the fetal organs and placenta. In a type IB or IIB, in which there is a disproportionate heart in one twin, perfusion of the other occurs through vascular connections or shared organs in a "parasitic" manner. Disparities in the proportion of the heart typically accompany disparities in fetal size and other organ development in a congruent manner. In other words, in a type IB, the twin partner with less of the heart will likely also have a less well developed body and other organs structures. Nevertheless, overall progressive growth in size occurs and the fetuses commonly remain stable throughout gestation.

Prenatal Management

Detailed analysis of the fetal anatomy is required in a conjoined twin in order to ascertain the possibility of a postnatal surgical separation.[6] The heart is often the key organ that dictates the potential for separation. Evaluation of the cardiovascular system in a conjoined twin can be one of the most challenging undertakings for the fetal echocardiographer. The anatomy can appear quite complex and confusing with unrecognizable structures unlike anything seen in a singleton fetus. A logical, stepwise approach is best. First, we recommend classification based on heart number and location as we have described. Then, a segmental approach is applied to each heart, or side of the heart for each twin, starting with venous return, atria, atrioventricular valve connections, ventricles, outflow tracts, and finally, great vessels. Each of these segments should be identified and structure and flow patterns understood for each twin.

Detailed assessment of the precise anatomy is ideally performed at 16 to 20 weeks' gestation; however, earlier scanning is recommended because sufficient anatomical information can be obtained to make general decisions about candidacy for separation.[7,8] To date, no successful separation of a type I single-heart amalgam has been reported.[1,9] Hence, identification of a type I single, shared heart is key in the early evaluation process. Furthermore, the number and location of the inferior venae cavae have importance as well. It is essential that the twin being considered for survival have a well-formed inferior vena cava draining to the heart because absence of such is prohibitive toward normal venous drainage, if the other twin is sacrificed. Evaluation should include detailed obstetrical ultrasound, fetal echocardiography, and fetal magnetic resonance imaging to obtain as much anatomical information as possible.

Because most conjoined twins are not candidates for surgery and termination is a common choice of families, early evaluation is essential. Termination of conjoined twins can be somewhat challenging in the second trimester because the size of the total fetal mass influences the method used; hence, the earlier the diagnosis, the better.

Prenatal counseling for the family carrying a fetus with conjoined twins is best done in a multidisciplinary setting with maternal-fetal medicine specialists, fetal cardiologists, surgeons, and social work/nursing support. If the heart is a type II and surgical separation is to be considered, extensive further preparation is necessary including cesarean section delivery at a center that can provide all of the necessary resources for postnatal evaluation and care.

Postnatal Physiology, Management, and Outcomes

Whereas the anatomy can be well ascertained using various imaging modalities in the patient with conjoined twins, postnatal physiology and viability are less predictable. Cesarean section delivery is indicated, which is typically performed no later than 35 to 36 weeks' gestation. Lung function can be unpredictable and is often limited by mechanical constraint owing to the position of the twins in relation to each other.

Depending upon the type of anatomy, some twins have stable hemodynamics without much intervention, whereas others may require prostaglandin infusion if there is critical obstruction present. In some, stability can be achieved and surgical intervention delayed, whereas in others, early separation is optimal.

Surgical treatment in conjoined twins involves separation, often with sacrifice of one of the twins in order to allow for successful reconstruction and survival of the other.[10,11] As previously mentioned, there are no survivors of type I, single-heart amalgam forms of conjoined twins. No matter how well repaired and functional such a heart may be after separation, the inability to fully reconstruct a normal chest and the markedly altered chest wall and lung mechanics ultimately lead to early demise.

In our series of 25 fetus pairs, surgical separation was undertaken in 5 sets: 1 type I and 4 type II. Survival of at least 1 twin was achieved only in type II, with two separate hearts. In fact, in type II, survival of both twins is possible if there is a normal heart or if the structural defect is amenable to surgical repair, as in our case of a type IIA in which transposition of the great arteries was successfully repaired after separation. If undertaken, these are major operations that require long operative times and multiple teams of physicians and surgeons. Recuperation can be quite prolonged. Decisions concerning elective separation in the stable set of conjoined twins must also be balanced against the possibility of survival without intervention. Such twin sets, however, may face a challenging life from a social and societal perspective.

Imaging Essentials and Important Points

- There are no survivors of conjoined twins with a single-heart amalgam (type I); hence, early identification of this type is essential for early counseling and decision making.
- Fetal echocardiographic imaging is important and quite challenging. A segmental approach should be applied. Plenty of time should also be allowed for imaging, and we commonly schedule such a patient for multiple time slots.
- Often, we will use a sketchpad and pencil while imaging in order to draw the segmental structures as they are delineated and understood.
- In type I, atria are commonly fused at the right atrial level; ventricles are commonly fused at the left ventricles. The left ventricles are typically positioned medially, with the right ventricles laterally.
- When evaluating a type I heart, a cardiac axis or "equator" can often be delineated as the possible site of fusion. However, this cardiac equator may not be in the same position as the anatomical dividing line between the twins.
- In assessing type II conjoined twins, the hearts may be separate; however, they may share a pericardium.
- When considering the possibility of separating conjoined twins, the presence of an inferior vena cava is essential for survival. Identification of the inferior vena cava is of utmost importance in the evaluation. Magnetic resonance imaging can be used to aid in delineation of this anatomy.

References

1. Andrews RE, McMahon CJ, Yates RW, et al. Echocardiographic assessment of conjoined twins. *Heart*. 2006;92:382-387.
2. Gerlis LM, Seo JW, Ho SY, Chi JG. Morphology of the cardiovascular system in conjoined twins: spatial and sequential segmental arrangements in 36 cases. *Teratology*. 1993;47:91-108.
3. Danford DA, McManus BM, Nielsen SM, Levine MG, Needelman HW. Definition of inseparably fused ventricular myocardium in thoracopagus: fetal echocardiographic utility and pathologic refinement. *Pediatr Cardiol*. 1993;14:242-246.
4. Gilbert-Barness E, Debich-Spicer D, Opitz JM. Conjoined twins: morphogenesis of the heart and a review. *Am J Med Genet A*. 2003;120A:568-582.
5. Poret H, Blanchard M, Lemseffer M, Royere D, Guerif F. Conjoined twins after intracytoplasmic sperm injection and transfer of a single day 2 embryo: case report. *Fertil Steril*. 2010;93:268.e7-268.e9.
6. Sanders SP, Chin AJ, Parness IA, et al. Prenatal diagnosis of congenital heart defects in thoracoabdominally conjoined twins. *N Engl J Med*. 1985;313:370-374.
7. Maggio M, Callan NA, Hamod KA, Sanders RC. The first-trimester ultrasonographic diagnosis of conjoined twins. *Am J Obstet Gynecol*. 1985;152:833-835.
8. Pajkrt E, Jauniaux E. First-trimester diagnosis of conjoined twins. *Prenat Diagn*. 2005;25:820-826.
9. McMahon CJ, Spencer R. Congenital heart defects in conjoined twins: outcome after surgical separation of thoracopagus. *Pediatr Cardiol*. 2006;27:1-12.
10. O'Neill JA Jr, Holcomb GW 3rd, Schnaufer L, et al. Surgical experience with thirteen conjoined twins. *Ann Surg*. 1988;208:299-312.
11. Mackenzie TC, Crombleholme TM, Johnson MP, et al. The natural history of prenatally diagnosed conjoined twins. *J Pediatr Surg*. 2002;37:303-309.

CASES

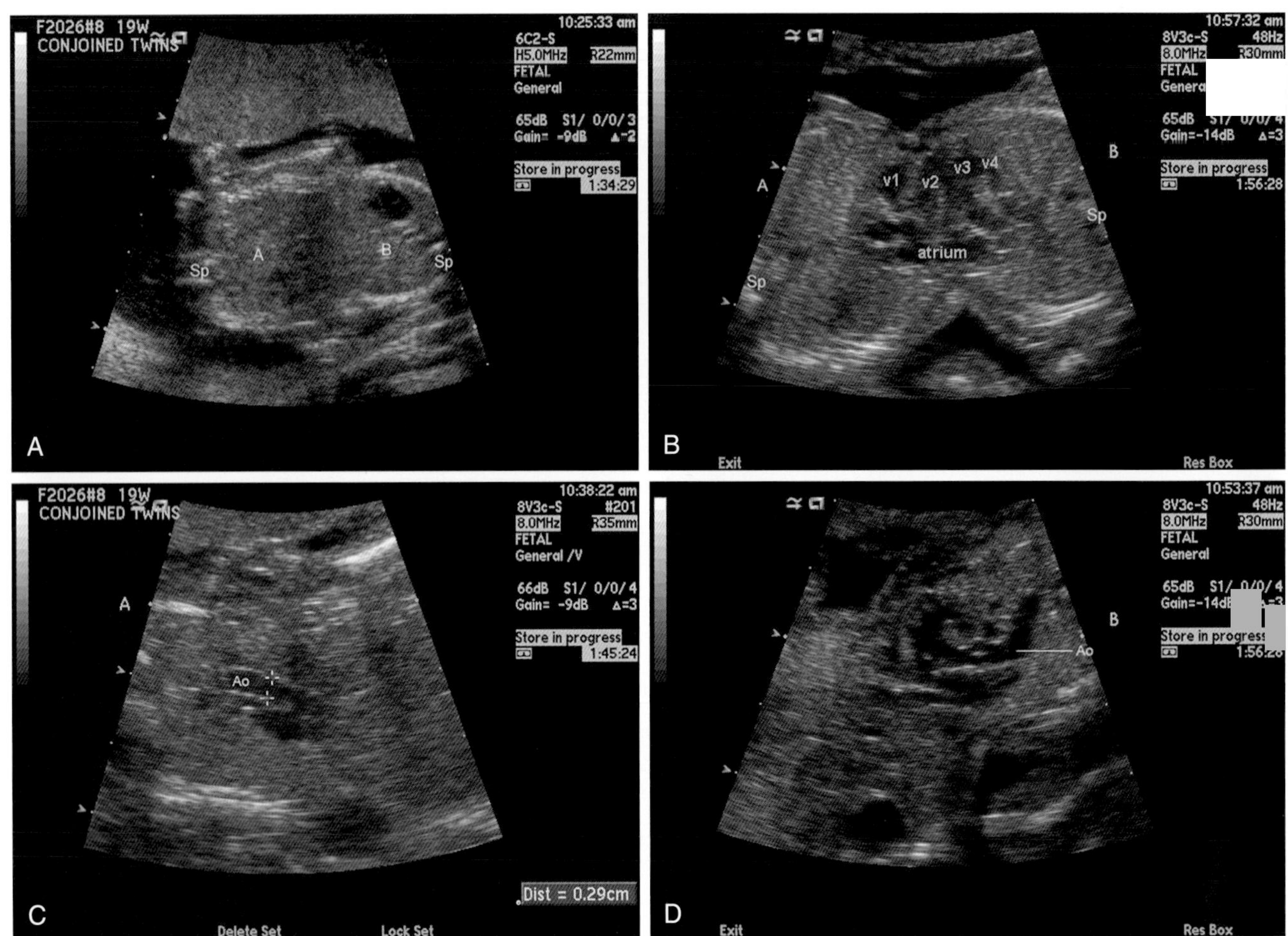

Case 34-1. (**A**) Conjoined twins at 19 weeks' gestation. The spines (Sp) are seen at opposite poles of 3 o'clock and 9 o'clock. Note the fusion centrally at the level of the liver. By common convention, we label the twin on the right "A" and the one on the left "B." The stomach on twin B is visualized. (**B**) Sweeping downward, a common heart is seen centrally located within the common, fused chest. This is a type IA in which there is a single-heart amalgam, centrally situated and equally distributed between the twins. Four ventricular cavities (v) are seen. There is an anatomical symmetry in this heart—the heart mass is central and the great vessels come off the poles in a similar fashion in each twin. (**C**) Angling toward twin A reveals the outflow tracts. There is a large aortic vessel (Ao) arising from the "outer" ventricle, which is a right ventricle. (**D**) Angling toward twin B reveals a large vessel, the aorta (Ao), arising from a morphological-appearing right ventricle. Hence, this twin's heart configuration is likely a double-outlet right ventricle.

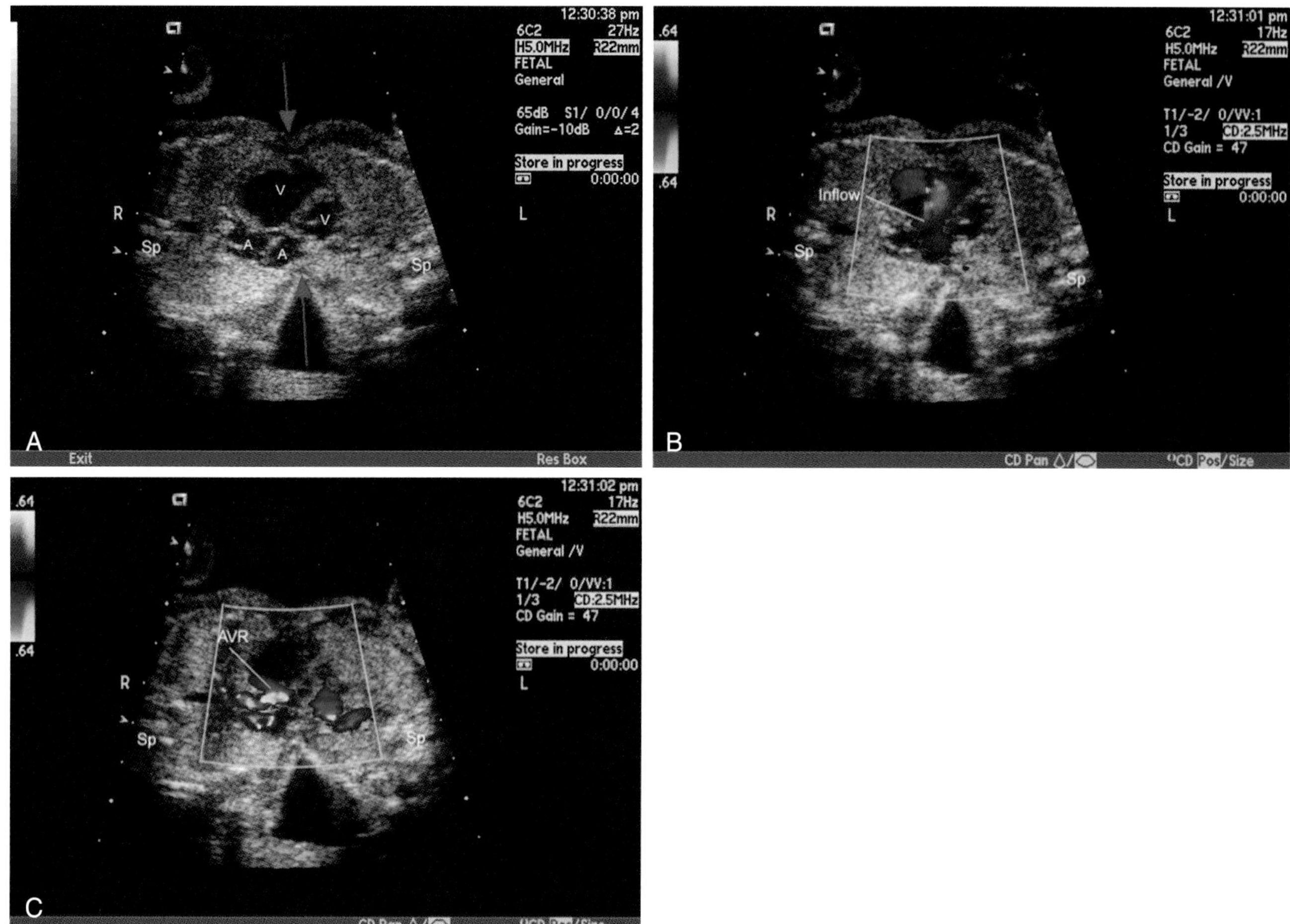

Case 34-2. **(A)** A case of thoracopagus with a single-heart amalgam between the twins. By following the planes at the site of fusion between the twins *(red arrows)*, one can see that the heart mass is situated more so into the chest cavity of the twin on the right side. There is an asymmetry in position of the single heart; hence, this is categorized as type IB. A, atria; V, ventricle. **(B)** Color imaging inflow demonstrates a dominant ventricle located more so to the right-sided twin. **(C)** Atrioventricular valve regurgitation (AVR) of the larger ventricle is present.

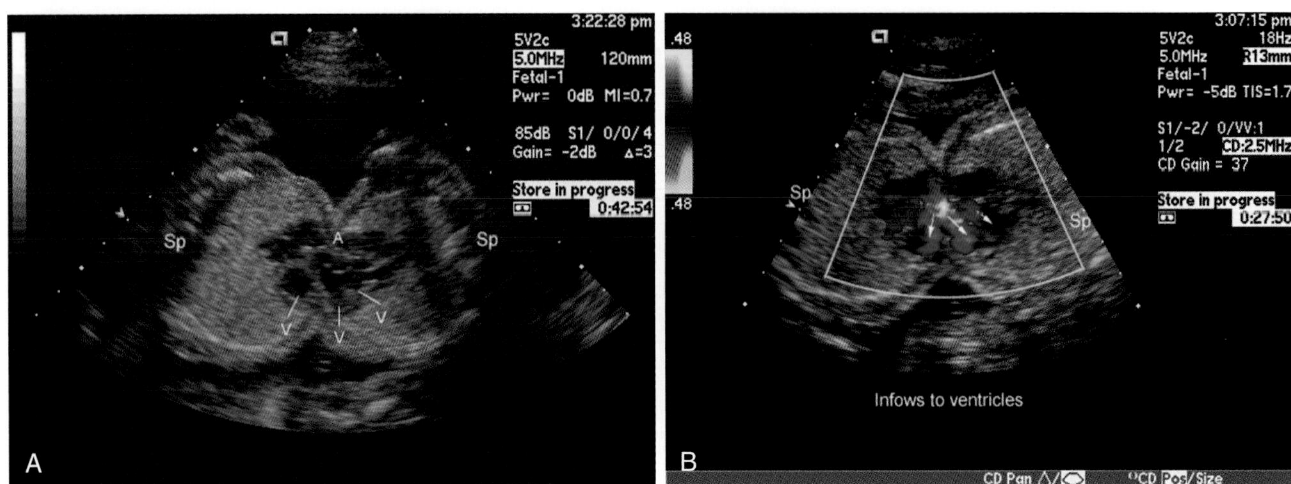

Case 34-3. **(A)** A case of type IA thoracopagus. A common centrally positioned heart with three ventricles is seen. **(B)** Color flow imaging delineates the inflow *(arrows)* across the inflows into the three ventricles.

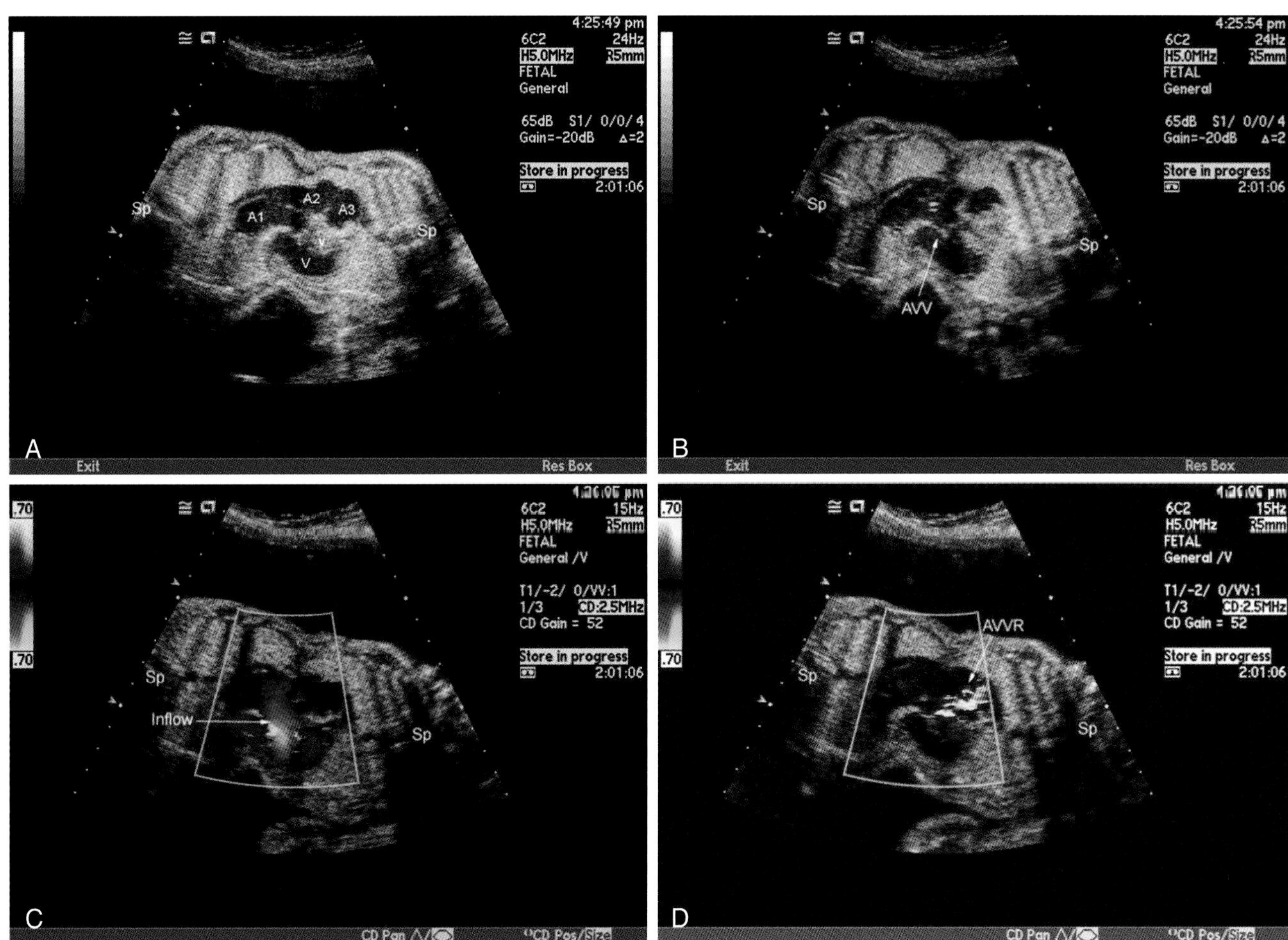

Case 34-4. **(A)** Thoracopagus type IB with three atria (A) and one dominant and one smaller ventricle (V). **(B)** There appears to be a large common atrioventricular valve (AVV) positioned over the larger and smaller leftward ventricle, suggesting an unbalanced atrioventricular canal as an element of this complex heart defect. **(C)** Color flow imaging of inflow across the common AVV. **(D)** Eccentric jet of significant atrioventricular valve regurgitation (AVVR).

35 Fetal Cardiomyopathy

Jack Rychik

Key Echocardiographic Features

- Investigate for heart size (cardiothoracic ratio).
- Investigate systolic function, qualitative and quantitative (myocardial performance index, shortening fraction).
- Look for evidence of pericardial effusion or hydrops.
- Look for atrioventricular valve regurgitation.
- Assess Doppler signals of ventricular inflow, ductus venosus, and umbilical vein.
- Measure peak systolic middle cerebral artery velocity when looking for fetal anemia as a possible explanation for cardiomegaly and high-output state.
- Calculation of combined cardiac output and serial follow-through can be instructive in cases of markedly low or markedly elevated cardiac output values.
- Assess Doppler flow patterns from umbilical artery and middle cerebral artery. Ratio of pulsatility indices reflects flow and overall fetal wellness or unwellness.

Table 35-1 Examples of Causes of Cardiomyopathy in the Fetus

CATEGORY	CAUSE
Dilated Cardiomyopathy	
Infection	Parvovirus Coxsackie virus Toxoplasma HIV Cytomegalovirus
Metabolic/genetic	Sialic acid storage disease X-linked cardiomyopathy Barth's syndrome Mitochondrial disorders Arterial calcinosis Noncompaction of the left ventricle
Anemia	Anti–C antibody Alpha-thalassemia (hemoglobin Bart's disease) Parvovirus
Other	Maternal autoimmune (lupus or Sjögren's disease) Tachyarrhythmias Renal disease Idiopathic (?)
Hypertrophic Cardiomyopathy	
Metabolic/genetic	Maternal diabetes mellitus Noonan's syndrome Glycogen storage (Pompe's disease) B lipase deficiency Cytochrome oxidase deficiency Familial hypertrophic cardiomyopathy
Other	Renal disease Twin-twin transfusion syndrome

HIV, human immunodeficiency virus.

Fetal cardiomyopathy is a disorder in which the heart muscle of the fetus is diseased and not functioning properly.[1-4] It makes up approximately 2% to 4% of all forms of cardiovascular disease seen in the fetus. Fetal cardiomyopathy can be classified into two categories. *Dilated cardiomyopathy (DCM)* is defined as the presence of ventricular chambers enlarged above normal and poor systolic function. *Hypertrophic cardiomyopathy (HCM)* is defined as abnormally thickened ventricular walls, in the absence of any structural abnormality that might explain the hypertrophy. Cardiomyopathy in the fetus can be due to a variety of causes such as infection, metabolic disease, genetic disorders of myocardial dysfunction, fetal anemia, or it is of unclear etiology and, therefore, labeled as *idiopathic*. Some examples of diseases causing fetal cardiomyopathy are listed in Table 35-1; however, a complete, exhaustive list is not possible because the potential etiologies and pathways to myocardial dysfunction are endless.

Dilated Cardiomyopathy

Etiologies

Infectious etiologies are the most likely cause for DCM in the fetus, with metabolic/genetic abnormalities a close second. Viral agents can cross the placenta and cause active fetal viral myocarditis.[5] The presence of an isolated large pericardial effusion in association with a dilated, poorly functioning heart indicates ongoing myocarditis and inflammation. Maternal history for an acute illness may be elicited, but commonly, no such event can be documented upon questioning. In viral myocarditis, dysfunction may resolve spontaneously or persist, suggesting myocardial damage.

Mutations in the tafazzin gene *(TAZ)* located on the X chromosome are responsible for a variety of X-linked cardiomyopathies that may present in the fetus.[6] Barth's syndrome is one such disorder in which there is DCM, cyclical neutropenia, and growth delay. Isolated noncompaction of the left ventricle (NCLV) can occur in an X-linked manner or may be seen without any particular genetic/chromosomal explanation.[7] In this disorder, there are deep crypts within the left ventricle (LV) apex and free wall, with the noncompacted region measuring at least twice the diameter of the compacted myocardium. It is a disease primarily of the LV because the right ventricle (RV) is normally noncompacted. NCLV manifests a wide range of clinical symptoms with some patients asymptomatic with good ventricular function and others with poor systolic function. NCLV can evolve over time into DCM with progressive wall thinning, ventricular dilation, and dysfunction.

Fetal anemias, either through viral suppression as with parvovirus or genetic hemoglobinopathy, can cause DCM.

Hemoglobin Bart's disease is the homozygous form of alpha-thalassemia in which oxygen-carrying capacity is severely diminished. Hemoglobin Bart's develops in fetuses with four-gene deletion alpha-thalassemia, in which no alpha chain of hemoglobin is produced. The gamma chains produced during fetal development combine to form gamma chain tetramers, which transport oxygen poorly. Most individuals with four-gene deletion thalassemia and consequent hemoglobin Bart's manifest severe hydrops fetalis and die in utero. This disorder was characterized at St. Bartholomew's Hospital in London; hence, the name *hemoglobin Bart's*. When hemoglobin Bart's disease is present, severe fetal hydrops and demise are nearly certain and can cause a "mirror syndrome" in the mother, placing her at risk as well.[8]

A rare, but striking, disorder known as *infantile arterial calcinosis* can be identified during fetal life. Fetal imaging demonstrates the appearance of a thick, echo-bright "icing" of calcification outlining the walls of the great vessels.[9] The disease is characterized by extensive calcification of medium and large arteries. Histologically, calcifications are seen to extend from the internal elastic lamina into the intima and media and are associated with giant cell reaction and smooth muscle proliferation. The aorta, main pulmonary arteries, or renal arteries can be affected. Myocardial dysfunction is common, presumably related to coronary calcification and myocardial ischemia. In addition, hypertension due to renal artery disease compounds the pathophysiology. Most cases lead to fetal hydrops and demise, or some fetuses make it to term with multiorgan system involvement but then manifest neonatal demise. Rarely, milder forms can be identified in infancy and may respond to chelating agents and diphosphonates.

Although most known for its effects on the conduction system, maternal autoimmune disorders such as lupus or Sjögren's disease can cause DCM.[1] Inflammation of the myocardium with dilation and dysfunction can occur in conjunction with destruction of conduction tissue or independently. Testing for SS-A and SS-B antibodies is warranted as part of the workup for DCM because most mothers carrying such fetuses can be completely asymptomatic without any hint of autoimmune disease. We, as well as others, have noticed an interesting echocardiographic phenomenon that seems to be indicative of possible maternal autoimmune disease. Some fetuses exposed to these antibodies will develop a unique echo-brightness to various regions of the myocardium, either at the atria, at the atrioventricular groove, or at the crux of the heart.[10,11] We suspect that this may represent ongoing regional inflammation, which leads to an increased ultrasound reflectivity.

Prenatal Diagnosis

In general, the fetus with DCM will exhibit dilation of the left, right, or both ventricles, with poor systolic function. Qualitative cardiomegaly can be seen upon fetal echocardiography and the cardiothoracic ratio will exceed 40%. Shortening fraction measurement can provide a quantitative sense of the degree of systolic dysfunction and will be less than 30%. Atrioventricular valve regurgitation is common, due to either annular dilation and poor valve leaflet coaptation or papillary muscle dysfunction. Pericardial effusion, in particular with infectious causes, can be seen. Diastolic abnormalities may occur simultaneously or, at times, precede the onset of systolic dysfunction. Abnormalities such as fusion of the diastolic inflow pattern across the tricuspid or mitral valves, absence or reversal of flow with atrial contraction in the ductus venosus, or venous pulsations all reflect elevated ventricular filling pressures.[12] Global measures of myocardial function are helpful in quantifying the degree of dysfunction. The myocardial performance index will be elevated, typically greater than 0.5, and can be used serially to assess for progression of disease. We have used the Doppler-derived combined cardiac output as a means to evaluate for the overall impact of dysfunction. Normal combined cardiac output is approximately 400 to 500 mL/kg/min of flow. In our experience, we have found that a value below 400 mL/kg/min reflects a decompensated state and suggests severe disease with poor outcome. Hydrops fetalis when associated with DCM indicates markedly elevated ventricular filling pressures and low cardiac output. The presence of hydrops fetalis bodes poorly for outcome, with a high likelihood of fetal or neonatal demise.[2] The detection of any ventricular dilation and dysfunction requires close serial evaluation because disease progression can be rapid in some cases.

Evaluation of the arterial vascular systems, the umbilical arterial (UA) and middle cerebral arterial (MCA) flow, offers important information in the fetus with DCM. As an indirect measure of the adequacy of cardiac output, the resistance of the MCA should normally always be higher than the UA, which reflects a healthy distribution of flow. Hence, MCA pulsatility index (PI) should be higher than UA PI. When cardiac output is diminished, there is a vasoregulatory attempt to increase blood flow to the cerebral circulation, and the MCA PI will drop below the UA PI value.[13] Serial evaluation of the UA and MCA PI values is, therefore, an important component of the overall fetal echocardiographic assessment of DCM. Furthermore, in conditions of fetal anemia, the MCA peak systolic velocity has been reported to be markedly elevated and can be a reliable measure of the degree of anemia (Figure 35-1).[14] As oxygen-carrying capacity diminishes with reduction in hemoglobin, there is a compensatory increase in cerebral volume of flow reflected by an increase in MCA peak systolic velocity. Assessment of MCA peak systolic velocity is of significant value because it can also be incorporated into the differential diagnostic assessment when trying to determine the etiology of DCM.

A useful scoring system for grading severity of fetal congestive heart failure has been developed. The

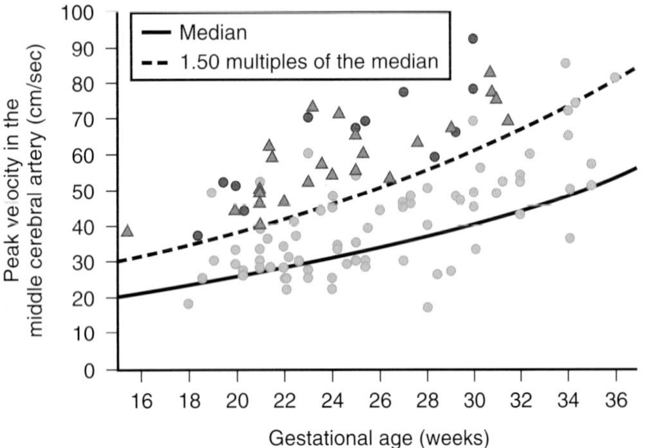

Figure 35-1. Relationship between peak systolic velocity in the middle cerebral artery and gestational age, derived from 111 fetuses at risk for anemia due to maternal red cell alloimunization. The *solid curve* indicates the median peak systolic velocity and the *dashed curve* indicates velocity values above 1.50 multiples of the median. The *yellow circles* indicate fetuses with no anemia; the *triangles* are fetuses with moderate-severe anemia; the *red circles* are fetuses with hydrops. (Data from Mari G, Deter RL, Carpenter RL, et al. Noninvasive diagnosis by Doppler ultrasonography of fetal anemia due to maternal red-cell alloimunization. *N Engl J Med.* 2000;342:9-14.)

cardiovascular profile score (CPS) comprises five categories of findings that, if abnormal, portray the degree of heart failure (Figure 35-2).[15,16] A normal heart would have a complete score of 10, and points are subtracted based on findings present. The categories include measures of degree of hydrops, venous Doppler, heart size, heart function, and umbilical arterial Doppler tracings. Studies have demonstrated the utility of the CPS in predicting outcome and correlation with other measures of cardiac performance such as the Tei index.[17] In our view, the CPS can be helpful, but we would caution the use of a general "heart failure" score when applying it for a specific disease process because each disease has its own unique pathophysiology. For example, in twin-twin transfusion syndrome, the pathophysiology and severity of disease may not lend itself toward findings that are specifically present in the CPS. Findings such as wall thickness and right-sided outflow tract obstruction, key elements of twin-twin transfusion syndrome, are not included in the CPS. In general, all of the elements of the CPS can be helpful tools to gauge the degree of fetal unwellness. However, it should not be used exclusively in the absence of other variables that may provide greater information concerning the state of a specific disease.

DCM should be distinguished from other causes of ventricular chamber enlargement and dysfunction. These abnormalities should be considered and investigated when working through the differential diagnosis for DCM. Venous anomalies can cause undue dilation of the RV, for example, as in interrupted inferior vena cava with continuation to the azygos vein, in which venous return is preferentially streamed toward the RV. Abdominal coarctation and aortic narrowing distal to the insertion of the ductus arteriosus will add undue afterload onto both ventricles and can cause dilation and dysfunction. Arteriovenous malformations or tumors such as sacrococcygeal teratoma can add volume load onto a normal myocardium, causing it to exhibit findings similar to those of DCM and fail. Cardiac output in these conditions will be increased and systolic function is usually preserved, at first, despite the presence of ventricular dilation. Obstructive uropathy such as posterior urethral valves can cause massive enlargement of the bladder leading to distal arterial obstruction, in particular along the iliac arteries, and a "functional coarctation" effect.

Management and Outcomes

Management of DCM in the fetus is disease-specific. Some forms of ventricular dysfunction, such as those related to a viral process, may self-resolve. In utero blood transfusion has been used for the fetus with anemia. Fetal cardiomyopathy related to maternal autoimmune disease may respond to anti-inflammatory steroid treatment. Whereas steroids will not resolve heart block once damage to the conduction system has occurred, squelching myocardial inflammation can preserve myocardial function and improve outcome. Dexamethasone at 4 to 8 mg daily administered maternally has been our drug of choice for treatment of this disease.

The use of digoxin to improve fetal heart function has once again become popularized of late.[18] Digoxin easily crosses the placenta, and although its mechanism of action is still after, over 100 years of use, poorly understood, it can have dramatic effects in improving hydrops and outcome in the fetus with heart failure.

Regardless of the implementation of therapy or not, close observation and serial fetal echocardiography are essential in monitoring the fetus with DCM. In one large series of 50 fetuses with DCM, 10 cases (20%) terminated the pregnancy; survival to delivery based on intention to treat was only 63%, survival at 28 days 43%, and survival at 1 year 38%.[2] The overall survival of nonhydropic fetuses was 50% compared with 18% for hydropic fetuses. Prognosis for DCM in the fetus is poor. Improvement awaits the development of more effective means of delivery of therapeutics. In some cases that survive to a viable gestational age, and depending upon the etiology of the DCM, cardiac transplantation can be an option to families with prenatal listing possible.[19]

Hypertrophic Cardiomyopathy

HCM is present when there is abnormal thickening of the heart in the absence of a structural obstructive lesion such aortic or pulmonic stenosis, which may be the cause. Hypertrophy can be concentric throughout the ventricle or localized to the septum. When present in the septum, such thickening itself may cause outflow tract obstruction, further promoting ventricular hypertrophy.

CARDIOVASCULAR PROFILE SCORE (10 POINTS = NORMAL)

	Normal	−1 point	−2 points
Hydrops	None (2 pts)	Ascites *or* pleural effusion *or* pericardial effusion	Skin edema
Venous Doppler (umbilical vein and ductus venosus)	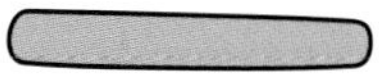 UV 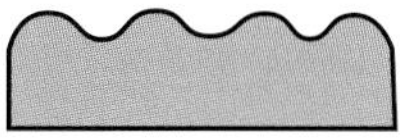 DV (2 pts)	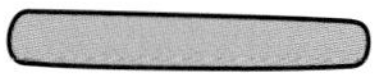 UV 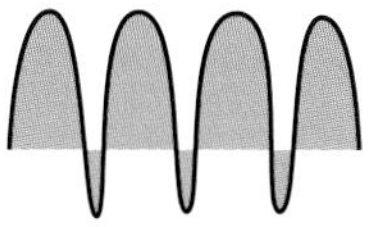 DV	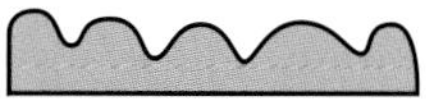 UV pulsations
Heart size (heart area/chest area)	>0.20 and <0.35 (2 pts)	0.35–0.50	>0.50 or <0.20
Cardiac function	Normal TV and MV RV/LV S.F. >0.28 Biphasic diastolic filling (2 pts)	Holosystolic TR *or* RV/LV S.F. <0.28	Holosystolic TR *or* TR d*P*/d*t* 400 *or* monophasic filling
Arterial Doppler (umbilical artery)	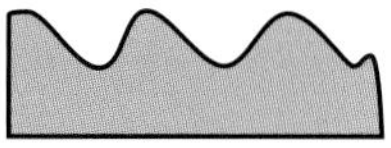 UA (2 pts)	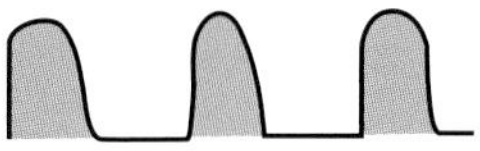 UA (AEDV)	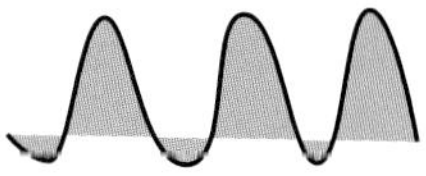 UA (REDV)

Figure 35-2. Grading system for the five elements of the cardiovascular profile score. The elements include assessment of hydrops, venous Doppler, heart size, cardiac function, and arterial Doppler. A fetus without evidence of heart failure will have a score of 10. Points are deducted based on specific findings that are present. AEDV, absent end-diastolic velocity; DV, ductus venosus; LV, left ventricle; MV, mitral valve; REDV, reversed end-diastolic velocity; RV, right ventricle; S.F., shortening fraction; TR, tricuspid regurgitation; TV, tricuspid valve; UA, umbilical artery; UV, umbilical vein.

Etiologies

A number of diseases can result in abnormal thickening of the fetal heart. Noonan's syndrome can manifest as septal hypertrophy with concomitant LV free wall hypertrophy. Increased nuchal translucency in the first trimester with a normal karyotype may be an early clue to the diagnosis of Noonan's syndrome, when septal thickening is noted in the second trimester. Pleural effusions and skin edema out of proportion to the degree of heart dysfunction may also be another clue.[20] Familial HCM can manifest in fetal life and can be suspected after a careful ascertainment of family history for cardiac disease or sudden death.[21] When suspected, genetic testing for the various familial subtypes is currently available.

The most common cause of HCM in the fetus is related to maternal diabetes mellitus.[1,22] Maternal gestational diabetes is on the rise as a consequence of the increasing prevalence of overweight and obese mothers in the United States today. Although conventionally thought to be an isolated disorder of glucose metabolism, diabetes is in reality a pervasive disorder of metabolic derangement affecting glucose, fatty acid, and protein processing with far-reaching effects on the developing fetus. Despite improvements in obstetrical and perinatal care, pregnancies associated with maternal diabetes carry a significantly higher risk of fetal and neonatal complications. With maternal diabetes, the risk of major congenital malformations is 2 to 10 times higher than normal pregnancies. There is a 3% to 5% risk of structural heart disease in the fetuses of diabetic mothers and approximately a 30% risk of HCM with disproportionate septal hypertrophy. Morphologic changes of myocardial hypertrophy can be detected by fetal echocardiography in midgestation and may progressively worsen to term. Although these changes tend to be more severe with poor maternal diabetic control, studies have shown structural myocardial changes and increased interventricular septal thickness even in fetuses with well-controlled maternal diabetes. Most cases of myocardial hypertrophy secondary to maternal diabetes are nonobstructive and tend to resolve in infancy following separation from the maternal metabolic stimulus. However, there are reports of sudden death in utero or stillbirth, attributed to this condition.

Prenatal Diagnosis

Systolic and diastolic cardiac function is usually preserved in fetuses with mild septal hypertrophy and well-controlled maternal diabetes. Septal thickness can be measured either by two-dimensional means or by M-mode with published references available based on gestational age.[23,24] Severe fetal HCM in the setting of maternal diabetes may be associated with significantly increased ventricular stiffness and diastolic dysfunction or outflow tract obstruction. Increased velocity of flow across the left ventricular outflow tract of greater than 1.2 m/sec is abnormal. Mitral regurgitation may be evident if the left ventricular outflow is narrowed. Frank congestive heart failure and fetal hydrops is a rare finding.

Contradictory data exist as to the presence of diastolic abnormalities in all fetuses exposed to a maternal environment of diabetes, even if well controlled. One study found an increased interventricular septal wall thickness in fetuses of well-controlled, asymptomatic diabetic mothers but no differences in systolic or diastolic parameters of function.[25] In another study, 26 fetuses from mothers with type 1 diabetes were compared with 30 age-matched normals in a serial fashion throughout gestation.[26] In the first trimester, there was evidence of poorer fetal cardiac diastolic function among the diabetic cohort as reflected by a lower mitral Doppler early/atrial velocity waveform ratio, a longer isovolumetric relaxation time, and a higher left myocardial performance index. In the third trimester, the fetal interventricular septum and the right ventricular free wall were thicker in the diabetic cohort. The authors concluded that altered cardiac function may precede cardiac structural changes in fetuses of type 1 diabetic pregnancy. Another study demonstrated a direct relationship between hemoglobinA_{1C} and degree of septal hypertrophy and an inverse relationship with parameters of cardiac performance.[27]

Management and Outcomes

Serial follow-up is indicated in the presence of abnormal septal thickening on fetal echocardiography. It is currently standard practice for performance of a detailed fetal echocardiographic evaluation in all pregnancies with diabetes, either pregestational or gestational at approximately 20 to 24 weeks. If abnormal septal thickening is present, or if there is a subsequent history of poor glycemic control, a follow-up evaluation is indicated.

For maternal diabetes–induced HCM, resolution of the myocardial hypertrophy is common after birth, but normalization may take weeks. Rarely, some neonates may require supportive measures if the HCM is severe. For nondiabetic HCM, postnatal workup should include a metabolic assessment as well as genetics evaluation.

Imaging Essentials and Important Points

- The fetal echocardiographer can use a variety of tools to assess the fetal heart that is suspected of dysfunction. Parameters can be separated into diastolic, systolic, or combined.
- Shortening fraction of the LV is one of the most elemental means of assessing systolic function. It can be measured in the long-axis or short-axis planes with the angle of insonation at 90 degrees to the septum and posterior wall of the LV.
- The CPS provides a general, quantitative means for measuring overall "unwellness"; however, individual parameters within the CPS, as well as others, may be better used when appropriately weighted and applied selectively based on the specific pathophysiology of the disease.
- When is atrioventricular valve regurgitation abnormal? With improved instrument sensitivity, mild degrees of tricuspid regurgitation are within normal limits. However, we would consider any mitral regurgitation abnormal. Holosystolic tricuspid regurgitation on pulse wave Doppler or a color Doppler jet that exceeds 25% of the right atrial area is clearly abnormal.
- Frequency of evaluation is a topic of energetic discussion among practitioners. No doubt, if there is evidence of dysfunction, serial weekly evaluation, if not more frequently, may be advised. However, there is no universal standard for screening for dysfunction, such as in maternal diabetes or autoimmune disease.
  - Maternal diabetes: It has been our style of practice to see patients with diabetes once at 20 to 26 weeks' gestation. If there is no structural heart disease and normal wall thickness, the patient is discharged from serial fetal echocardiography, unless there is glycemic instability or if the referring obstetrician is suspicious for some new concern.
  - Maternal autoimmune disease: With maternal documentation of disease such as lupus or Sjögren's or the presence of maternal antibodies, we will screen the fetus every 2 weeks from the beginning of the second trimester (14-16 wk) until 28 weeks' gestation, at which point the likelihood for fetal disease is markedly diminished.

References

1. Pedra SR, Smallhorn JF, Ryan G, et al. Fetal cardiomyopathies: pathogenic mechanisms, hemodynamic findings, and clinical outcome. *Circulation*. 2002;106:585-591.
2. Sivasankaran S, Sharland GK, Simpson JM. Dilated cardiomyopathy presenting during fetal life. *Cardiol Young*. 2005;15:409-416.
3. Schmidt KG, Birk E, Silverman NH, Scagnelli SA. Echocardiographic evaluation of dilated cardiomyopathy in the human fetus. *Am J Cardiol*. 1989;63:599-605.
4. Yinon Y, Yagel S, Hegesh J, et al. Fetal cardiomyopathy—in utero evaluation and clinical significance. *Prenat Diagn*. 2007;27:23-28.
5. Ramirez MM, Mastrobattista JM. Diagnosis and management of human parvovirus B19 infection. *Clin Perinatol*. 2005;32:697-704.
6. Brady AN, Shehata BM, Fernhoff PM. X-linked fetal cardiomyopathy caused by a novel mutation in the *TAZ* gene. *Prenat Diagn*. 2006;26:462-465.
7. Richards A, Mao CY, Dobson NR. Left ventricular noncompaction: a rare cause of hydrops fetalis. *Pediatr Cardiol*. 2009;30:985-988.
8. Nakayama R, Yamada D, Steinmiller V, Hsia E, Hale RW. Hydrops fetalis secondary to Bart hemoglobinopathy. *Obstet Gynecol*. 1986; 67:176-180.
9. Chong CR, Hutchins GM. Idiopathic infantile arterial calcification: the spectrum of clinical presentations. *Pediatr Dev Pathol*. 2008;11: 405-415.
10. Kaur A, Lai WW. Echogenic atria in a fetus. *Ultrasound Obstet Gynecol*. 2007;30:351-353.
11. Cuneo BF, Strasburger JF, Niksch A, Ovadia M, Wakai RT. An expanded phenotype of maternal SSA/SSB antibody-associated fetal cardiac disease. *J Matern Fetal Neonatal Med*. 2009;22:233-238.
12. Gudmundsson S, Huhta JC, Wood DC, Tulzer G, Cohen AW, Weiner S. Venous Doppler ultrasonography in the fetus with nonimmune hydrops. *Am J Obstet Gynecol*. 1991;164:33-37.
13. Hecher K, Campbell S, Doyle P, Harrington K, Nicolaides K. Assessment of fetal compromise by Doppler ultrasound investigation of the fetal circulation. Arterial, intracardiac, and venous blood flow velocity studies. *Circulation*. 1995;91:129-138.
14. Imbar T, Lev-Sagie A, Cohen S, Yanai N, Yagel S. Diagnosis, surveillance, and treatment of the anemic fetus using middle cerebral artery peak systolic velocity measurement. *Prenat Diagn*. 2006; 26:45-51.
15. Huhta JC. Guidelines for the evaluation of heart failure in the fetus with or without hydrops. *Pediatr Cardiol*. 2004;25:274-286.
16. Huhta JC. Fetal congestive heart failure. *Semin Fetal Neonatal Med*. 2005;10:542-552.
17. Falkensammer CB, Paul J, Huhta JC. Fetal congestive heart failure: correlation of Tei-index and cardiovascular-score. *J Perinat Med*. 2001;29:390-398.
18. Patel D, Cuneo B, Viesca R, Rassanan J, Leshko J, Huhta J. Digoxin for the treatment of fetal congestive heart failure with sinus rhythm assessed by cardiovascular profile score. *J Matern Fetal Neonatal Med*. 2008;21:477-482.
19. Pollock-Barziv SM, McCrindle BW, West LJ, Dipchand AI. Waiting before birth: outcomes after fetal listing for heart transplantation. *Am J Transplant*. 2008;8:412-418.
20. Nisbet DL, Griffin DR, Chitty LS. Prenatal features of Noonan syndrome. *Prenat Diagn*. 1999;19:642-647.
21. Stewart PA, Buis-Liem T, Verwey RA, Wladimiroff JW. Prenatal ultrasonic diagnosis of familial asymmetric septal hypertrophy. *Prenat Diagn*. 1986;6:249-256.
22. Hornberger LK. Maternal diabetes and the fetal heart. *Heart*. 2006;92:1019-1021.
23. Tan J, Silverman NH, Hoffman JI, Villegas M, Schmidt KG. Cardiac dimensions determined by cross-sectional echocardiography in the normal human fetus from 18 weeks to term. *Am J Cardiol*. 1992;70:1459-1467.
24. Allan LD, Joseph MC, Boyd EG, Campbell S, Tynan M. M-Mode echocardiography in the developing human fetus. *Br Heart J*. 1982;47:573-583.
25. Jaeggi ET, Fouron JC, Proulx F. Fetal cardiac performance in uncomplicated and well-controlled maternal type I diabetes. *Ultrasound Obstet Gynecol*. 2001;17:311-315.
26. Russell NE, Foley M, Kinsley BT, Firth RG, Coffey M, McAuliffe FM. Effect of pregestational diabetes mellitus on fetal cardiac function and structure. *Am J Obstet Gynecol*. 2008;199:312.e1-312.e7.
27. Gardiner HM, Pasquini L, Wolfenden J, Kulinskaya E, Li W, Henein M. Increased periconceptual maternal glycated haemoglobin in diabetic mothers reduces fetal long axis cardiac function. *Heart*. 2006;92:1125-1130.

CASES

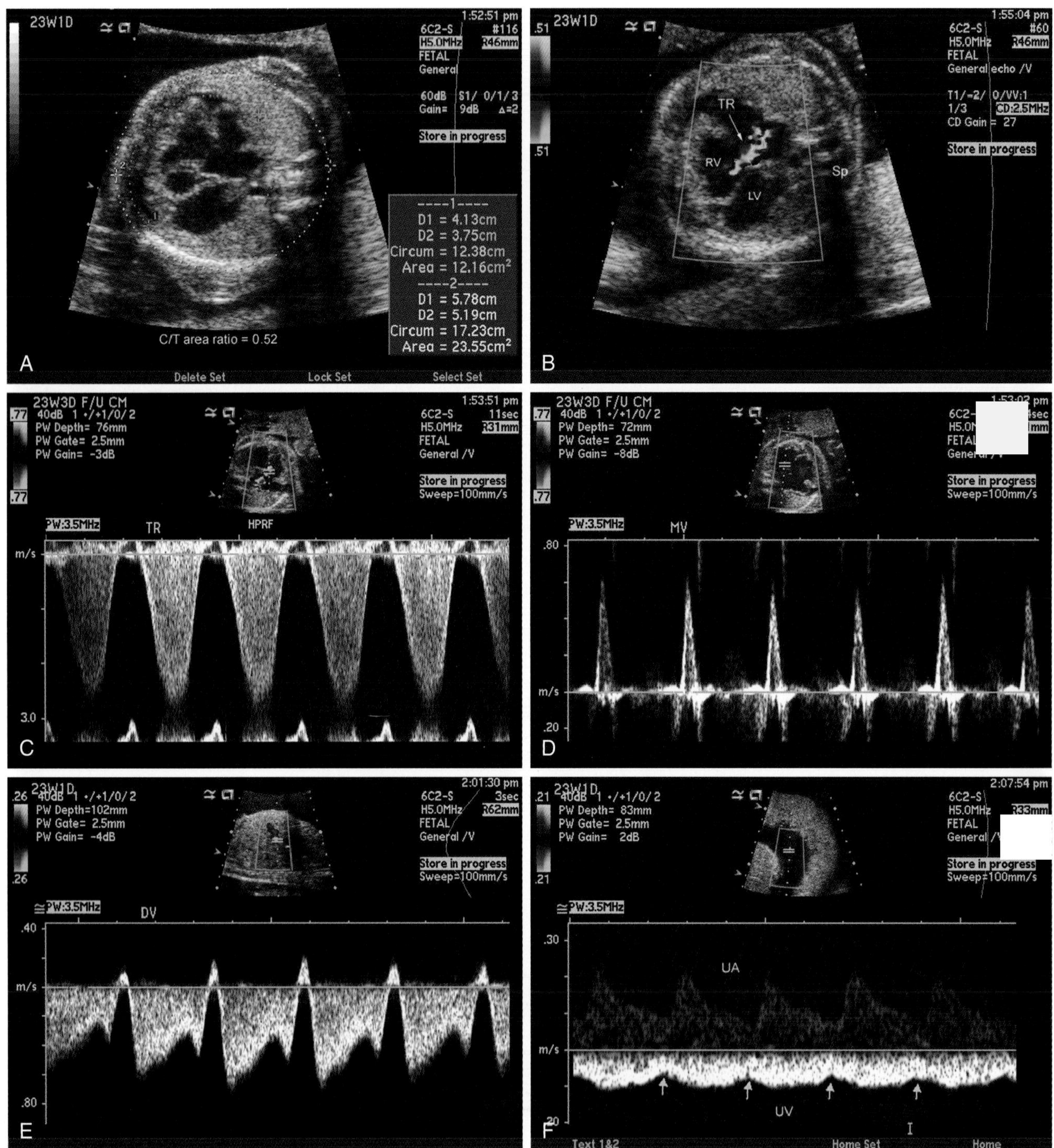

Case 35-1. **(A)** Fetus at 23 weeks' gestation with cardiomyopathy of unknown etiology, likely viral. There is cardiomegaly with cardiothoracic area (C/T) ratio = 0.52. There is also a small pericardial effusion. **(B)** There is a moderate degree of tricuspid regurgitation (TR). LV, left ventricle; RV, right ventricle; Sp, spine. **(C)** Pulse wave Doppler of tricuspid regurgitant jet. The peak velocity is less than 3 m/sec, suggesting a relatively low intracavitary RV peak systolic pressure. **(D)** Doppler wave inflow across the mitral valve (MV). There is a single-peak fused inflow pattern, suggesting abnormal LV diastolic compliance. **(E)** Pulse wave Doppler sampling in the ductus venosus (DV) with prominent reversal at atrial contraction. This pattern suggests abnormal right-sided compliance and diastolic dysfunction. **(F)** Pulse wave Doppler sampling in the umbilical cord. There are pulsations in the umbilical vein (UV; *arrows*), suggesting a significant impediment to right-sided relaxation and significant diastolic dysfunction. UA, umbilical artery.

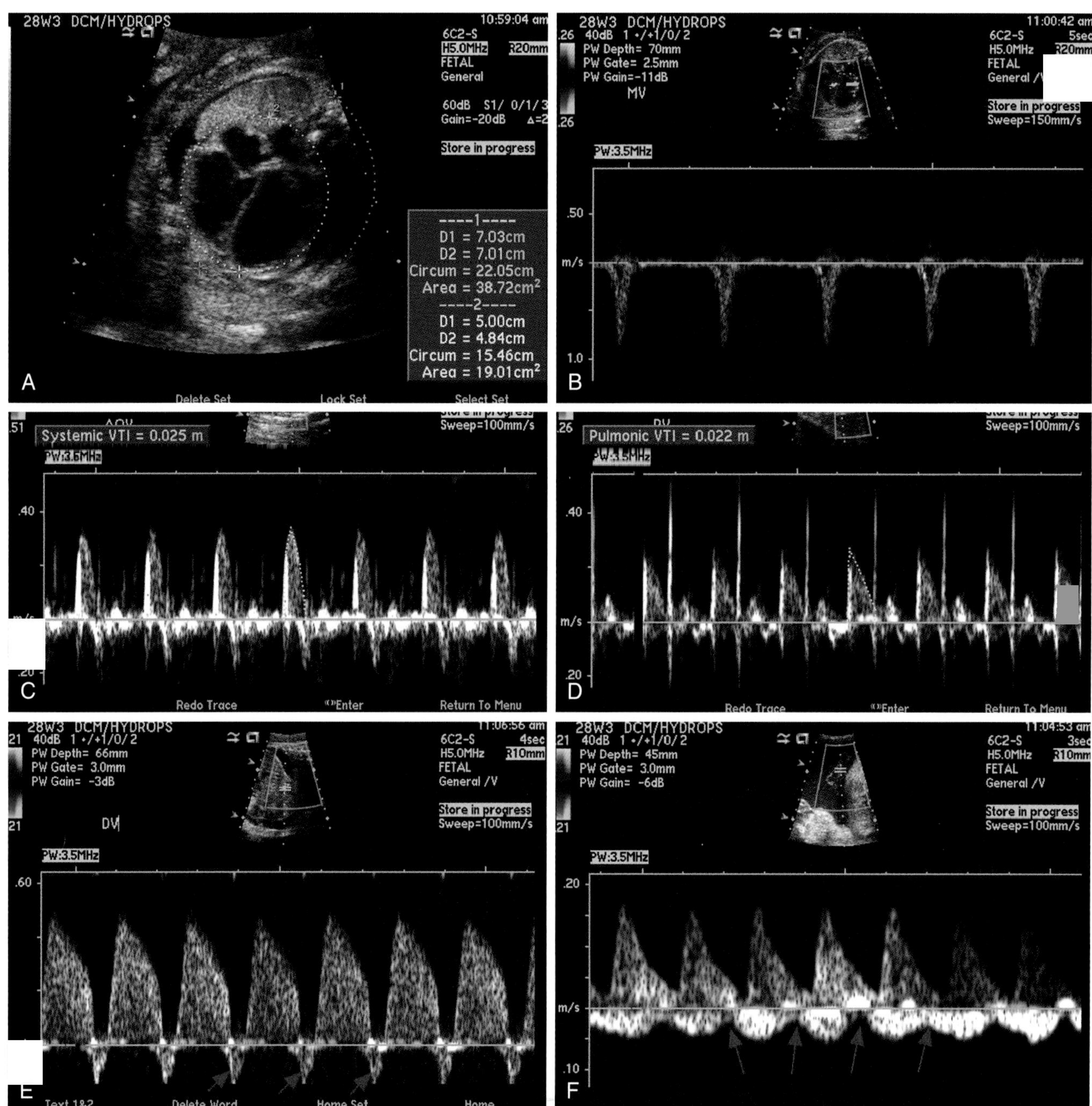

Case 35-2. **(A)** Fetus at 32 weeks' gestation with dilated cardiomyopathy of unknown etiology. The heart is markedly enlarged with C/T ratio greater than 50%. **(B)** Abnormal single-peak Doppler inflow pattern across the MV, suggesting diastolic dysfunction and elevated diastolic pressure. **(C)** Doppler flow across the aortic valve. There is very low velocity and a narrow systolic waveform, indicating low stroke volume. **(D)** Doppler flow across the pulmonic valve. Similar to the aortic flow, there is very low velocity and a narrow systolic waveform, indicating low stroke volume. Overall combined cardiac output for this fetus was approximately 300 mL/kg/min (normal 400-500 mL/kg/min). VTI, velocity-time integral. **(E)** Doppler sampling in the DV. There is reversal with atrial contraction *(arrows)*, suggesting diastolic dysfunction. **(F)** Doppler sampling in the umbilical cord. There are venous pulsations *(arrows)* in the UV, further suggesting severe diastolic dysfunction. Hydrops fetalis ensued within days and there was in utero fetal demise at 30 weeks' gestation.

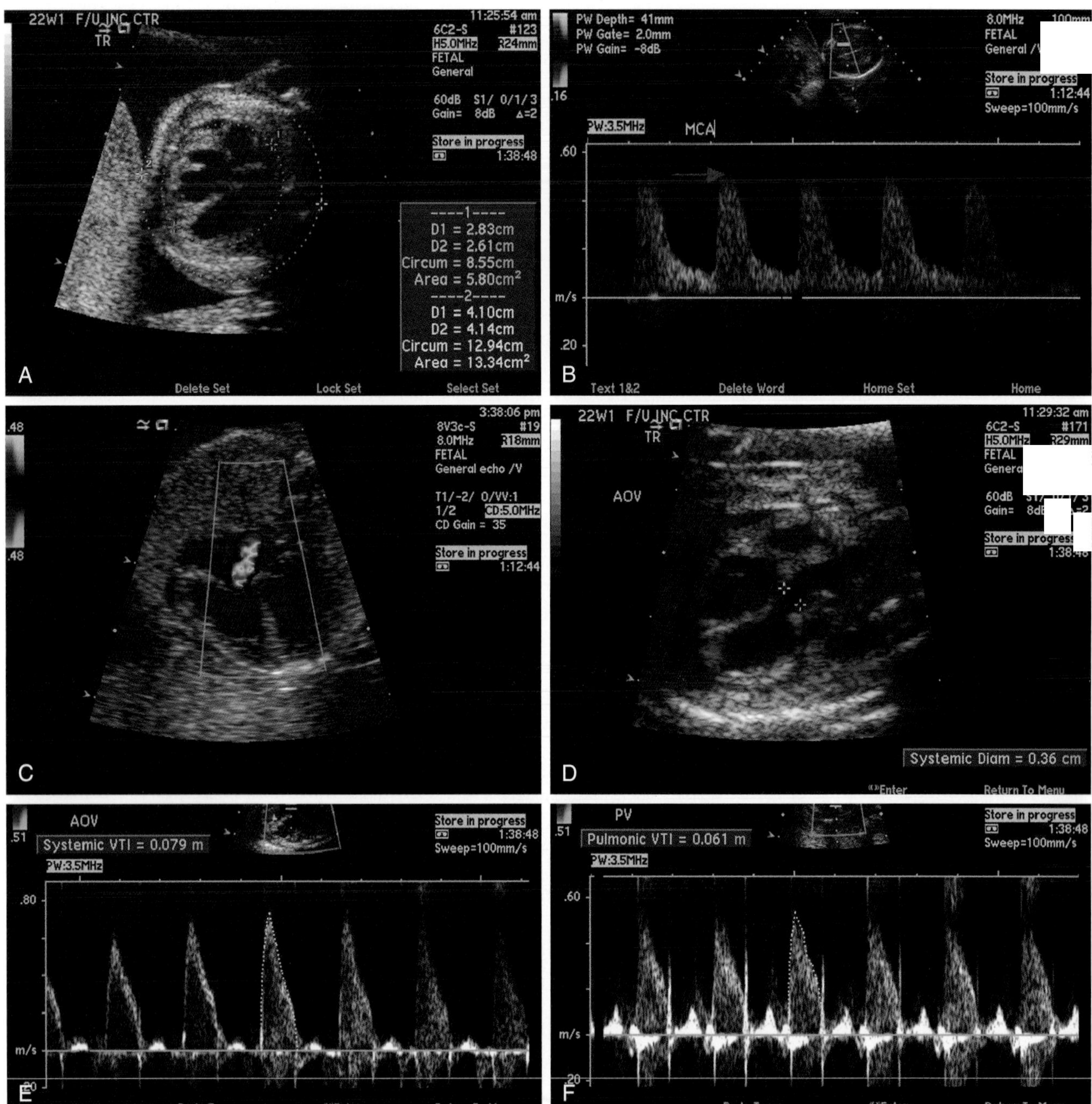

Case 35-3. **(A)** A case of a fetus presenting at 22 weeks' gestation with mild cardiomegaly. Upon further questioning, it became apparent that both parents have a history of thalassemia. **(B)** Doppler sampling in the middle cerebral artery (MCA) revealed an increased peak systolic velocity (*arrow*) of approximately 50 cm/sec. This value is above the normal range for a fetus at 22 weeks' gestation (see Figure 35-1). This finding suggested the presence of anemia and high-output state. The fetus was identified as having hemoglobin Bart's disease. **(C)** Color flow imaging demonstrates moderate tricuspid regurgitation. **(D)** Measurement of the aortic annulus for calculation of left-sided cardiac output. AOV, aortic valve. **(E)** Doppler tracing of aortic flow waveform for calculation of the VTI for left-sided cardiac output. **(F)** Doppler tracing of pulmonic flow waveform for calculation of the VTI for right-sided cardiac output. The combined cardiac output exceeded 700 mL/kg/min, consistent with a high-output state secondary to anemia.

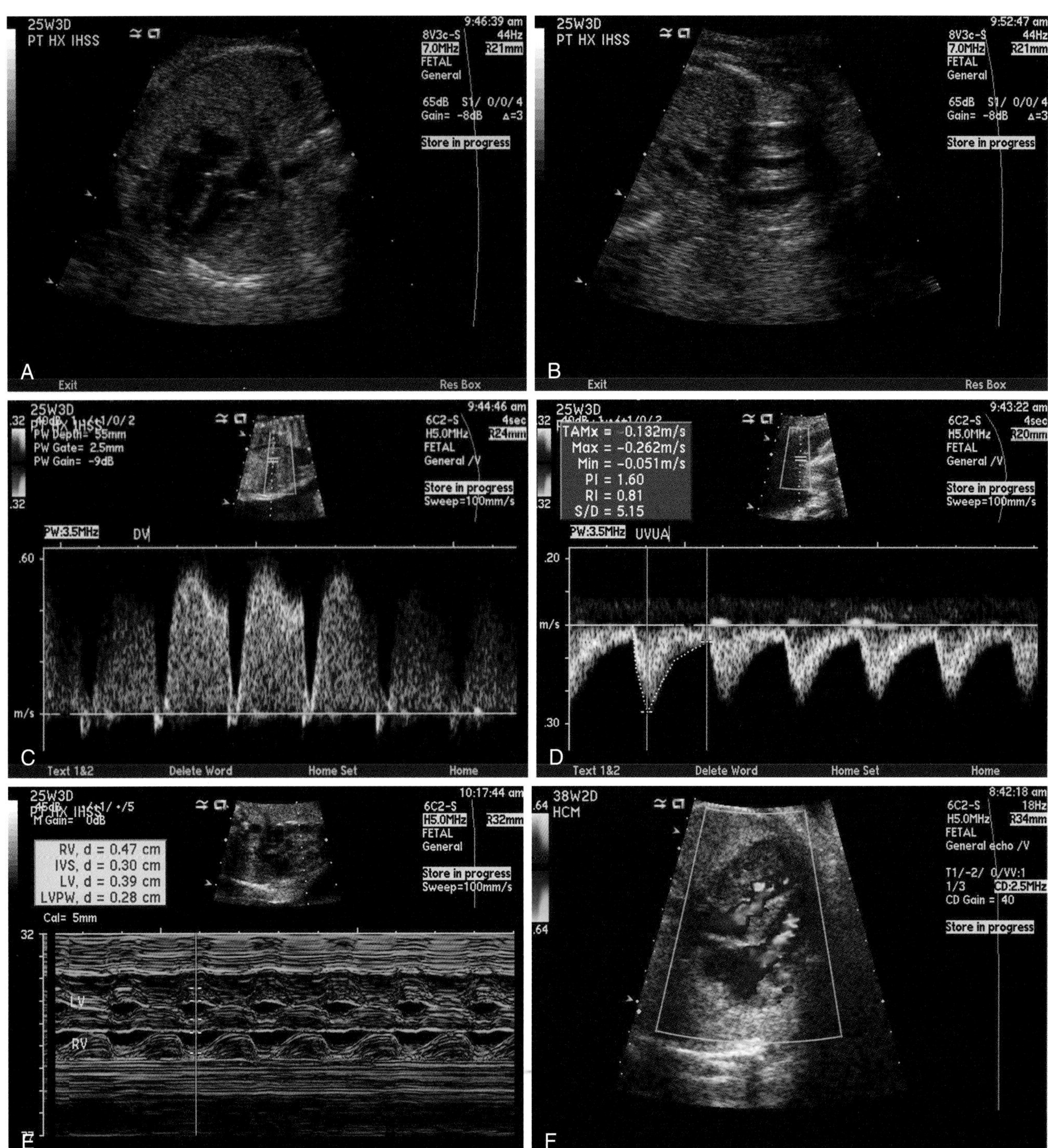

Case 35-4. (**A**) Patient presented at 25 weeks' gestation for fetal screening. The mother of the fetus has a history of hypertrophic cardiomyopathy, operated upon in the first year of life. She also has evidence of multiple lentigines and congenital deafness. Four-chamber view of the fetal heart demonstrates no cardiac enlargement and no significant thickening in this view. (**B**) The short-axis view demonstrates some hypertrophy with septal thickening. (**C**) Doppler interrogation of the ductus venosus (DV) is abnormal and demonstrates decreased flow with atrial contraction suggesting altered ventricular compliance. (**D**) Umbilical artery (UA) and umbilical vein (UV) flow are normal. (**E**) M-mode tracing at the level of the mid-ventricular septum further demonstrates some myocardial hypertrophy. LV, left ventricle; RV, right ventricle. (**F**) With early, subtle findings of overall myocardial thickening and the family history of hypertrophic cardiomyopathy, close follow-up with serial fetal echocardiography was undertaken. In this follow-up study at 38 weeks' gestation, color flow imaging in the four-chamber view shows global wall thickening with somewhat small cavity volumes.

Continued

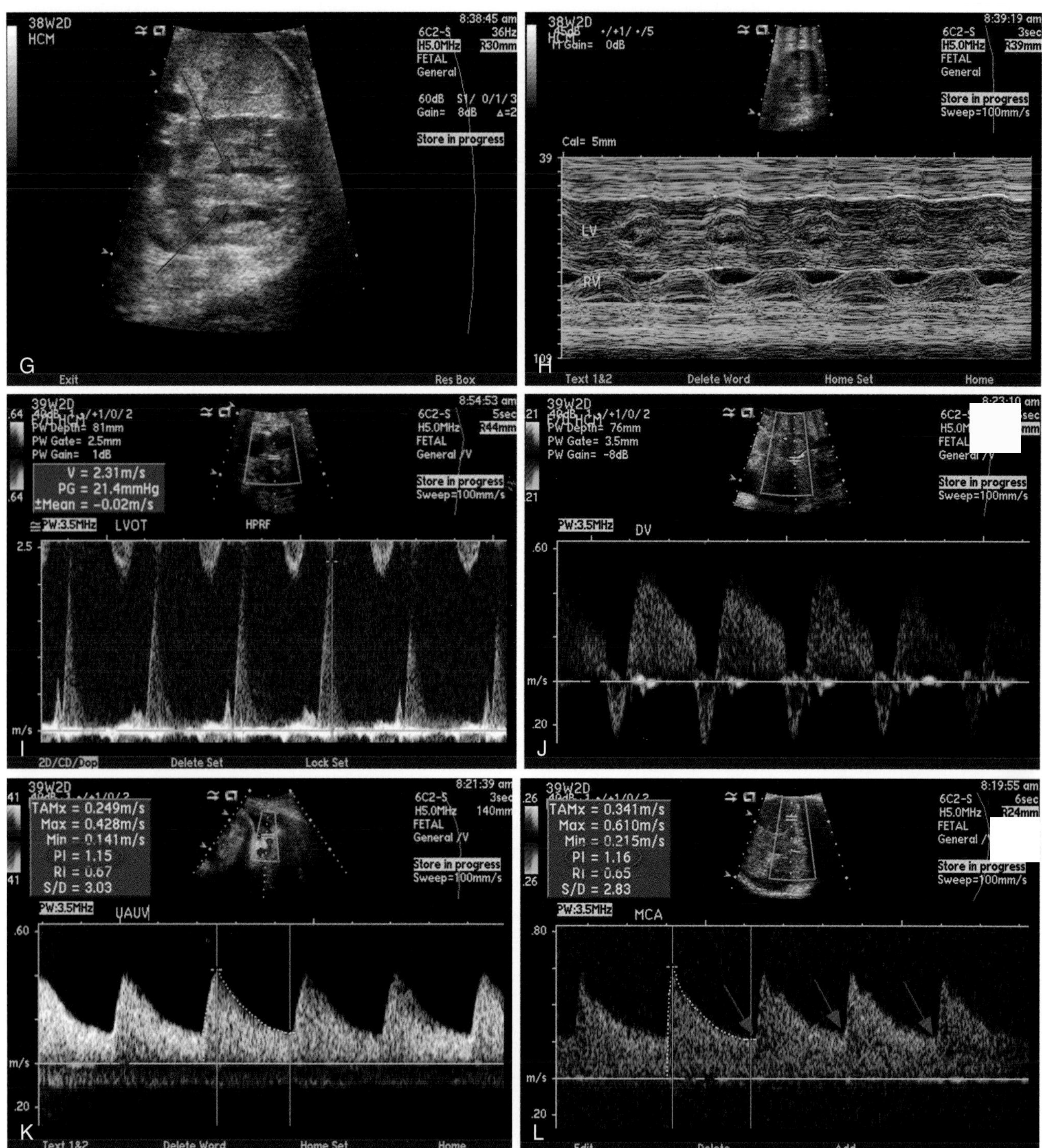

Case 35-4, cont'd **(G)** Short-axis view reveals the degree of diffuse severe myocardial hypertrophy. The *arrows* denote significant septal wall thickening. **(H)** M-mode tracing shows severe hypertrophy with near cavity obliteration in systole. **(I)** Doppler flow tracing across the left ventricular outflow tract (LVOT) demonstrates a very narrow waveform with rapid acceleration, consistent with dynamic outflow tract obstruction. **(J)** Doppler imaging of the DV now demonstrates reversal of flow with atrial contraction indicating progressive worsening of RV diastolic function. **(K)** Umbilical venous flow is normal. UA pulsatility index (PI) is 1.15. **(L)** MCA PI is 1.16, essentially identical to the UA PI. Note the increased diastolic flow *(arrows)* suggestive of cerebrovascular vasodilation. This may be related to decreased left-sided cardiac output as a consequence of limited LV filling and outflow tract obstruction.

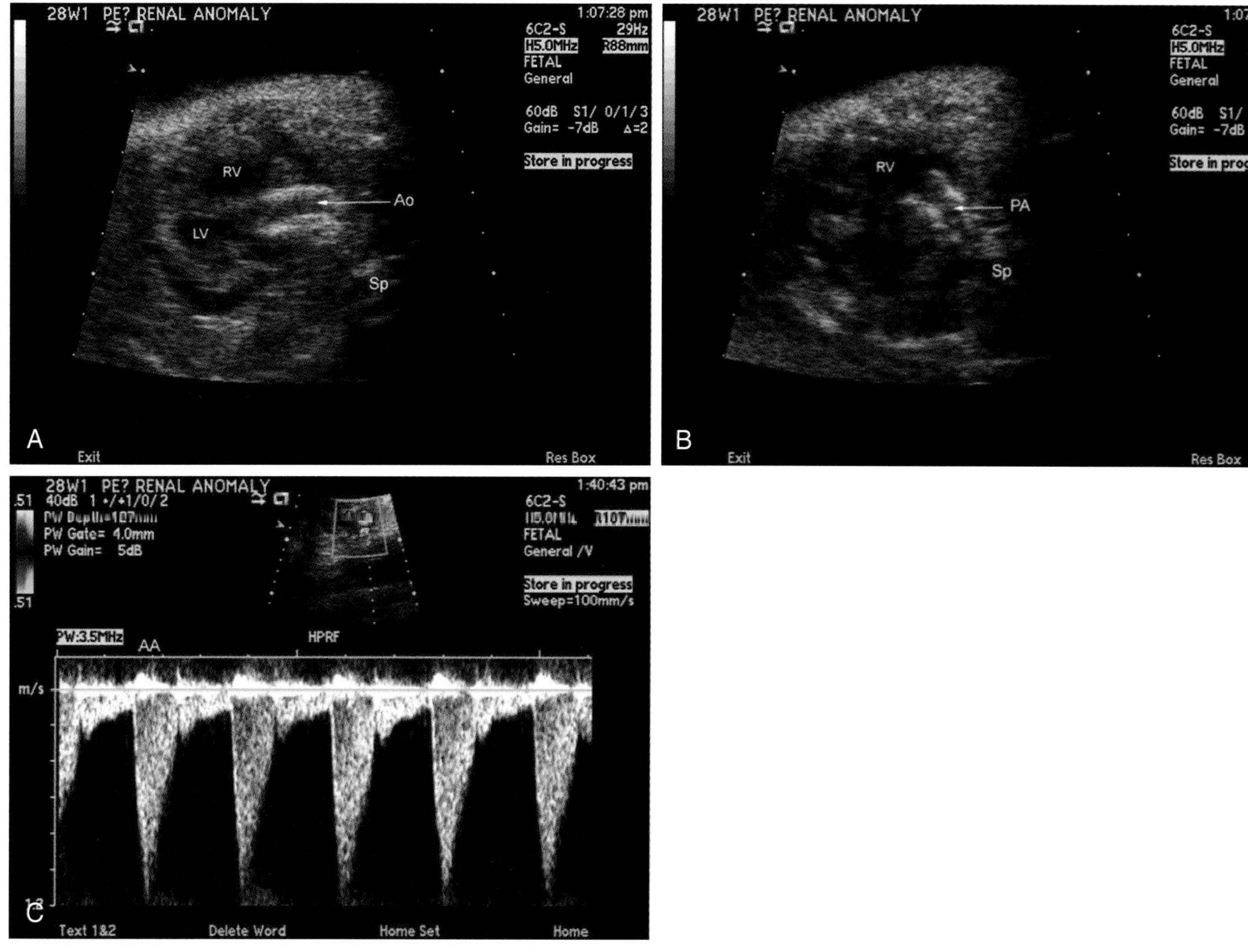

Case 35-5. **(A)** A rare case of arterial calcinosis. Note the echo-bright walls of the ascending aorta (Ao). There is a small pericardial effusion. **(B)** The main pulmonary artery (PA) is also involved and its walls are outlined by a layer of calcium. **(C)** Loss of elasticity and distensibility due to calcium deposition in the walls of the aorta cause a flow disturbance and increased peak velocity. AA, ascending aorta.

36

Abnormalities of the Ductus Arteriosus

Jack Rychik

Key Echocardiographic Features

- Identify the presence, position, and location of the ductus arteriosus as originating from the confluence of the branch pulmonary arteries off of the main pulmonary artery and inserting into the descending aorta distal to the left subclavian.
- Identify the shape and contour of the ductus arteriosus and the ductal arch.
- Perform Doppler interrogation of the ductus arteriosus and determine the direction of flow (normally antegrade from pulmonary artery to aorta).
- Assess the ductus arteriosus for evidence of constriction via two-dimensional imaging, color flow imaging, and Doppler interrogation.
- If there is evidence for constriction of the ductus arteriosus, assess the right ventricle for any hypertrophy or dysfunction and assess the tricuspid valve for any regurgitation and right ventricular pressure estimate.
- When there is structural heart disease, take particular note of the direction of flow across the ductus arteriosus within the context of the presence or absence of pulmonic or aortic obstruction.

The ductus arteriosus (DA) is a structure that connects the pulmonary artery to the descending aorta and is the conduit for blood exiting the right ventricle (RV) to the aorta. The DA has a very characteristic shape and contour that directs flow between the RV and the aorta. Sixty percent of the total fetal cardiac output exits the RV with the majority diverted down the DA. A relatively small amount of blood flow enters the branch pulmonary arteries to perfuse the developing pulmonary vasculature and nourish the immature lung parenchyma. The amount of blood entering the lungs increases with gestation, with approaching up to 25% of the cardiac output perfusing the branch pulmonary arteries near term.[1]

Structural abnormalities of the DA exist and can have a significant impact on fetal blood flow patterns. Impediment to flow across the DA not only affects downstream blood delivery to the descending aorta but may also alter flow into the branch pulmonary arteries or create alterations in flow patterns upstream such as at the atrial level. These changes in flow can influence cardiovascular development leading to various pathological conditions.

Structural abnormalities can include (1) constriction or premature closure of the DA, (2) agenesis of the DA, or (3) aneurysm of the DA.

Constriction or Premature Closure of the Ductus Arteriosus

Anatomy, Development, and Prenatal Physiology

Constriction or complete premature closure of the DA is an unusual phenomenon with potentially devastating consequences.[2–5] Premature closure of the DA results in an undue afterload on the RV because the pathway to the descending aorta is obliterated and pulmonary vascular resistance is naturally very high. It is associated with right ventricular hypertrophy and tricuspid regurgitation. RV pressure can be increased to levels higher than normal. Right ventricular hypertrophy alters ventricular compliance, which induces more right-to-left shunting at the atrial level, with reduction in volume delivered to the RV and pulmonary arteries.[6] As a result, blood flow patterns to the lungs are markedly affected with increased pulmonary artery pressure leading to the potential for development of pulmonary vascular disease.[5] An outline for possible outcomes after premature closure of the ductus arteriosus has been proposed (Figure 36-1).

Constriction of the DA is likely a more common, fleeting event than is complete premature closure, and hence, it is unknown how often it takes place. Constriction or temporary "spasm" of the DA, with relaxation and return to normal caliber, is possible.

Constriction or premature closure of the DA is due to known extrinsic agents that cause ductal constriction, or it is "idiopathic," which essentially means it is likely also caused by some extrinsic agent; however, we cannot identify what that agent may be.[7] Nonsteroidal anti-inflammatory drugs such as indomethacin, as well as salicylates, are well-known constrictors of the fetal DA.[8] In our experience, we have also found that maternal intake of sympathomimetics, such as those contained in over-the-counter cold remedies, may predispose to DA constriction. Colleagues in South America described fetal constriction of the DA with excessive intake of "maté" beverage, a popular, hot drink derived from the steeping of yerba maté leaves. Furthermore, we once identified serious constriction of the DA in a native African woman. Upon questioning, she revealed the use of a cream derived from local African plants, which was being applied to her gravid abdomen. The purpose of the cream, extremely popular in her native Kenya, is to improve the abdominal skin condition and prevent the development of unsightly stretch marks after birth. Of course, the precise herbal contents of this cream are unknown. These anecdotes convey the point that constriction of the DA can be influenced by a myriad of agents, most of which are unknown to the medical practitioner.

The consequences of prenatal ductal constriction are primarily changes in the morphology of the RV with myocardial thickening and development of tricuspid regurgitation. Systolic dysfunction and right-sided heart

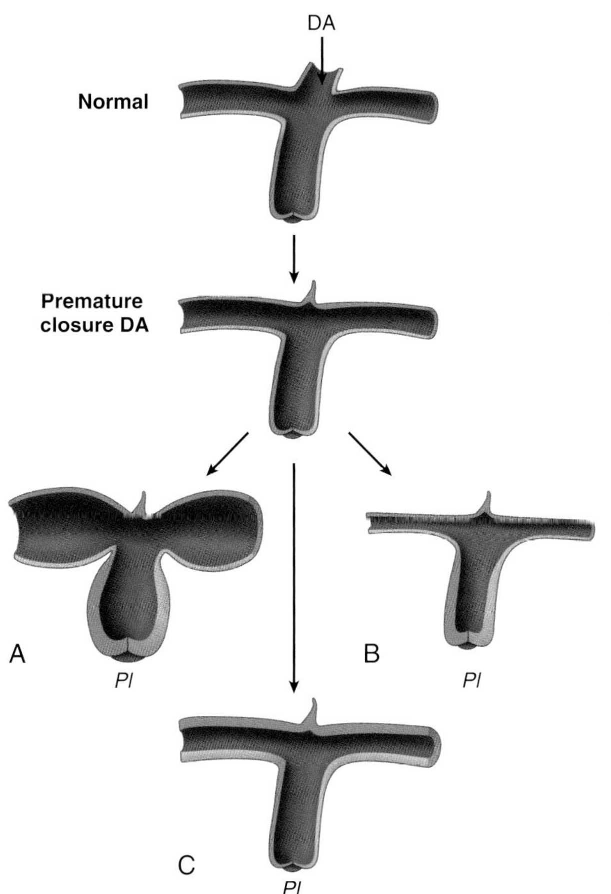

Figure 36-1. Schema of possible outcome following premature closure of the ductus arteriosus (DA) as per Gewillig and coworkers. Premature closure of the DA can be associated with (**A**) aneurysmal dilation of the branch pulmonary arteries and severe pulmonary insufficiency (PI) and pulmonic valve thickening/stenosis with neonatal airway compression and respiratory insufficiency; (**B**) isolated pulmonic valve stenosis and insufficiency without branch pulmonary artery dilation with neonatal pulmonary valve disease and/or right ventricular hypertrophy and/or hypoplasia; or (**C**) development of pulmonary vascular disease with neonatal pulmonary hypertension, right ventricular hypertrophy, and right ventricular dysfunction. (Redrawn from Gewillig M, Brown SC, De Catte L, et al. Premature foetal closure of the arterial duct: clinical presentations and outcome. *Eur Heart J.* 2009;30:1530-1536.)

failure ensues, possibly leading to fetal hydrops.[9-11] Longstanding constriction or complete premature closure can lead to right ventricular hypertrophy, right ventricular hypoplasia with pulmonary valve stenosis, or even atresia, the latter being related to chronic diversion of blood away from the right-sided structures. Persistent pulmonary hypertension in the newborn due to abnormal pulmonary vascular development is the most feared consequence and can be difficult to manage.[5]

Prenatal Diagnosis

Constriction of the DA is oftentimes first suspected when there is fetal echocardiographic evidence for ventricular size discrepancy, with a dilated and hypertrophied RV in comparison with the left ventricle. Greater than mild tricuspid regurgitation is common, but not necessarily present in all cases. Inspection in the region of the DA will reveal a narrowed structure. Color Doppler flow will demonstrate a high-velocity jet emanating from the orifice of the constricted DA directed into the descending aorta. Doppler echocardiography will reveal an increased systolic and diastolic velocity.[12] The pulsatility index (PI) will be decreased. The PI for a normal DA is typically 2.0 to 2.5, whereas in the constricted DA, it is typically less than 1.8. In a reported series of 22 fetuses with constriction of the DA due to indomethacin treatment, the average DA PI was 1.25.[13]

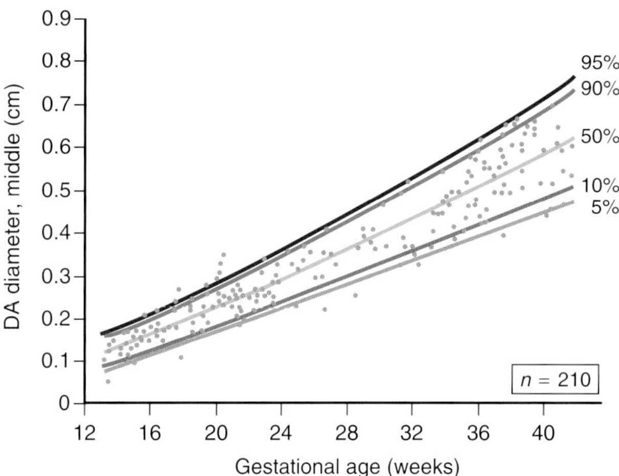

Figure 36-2. The midportion diameter of the ductus arteriosus in the structurally normal heart increases with gestational age. (Data from Mielke G, Benda N. Reference range for two-dimensional echocardiographic examination of the fetal ductus arteriosus. *Ultrasound Obstet Gynecol.* 2000;15:219-225.)

Two-dimensional measures of the DA have been described; however, such measurements can be difficult to obtain. The width diameter of the DA increases with gestation (Figure 36-2).[14]

Management and Outcomes

Identification of a constricted DA, or premature closure, warrants close serial scrutiny with fetal echocardiography for any deleterious consequences. Right ventricular dysfunction with severe tricuspid regurgitation and development of hydrops is possible. Serial assessment looking for fusion of the normal dual peak inflow pattern across the tricuspid valve, increased reversal of ductus venosus flow with atrial contraction, and umbilical venous pulsations is required, because these may herald the onset of heart failure and hydrops. Careful history taking may reveal an inciting agent, which should be eliminated. In cases of impending hydrops or severe right ventricular dysfunction, early delivery should be considered. Delivery will result in opening of the pulmonary vasculature and relief of right ventricular afterload. The neonate can then be further treated with pulmonary vasodilating agents such as nitric oxide. Postnatal diagnosis is often made of premature closure of the DA when there is marked cyanosis, a small right ventricular cavity with thickened ventricular myocardium, and the absence of visualization of a patent DA within the first 24 hours of life.

Outcome depends upon the degree, duration, and developmental stage at which DA constriction has taken place. In mild cases, elimination of the inciting agent can result in complete normalization without any further consequences. In severe cases, when pulmonary vascular disease is present, death can occur with placental separation despite aggressive intervention. An intriguing additional notion has recently been raised. Based on the theory of "fetal origins" of adult-onset cardiovascular disease (Barker's hypothesis), it is plausible that "primary" pulmonary hypertension, a disease whose origins are poorly understood, may be founded in the altered fetal flow patterns of ductal constriction leading to a developmental predisposition to this disorder.

Agenesis of the Ductus Arteriosus

Anatomy, Development, and Prenatal Physiology

Absence or agenesis of the DA is typically associated with congenital heart disease. It is most commonly associated with tetralogy of Fallot and absent pulmonary valve leaflet syndrome.[15] In a structurally normal heart, nonvisualization of the DA is more likely to be premature closure, implying the presence of a DA at some point in the past. Agenesis of the DA in association with structural heart disease likely reflects an early developmental abnormality, in which no DA formed or it disappeared very early in gestation.

Agenesis of the DA in association with absent pulmonary valve is well described (see Chapter 12). When seen with other anomalies, it reflects a very serious potential abnormality of lung development and is extremely rare with very poor outcome. We have seen a case of complex single ventricle with pulmonary stenosis, main pulmonary artery hypoplasia, small branch pulmonary arteries, and complete absence of the DA. No aortopulmonary collaterals were identified. The infant succumbed to severe hypoxemia at birth.

Diagnosis, Management, and Outcomes

Nonvisualization of the DA should prompt a search for a right-sided DA. In the normal, a left aortic arch will have a left-sided DA originate adjacent to the origin of the left pulmonary artery and insert into the descending aorta. However, in a left aortic arch and a right-sided DA, it will travel in the right mediastinum and connect between the central portion of the main pulmonary artery and the base of the innominate artery.

Unfortunately, there is no effective treatment for agenesis of the DA in association with structural heart disease and in which there is an abnormality of pulmonary vascular development. Poor outcome is likely in this scenario.

Aneurysm of the Ductus Arteriosus

Anatomy, Development, and Prenatal Physiology

Aneurysm of the ductus arteriosus (ADA) is defined as a tortuous DA with a diameter that is greater than 95% expected for gestational age. In the past, this anomaly was believed to signify a serious problem, because there are reports of ADA rupture, thrombus formation with thromboembolism, and compression of adjacent structures possible. However, this likely represents a presentation bias of only symptomatic patients with ADA. As imaging tools and knowledge of this anomaly have become more sophisticated, it appears that ADA occurs more frequently and may be benign in most cases with self-resolution.

In a reported series of 200 fetal echocardiograms, saccular or fusiform dilation of the midportion of the DA with a diameter measurement of greater than 95% for gestational age was seen in 1.6% of cases.[16] An association with Marfan's syndrome and Ehlers-Danlos syndrome has been suggested.

The histological makeup of the DA is quite different from its surrounding vascular tissue. There is a distinct elastic laminae and a medial layer of muscularity. In the third trimester of gestation, endothelial cushions normally develop in the DA, which form the foundation for future closure. Histological assessment of patients with ADA has revealed absence of endothelial cushion formation and/or interruption of the elastic laminae.[16] Subjects with connective tissue disorders may, therefore, be at greater risk for development of ADA.

Prenatal Diagnosis, Management, and Outcomes

The ductal arch should be evaluated in every fetus undergoing fetal echocardiography. The contour and angulation of the DA changes with gestation, with it taking a higher-arched course with increasing curvature and more of an acutely angled turn late in the third trimester.[17] Nevertheless, the diameter of the DA should never be visually much larger than the main pulmonary artery segment from which it originates. When it appears subjectively larger, measurements should be made and compared with published standards (see Figure 36-2). If enlarged, follow-up fetal echocardiography is indicated.

No prenatal treatment is indicated. At birth, postnatal echocardiography should be performed to assess the anatomy. Chest magnetic resonance imaging (MRI) or computed tomography (CT) scanning may be helpful in defining the three-dimensional relationship of the ADA to adjacent structures and identifying thrombus, if present.

Many cases of ADA resolve spontaneously with normal spontaneous closure of the DA in the first few days to weeks of life with no further consequences.[18] Surgical resection should be considered if there is a patent DA and ADA present beyond the neonatal period (3 mo of age), an associated connective tissue disorder, evidence of thrombus or thromboembolism, or compression and compromise of adjacent vascular or airway structures. Full resection of the diseased tissue is necessary to prevent late development of aneurysm formation in either the pulmonary artery or the aorta. This may require cardiopulmonary bypass and a sternotomy approach as opposed to the typical ductal ligation approach performed through the chest in a lateral thoracotomy.

Imaging Essentials and Important Points

- Evaluation of the ductal arch and its geometry is an essential part of the fetal echocardiographic examination. The contour of the DA in the normal heart differs from when there is structural heart disease.
  - When there is limitation to pulmonary blood flow (pulmonary stenosis or atresia), the DA is smaller than normal and will have a hooked appearance arising from the underside of the arch as it inserts into the confluence of the pulmonary arteries.
  - When there is limitation to systemic blood flow (hypoplastic left heart syndrome), the DA will appear larger than normal and will curve gently from its origin on the main pulmonary artery to the descending aorta.
- In transposition of the great arteries, the DA should be carefully scrutinized because it may be smaller than normal. When very small, this may indicate pulmonary vascular changes and can lead to profound neonatal hypoxemia at birth.[19]
- When ductal constriction is present, the Doppler flow pattern across the DA has the appearance of a "coarctation" of the vessel with increased systolic velocity and increased diastolic velocity as well with a characteristic "run-off" pattern appearance.
- In the structurally normal heart, ductal constriction is probably a more common phenomenon than we think. If there is a color jet in the descending aorta suggesting DA constriction and the DA PI is abnormally diminshed, follow-up examination is warranted to make sure the process does not progress. However, if the RV looks normal in function and is without hypertrophy or tricuspid regurgitation, the prognosis is quite good and the constriction is likely a transient phenomenon.

References

1. Rasanen J, Wood DC, Weiner S, Ludomirski A, Huhta JC. Role of the pulmonary circulation in the distribution of human fetal cardiac output during the second half of pregnancy. *Circulation.* 1996;94:1068-1073.
2. Huhta JC, Moise KJ, Fisher DJ, Sharif DS, Wasserstrum N, Martin C. Detection and quantitation of constriction of the fetal ductus arteriosus by Doppler echocardiography. *Circulation.* 1987; 75:406-412.
3. Takahashi Y, Harada K, Ishida A, Tanaka T, Tsuda A, Takada G. Doppler echocardiographic findings of indomethacin-induced occlusion of the fetal ductus arteriosus. *Am J Perinatol.* 1996; 13:15-18.
4. Hofstadler G, Tulzer G, Altmann R, Schmitt K, Danford D, Huhta JC. Spontaneous closure of the human fetal ductus arteriosus—a cause of fetal congestive heart failure. *Am J Obstet Gynecol.* 1996; 174:879-883.
5. Gewillig M, Brown SC, De Catte L, et al. Premature foetal closure of the arterial duct: clinical presentations and outcome. *Eur Heart J.* 2009;30:1530-1536.
6. Harada K, Rice MJ, McDonald RW, et al. Doppler echocardiographic evaluation of ventricular diastolic filling in fetuses with ductal constriction. *Am J Cardiol.* 1997;79:442-446.
7. Trevett TN Jr, Cotton J. Idiopathic constriction of the fetal ductus arteriosus. *Ultrasound Obstet Gynecol.* 2004;23:517-519.
8. Moise KJ Jr, Huhta JC, Sharif DS, et al. Indomethacin in the treatment of premature labor. Effects on the fetal ductus arteriosus. *N Engl J Med.* 1988;319:327-331.
9. Harada K, Rice MJ, Shiota T, McDonald RW, Reller MD, Sahn DJ. Two-dimensional echocardiographic evaluation of ventricular systolic function in human fetuses with ductal constriction. *Ultrasound Obstet Gynecol.* 1997;10:247-253.
10. Mori Y, Rice MJ, McDonald RW, et al. Evaluation of systolic and diastolic ventricular performance of the right ventricle in fetuses with ductal constriction using the Doppler Tei index. *Am J Cardiol* 2001;88:1173-1178.
11. Kondo T, Kitazawa R, Noda-Maeda N, Kitazawa S. Fetal hydrops associated with spontaneous premature closure of ductus arteriosus. *Pathol Int.* 2006;56:554-557.
12. Mielke G, Benda N. Blood flow velocity waveforms of the fetal pulmonary artery and the ductus arteriosus: reference ranges from 13 weeks to term. *Ultrasound Obstet Gynecol.* 2000;15:213-218.
13. Tulzer G, Gudmundsson S, Sharkey AM, Wood DC, Cohen AW, Huhta JC. Doppler echocardiography of fetal ductus arteriosus constriction versus increased right ventricular output. *J Am Coll Cardiol.* 1991;18:532-536.
14. Mielke G, Benda N. Reference ranges for two-dimensional echocardiographic examination of the fetal ductus arteriosus. *Ultrasound Obstet Gynecol.* 2000;15:219-225.
15. Emmanoulides GC, Thanopoulos B, Siassi B, Fishbein M. "Agenesis" of ductus arteriosus associated with the syndrome of tetralogy of Fallot and absent pulmonary valve. *Am J Cardiol.* 1976;37: 403-409.
16. Dyamenahalli U, Smallhorn JF, Geva T, et al. Isolated ductus arteriosus aneurysm in the fetus and infant: a multi-institutional experience. *J Am Coll Cardiol.* 2000;36:262-269.
17. Benson CB, Brown DL, Doubilet PM, DiSalvo DN, Laing FC, Frates MC. Increasing curvature of the normal fetal ductus arteriosus with advancing gestational age. *Ultrasound Obstet Gynecol.* 1995;5:95-97.
18. Tseng JJ, Jan SL. Fetal echocardiographic diagnosis of isolated ductus arteriosus aneurysm: a longitudinal study from 32 weeks of gestation to term. *Ultrasound Obstet Gynecol.* 2005;26:50-56.
19. Maeno YV, Kamenir SA, Sinclair B, van der Velde ME, Smallhorn JF, Hornberger LK. Prenatal features of ductus arteriosus constriction and restrictive foramen ovale in D-transposition of the great arteries. *Circulation.* 1999;99:1209-1214.

CASES

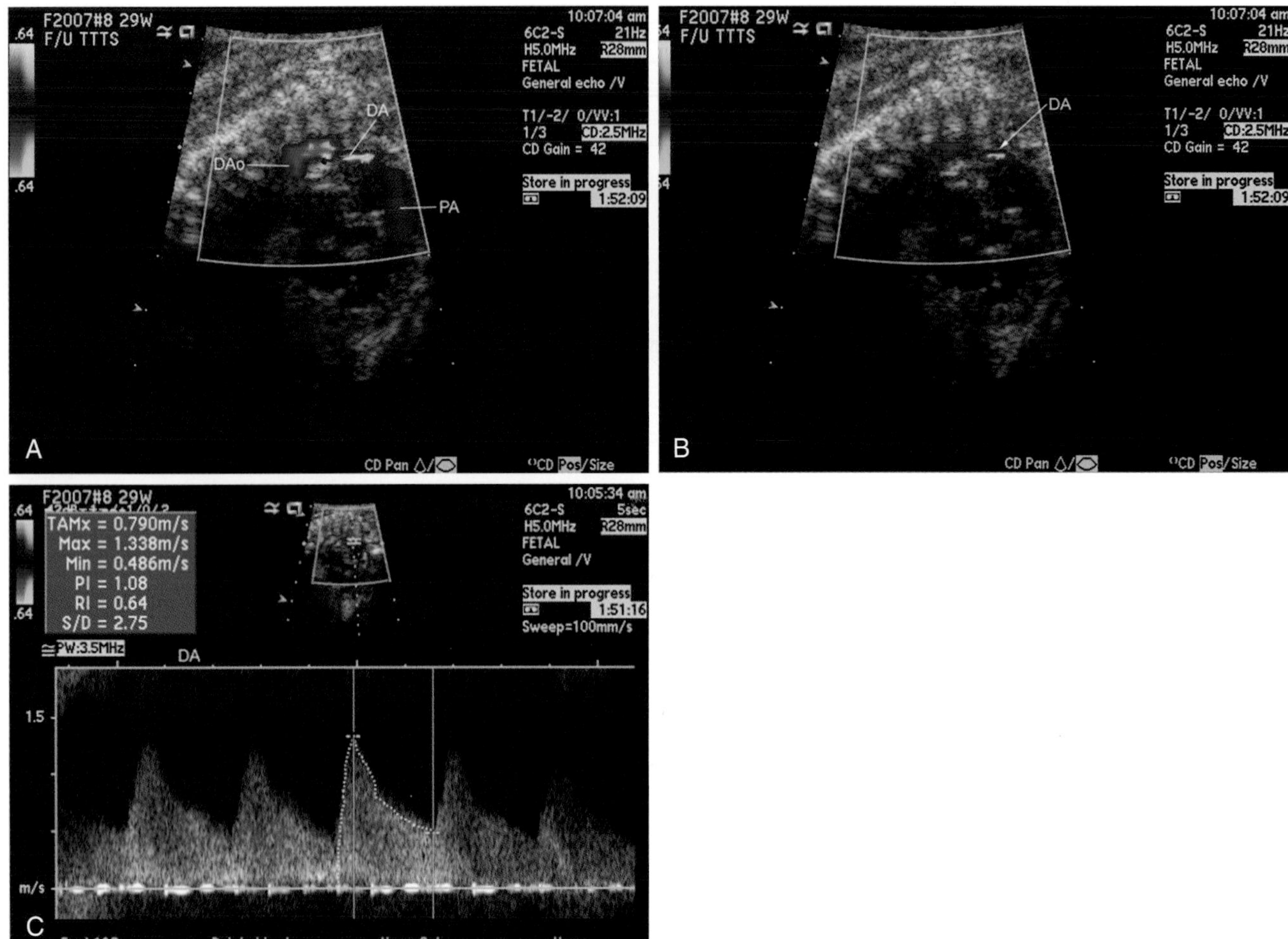

Case 36-1. **(A)** A case of ductal constriction secondary to maternal nonsteroidal anti-inflammatory intake. Ductal arch view demonstrates the pulmonary artery (PA) ascending toward the transducer (red) and the descending aorta (DAo) in *blue* with speckled color aliasing of the ductus arteriosus (DA) connection between the two. The DA should normally be no smaller than the main pulmonary artery segment or DAo. **(B)** Another frame from color flow imaging demonstrates marked near-pinhole narrowing of the DA. **(C)** Doppler interrogation at the site of constricted DA. There is a classic "saw-tooth" run-off pattern with increased diastolic flow, similar to what is frequently seen in the presence of a coarctation of the aorta in a child. The calculated pulsatility index (PI) is low at 1.08.

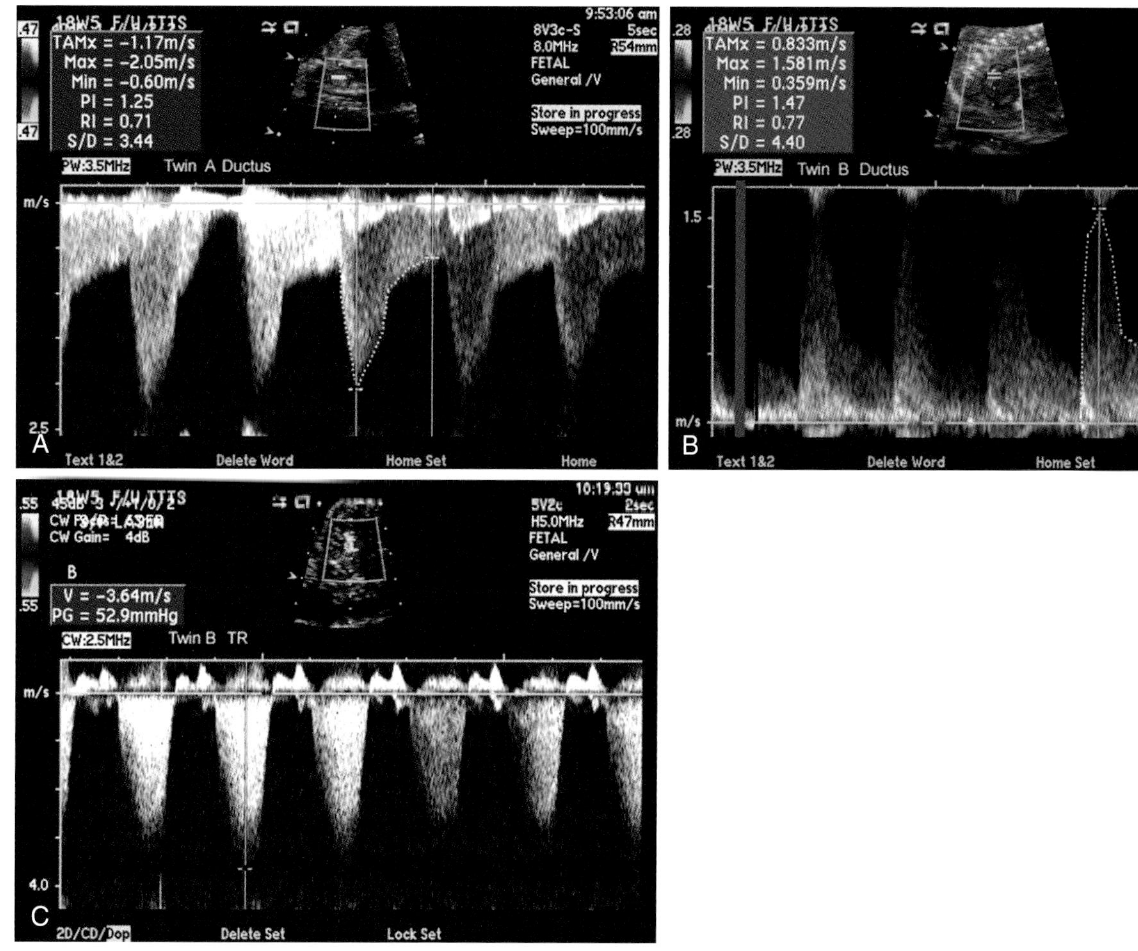

Case 36-2. **(A)** A case of twin-twin transfusion syndrome 24 hours after laser therapy in which the mother has been treated with indomethacin to prevent contractions and labor. Imaging of the ductal arch in the recipient twin. Ductal constriction is noted based on a Doppler interrogation assessment revealing a diastolic run-off pattern with PI of 1.25. **(B)** Ductal arch imaging with Doppler interrogation in the donor twin. Note that this fetus also has evidence for ductal constriction with diastolic run-off pattern and PI of 1.47. **(C)** The donor twin (twin B) has new-onset tricuspid regurgitation (TR) in relation to constriction of the DA, with elevated intracavitary right ventricular pressure greater than 50 mm Hg. Following discontinuation of indomethacin, ductal constriction and TR fully resolved.

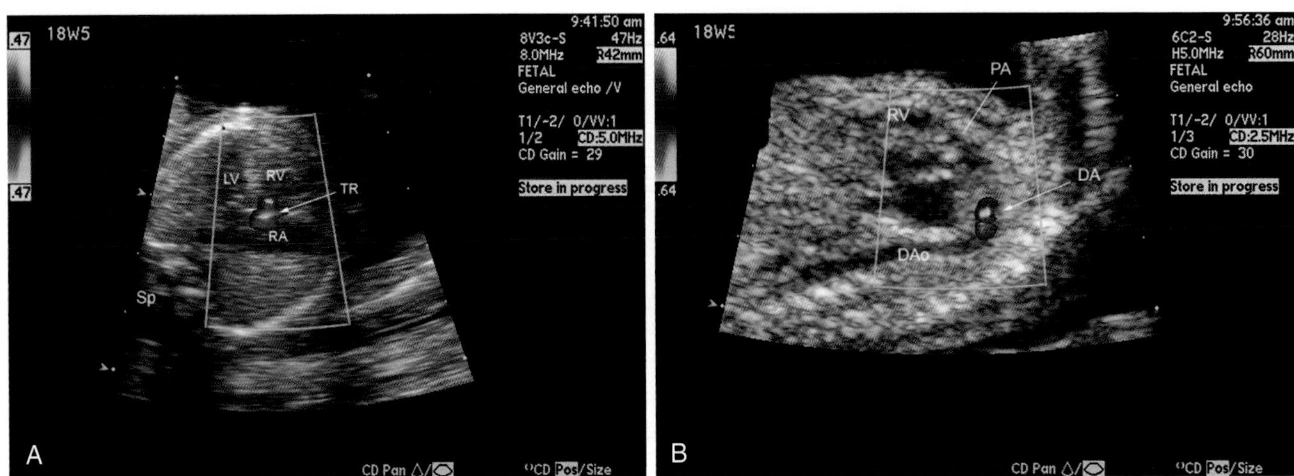

Case 36-3. **(A)** Fetus referred at 18 weeks and 5 days for unexplained TR. The tricuspid valve structure is normal. LV, left ventricle; RA, right atrium; RV, right ventricle; Sp, spine. **(B)** Examination of the DA reveals aliasing of flow with constriction of the DA. Follow-up 1-week later revealed complete resolution of the TR and spontaneous relief of ductal constriction. The cause for ductal constriction in this fetus was never discovered. PA, pulmonary artery.

37

Agenesis of the Ductus Venosus

Jack Rychik

Key Echocardiographic Features

- Trace and identify the insertion of the umbilical vein into the fetus and follow its course to the heart.
- Determine whether the umbilical vein connects to the liver (i.e., portal or hepatic venous system) or connects extrahepatically (i.e., to a systemic vein or coronary sinus or directly to the heart).
- Assess for heart size via the cardiothoracic ratio.
- Assess for systolic function.
- Assess for the presence and grade of atrioventricular valve regurgitation.
- Look for signs of pleural effusion, pericardial effusion, or hydrops as a consequence of heart failure due to volume overload.
- Determination of combined cardiac output can be helpful in serial evaluation.

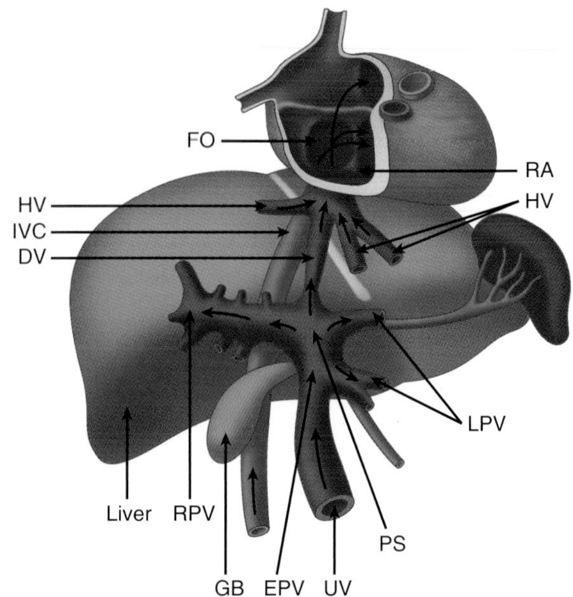

Figure 37-1. Schematic representation of the fetal umbilical, portal, and hepatic circulations. The color indicates the degree of oxygen content *(red* = high; *purple* = medium; *blue* = low). The *arrows* indicate the direction of blood flow. DV, ductus venosus; EPV, extrahepatic portal vein; GB, gallbladder; FO, foramen ovale; HV, hepatic veins; IVC, inferior vena cava; LPV, left portal vein; PS, portal sinus; RA, right atrium; RPV, right portal vein; UV, umbilical vein. (From Mavrides E, Moscoso G, Carvalho JS, Campbell S, Thilaganathan B. The anatomy of the umbilical, portal and hepatic venous systems in the human fetus at 14-19 weeks of gestation. *Ultrasound Obstet Gynecol.* 2001;18: 598-604.)

Anatomy and Anatomical Associations

The ductus venosus (DV) is a short, hourglass-shaped venous structure that shunts umbilical venous return to the fetal heart. It is part of a collection of vessels located beneath the diaphragm that is involved in carrying placental venous return back to the fetus. The anatomical arrangement of venous return from the placenta is designed to optimize streaming of flow of the most highly oxygenated blood to the most essential developing organs. A review of the venous anatomy leading from the placenta to the fetal heart is important in order to understand the implications of absence or agenesis of the DV.[1-3]

Figure 37-1 demonstrates this unique and complex anatomy. Venous return from the placenta to the fetus can be conceptualized with the liver as the primary focal point. There are (1) afferent veins—the umbilical and portal veins and (2) efferent veins—the hepatic veins and subdiaphragmatic vestibulum, going toward and emerging from the liver, respectively.

The umbilical vein enters the fetal abdomen within the falciform ligament and ascends steeply toward the liver where it runs along its inferior surface. The umbilical vein then joins a confluence of vessels termed the *portal sinus.* The portal sinus is a vascular space and is a conglomeration of structures including (1) the intrahepatic portal vein, made up of the left and right portal veins, (2) the extrahepatic portal vein comprising the splenic and mesenteric veins, and (3) the DV. Blood flows into the portal sinus from the umbilical vein and is then dispersed into the liver via the afferent system of the portal veins. Blood exits the liver parenchyma via the efferent system of hepatic veins, which coalesce into a subdiaphragmatic vestibulum or chamber together with the inferior vena cava, just prior to entry into the right atrium.

Because the umbilical vein is closer to the left portal vein than to the right, the left portal vein and left lobe of the liver receive relatively highly oxygenated blood. The extrahepatic portal vein carries poorly oxygenated blood and it enters closer to the right portal vein. Oxygen consumption within the liver is relatively low, and as the blood entering the left lobe of the liver is preferentially streamed from the umbilical vein, blood exiting the left hepatic vein is relatively highly oxygenated in comparison with the right hepatic vein.

The DV can be thought of as a structure that acts as a bypass, or shunt, between the afferent and the efferent venous systems. The DV originates from the superior aspect of the portal sinus and constricts slightly as it heads cephalad. An important point to recognize is that there is no anatomical continuity between the umbilical vein and the DV, but in fact, the latter originates from the portal sinus. However, its ostium is aligned with the outlet of the umbilical vein; hence, it carries richly oxygenated blood. The DV has a pinched appearance and is slightly constricted relative to the proximal portal sinus and umbilical vein. This acts to increase kinetic energy and accelerate flow, thereby directing a stream of highly oxygenated blood through the subdiaphragmatic vestibulum angled toward the foramen ovale. There is debate as to whether or not a muscular sphincter is associated with the DV. Histopathological analysis demonstrates the presence of endothelial corrugations and innervated smooth muscle, which supports the hypothesis that the DV is an actively regulated vessel with the capacity to rapidly change diameter along its entire length in response to certain stimuli.[4] The left hepatic vein also carries highly oxygenated blood and runs parallel with the DV, whereas the right hepatic vein runs parallel with the inferior vena cava. Hence, left hepatic venous effluent also contributes somewhat to the preferential streaming of oxygenated blood to the foramen ovale and left side of the heart. Color Doppler studies have shown an interesting symmetry in that the left-sided DV and left portal vein axis carries relatively highly oxygenated blood, and the inferior vena cava and right portal vein axis carries relatively poorly oxygenated blood that is directed more rightward into the right atrium.

Perhaps somewhat underappreciated is the fact that the DV does not carry the full complement of umbilical venous return. Placental venous return is shared by the DV and the portal-hepatic venous system. In essence, the liver and the DV are partners in guarding placental venous return to the fetus. One function of the DV is to divert umbilical venous blood away from the liver. The DV can be considered a physiological "resistance valve"—when tone is high, blood is shunted into the liver; when tone is relaxed, more blood passes through it directed toward the foramen ovale. It is believed that, early in gestation, up to 50% of the umbilical venous return is shunted through the DV, which decreases to 20% to 30% in the latter half of the third trimester.[5] The amount of blood shunted through the DV can change under conditions of stress. During periods of hypoxemia or placental insufficiency, a greater proportion of umbilical venous return is shunted through the DV. This appears to be an adaptive mechanism aimed at preserving preferential streaming and delivery of richly oxygenated blood to the left side of the heart at times of greatest need.[6]

A substantial amount of blood is directed through the liver before it reaches the fetal heart; the proportion directed into the liver increases with gestational age. The significance of this phenomenon, particularly in terms of development of the liver—or conversely and perhaps more important, the contribution of the liver to overall fetal development by release of biologically active elements into its venous effluent—is still unclear and worthy of investigation.

Absence, or agenesis, of the DV results in two general alternate pathways of umbilical venous return: (1) intrahepatic, in which the umbilical vein connects to the portal system, usually the left portal vein, or (2) extrahepatic, in which the umbilical vein connects to a venous structure outside of the liver such as the femoral veins, iliac veins, inferior vena cava, coronary sinus, or atria. Regardless of the type, agenesis of the DV results in a loss of the preferential streaming phenomenon of umbilical venous return across the foramen ovale to the left heart. In the intrahepatic type, umbilical venous return is still "washed" through the liver and blood must make its way through the hepatic microcirculation before ending up in the heart. The hepatic vasculature then acts as a "resistor" to umbilical venous return, in a similar fashion to the DV. Absence of such a resistor can result in unimpeded umbilical venous return and a potential torrent of placental blood flow flooding the fetal circulation. Such is the case when the umbilical vein connects in an extrahepatic manner.

Frequency, Genetics, and Development

Agenesis of the DV is thought to be a rare disorder; however, we have found in our own experience that it is more common than previously appreciated, in particular the intrahepatic umbilical venous return subtype, in which hemodynamics are only minimally disturbed. However, when there is agenesis of the DV, there is a relatively high degree of association with structural abnormalities of the heart or chromosomal/genetic syndromes.[7] Noonan's syndrome has been identified in a number of cases. Careful genetics evaluation is indicated when agenesis of the DV is identified in the fetus.

Prenatal Physiology

Absence of the "resistance valve" to umbilical venous return as seen in agenesis of the DV with extrahepatic connection can lead to massive volume overload of the heart and the development of hydrops.[8-13] The frequent association of hydrops with agenesis of the DV can certainly be purely related to the hemodynamics because combined cardiac output is markedly elevated in some cases. However, at times, the degree of hydrops can seem out of proportion to the magnitude of volume overload. One explanation is the high association of genetic/chromosomal anomalies in which inherent abnormalities of the lymphatic system may play a role. Another plausible theory is that diversion of the umbilical venous return away from the liver alters fetal development[14] or perhaps prevents the deposition of some critically important agent into the placental venous return that prevents development of hydrops in the fetus.

Prenatal Management

Little, if any, intervention is necessary in cases of intrahepatic umbilical venous return type of agenesis of the DV, except for careful investigation for additional congenital anomalies and genetic/chromosomal defects. For the extrahepatic type, anticongestive medication such as digoxin may play a role; however, early delivery and elimination of the placental volume load may be the only option, if impending demise is apparent.

Serial evaluation via fetal echocardiography is indicated when there is extrahepatic umbilical venous connection and agenesis of the DV. The inferior vena cava may be enlarged and substantially out of proportion to the superior vena cava. Heart size and cardiothoracic ratio will be increased, as will all peak velocities across the atrioventricular and semilunar valves. Ventricular dilation can lead to atrioventricular annular dilation, poor valve coaptation, and the development of regurgitation, which can further add to the volume load. Combined cardiac output should be measured via Doppler techniques, with normal values being 400 to 500 mL/kg/min. Combined cardiac output values above 750 to 800 mL/kg/min are of concern and may require early delivery to prevent hydrops.

Postnatal Management and Outcomes

With increased recognition and understanding of the nature of agenesis of the DV, perinatal outcome has improved. Long-term outcome is dictated by the presence of associated anomalies and genetic/chromosomal problems. In the short-term, soon after birth, prenatal pathways of umbilical venous return through the portal system and hepatic channels may act as a source for abnormal shunting after birth. Persistent cardiomegaly and signs of volume overload after birth should raise suspicion for a portosystemic shunt, possibly due to an ill-recognized agenesis of the DV before birth. Such defects may require catheterization delineation through angiography and can be occluded through various devices.[15]

Anomalous umbilical venous return and diversion of blood away from its natural course through the liver and across the foramen ovale may have subtle long-term effects, which are not yet not fully recognized or understood. Long-term follow-up of these individuals is warranted.

Imaging Essentials and Important Points

- In a sagittal tomographic cut across the liver, the abdominal entry site of the umbilical vein will align with the DV. The DV is identified as the vascular portion of the pathway from the intra-abdominal umbilical vein toward the heart in which turbulence is easily seen on color Doppler imaging. This turbulence is created by the natural narrowing of the DV and is helpful in indicating the site for examination and Doppler sampling.
- Agenesis of the DV is suspected when there is no clearly evident linear continuity between the umbilical vein and the vascular entry into the right atrium. If by following the path of umbilical venous return, one must take a number of twists and turns through the liver itself before reaching the heart, agenesis of the DV with intrahepatic continuity of the umbilical vein should be suspected.
- Unexplained cardiomegaly, ventricular enlargement, or inferior vena caval dilation should prompt suspicion of agenesis of the DV with extrahepatic umbilical venous connection.
- Serial combined cardiac output assessment is of value when monitoring the fetus with agenesis of the DV with extrahepatic umbilical venous connection. Such patients should be monitored in a manner similar to those with arteriovenous malformation.

References

1. Mavrides E, Moscoso G, Carvalho JS, Campbell S, Thilaganathan B. The anatomy of the umbilical, portal and hepatic venous systems in the human fetus at 14-19 weeks of gestation. *Ultrasound Obstet Gynecol*. 2001;18:598-604.
2. Kiserud T. Naming veins: by morphology, physiology or sociology. *Ultrasound Obstet Gynecol*. 2001;18:562-563.
3. Kiserud T, Acharya G. The fetal circulation. *Prenat Diagn*. 2004;24:1049-1059.
4. Mavrides E, Moscoso G, Carvalho JS, Campbell S, Thilaganathan B. The human ductus venosus between 13 and 17 weeks of gestation: histological and morphometric studies. *Ultrasound Obstet Gynecol*. 2002;19:39-46.
5. Kiserud T. Physiology of the fetal circulation. *Semin Fetal Neonatal Med*. 2005;10:493-503.
6. Kiserud T, Stratford L, Hanson MA. Umbilical flow distribution to the liver and the ductus venosus: an in vitro investigation of the fluid dynamic mechanisms in the fetal sheep. *Am J Obstet Gynecol*. 1997;177:86-90.
7. Volpe P, Marasini M, Caruso G, et al. Prenatal diagnosis of ductus venosus agenesis and its association with cytogenetic/congenital anomalies. *Prenat Diagn*. 2002;22:995-1000.

8. Berg C, Kamil D, Geipel A, et al. Absence of ductus venosus—importance of umbilical venous drainage site. *Ultrasound Obstet Gynecol*. 2006;28:275-281.
9. Hajdu J, Marton T, Kozsurek M, et al. Prenatal diagnosis of abnormal course of umbilical vein and absent ductus venosus—report of three cases. *Fetal Diagn Ther*. 2008;23:136-139.
10. Hoppen T, Hofstaetter C, Plath H, Kau N, Bartmann P. Agenesis of the ductus venosus and its correlation to hydrops fetalis. *J Perinat Med*. 2000;28:69-73.
11. Jaeggi ET, Fouron JC, Hornberger LK, et al. Agenesis of the ductus venosus that is associated with extrahepatic umbilical vein drainage: prenatal features and clinical outcome. *Am J Obstet Gynecol*. 2002;187:1031-1037.
12. Perles Z, Nir A, Nadjari M, Ergaz Z, Raas-Rothschild A, Rein AJ. Absent ductus venosus in the fetus: review of the literature and first report of direct umbilical venous drainage to the coronary sinus. *Fetal Diagn Ther*. 2003;18:247-251.
13. Sau A, Sharland G, Simpson J. Agenesis of the ductus venosus associated with direct umbilical venous return into the heart—case series and review of literature. *Prenat Diagn*. 2004;24:418-423.
14. Takeuchi M, Nakayama M, Tamura A, Kitajima H. Hydrops fetalis due to agenesis of the ductus venosus: new hepatic histological features. *Pediatr Dev Pathol*. 2009;12:239-243.
15. Cho YK, Chang NK, Ma JS. Successful transcatheter closure of a large patent ductus venosus with the Amplatzer vascular plug II. *Pediatr Cardiol*. 2009;30:540-542.

CASES

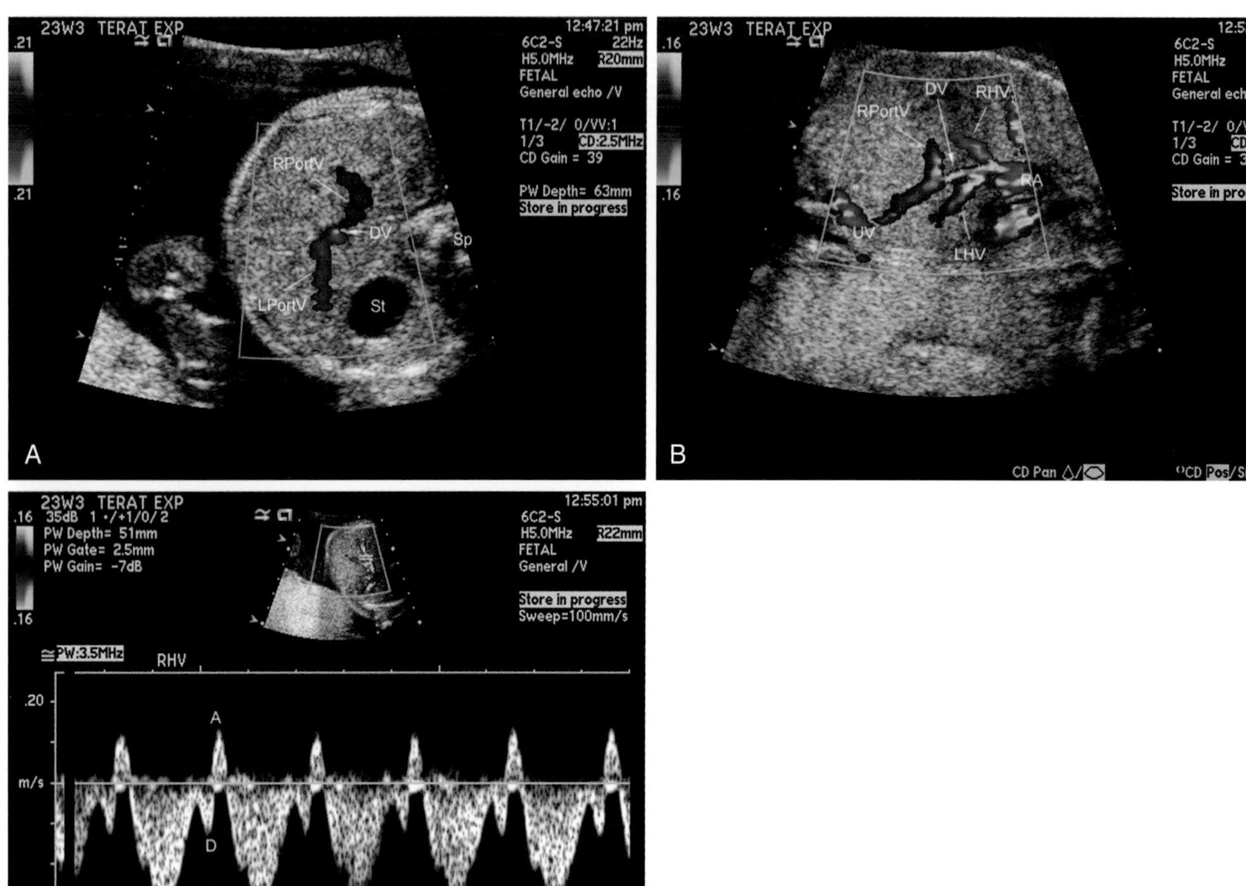

Case 37-1. (A) Color flow imaging delineation of normal anatomy and normal vascular connections of the ductus venosus. Transverse view at the level of the abdomen demonstrates the stomach (St) on the left and anterior to the spine (Sp). The ductus venosus (DV) is seen in short-axis view as a high-velocity region of flow as it travels through the portal system. Both the right (RPortV) and the left (LPortV) portal veins are seen. (B) Long-axis splayed-out view of the normal anatomy and normal vascular connections of the DV. The DV receives the umbilical venous flow and acts as a bridge between the portal venous system (PortV) and the hepatic venous system. Seen well are the RPortV and the right (RHV) and left (LHV) hepatic veins as they join together in their entry into the right atrium (RA). One can appreciate from this image that in the absence of a DV, so long as the umbilical vein (UV) connects to the liver, UV flow will drain fully into the PortV and out through the hepatic venous system before making its way to the RA. The liver parenchyma and microvasculature itself will continue to function as a "resistor" to control umbilical venous return. Without this "resistor" as when the UV connects in an extrahepatic manner such as to the inferior vena cava, a torrent of umbilical venous return will flood the heart, causing volume-overload failure. (C) Doppler pattern of flow in the RHV. Note the triphasic pattern with reversal of flow with atrial contraction. Reversal of flow is not normally seen in the DV.

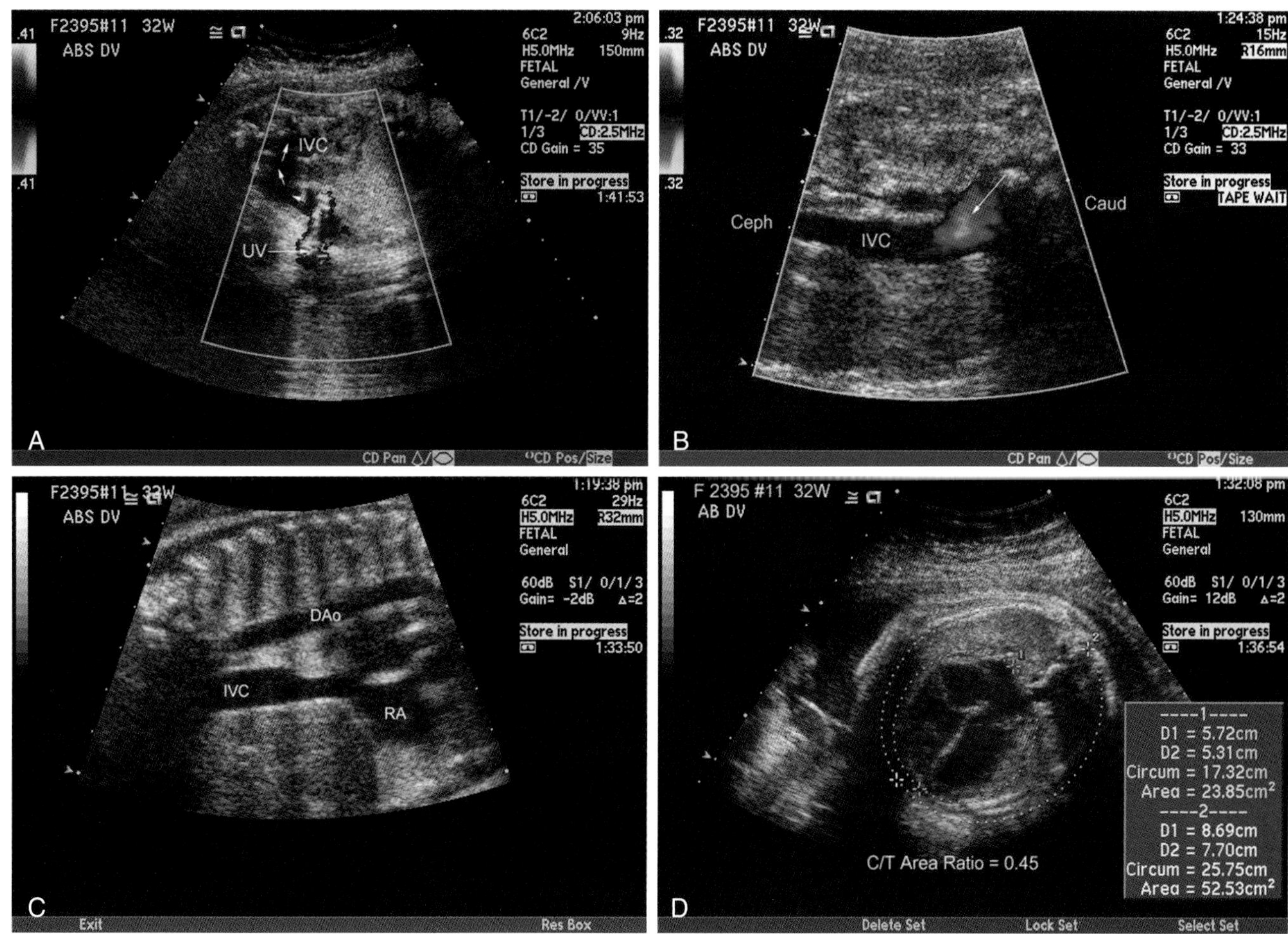

Case 37-2. **(A)** Color flow image of entry of the UV directly into the inferior vena cava (IVC). **(B)** Long-axis view of the entry site of the UV *(arrow)* into the IVC. **(C)** Note the dilation of the IVC, which is larger in diameter than the descending aorta (DAo). The IVC is carrying a much larger degree of blood than normal. Umbilical venous return is unhampered as it returns from the placenta to the fetus and is flooding the fetal circulatory system. **(D)** As a consequence of the torrent of volume overload, the heart is enlarged with cardiothoracic (C/T) ratio of 0.45.

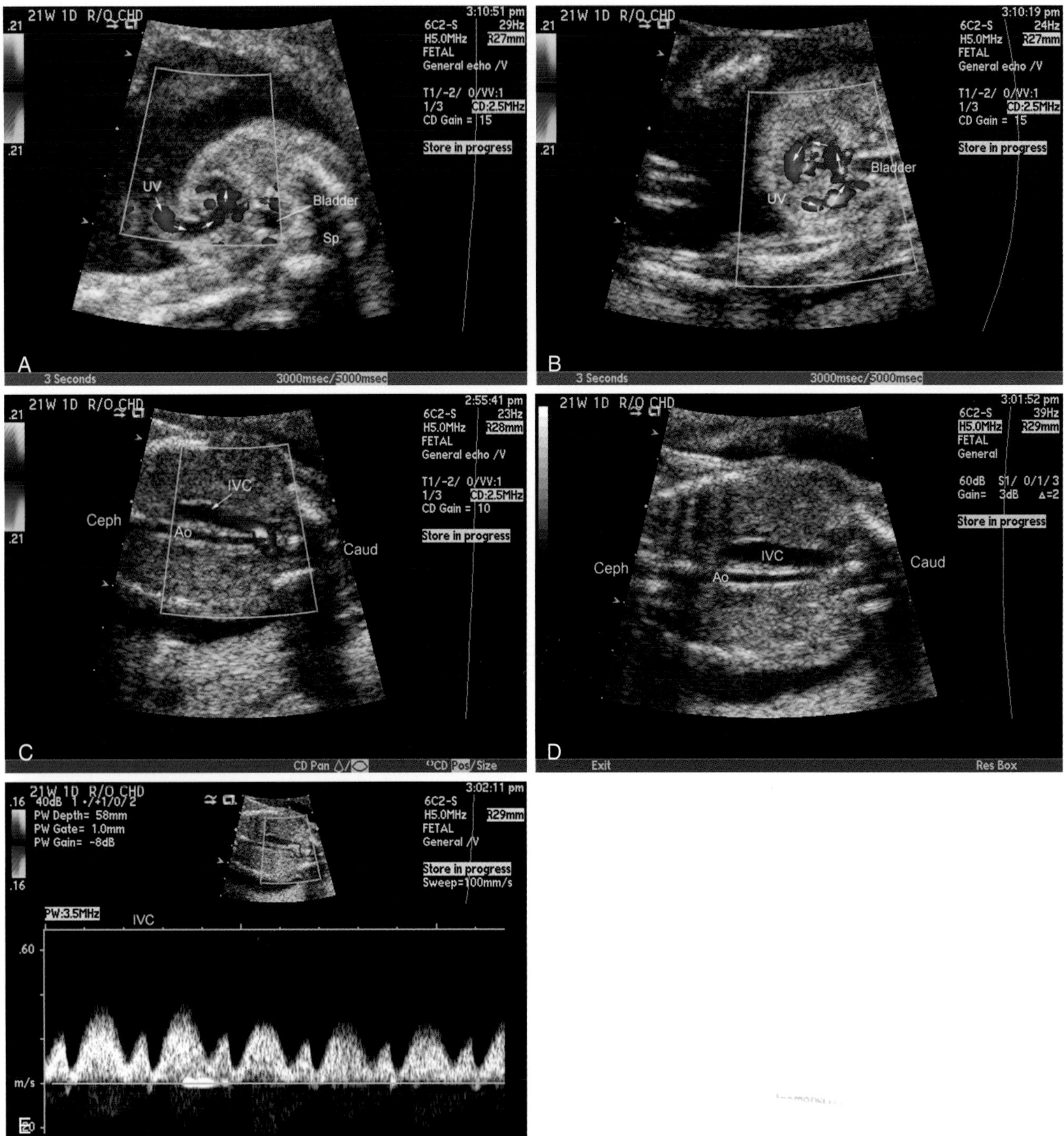

Case 37-3. **(A)** Case of UV entry directly into the femoral vein of the fetus. **(B)** Trajectory of umbilical venous connection to the fetal femoral vein. **(C)** Entry into the IVC. **(D)** Dilated IVC. Ao, aorta. **(E)** Doppler flow pattern at the iliac vein–IVC connection. This flow pattern is seen throughout the lower systemic venous return as the overall volume of return is increased.

Disorders and Anomalies Secondarily Affecting the Cardiovascular System in the Fetus

38

Twin-Twin Transfusion Syndrome

Jack Rychik

Key Echocardiographic Features

- Monochorionic pregnancy with size discrepancy between twins.
- For the smaller donor, heart function appears ostensibly normal with small ventricular cavity volumes and hyperdynamic systolic function.
- Umbilical artery impedance (pulsatility index) can be higher than normal.
- For the larger recipient, a number of cardiovascular findings are common including:
  - Cardiomegaly.
  - Ventricular hypertrophy.
  - Poor systolic function.
  - Atrioventricular valve regurgitation.
  - Abnormalities of Doppler flow suggesting poor right ventricular compliance and diastolic dysfunction such as reversal in the ductus venosus and umbilical venous pulsations.
  - Abnormalities of Doppler inflow across the tricuspid and mitral valves, namely formation of a single-peak inflow.
  - Pulmonary insufficiency.
  - Right ventricular outflow tract obstruction manifested as a smaller than normal pulmonary artery relative to the aorta, "functional" pulmonary atresia, or frank anatomical pulmonary atresia.
  - Reversal of flow in the ductus arteriosus in the presence of right ventricular outflow tract obstruction.
- Look for signs of hydrops in the recipient.

Anatomy and Anatomical Associations

The twin-twin transfusion syndrome (TTTS) is a disorder that occurs in monochorionic multiple pregnancies. Placental vascular connections provide the substrate for exchange of volume and mediators between twin fetuses, which leads to a host of abnormal findings for both. One twin, the recipient, is larger, manifests polyhydramnios, and develops cardiovascular changes reflective of volume load and ventricular hypertrophy leading to cardiomyoapthy. The other twin, the donor, is smaller, manifests oligohydramnios, and develops hypovolemia and increased vascular tone. The term "transfusion syndrome" is a bit of a misnomer and an oversimplification of the pathophysiological process because hemoglobin levels measured in the twin partners are usually not different from each other. However, volume exchange between the twins prompts a cascade of events that results in profound physiological changes for both.

Overall, TTTS manifests significant morbidity and mortality and is fatal to one or both twins in over 90% of cases if not treated in some manner.[1]

Frequency, Genetics, and Development

TTTS is seen in approximately 15% of monochorionic twin pregnancy. With increasing use of reproductive technologies, twinning in general is occurring more frequently in the human population. Hence, screening for TTTS, the means of accurate detection, an improved understanding, and the actual number of patients with this disorder are all on the rise.

TTTS is a "placental vasculopathy" and is a disorder that can be considered primarily of cardiovascular origins.[2] In the normal monochorionic pregnancy, multiple placental vascular connections naturally allow for exchange between the twin partner circulations. Exchange takes place at arterial-to-venous connections with equilibration of net flow at arterial-to-arterial connections. The arterial-to-arterial connections compensate for any net flow from one twin to the other and keep the relative circulatory volumes stable. However, if there are an inadequate number of such arterial-to-arterial connections, equilibration is hampered and flow due to arterial-to-venous connections predominates, resulting in volume load to one twin and volume depletion to the other. TTTS is presumed due to an inadequate number of such arterial-to-arterial connections.[3] Furthermore, abnormalities of donor cord insertion have been described as a possible precursor to TTTS. Insertion of the donor umbilical cord onto the edge of the placenta with reduction in vascular territory or the velamentous insertion of the cord onto the placenta (*velamentous insertion* means that the veins, unprotected by Wharton's jelly, traverse the membranes before they come together into the umbilical cord) may predispose to creating disparity in blood flow between the twins.[4]

There are no current data to suggest a genetic basis to TTTS. In a recent large review of karyotype of fetuses undergoing therapy for TTTS, only 1% of 600 fetuses were found to have abnormalities including Turner's syndrome (46,XO) and 47, XYY.[5] The authors concluded that abnormal karyotype in TTTS is no different than what is seen in the general population.

Prenatal Physiology

The pathophysiology of TTTS and its cardiovascular manifestations are not fully understood. However, based on observable findings, a working plausible hypothesis has been generated.[6] With net transfer of volume between the donor twin and the recipient, a cascade of events

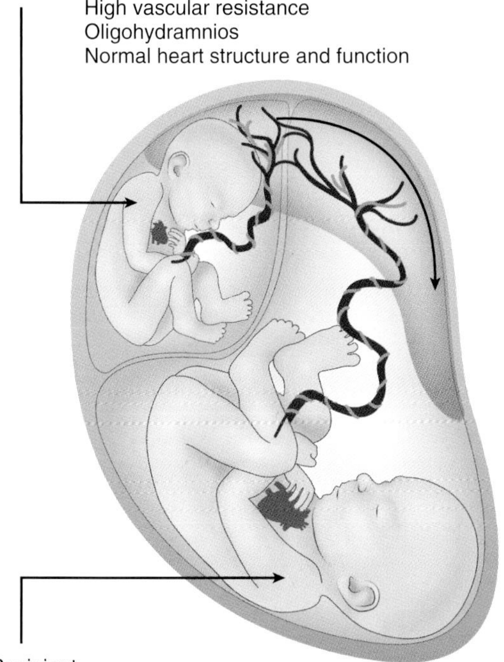

Figure 38-1. The proposed pathophysiology of twin-twin transfusion syndrome. The smaller donor experiences hypovolemia and as a consequence releases vasoconstrictive mediators to maintain perfusion. Through placental vascular connections, both volume and these vasoactive mediators are transmitted to the larger recipient, leading to myocardial remodeling and cardiomyopathy.

takes place (Figure 38-1). First, the donor twin experiences progressive hypovolemia. The normal response to hypovolemia is an increase in systemic vascular resistance, in order to preserve perfusion pressure. In order to achieve this goal, a host of mediators are released, such as endothelin-1.[7] The renin-angiotensin system is up-regulated with release of angiotensin II. Observation of the donor twin reveals a small heart size, with underfilled ventricular cavities, and a hyperdynamic state with ostensibly good systolic ventricular function. Urine production is diminished, visualization of the bladder may be limited, and oligohydramnios occurs. The recipient twin experiences an increase in volume load, but in addition to a transfer of volume, it also receives the various vasoactive mediators released by the donor.[8] Recent data also suggests renin-angiotensin release from a portion of the recipient placenta may also contribute.[9] In essence, these mediators compound the pathological response of the recipient's cardiovascular system to the volume load. Observation of the recipient reveals ventricular dilation and marked hypertrophy. Progressive cardiomegaly, atrioventricular valve regurgitation, and development of a characteristic cardiomyopathy ensue. Increase in fetal brain natriuretic peptide (BNP) as a consequence of these cardiomyopathic changes has been found in recipients.[10] Angiotensin II in combination with increase in preload are the likely agents responsible for what can be observed as a relatively rapid changeover from a normal size and normal functioning heart to a dilated, hypertrophied and poorly functioning heart, all in a matter of weeks.

TTTS can be seen as early as 14 to 16 weeks' gestation. The cardiovascular changes can be observed to take place with rapid progression from 18 to 28 weeks. Besides the changes of ventricular dilation, hypertrophy, and dysfunction, diastolic changes in myocardial compliance can be seen early in the process and are reflected by changes in ventricular filling parameters such as the E:A wave ratio across the tricuspid or mitral valves. Right-sided changes always precede, and are more severe, than left-sided changes. Initially, cardiac output in the recipient is increased relative to the donor. As the process progresses and systolic and diastolic dysfunction sets in, cardiac output diminishes. Measures of ventricular performance such as the myocardial performance index are abnormal in TTTS and reflect both systolic and diastolic dysfunction.[11,12]

If TTTS is left unchecked, severe ventricular dysfunction can progress to development of hydrops and fetal demise. In addition, a subset of recipient twins, approximately 10%, develop pulmonic stenosis and right ventricular outflow tract obstruction (RVOTO).[13,14] This has been referred to as the development of "acquired" congenital heart disease, a fascinating phenomenon that reflects the potential plasticity of the human heart to convert from normal to a form of structural heart disease, in response to flow dynamics, loading conditions, and mediator release during a vulnerable time of gestation.

Recipient cardiomyoapthy can lead to impaired cerebral perfusion and neurological insult.[15] Severe hypovolemia and oliguria in the donor can also result in poor growth. Umbilical arterial flow in the donor is altered as placental vascular resistance is elevated. This is reflected in the findings of either absent or at times reversed umbilical diastolic arterial flow, an ominous sign suggesting impaired placental flow. Death of one twin in untreated TTTS is common. Because there are vascular connections within the placenta uniting the two circulations, death of a twin results in creation of a vascular sink that can acutely drain volume from the surviving co-twin. Such sudden hypoperfusion can also lead to neurological insult or secondary demise in the survivor; hence, the fates of both twins in TTTS are interrelated.

Prenatal Management

Fetal treatment for TTTS is currently possible and very effective. But who is to be treated, and how is the

Table 38-1 Quintero's Scoring System to Gauge Disease Severity

QUINTERO STAGE	FINDINGS
I	Twin size discrepancy and polyhydramnios + oligohydramnios sequence
II	Absent bladder filling in donor
III	"Critical Doppler abnormalities" (UA, UV, and ductus venosus)
IV	Fetal hydrops
V	Fetal demise

UA, umbilical artery; UV, umbilical vein.

Table 38-2 Children's Hospital of Philadelphia Twin-Twin Transfusion Syndrome Cardiovascular Score

Ventricular Elements			
Cardiac enlargement	None (0)	Mild (1)	>Mild (2)
Systolic dysfunction	None (0)	Mild (1)	>Mild (2)
Ventricular hypertrophy	None (0)	Present (1)	
Valve Function			
Tricuspid regurgitation	None (0)	Mild (1)	>Mild (2)
Mitral regurgitation	None (0)	Mild (1)	>Mild (2)
Venous Doppler			
Tricuspid inflow	Two peaks (0)	One peak (1)	
Mitral inflow	Two peaks (0)	One peak (1)	
Ductus venosus	All forward (0)	Decreased (1)	Reversal (2)
UV pulsation	None (0)	Present (1)	
Great Vessel Analysis			
Outflow tracts	PA > Ao (0)	PA = Ao (1)	PA < Ao (2) RVOTO (3)
Pulmonary insufficiency	None (0)	Present (1)	
Umbilical Artery Flow in Donor			
UA Doppler	Normal (0)	Decreased diastolic flow (1)	Absent of reversed diastolic flow (2)

Ao, aorta; PA, pulmonary artery; RVOTO, right ventricular outflow tract obstruction.

spectrum of the disease best described? The basic criteria for diagnosis of TTTS are

1. Monochorionic pregnancy.
2. Size discrepancy of at least 10% between the twins.
3. Oligohydramnios in the smaller twin and polyhydramnios in the larger twin.

A scoring system to gauge disease severity in TTTS exists. Quintero and coworkers developed a five-stage system based on clinical and ultrasound findings (Table 38-1).[16] This system has been extremely useful in guiding therapy and response to therapy.

Because TTTS is inherently a cardiovascular disorder, we have argued that the Quintero system is inadequate in fully describing and characterizing the complement of cardiovascular sequelae that exists. Based on observations made in hundreds of twin pairs that have been referred to our center at Children's Hospital of Philadelphia (CHOP), we have developed a disease specific cardiovascular scoring system for TTTS (Table 38-2).[17] The CHOP TTTS Cardiovascular Score assesses five different domains of cardiovascular function, with grades given for various abnormal findings. Four of the domains relate to cardiovascular findings in the recipient twin, and the final domain addresses the donor umbilical artery flow. No structural cardiac changes are typically seen in the donor; however, there is commonly evidence of elevated placental resistance manifested as a decreased or reverse flow in diastole when sampling in the umbilical artery.[18] In particular, one of the domains in the recipient addresses the issue of RVOTO. Normally, the pulmonary artery should always be larger than the aorta. We have observed that, in some recipient twins, the pulmonary artery is either the same size or smaller than the aorta, this in advance of the findings of frank pulmonary or right ventricular outflow tract stenosis. This suggests a spectrum of right-sided obstruction, starting with very subtle differences. Furthermore, pulmonary valve insufficiency suggesting early functional change is present in some recipients as well, in advance of frank pulmonary stenosis of outflow tract obstruction. We have, therefore, incorporated these variables in our evaluation system.

The five domains and the point values for the various elements of the CHOP TTTS Cardiovascular Score are:

1. **Ventricular characteristics** such as ventricular hypertrophy (absent = 0, present = 1), ventricular dilation (cardiothoracic ratio >0.33 = 1, >0.5 = 2), and systolic dysfunction (absent = 0, mild dysfunction = 1, more than mild dysfunction = 2).
2. **Atrioventricular Valvar function**, with assessment of tricuspid regurgitation (absent = 0, mild = 1, greater than mild = 2) and mitral regurgitation (absent = 0, mild = 1, greater than mild = 2).
3. **Venous Doppler findings** that reflect diastolic performance such as tricuspid inflow pattern (normal two-peak inflow = 0, abnormal single-peak inflow = 1) and mitral inflow pattern normal two-peak inflow = 0, abnormal single-peak inflow = 1); ductus venosus flow (normal all forward = 0, decreased forward flow with atrial contraction = 1, reversal of flow with atrial contraction = 2); and umbilical vein pulsations (normal absent = 0, present = 1).

4. **Great vessel analysis** looking at the ratio of size of the pulmonary artery to the aorta (normal pulmonary artery larger than the aorta = 0, pulmonary artery appearing close to the aorta in size, suggesting abnormal smallness = 1, pulmonary artery measures smaller than the aorta = 2, pulmonary stenosis or RVOTO = 3); and looking at grade of pulmonary insufficiency (none = 0, present = 1).
5. **Umbilical arterial flow in the donor** (normal flow with ample diastolic flow = 0, decreased diastolic flow reflecting elevated placental vascular resistance = 1, absent or reversed diastolic flow reflecting severely elevated placental vascular resistance = 2).

The higher the score, the greater the cardiovascular burden of disease, with a maximum score of 20 points possible. Patients can be categorized into quartiles with cardiovascular severity grades offered: score 1-5 = severity grade I; score 6-10 = severity grade II; score 11-15 = severity grade III; score 16-20 = severity grade IV.

A comparison of the Quintero scoring system with the CHOP score reveals some overlap but also substantial discrepancy in that many subjects with relatively low Quintero scores often have higher cardiovascular severity grades, reflecting the inadequate nature of the Quintero system to accurately capture and describe the cardiovascular phenomenon taking place in TTTS (Figure 38-2).

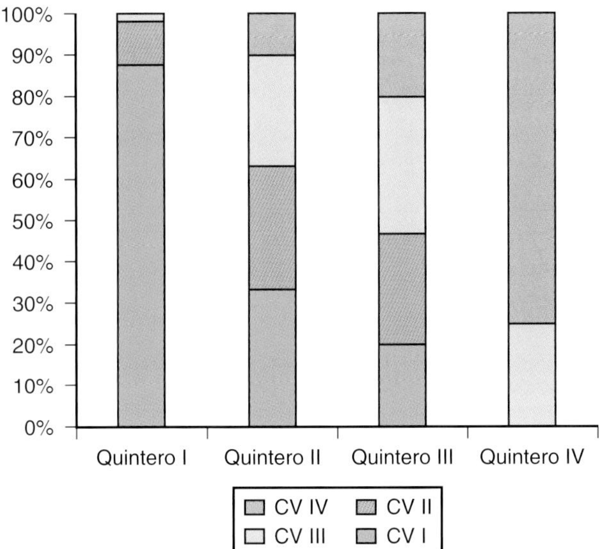

Figure 38-2. Graphic display of the relationship between the Quintero stage and the presence of cardiovascular manifestations for 150 twin pairs with twin-twin transfusion syndrome. The Children's Hospital of Philadelphia (CHOP) Cardiovascular Score (range 1-20) was divided into quartiles with score of 1-5 = CV I; 6-10 = CV II; 11-15 = CV III; and 16-20 = CV IV. Note that for Quintero stage I, 12% of subjects exhibited CV II grade manifestations, and for Quintero II, 65% of subjects exhibited cardiovascular manifestations of CV II or higher. Recall that neither of these Quintero stages, I or II, include any cardiac findings because "critical Doppler" findings are described only for Quintero stage III. This suggests that the Quintero grading system misses a significant amount of cardiovascular pathology and is insufficient in characterizing the cardiovascular system in twin-twin transfusion syndrome.

A number of treatment options are available for in utero management of TTTS. If the disease is severe and far along and the demise of one twin is anticipated, a selective termination with the goal of saving the co-twin is appropriate to consider. Such a procedure can be done using an ultrasound bipolar cord cauterization technique and is relatively safe with good outcomes for the surviving twin.[19]

Amnioreduction has been an effective means for creating maternal comfort by relieving the pressure of excess fluid accumulation. In addition, the removal of fluid has resulted in physiological changes in some cases. Theoretically, reduction in intra-amniotic pressure by fluid removal may alleviate compression of placental vasculature thereby improving blood flow and exchange between the twins. There are reports of amnioreduction reversing the TTTS process; however, overall, this proved not to be a very reliable strategy.[20]

Laser photocoagulation (LP) of placental vascular connections is currently the treatment of choice for TTTS.[21] Because the origins of the disease derive from net flow across connections between the two circulations, it makes sense that interruption of such connections will offer the best hope for successful outcome. LP is superior to amnioreduction and has dramatically improved the survival of twins in the TTTS. Morbidity has also been diminished by the widespread use of LP. We have applied the CHOP TTTS score to patients before and after LP in order to gauge the response to therapy from the cardiovascular perspective. In a series of 54 patients treated with LP, the score was cut in half within 1 week after treatment from 9 ± 5 before treatment to 4 ± 3 after treatment. In addition, when we analyzed each of the components of the score, we found a decrease in all elements; however, the greatest degree of change appeared to be in the diastolic parameters (Figure 38-3). For example, the finding of single-peak inflow across the tricuspid valve normalized by 50% and the finding of single-peak inflow across the mitral valve was normalized by 86%. Both ductus venosus flow and umbilical venous flow parameters improved substantially (Figures 38-4 to 38-6). Most interesting was the discovery that outflow tract abnormalities, primarily the size ratio of the pulmonary artery to the aorta, normalized by 73%; somewhat surprising as an element related to a structural change should take much longer to normalize than a Doppler flow change. Perhaps this phenomenon suggests that some of the diminution in pulmonary artery size is related to the dramatic diastolic changes in compliance that take place in the right ventricle of the recipient in TTTS. Stiffness of the right ventricle may be associated with a stiffness or constriction of the right ventricular outflow tract. Perhaps this is volume related or mediated through some other biological process. What is known is that once clear evidence for pulmonary valvar stenosis with thickened nonmobile leaflets or anatomical valvar atresia is present, LP does not affect a change in these findings. It appears as if the

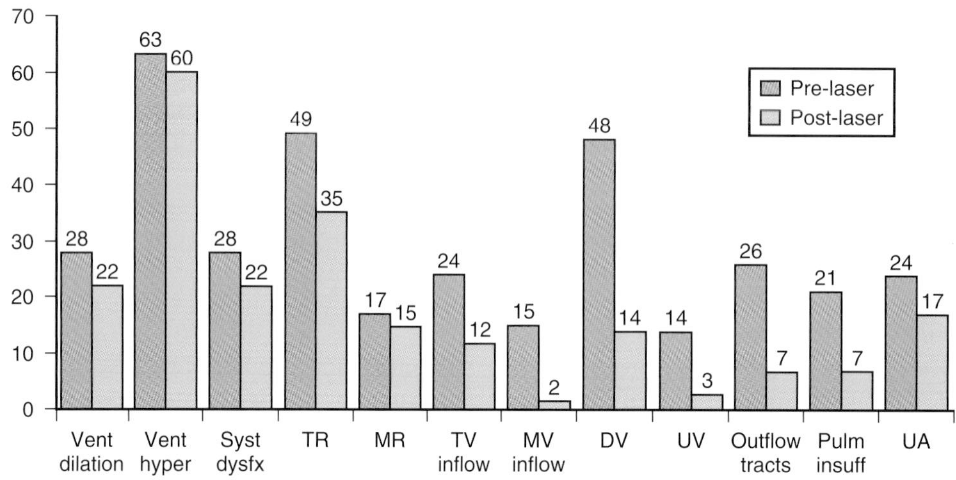

Figure 38-3. Bar graph display of pre-laser *(purple)* and post-laser *(green)* aggregate scores for the various elements of the CHOP Cardiovascular Score for twin-twin transfusion syndrome. Post-laser scores are within 1 week after therapy. There is a decrease in all elements of the score; however, the greatest degree of change appears to take place in the diastolic elements such as tricuspid valve (TV) inflow, mitral valve (MV) inflow, ductus venosus (DV), and umbilical vein (UV) Doppler flow patterns. Note as well that the degree of right ventricular outflow tract obstruction improved post-laser. hyper, hypertrophy; MR, mitral regurgitation; Pulm Insuff, pulmonary insufficiency; Syst Dysfx, systolic dysfunction; TR, tricuspid regurgitation; Vent, ventricular; UA, umbilical artery.

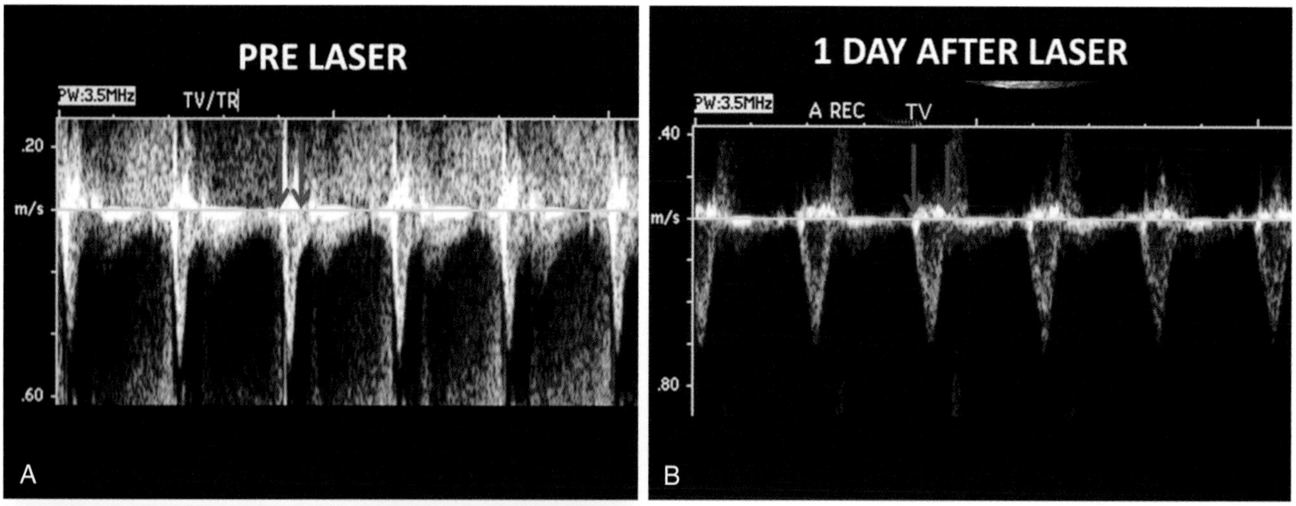

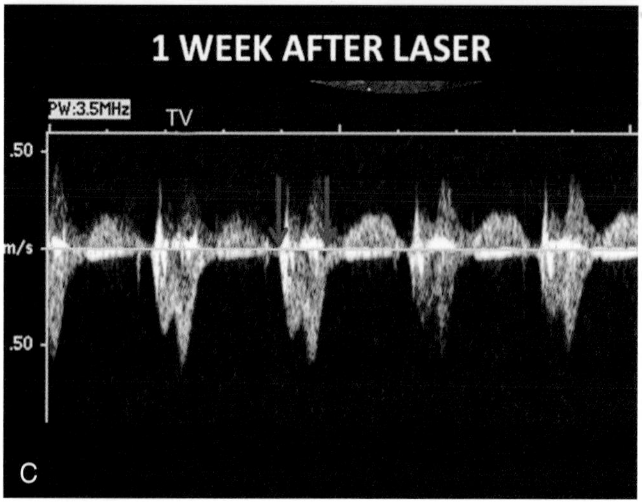

Figure 38-4. Serial Doppler flow assessment of changes in the recipient twin heart reflecting myocardial compliance before and after laser photocoagulation therapy for twin-twin transfusion syndrome. **(A)** Pre-laser inflow pattern across the tricuspid valve (TV). Note a very narrow inflow waveform, with a very short diastolic filling time. This short filling time contributes to impaired ventricular volume filling and decreased stroke volume and ejection volume across the pulmonary valve. TR, tricuspid regurgitation. **(B)** One day after laser therapy. Note the increase in diastolic filling times, designated by the *arrows.* A single peak inflow pattern is still present. **(C)** One week after laser therapy. There is further extension of the filling time, with complete normalization of the inflow to a two-peak pattern.

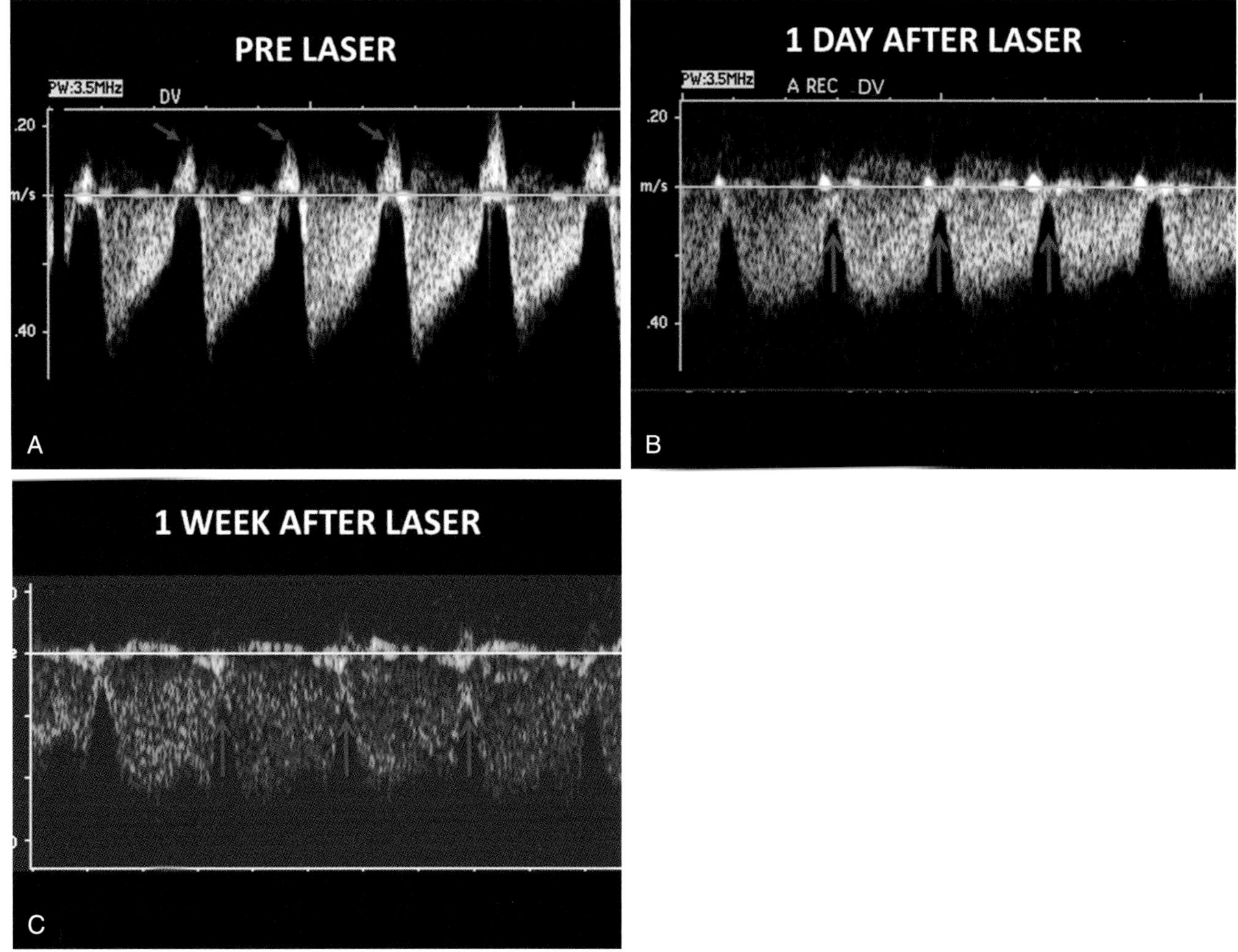

Figure 38-5. (A) Ductus venosus (DV) flow pattern before laser therapy. There is reversal of flow with atrial contraction suggesting a very poorly compliant right ventricle with diastolic dysfunction. (B) DV flow pattern at 1 day after laser therapy demonstrates improvement with antegrade but diminished flow with atrial contraction. (C) At 1 week after laser therapy, the DV demonstrates normal flow pattern. *Arrows* point to flow during atrial contraction.

early precursors for right-sided obstruction (i.e., pulmonary artery size smaller than aorta) are amenable to reversal as is the finding of "functional" pulmonary atresia in which there is pulmonic insufficiency but no antegrade flow across. However, once a fixed structural change such as anatomical pulmonary atresia is evident, the heart is no longer plastic and responsive to the physiological effects of LP.

Other investigators have found an improvement in recipient ventricular performance as evidenced by an improvement in the myocardial performance index after LP, with the time frame of 1 month until complete normalization can be seen.[22,23]

Although our understandings of the pathophysiology are limited, the positive effects of LP on TTTS are significant and an important contribution to the management of this disorder. Questions of when to apply LP therapy still exist. For example, would all cases of TTTS, even those with Quintero stage 1 findings, do better with LP than amnioreduction or expectant observation? Further investigational work in this area is warranted.[24]

Postnatal Physiology and Management

LP has improved the status of many twin pairs with TTTS who would otherwise be quite ill at birth. Regression of disease is common after LP; however, some infants require attention at birth. Twins in general are at risk for prematurity, and even more so those who have been exposed to a laparascopic procedure such as LP. Echocardiographic evaluation in the newborn period is important for those who have had prenatal treatment. There is an increased risk of persistent pulmonary hypertension of the newborn in survivors of TTTS.[25] Residual

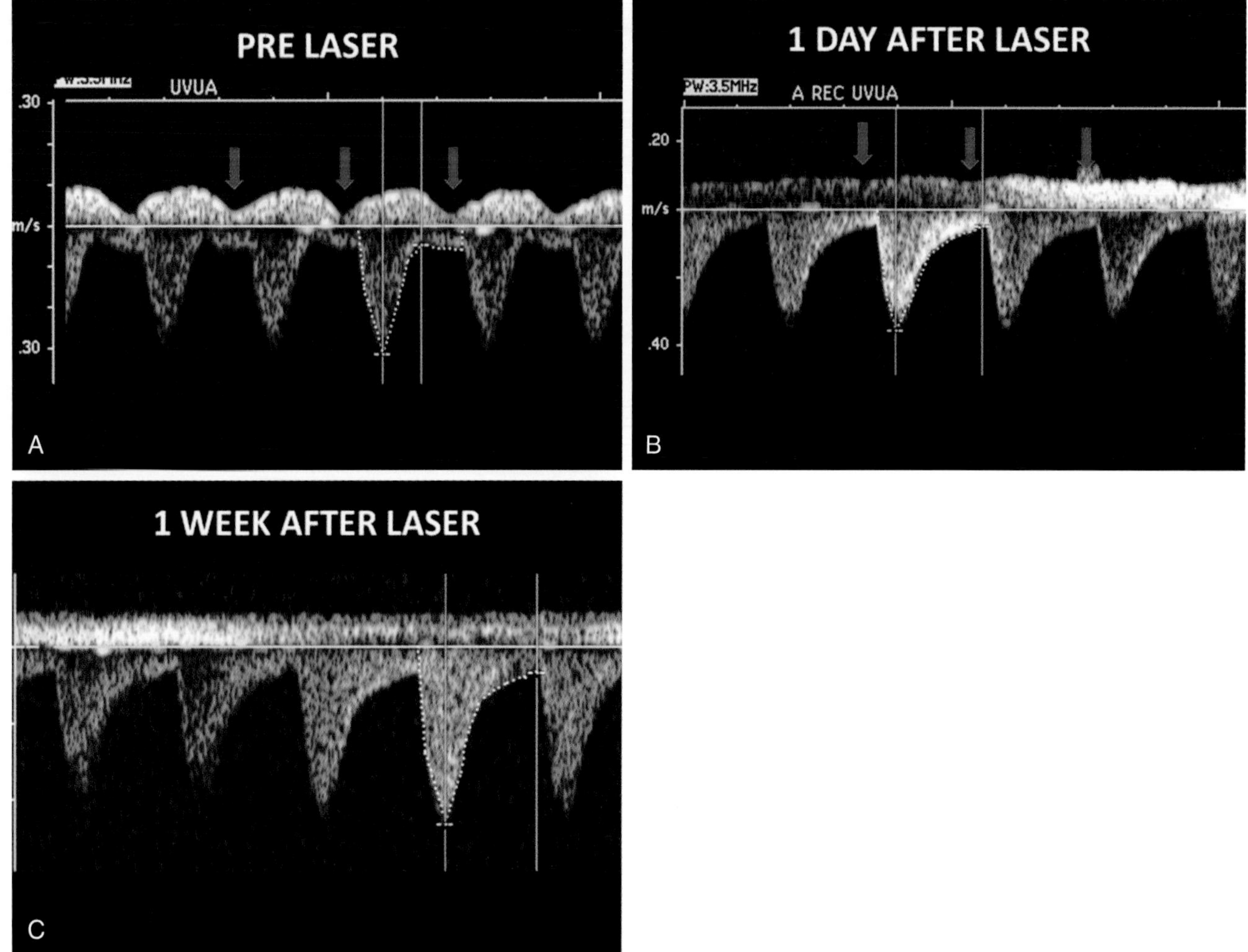

Figure 38-6. (A) Doppler sampling of the umbilical cord before laser therapy demonstrates umbilical venous pulsations. *Arrows* point to decreased flow during atrial contraction. UA, umbilical artery; UV, umbilical vein. (B) At 1 day after laser therapy, there are only mild undulations *(arrows)* in the umbilical venous flow pattern. (C) At 1 week after laser therapy, umbilical venous flow is normal without any pulsations.

ventricular dysfunction should be treated if present. It is not uncommon to see evidence of a thickened heart or residual tricuspid regurgitation. Infants born with "acquired" congenital heart disease may require treatment, through either balloon valvuloplasty or surgery, as indicated. The infants who acquire right-sided obstruction behave no differently than those who have the pure "congenital" form of the disease.[26]

Outcomes

Outcome has dramatically improved with the growth of application of LP.[27] Currently, LP yields survival of at least one twin in 85% to 90% of cases. Neurological deficits have also been substantially reduced.[28] Long-term cardiovascular manifestations in this population are yet to be fully documented.[29] Abnormalities in vascular reactivity and endothelial function have been described and may be improved upon by LP therapy.[30] Endothelial dysfunction set early in human development may have profound negative long-term effects on adult cardiovascular health.[31] Barker[32] has proposed the hypothesis of "fetal origins" of adult disease, in that cardiovascular health may to a substantial degree be predetermined by prenatal factors such as fetal cardiovascular milieu. Considering the degree of cardiovascular derangement in TTTS, survivors of this process may be at significant risk as they grow into adulthood. Long-term follow-up studies are warranted to answer these questions.

Imaging Essentials and Important Points

- Systematic and serial evaluation of patients with potential TTTS, before and after treatment, is essential in the management and in gauging response to therapy.
- The CHOP TTTS Cardiovascular Score has been helpful in the differential diagnosis of TTTS. Distinguishing TTTS from a situation of monochorionic twins in which the smaller one has intrauterine growth restriction but in fact no TTTS exists, can be a challenge. We have found that, whereas Quintero staging may gauge suspicion of TTTS, if there are absolutely no cardiovascular findings whatsoever in the recipient as proposed by the CHOP score, TTTS is either unlikely or is at a very early stage. Follow-up is necessary to help make the diagnosis and determine the course.
- When questions arise as to the presence of a particular element within the score such as a single- or double-peak inflow across the tricuspid valve, decreased ductus venosus flow with atrial contraction, or the presence or absence of ventricular hypertrophy, a comparison can be made between the donor and the recipient findings. These findings should be similar between the two co-twins if TTTS is not active. Comparison of Doppler tracings or two-dimensional images between the twins will allow for better judgment as to the presence or absence of particular elements of the score.
- Judging the grade of atrioventricular valve regurgitation can be quite subjective. We have found the index of the ratio of the maximal color jet area of regurgitation to the area of the atrium to be an effective and consistent general guideline. If the ratio is less than 25%, the degree of regurgitation is mild (would receive 1 point on the score); if greater than 25%, the degree of regurgitation is greater than mild (would receive 2 points on the score).
- Other variables not included in the CHOP TTTS Cardiovascular Score should also be investigated and noted. For example, we have seen cases of "functional" pulmonary atresia in the recipient, where the pulmonary valve does not open in systole but measures smaller than the aorta and there is pulmonary insufficiency with reversal of flow in the ductus arteriosus to compensate for the lack of antegrade flow into the pulmonary arteries. Following treatment with LP, antegrade flow across the pulmonary valve was generated. Features such as flow direction in the ductus arteriosus and flow across the pulmonary valve should be documented and monitored serially.
- The findings of hydrops are quite ominous in TTTS and hint at impending demise if left untreated or, at times, even if treated. Presence of pericardial effusions, pleural effusions, or ascites should be well noted.
- Abnormal findings in the donor twin after LP are common. We have found evidence for dilation, atrioventricular valve regurgitation, and pericardial effusion early after LP; however, many of these findings resolve over time. Frank reversal of the process with the donor taking on the role of a recipient with increased volume load, and so on, has been reported.
- Fetal echocardiographic evaluation of TTTS can be quite time consuming. The degree of detailed information needed to properly manage these patients can be quite daunting. We suggest scheduling protected time of at least 60 to 90 minutes for fetal echocardiography in these cases. Efficiency is achieved through experience, and one must go through a learning curve with continued practice in order to become proficient in assessing this complex disorder.

References

1. Habli M, Lim FY, Crombleholme T. Twin-to-twin transfusion syndrome: a comprehensive update. *Clin Perinatol.* 2009;36:391-416, x.
2. Bajoria R, Wigglesworth J, Fisk NM. Angioarchitecture of monochorionic placentas in relation to the twin-twin transfusion syndrome. *Am J Obstet Gynecol.* 1995;172:856-863.
3. Galea P, Jain V, Fisk NM. Insights into the pathophysiology of twin-twin transfusion syndrome. *Prenat Diagn.* 2005;25:777-785.
4. Fries MH, Goldstein RB, Kilpatrick SJ, Golbus MS, Callen PW, Filly RA. The role of velamentous cord insertion in the etiology of twin-twin transfusion syndrome. *Obstet Gynecol.* 1993;81:569-574.
5. Vialard F, Salomon LJ, Winer N, Bussieres L, Molina Gomes D, Ville Y. Fetal karyotype in feto-fetal transfusion syndrome: a 7-year experience. *Prenat Diagn.* 2009;29:804-805.
6. Mahieu-Caputo D, Meulemans A, Martinovic J, et al. Paradoxic activation of the renin-angiotensin system in twin-twin transfusion syndrome: an explanation for cardiovascular disturbances in the recipient. *Pediatr Res.* 2005;58:685-688.
7. Bajoria R, Sullivan M, Fisk NM. Endothelin concentrations in monochorionic twins with severe twin-twin transfusion syndrome. *Hum Reprod.* 1999;14:1614-1618.
8. Mahieu-Caputo D, Dommergues M, Delezoide AL, et al. Twin-to-twin transfusion syndrome. Role of the fetal renin-angiotensin system. *Am J Pathol.* 2000;156:629-636.
9. Galea P, Barigye O, Wee L, Jain V, Sullivan M, Fisk NM. The placenta contributes to activation of the renin angiotensin system in twin-twin transfusion syndrome. *Placenta.* 2008;29:734-742.
10. Bajoria R, Ward S, Chatterjee R. Natriuretic peptides in the pathogenesis of cardiac dysfunction in the recipient fetus of twin-twin transfusion syndrome. *Am J Obstet Gynecol.* 2002;186:121-127.
11. Szwast A, Tian Z, McCann M, et al. Impact of altered loading conditions on ventricular performance in fetuses with congenital cystic adenomatoid malformation and twin-twin transfusion syndrome. *Ultrasound Obstet Gynecol.* 2007;30:40-46.

12. Michelfelder E, Gottliebson W, Border W, et al. Early manifestations and spectrum of recipient twin cardiomyopathy in twin-twin transfusion syndrome: relation to Quintero stage. *Ultrasound Obstet Gynecol*. 2007;30:965-971.
13. Lougheed J, Sinclair BG, Fung Kee Fung K, et al. Acquired right ventricular outflow tract obstruction in the recipient twin in twin-twin transfusion syndrome. *J Am Coll Cardiol*. 2001;38: 1533-1538.
14. Barrea C, Alkazaleh F, Ryan G, et al. Prenatal cardiovascular manifestations in the twin-to-twin transfusion syndrome recipients and the impact of therapeutic amnioreduction. *Am J Obstet Gynecol*. 2005;192:892-902.
15. Quarello E, Molho M, Ville Y. Incidence, mechanisms, and patterns of fetal cerebral lesions in twin-to-twin transfusion syndrome. *J Matern Fetal Neonatal Med*. 2007;20:589-597.
16. Quintero RA, Morales WJ, Allen MH, Bornick PW, Johnson PK, Kruger M. Staging of twin-twin transfusion syndrome. *J Perinatol*. 1999;19:550-555.
17. Rychik J, Tian Z, Bebbington M, et al. The twin-twin transfusion syndrome: spectrum of cardiovascular abnormality and development of a cardiovascular score to assess severity of disease. *Am J Obstet Gynecol*. 2007;197:392.e1-392.e8.
18. Kontopoulos EV, Quintero RA, Chmait RH, Bornick PW, Russell Z, Allen MH. Percent absent end-diastolic velocity in the umbilical artery waveform as a predictor of intrauterine fetal demise of the donor twin after selective laser photocoagulation of communicating vessels in twin-twin transfusion syndrome. *Ultrasound Obstet Gynecol*. 2007;30:35-39.
19. Ilagan JG, Wilson RD, Bebbington M, et al. Pregnancy outcomes following bipolar umbilical cord cauterization for selective termination in complicated monochorionic multiple gestations. *Fetal Diagn Ther*. 2008;23:153-158.
20. Crombleholme TM, Shera D, Lee H, et al. A prospective, randomized, multicenter trial of amnioreduction vs selective fetoscopic laser photocoagulation for the treatment of severe twin-twin transfusion syndrome. *Am J Obstet Gynecol*. 2007;197:396.e1-396.e9.
21. Senat MV, Deprest J, Boulvain M, Paupe A, Winer N, Ville Y. Endoscopic laser surgery versus serial amnioreduction for severe twin-to-twin transfusion syndrome. *N Engl J Med*. 2004;351:136-144.
22. Habli M, Michelfelder E, Livingston J, et al. Acute effects of selective fetoscopic laser photocoagulation on recipient cardiac function in twin-twin transfusion syndrome. *Am J Obstet Gynecol*. 2008;199: 412.e1-492.e6.
23. Van Mieghem T, Klaritsch P, Done E, et al. Assessment of fetal cardiac function before and after therapy for twin-to-twin transfusion syndrome. *Am J Obstet Gynecol*. 2009;200:400.e1-400.e7.
24. Wagner MM, Lopriore E, Klumper FJ, Oepkes D, Vandenbussche FP, Middeldorp JM. Short- and long-term outcome in stage 1 twin-to-twin transfusion syndrome treated with laser surgery compared with conservative management. *Am J Obstet Gynecol*. 2009;201: 286.e1-286.e6.
25. Delsing B, Lopriore E, Blom N, Te Pas AB, Vandenbussche FP, Walther FJ. Risk of persistent pulmonary hypertension of the neonate in twin-to-twin transfusion syndrome. *Neonatology*. 2007;92:134-138.
26. Nizard J, Bonnet D, Fermont L, Ville Y. Acquired right heart outflow tract anomaly without systemic hypertension in recipient twins in twin-twin transfusion syndrome. *Ultrasound Obstet Gynecol*. 2001;18:669-672.
27. Odibo AO, Caughey AB, Grobman W, Stamilio DM, Ville Y. Selective laser photocoagulation versus serial amniodrainage for the treatment of twin-twin transfusion syndrome: a cost-effectiveness analysis. *J Perinatol*. 2009;29:543-547.
28. Lenclen R, Ciarlo G, Paupe A, Bussieres L, Ville Y. Neurodevelopmental outcome at 2 years in children born preterm treated by amnioreduction or fetoscopic laser surgery for twin-to-twin transfusion syndrome: comparison with dichorionic twins. *Am J Obstet Gynecol*. 2009;201:291.e1-291.e5.
29. Herberg U, Gross W, Bartmann P, Banek CS, Hecher K, Breuer J. Long term cardiac follow up of severe twin to twin transfusion syndrome after intrauterine laser coagulation. *Heart*. 2006;92: 95-100.
30. Gardiner HM, Taylor MJ, Karatza A, et al. Twin-twin transfusion syndrome: the influence of intrauterine laser photocoagulation on arterial distensibility in childhood. *Circulation*. 2003;107: 1906-1911.
31. Cheung YF, Taylor MJ, Fisk NM, Redington AN, Gardiner HM. Fetal origins of reduced arterial distensibility in the donor twin in twin-twin transfusion syndrome. *Lancet*. 2000;355:1157-1158.
32. Barker DJ. The fetal and infant origins of disease. *Eur J Clin Invest*. 1995;25:457-463.

CASES

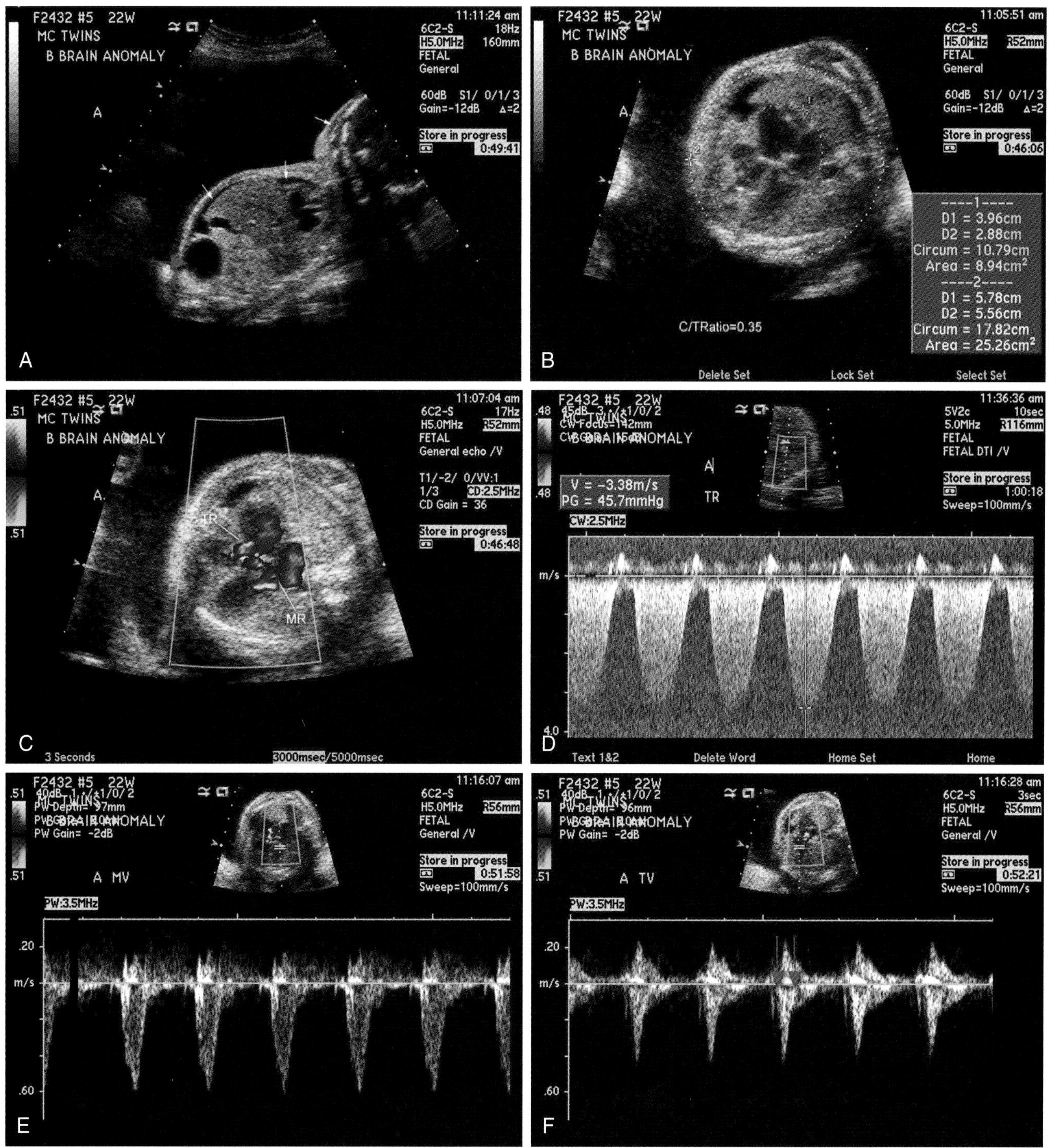

Case 38-1. **(A)** A case of twin-twin transfusion syndrome (TTTS) and imaging of the recipient twin at 22 weeks' gestation. There is evidence for hydrops fetalis by the presence of ascites, pleural effusion, and scalp edema *(white arrows)*. There is a large dilated urinary bladder *(red arrow)*, reflecting a volume overload state. **(B)** There is mild cardiomegaly with a cardiothoracic area ratio that is slightly greater than 0.33. **(C)** Color flow imaging. There is severe tricuspid regurgitation (TR) and severe mitral regurgitation (MR) as the regurgitant jets essentially fill nearly the entire right and left atria, respectively. **(D)** Pulse wave Doppler of the TR jet reveals a peak velocity of 46 mm Hg, suggesting elevated intracavitary right ventricular pressure in this recipient fetus. There is no obstruction to flow across the right ventricular outflow tract; hence, this demonstrates the presence of elevated pressure as an important component of the recipient twin pathophysiology in TTTS. **(E)** Doppler inflow across the mitral valve (MV) reveals a single peak, which reflects abnormal compliance and a "stiff" ventricle with diastolic dysfunction. **(F)** Doppler inflow across the tricuspid valve (TV) reveals a single peak, which reflects abnormal compliance and a "stiff" ventricle with diastolic dysfunction. The *red arrows* delineate the narrow waveform for tricuspid inflow and the remarkably diminished amount of time in which the ventricle fills with blood flow. Poor filling promotes poor forward flow in systole across the pulmonary valve and a diminished right ventricular cardiac output.

Continued

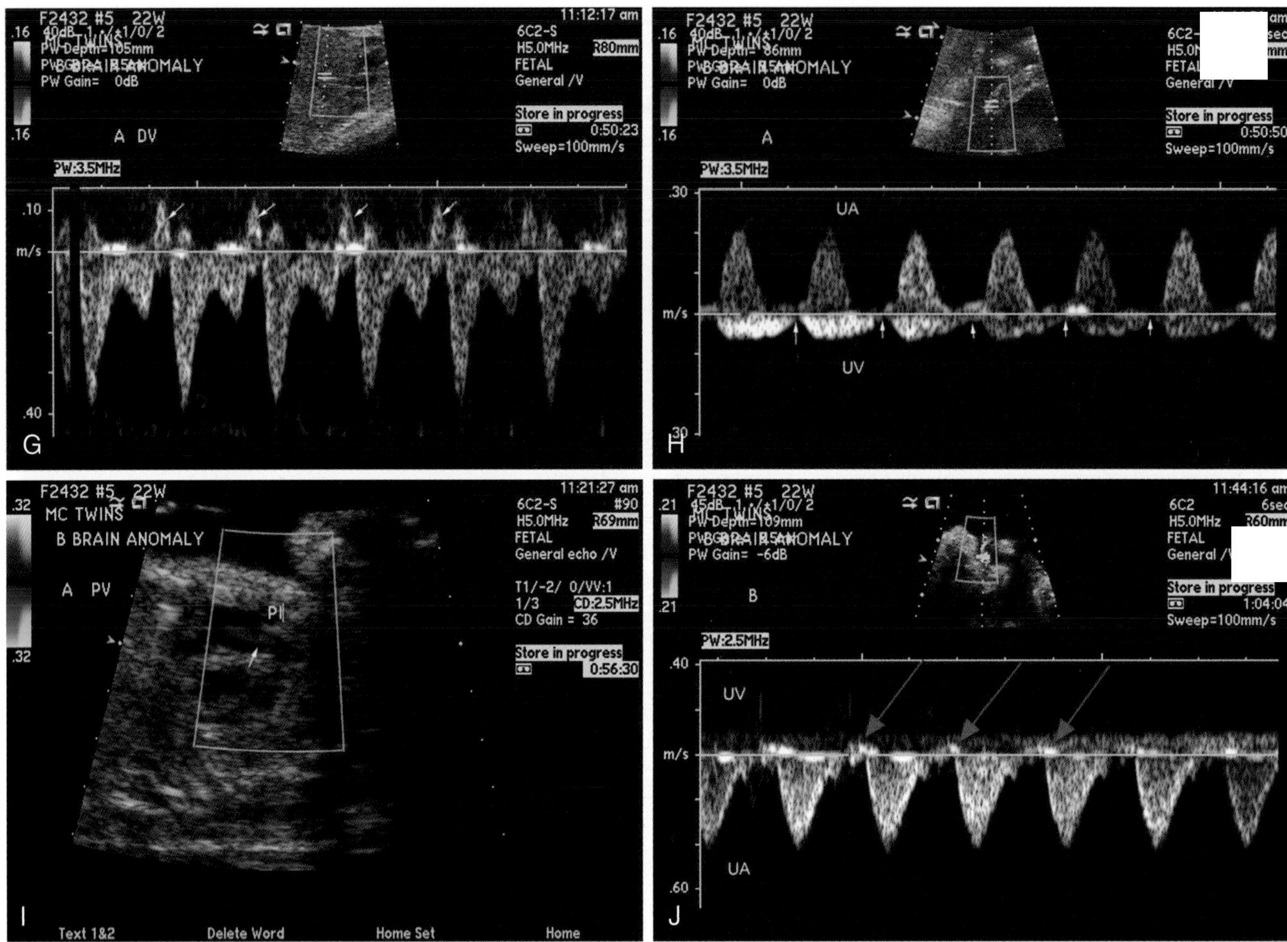

Case 38-1, cont'd (G) Doppler interrogation of the ductus venosus (DV). There are prominent A waves with reversal, suggesting a very poorly compliant right ventricle. (H) Doppler sampling within the umbilical cord of the recipient twin. There are umbilical venous pulsations *(arrows)*. UA, umbilical artery; UV, umbilical vein. (I) The pulmonic valve (PV) is open with forward flow and no pulmonary stenosis. The valve appears normal in structure and makeup; however, there is prominent pulmonic insufficiency *(arrow)*. (J) Doppler sampling of the donor umbilical cord. There is diastolic reversal of flow with arterial waveforms of reversal *(arrows)* seen through the umbilical venous flow. This reflects very high placental resistance as witnessed by the donor fetus.

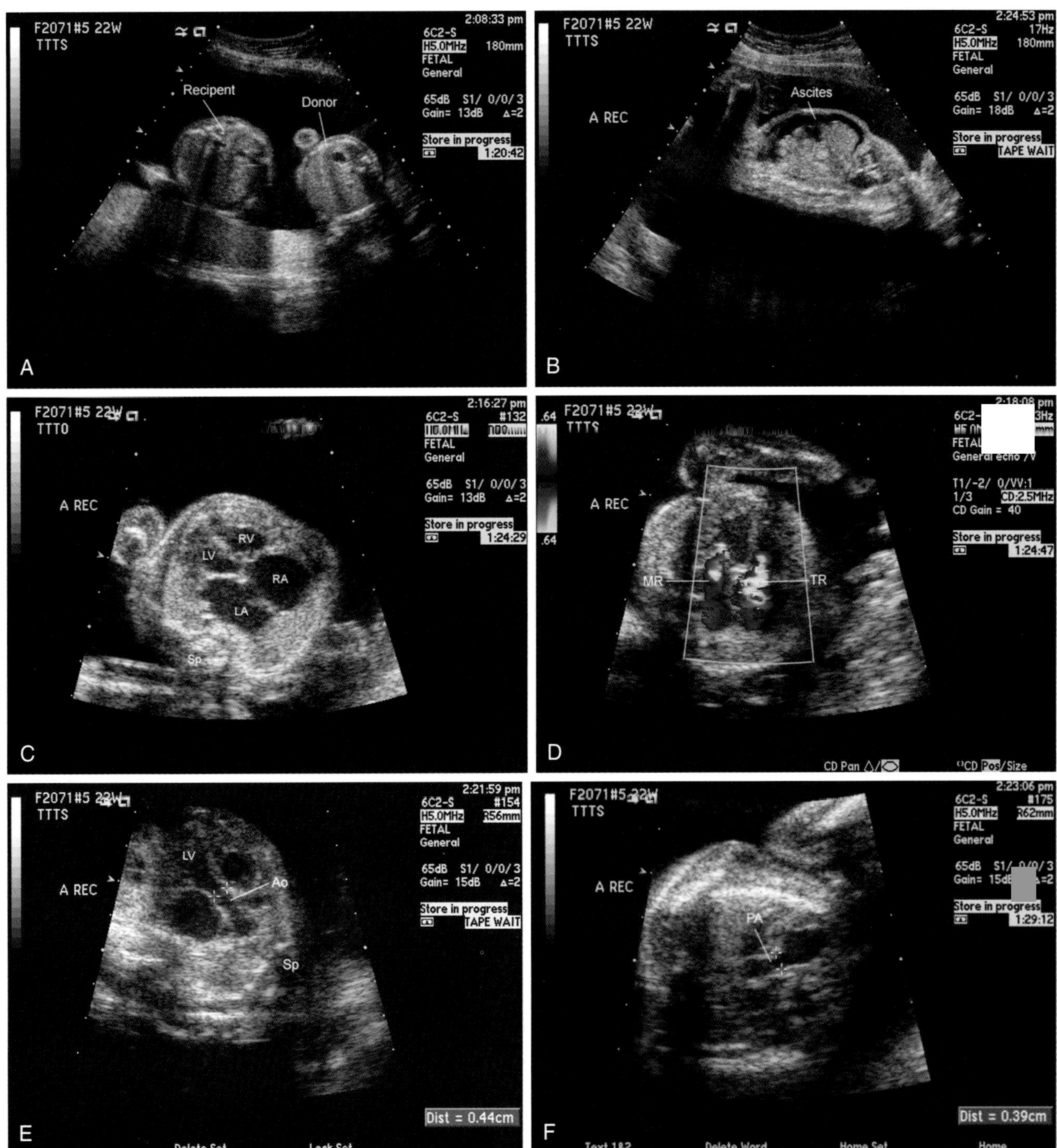

Case 38-2. (**A**) TTTS at 22 weeks' gestation. Note the size discrepancy between the smaller-appearing donor and the larger recipient. (**B**) Prominent ascites is seen in the recipient. (**C**) Four-chamber view of the recipient heart. Note the dilated left atrium (LA) and right atrium (RA). In fact, the atrial cavity volumes look to be larger than the ventricular cavities. Atrial dilation can be due to poor ventricular compliance with diastolic dysfunction, atrioventricular valve regurgitation, or the combination of both. LV, left ventricle; RV, right ventricle. (**D**) There is severe mitral (MR) and tricuspid (TR) regurgitation. (**E**) The aortic annulus measures 4.4 mm in diameter. Ao, aorta; Sp, spine. (**F**) The pulmonary annulus (PA) is smaller than the aortic annulus and measures 3.9 mm in diameter. This is an abnormality in that the pulmonary artery should normally always be larger than the aorta.

Continued

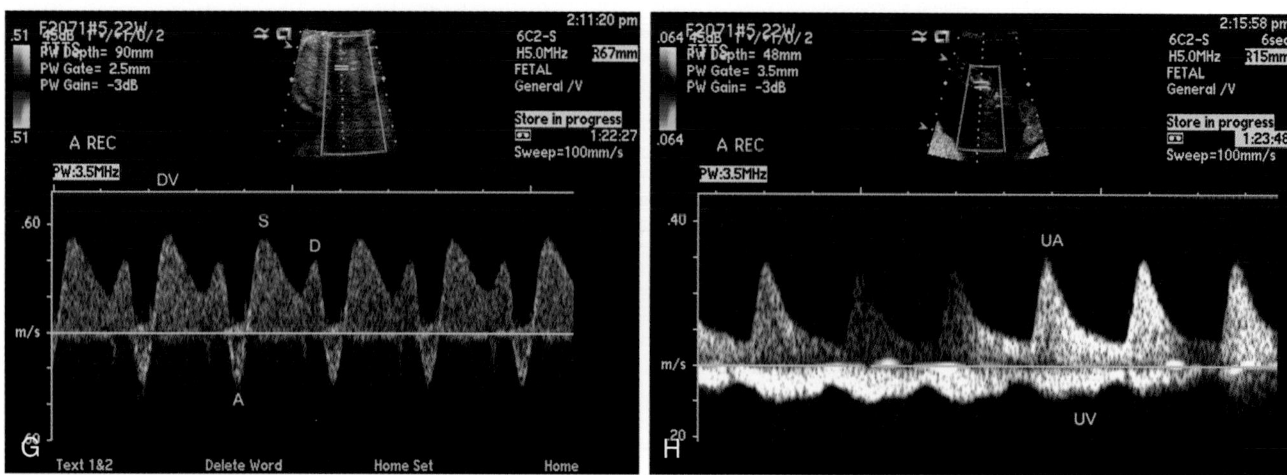

Case 38-2, cont'd **(G)** There is abnormal reversal of flow with atrial contraction in the ductus venosus (DV), suggesting right-sided diastolic dysfunction. **(H)** Doppler interrogation of the umbilical cord reveals umbilical venous pulsations, further suggesting severe diastolic dysfunction. Note the timing of decrease in the umbilical venous flow is during ventricular diastole, not systole, because it corresponds not with the peak velocity of umbilical arterial flow (systole) but rather with the diastolic portion of the arterial waveform. Hence, umbilical venous diminution in flow is unlikely related to suppression of forward flow from tricuspid regurgitation—a systolic phenomenon—but is rather likely due to ventricular "stiffness" and diastolic dysfunction. UA, umbilical artery; UV, umbilical vein.

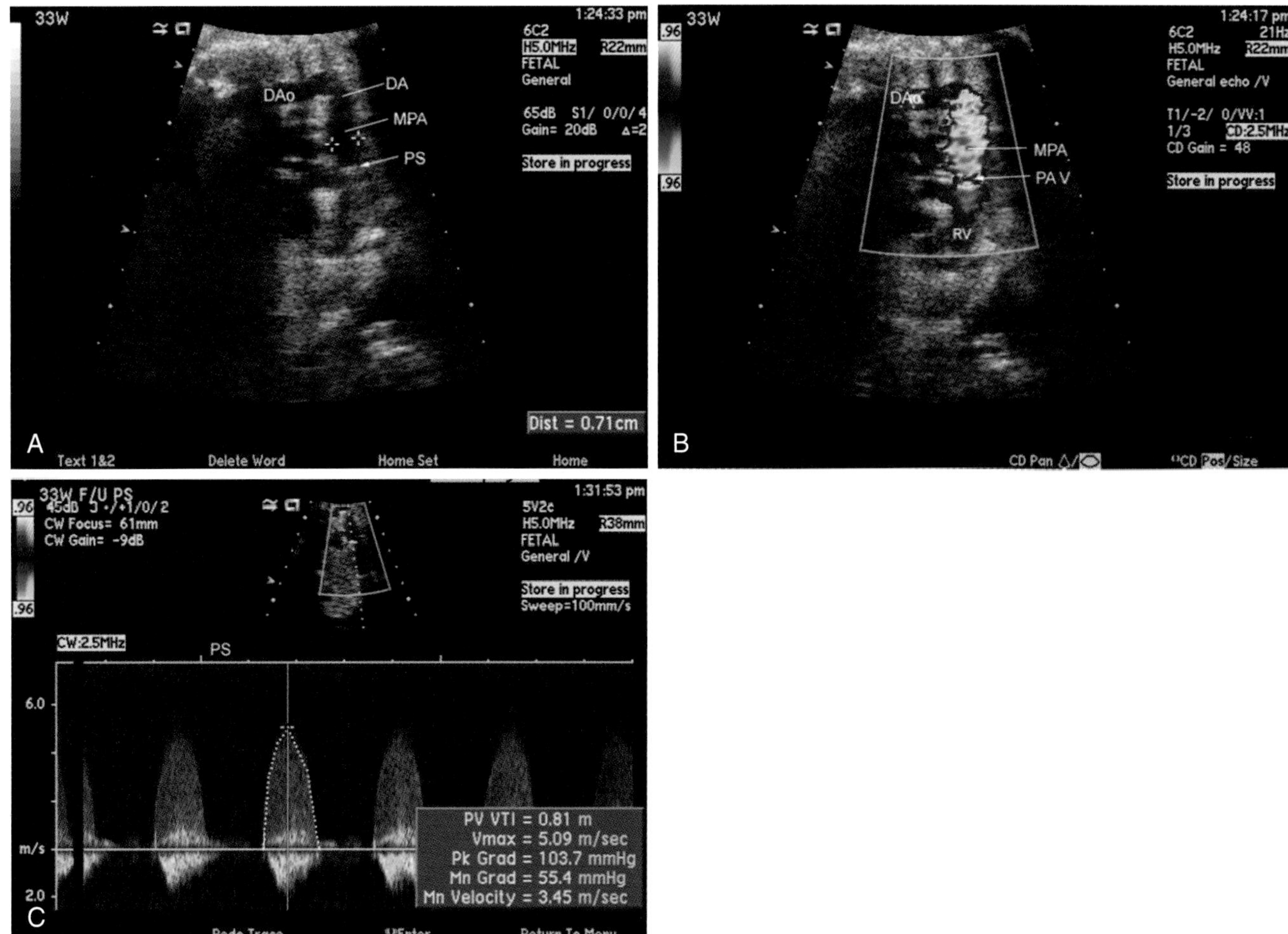

Case 38-3. **(A)** Recipient twin with TTTS who has developed valvar pulmonic stenosis (PS). A case of "acquired" congenital heart disease. DA, ductus arteriosus; DAo, descending aorta; MPA, main pulmonary artery. **(B)** Color flow imaging reveals turbulence of flow that starts at the level of the pulmonary valve (PAV) and is propagated into the main MPA and the DA. RV, right ventricle. **(C)** Pulse wave Doppler interrogation just above the pulmonic valve. Peak velocity is over 5 m/sec, with an estimate peak instantaneous gradient of over 100 mm Hg across the PAV.

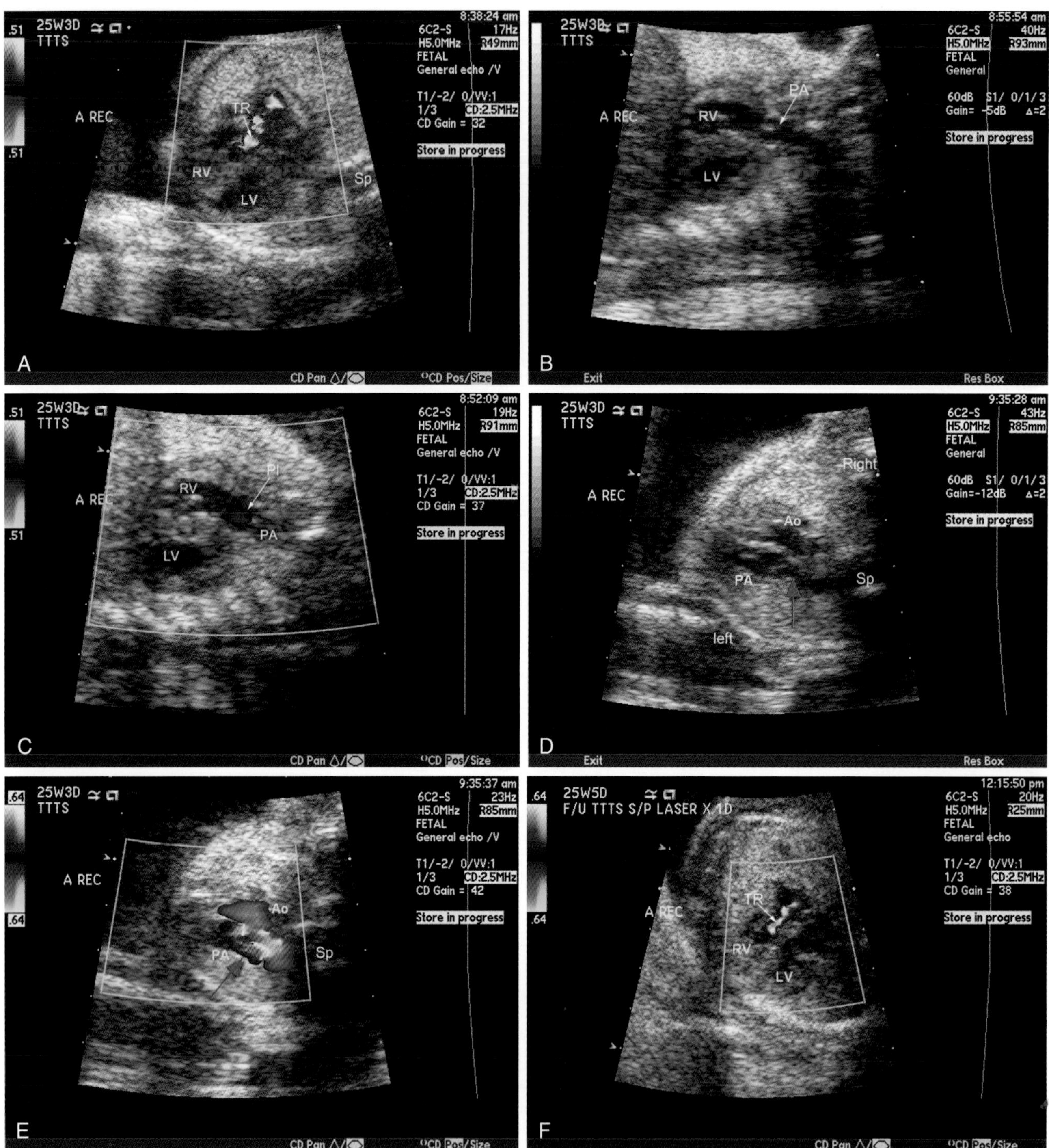

Case 38-4. **(A)** These images represent the serial findings in a recipient in whom there was reversal of "functional" pulmonary atresia after laser therapy. Significant tricuspid regurgitation (TR) is present. LV, left ventricle; RV, right ventricle; Sp, spine. **(B)** Pre-laser. In systole, the pulmonary valve did not appear to open and no antegrade flow was noted into the pulmonary artery (PA). **(C)** Pre-laser. In diastole, a red jet of pulmonary insufficiency (PI) is seen, demonstrating that the pulmonary valve is anatomically patent, but yet there is no antegrade flow across the valve in systole. This is "functional" pulmonary atresia. **(D)** Pre-laser. High mediastinal view with two-dimensional imaging demonstrates the aorta (Ao) and pulmonary artery (PA). The *arrow* points to the ductus arteriosus connection to the PA. **(E)** Pre-laser. High mediastinal view with color flow imaging. There is retrograde flow from the ductus arteriosus into the PA, confirming the absence of antegrade flow across the pulmonary valve. **(F)** One day after laser. The degree of TR has diminished.

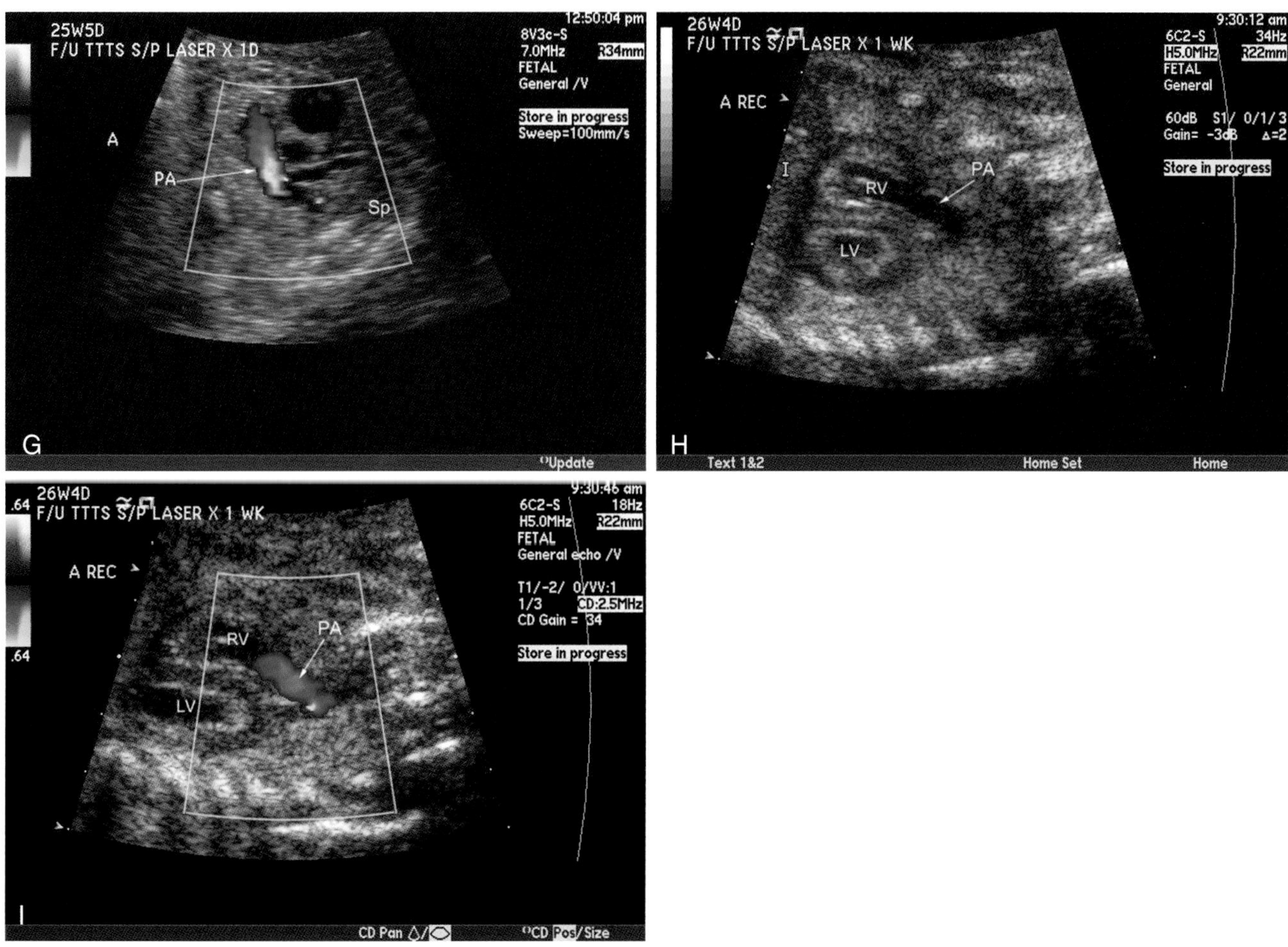

Case 38-4, cont'd (G) One day after laser. There is evidence for antegrade flow across the PA. (H) One week after laser. The pulmonary valve is now seen to open in systole. (I) One week after laser. Color flow imaging demonstrates unobstructed flow across the pulmonary valve into the PA. There is no longer any indication of "functional" pulmonary atresia.

39

Twin Reverse Arterial Perfusion

Donna A. Goff

Key Echocardiographic Features

- Presence of monochorionic pregnancy in which one twin has a primitive, ineffective heart.
- Direction of flow in the umbilical artery is from placenta to fetus in the acardiac-acephalic twin (twin reverse arterial perfusion).
- The normal "pump" twin can develop cardiomegaly, atrioventricular valve regurgitation, and signs of heart failure due to increased work and volume load.
- Serial assessment of combined cardiac output in the normal "pump" twin can be helpful in monitoring for increasing burden of cardiac work.

Anatomy and Anatomical Associations

Twin reversal arterial perfusion (TRAP) sequence is a rare anomaly that occurs in 1 in 35,000 pregnancies and in 1% of monochorionic twin pregnancies. In TRAP, there is a normal twin and one that is malformed without a functioning heart, each connected to the other through a common placenta, sharing vascular connections (Figure 39-1). The normal twin is called the *pump* twin and the affected one is the *acardiac* twin. The nonfunctional heart can range in spectrum from a rudimentary heart tube or markedly abnormal single ventricle that is beating to a complete lack of any cardiac structure. Because the affected twin has a nonfunctioning heart, the normal twin pumps blood through superficial arterial-arterial placental anastomoses to the affected twin. Deoxygenated blood from the affected or acardiac twin then returns to the placenta via its umbilical vein and through venous anastomoses traverses to the normal pump twin. As a result, the normal pump twin's heart experiences an increased cardiovascular workload, which can result in heart failure, hydrops, and death.[1]

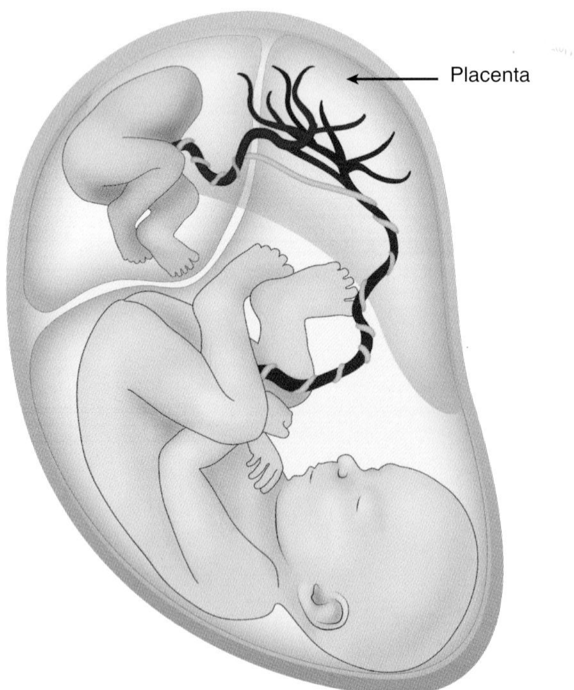

Figure 39-1. Twin reversed arterial perfusion (TRAP) sequence.

Although the pump twin is anatomically normal, a wide spectrum of anatomical pathology has been described in the acardiac twin from an amorphous mass of tissue to development of the semblance of a thorax and extremities and, occasionally, part of the cranium. There may be complete lack of cardiac structure (holocardius) to a malformed cardiac structure (hemicardius) with a heartbeat. The original classification for these developmental anomalies was based on examination of pathological specimens that lacked a cardiac structure (holocardius).[2] Four different categories were noted: (1) *acardius acephalus* is the most common form seen with a well-developed pelvis and lower extremities along with no head or skull, no thoracic organs, and often no arms, (2) *acardius anceps* has a well-developed body and extremities but only a partially formed head and face, (3) *acardius amorphous* is a shapeless mass with no recognizable organs, and (4) *acardius acormus,* which is the rarest, has development of only the head.[2,3] With the advent of ultrasound imaging, there is improvement in the understanding of the anatomical pathology of the acardiac twin. No abnormalities have been reported in the cardiac structure of the normal twin.[3,4]

Frequency, Genetics, and Development

Acardiac twinning is a rare anomaly that complicates 1% of monochorionic twin pregnancies and occasionally is observed in triplet or quadruplets. It is seen in 1 in 35,000 pregnancies overall.[2]

Because this is a rare pathology, most of the data in the literature are case reports.[5–9] Although it is clear that there are abnormal flow patterns as a result of superficial placental anastomoses between the normal and the malformed twin, it is unclear whether there is a primary developmental abnormality or that abnormal flow leads to abnormal cardiac morphogenesis.

In one of the largest cohorts studied, 46/49 (94%) cases were twin gestations with 2 cases occurring in triplet pregnancies and 1 in quadruplets.[4] In an analysis of 184 case reports of acardiac fetuses in the literature from 1960 to 1991, 92% were twins and 8% were triplets; 74% were monochorionic diamniotic with 24% monochorionic monoamniotic and 2% dichorionic diamniotic.[3] The acardiac fetus usually has a two-vessel cord (66%) and is most likely to develop structures that are supplied by lower aortic arteries. Of 33 acardiac fetuses that had karyotyping, 11 were abnormal (33%) consisting of monosomy, trisomy, deletions, mosaics, and polyploidy, whereas 3/34 pump fetuses were abnormal (trisomy). The only associated abnormalities are rare findings of omphalocele.[3]

Prenatal Physiology

In monochorionic pregnancies, placental vascular anastomoses normally occur between both fetuses. In pregnancies with an acardiac twin, there are abnormal superficial anastomoses both arterial and venous that allow the pump twin to supply blood for both fetuses. One of the most unique aspects of TRAP physiology is the retrograde perfusion of the acardiac twin via its umbilical artery, with hypoxic blood preferentially perfusing the caudal structures of the twin. Return of flow to the placenta is via the umbilical vein, the opposite direction of what is seen in the normal. This blood then traverses through the venous anastomoses to the pump twin. The pump twin's heart experiences an increased workload secondary to pumping blood retrograde to the acardiac twin while also receiving additional deoxygenated blood from the placenta. As a result, the pump twin over time can develop congestive heart failure (CHF).[1]

One report in the literature is of interest because it describes the natural progression of disease. A case of acardiac twins was followed with sequential ultrasounds from initial diagnosis at 16 weeks. The fetal echocardiogram at 30 weeks demonstrated only right and left ventricular hypertrophy. A subsequent echocardiogram 5 days later demonstrated right atrial dilation and mild tricuspid regurgitation with marked progression of these findings only a few days later leading to delivery of the fetus, suggesting the potential for rapid onset of cardiovascular deterioration. A postnatal echocardiogram, following removal of the volume load, showed resolution of the previous abnormalities.[10]

Prenatal Management

Predictors of poor outcome in acardiac twin pregnancies include greater than 50% ratio between the acardiac/pump twin's weights, polyhydramnios and CHF in the normal twin. Without intervention, mortality has been reported as high as 50% to 75%.[3,4] Many fetal therapies have been proposed including cord occlusion. Radiofrequency ablation and[11] laser coagulation of the acardiac twin's umbilical cord and laser coagulation of placental anastomoses[12] are a few techniques used.

Postnatal Physiology

In the current era, pregnancies with TRAP that are at risk for hemodynamic compromise of the pump (normal) twin have fetal intervention performed, whereas others have expectant management. In some cases, after intervention, there may be preterm delivery, which must be considered in the decision making. If the pump twin has inadequate time for cardiovascular function to improve, the neonate may present with low cardiac output requiring inotropic support. Otherwise, normal physiology for preterm or term neonates is expected.

Postnatal Management

Pump twins that have cardiovascular compromise and are delivered early should be assessed clinically for low cardiac output secondary to cardiac dysfunction and treated with inotropes and afterload reduction to improve perfusion. A postnatal echocardiogram should be performed to evaluate for systolic and diastolic function.

Outcomes

Limited data are available regarding predictors of outcome. In a study of 49 acardiac twin pregnancies, the acardiac/pump twin body size ratio that was determined postnatally was used to predict outcomes. If the body size ratio was greater than 70%, the incidence of preterm delivery was 90%, polyhydramnios was present in 40%, and CHF in the normal twin was seen in 30%. When the body size ratio was less than 70%, the incidence of preterm delivery was 75%, polyhydramnios was present in 30%, and CHF was seen in only 10%. If the acardiac/pump twin size ratio was less than 50%, outcomes were better with the incidence of preterm delivery of 35%, polyhydramnios 18%, and CHF 0%.[4] Although the weights were determined postnatally, this ratio of less than 50% is used by some as an indication for intervention in the current era.

Limited studies have assessed whether echocardiographic data can predict adverse outcomes. Umbilical artery resistance indexes of the acardiac twin were compared with the normal twin in six acardiac twin pregnancies. Those pregnancies with poorer outcome had a smaller difference between resistive indexes, but these data did not reach statistical significance.[13] In 10 acardiac twin cases, adverse outcomes (cardiac failure, delivery before 30 weeks, death) were associated with lower umbilical artery pulsatility index (PI) in the acardiac twin, increased left ventricular shortening fraction (LVSF) in the pump twin during the second trimester and rapidly growing acardiac mass. All these variables are associated with increase cardiovascular workload in the fetus.[14]

In order to improve identification of acardiac twins that may have adverse outcomes, a classification system was developed based on the ratio of size of acardiac to size of pump twin along with echocardiographic determinants of the pump twin's cardiovascular status. Based on the acardiac-to-pump twin size ratio, the twins were divided into type I for a ratio of less than 50% and type II for greater than 50%. The groups were then further subdivided by the presence of cardiovascular compromise in the pump twin determined by a variety of ultrasound characteristics including moderate to severe polyhydramnios, cardiomegaly, or pericardial effusion or abnormal Doppler signals, specifically tricuspid regurgitation, reverse flow in the ductus venosus, umbilical vein pulsation, or increased middle cerebral artery pulsation. Intervention was suggested for those with body size ratios greater than 50% and data suggesting cardiovascular compromise of the pump twin. This classification, however, has not been validated with outcomes.[1]

Multiple techniques involving umbilical cord occlusion such as ligating the cord, ligation and transection of the cord, photocoagulation, or radiofrequency ablation have been evaluated. Because the cohorts are small, it has been difficult to ascertain differences between various techniques of umbilical cord occlusion.

In one TRAP cohort of 74 patients, there were 64 surgical candidates with 51 patients undergoing a variety of umbilical cord occlusion techniques and 14 patients followed by expectant management. The criteria for undergoing umbilical cord occlusion were abdominal circumference of the acardiac fetus that was more than or equal to that of the pump twin, polyhydramnios (maximum vertical pocket ≥8 cm), abnormal Doppler studies or hydrops of pump twin, or monoamniotic twins. Perinatal survival in the interventional group was significantly improved with 78.5% survival (22/28) if the dividing membrane was not disrupted. Preterm delivery was common, with an average gestational age of 30 weeks.[12]

Outcomes after radiofrequency ablation in 27 monochorionic-diamniotic pregnancies (one of these was a triplet pregnancy) and 2 monochorionic-monoamniotic pregnancies demonstrates an overall survival of 86% (25/29) with mean gestation of 34.6 weeks at delivery. Evaluating only the monochorionic-diamniotic twin pregnancies, there is a 92% (24/26) survival.[11]

Currently, there are no published data on the long-term outcomes of survivors of the TRAP sequence. One important question is whether the normal twin is at increased risk for neurological sequelae, perhaps similar to that which has been described after intervention for twin-twin transfusion syndrome.[15] In the TRAP cohort described previously neurological complications, specifically grade III intraventricular hemorrhage and posthemorrhage hydrocephalus, were noted in the neonatal period in 2/51 patients in the intervention group.[12] It is unclear whether there are more subtle findings that may become apparent with long-term follow-up. As appropriate identification and improved fetal management for TRAP take place in the coming years, there will be further opportunity to evaluate the long-term outcome of this unique disorder.

Imaging Essentials and Important Points

- Sampling in the umbilical cord of both twins will demonstrate the unusual flow patterns in the acardiac twin. There will be retrograde flow from the placenta to the affected twin.
- In the acardiac twin, it is sometimes possible to identify a very rudimentary, primitive heart mass with an atrium and ventricle delivering blood into the aorta. Flow in the aortic arch is retrograde from abdomen and umbilical artery insertion, cephalad toward the heart.
- Assessment of the pump twin should involve analysis of measures that reflect undue cardiovascular burden. The following parameters are helpful:
  - An important parameter we have found very useful is a Doppler-derived estimate of combined cardiac output. Because this is essentially a disorder of high-output failure, similar to an arteriovenous malformation, serial combined cardiac output measures can be helpful in heralding heart failure.
  - Heart size and degree of cardiomegaly.
  - Tricuspid and mitral valve regurgitation.
  - Systolic function, based on qualitative assessment of wall motion.
  - Diastolic function as determined by Doppler flow patterns in the ductus venosus and umbilical vein.
  - Presence or absence of polyhydramnios, pericardial effusion, or hydrops.

References

1. Wong AE, Sepulveda W. Acardiac anomaly: current issues in prenatal assessment and treatment. *Prenat Diagn*. 2005;25:796-806.
2. Napolitani FD, Schreiber I. The acardiac monster: a review of the world literature and presentation of 2 cases. *Am J Obstet Gynecol*. 1960;80:582-589.
3. Healey MG. Acardia—predictive risk-factors for the co-twins survival. *Teratology*. 1994;50:205-213.
4. Moore TR, Gale S, Benirschke K. Perinatal outcome of 49 pregnancies complicated by acardiac twinning. *Am J Obstet Gynecol*. 1990; 163:907-912.
5. Driggers RW, Blakemore KJ, Bird C, et al. Pathogenesis of acardiac twinning: clues from an almost acardiac twin. *Fetal Diagn Ther*. 2002;17:185-187.
6. Ersch J, Stallmach T. Cardiac regression sequence: reversal of blood flow is diagnostic but not causative in an acardiac fetus. *Early Hum Dev*. 1998;52:81-85.
7. Kamitomo M, Kouno S, Ibuka K, et al. First-trimester findings associated with twin reversed arterial perfusion sequence. *Fetal Diagn Ther*. 2004;19:187-190.
8. Malhotra N, Sinha A, Deka D, et al. Twin reversed arterial perfusion: report of four cases. *J Clin Ultrasound*. 2004;32:411-414.
9. Mohanty C, Mishra OP, Singh CP, et al. Acardiac anomaly spectrum. *Teratology*. 2000;62:356-359.

10. Osborn P, Gross TL, Shah JJ, et al. Prenatal diagnosis of fetal heart failure in twin reversed arterial perfusion syndrome. *Prenat Diagn.* 2000;20:615-617.
11. Lee H, Wagner AJ, Sy E, et al. Efficacy of radiofrequency ablation for twin-reversed arterial perfusion sequence. *Am J Obstet Gynecol.* 2007;196:459.
12. Quintero RA, Chmait RH, Murakoshi T, et al. Surgical management of twin reversed arterial perfusion sequence. *Am J Obstet Gynecol.* 2006;194:982-991.
13. Dashe JS, Fernandez CO, Twickler DM. Utility of Doppler velocimetry in predicting outcome in twin reversed-arterial perfusion sequence. *Am J Obstet Gynecol.* 2001;185:135-139.
14. Brassard M, Fouron JC, Leduc L, et al. Prognostic markers in twin pregnancies with an acardiac fetus. *Obstet Gynecol.* 1999;94:409-414.
15. Rossi AC, D'Addario V. Laser therapy and serial amnioreduction as treatment for twin-twin transfusion syndrome: a meta-analysis and review of literature. *Am J Obstet Gynecol.* 2008;198:147-152.

CASES

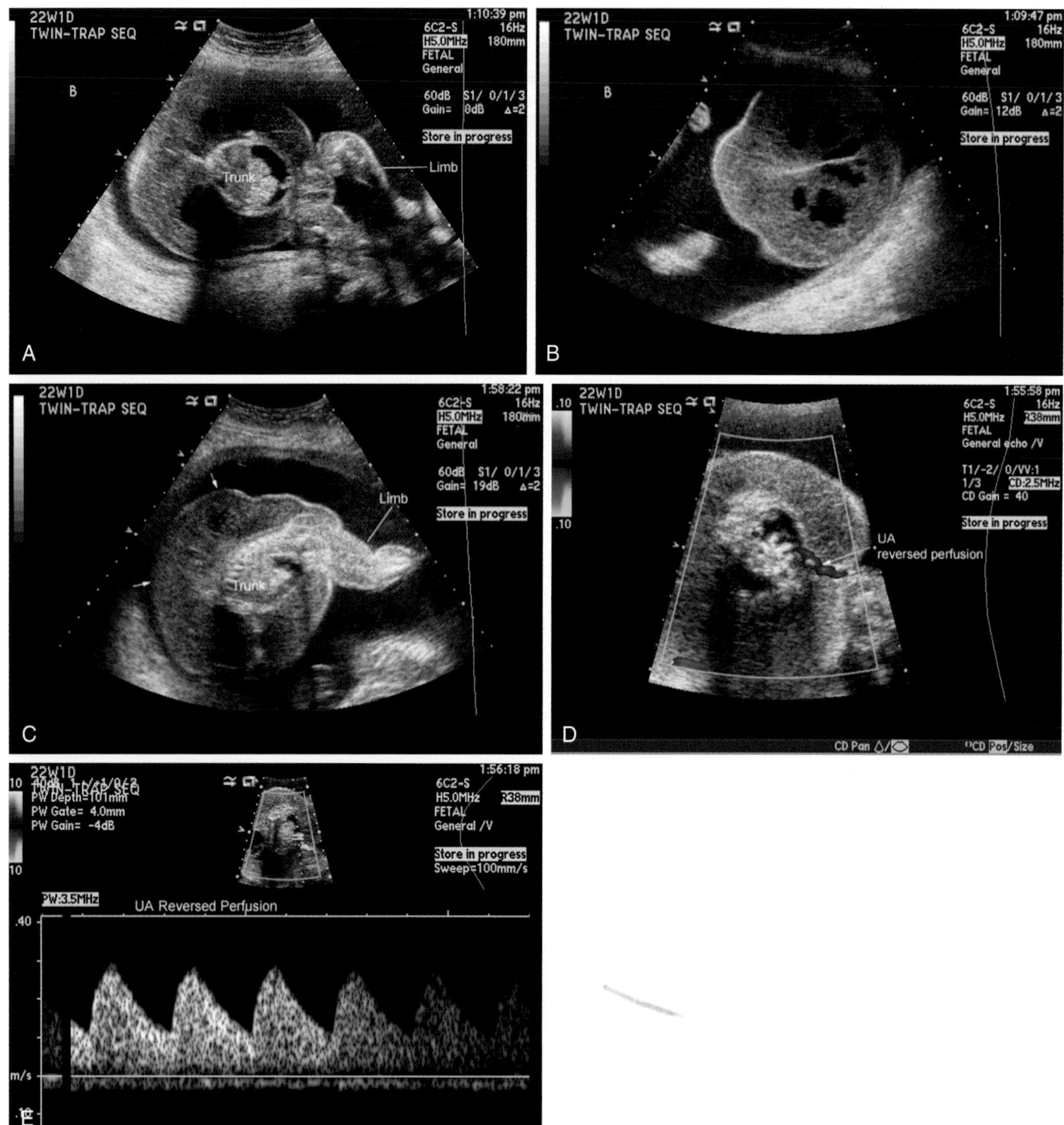

Case 39-1. **(A)** A case of twin reversed arterial perfusion (TRAP) sequence at 22 weeks' gestation shows the acardiac-acephalic twin. Note the relatively well developed lower limbs. The trunk consists of a central "coelomic" type cavity with no well-defined cardiac structure. Spongy fluid-filled tissue surrounds the trunk cavity. **(B)** The "caput" region of the acardiac-acephalic mass demonstrates primitive brain ventricles; however, there is no well-defined head or brain tissue and no distinction of a headlike structure from the trunk. **(C)** Long-axis view of the body of the acephalic-acardiac twin. The spine is seen as well as a lower limb. Note the substantial edematous *(arrows)* tissue above the spine. **(D)** The umbilical artery is the "feeder" artery perfusing the tissue of this twin. Perfusion is retrograde from placenta to fetus and is driven by pulsatile flow from the "pump" twin. UA, umbilical artery. **(E)** Pulsatile UA flow from the normal twin to the body of the acephalic-acardiac twin through the shared placenta.

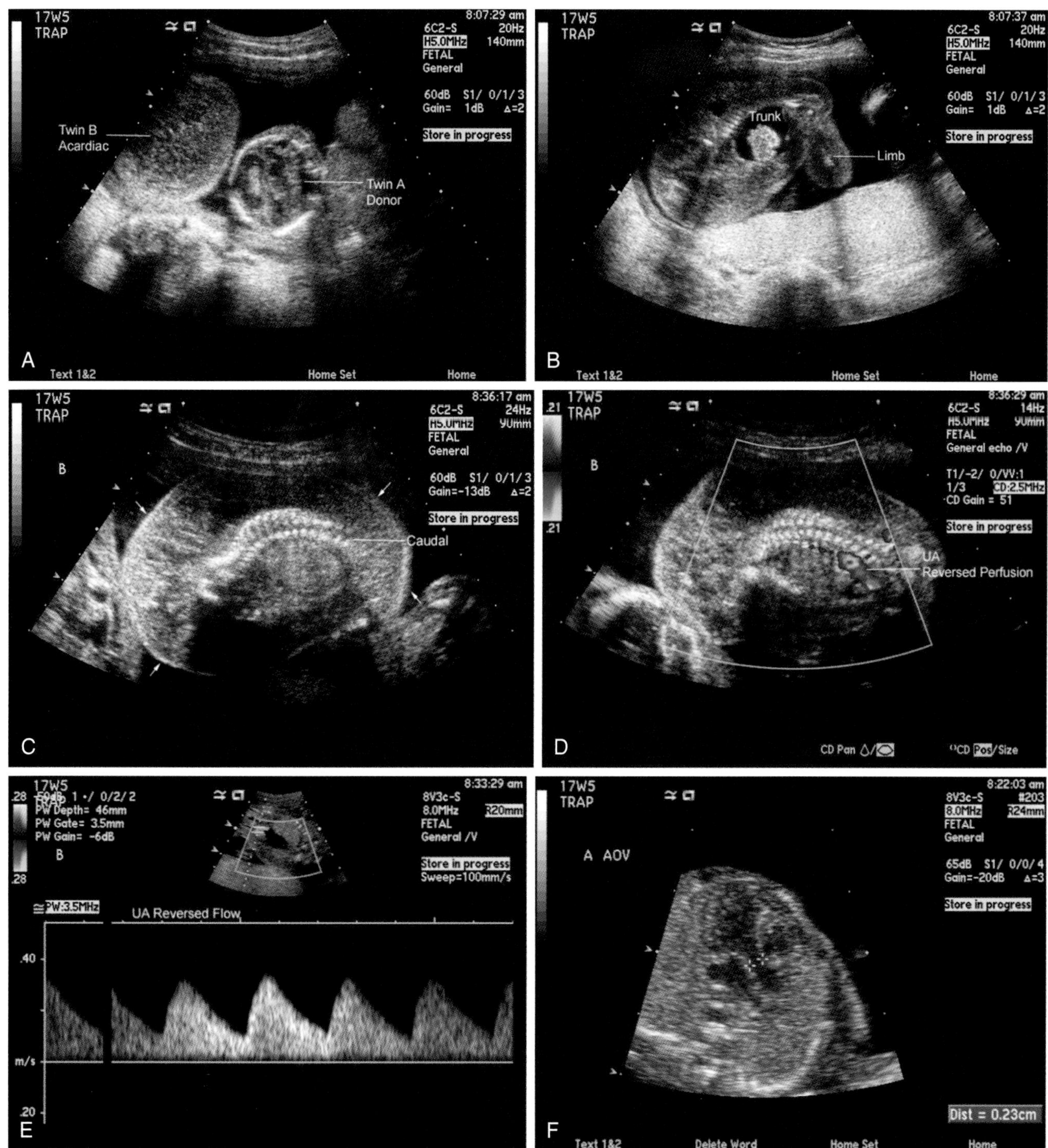

Case 39-2. **(A)** A case of TRAP at 17 weeks and 5 days' gestation. Note the normal contours of the head of the "pump" twin and the abnormal large "caput" of the acardiac twin. **(B)** Acardiac twin with a primitive cardiac mass located within a fluid-filled cavity. There is no cardiac pulsatile activity. The fetal tissues are solely dependent upon perfusion from the partner "pump" twin. **(C)** Edematous spongy tissue *(arrows)* surrounds the spine and body of this acardiac-acephalic twin. **(D)** Reversed flow retrograde from the umbilical artery (UA) to the descending aorta. **(E)** Doppler sampling of the umbilical artery demonstrates reversal of flow from placenta to the fetus. **(F)** Imaging of the "pump" twin with normal anatomy that is tasked with the burden of perfusing the acephalic-acardiac twin. Cardiac output for this twin can be markedly elevated. We routinely estimate cardiac output in a serial manner in these fetuses as a means of assessing wellness. Aortic annulus diameter is measured. AOV, aortic valve.

Continued

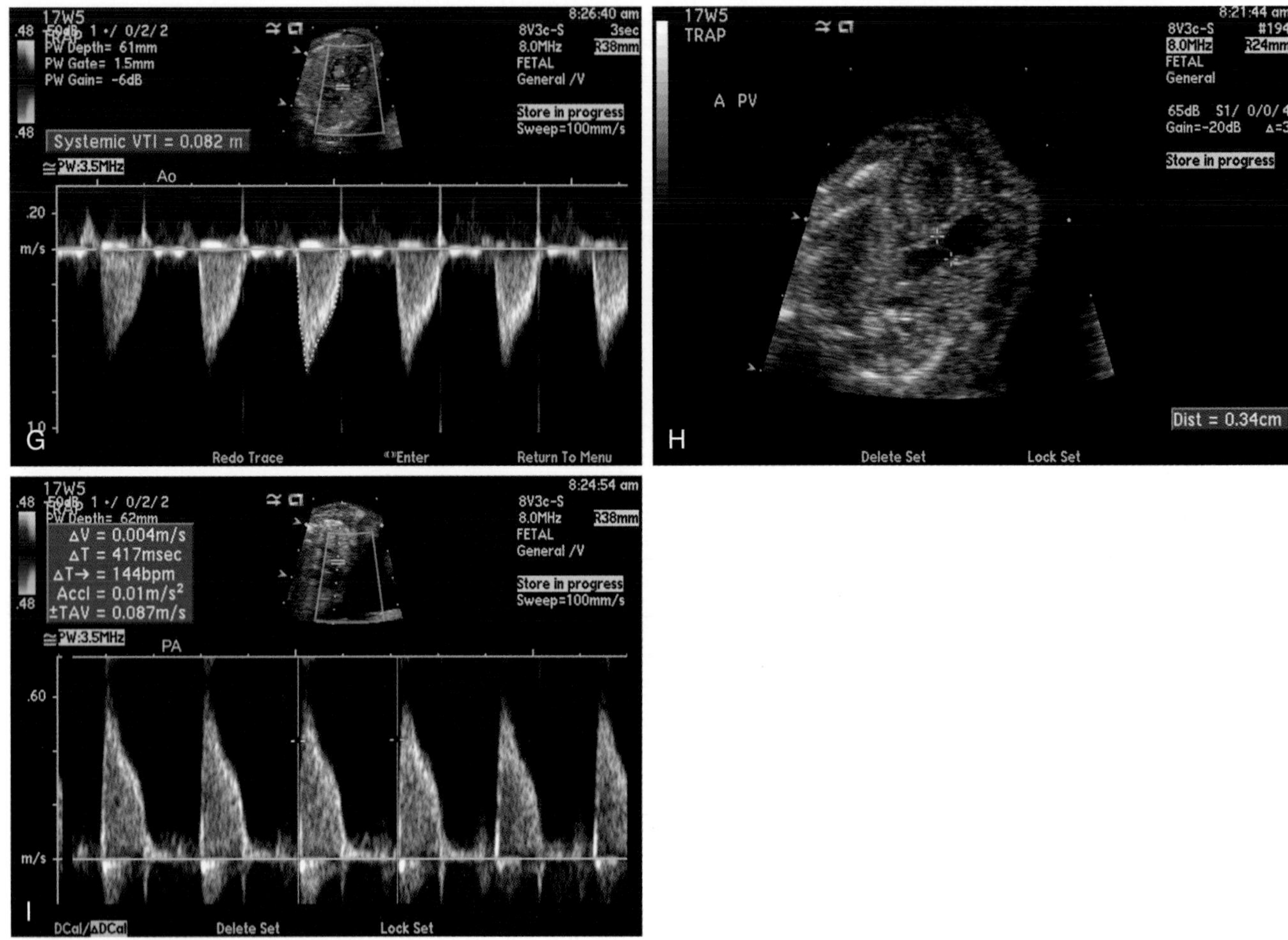

Case 39-2, cont'd **(G)** Doppler sampling at the level of the AOV. The velocity-time integral is obtained by tracing the waveform. This is used to calculate left-sided cardiac output. **(H)** Pulmonary annulus diameter is measured. PV, pulmonary valve. **(I)** Doppler sampling at the level of the PV. Velocity-time integral is obtained by tracing the waveform, and heart rate can be obtained. In this case, the combined right- and left-sided cardiac output was moderately elevated at 600 ml/kg/min. PA, pulmonary annulus.

40

Sacrococcygeal Teratoma

Jack Rychik

Key Echocardiographic Features

- Look for signs of fetal hydrops such as pericardial effusion, pleural effusion, ascites, or scalp edema.
- Assess heart size through cardiothoracic ratio measures.
- Evaluate ventricular systolic function.
- Assess size of the inferior vena cava (which may enlarge due to lower body increased venous return).
- Evaluate for tricuspid and mitral valve regurgitation.
- Assess umbilical arterial Doppler flow pattern, with particular attention to the diastolic component.
- Evaluate ductus venosus flow pattern.
- Evaluate umbilical venous flow pattern.
- Calculate the combined cardiac output measures and follow serially at regular intervals.

Anatomy, Frequency, and Development

Sacrococcygeal teratoma (SCT) is a tumor originating from the sacral-coccygeal region of the body. It is defined as a neoplasm composed of all three primordial tissue germ layers or a neoplasm formed from multiple tissues that are foreign to that part of the body, lacking in any organ specificity.[1] SCT is believed to arise from totipotent somatic cells in the caudal region of the developing embryo, which in some manner, escape the normal inductive influences of controlled differentiation and evolve into a growing mass of tissue. These tumors can grow wildly into enormously large structures with potential for invasion into the pelvic and abdominal cavities.[2]

Although rare, SCT is the most common tumor seen in the fetus and neonate. The reported incidence is 1 in 35,000 to 40,000 live births. The natural history of prenatally diagnosed SCT differs from that of postnatally diagnosed SCT. Malignant degeneration is the primary cause of death in the postnatal SCT, which is a rare phenomenon in the fetus. The high mortality rate of fetal SCT is attributed to the effects of tumor mass on dystocia, preterm labor due to secondary polyhydramnios, and fetal hydrops and placentomegaly related to the cardiovascular effects of high-output failure.[2–4] There are also reports of spontaneous rupture or hemorrhage with subsequent fetal anemia.[5]

Prenatal Physiology and Diagnosis

SCT can grow substantially and achieve a massive size (Figure 40-1). The impact of SCT on the fetal cardiovascular system is due to the highly vascularized nature of the tumor. As the tumor grows, so does its vascular supply. In addition, the tumor mass itself can be inherently highly vascularized with multiple arterial to venous connections, effectively creating a giant arteriovenous malformation (AVM).

Fetal SCT influences prenatal cardiovascular physiology in a number of ways.[6] Perfusion of the vascularized mass results in an increase in total fetal circulating blood volume and increased preload to the heart. The heart accommodates the volume load by compensatory dilation and increase in myocardial mass. Furthermore, the SCT mass can act as a low vascular resistance "sink." Because the arterial blood supply originates from the iliac region of the descending aorta, the SCT may compete with blood flow to the placenta. Placental vascular resistance is normally very low; however, if the SCT mass is large and highly vascularized, its resistance may be lower than that of the placenta, creating a "steal" phenomenon, shunting blood away from the placenta.

Overall, the deleterious impact of SCT is in creating a state of high-output heart failure, because the fetal heart tries to compensate for the massively increased volume load. Ventricular dilation can lead to atrioventricular annular dilation and induce atrioventricular valve regurgitation, further exacerbating the volume load. As the heart fails, atrial pressures rise and hydrops ensues. When present, hydrops in a fetus with SCT typically leads to in utero demise, unless prenatal intervention is undertaken.

SCT size and makeup can be assessed by ultrasound and magnetic resonance imaging techniques (Figure 40-2). Large tumors may consist mostly of cystic structures, which may have little vascularization or the degree of vascularization may be quite high, heralding the possibility of high-output heart failure.

Fetal echocardiography plays a key role in the evaluation and serial surveillance of the fetus with SCT.[7] Heart size should be assessed by measurement of cardiothoracic ratio. Overall ventricular systolic function should be noted. Inferior vena cava dilation is common, because lower body venous return is increased. Flow patterns in the ductus venosus and umbilical vein may reflect increased atrial pressure and worsening heart failure. Doppler evaluation of the umbilical artery will reveal a decrease in diastolic flow, or perhaps even reversal of flow, if there is a substantial competitive steal away from the placenta into the SCT.[8] Because the essence of the pathophysiology of SCT relates to high-output failure, Doppler derived measures of cardiac output are very important.[9,10] By measuring the diameter across the aortic and pulmonary valves and sampling blood flow using

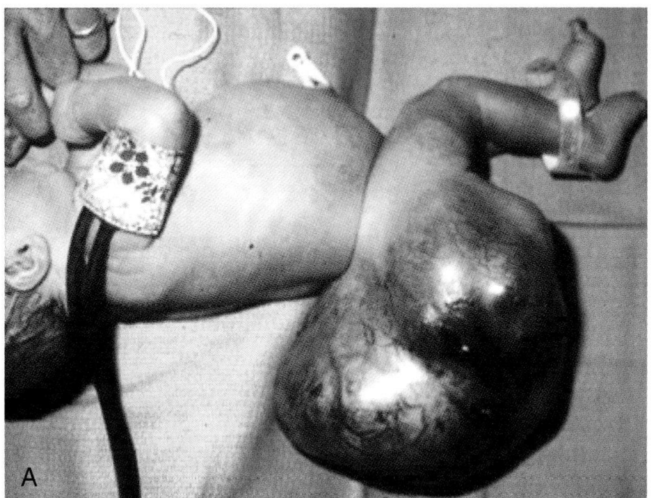

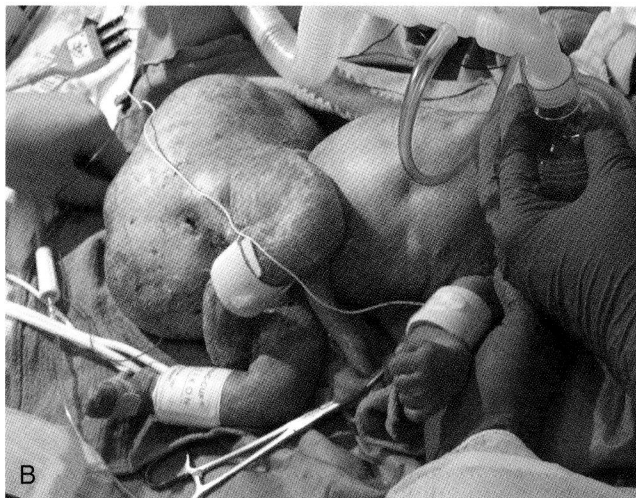

Figure 40-1. (A) Newborn with large sacrococcygeal teratoma (SCT). Note the areas of hemorrhage and infarction in the mass. (B) Newborn with large SCT moments after birth in the delivery room.

Doppler interrogation, one may calculate the individual ventricular and combined cardiac outputs by the formula: cardiac output = valvar cross-sectional area (3.14 × radius^2) × velocity-time integral of flow across the valve × heart rate. Indexed combined cardiac output in the normal fetus is relatively stable throughout gestation and is approximately 400 to 500 mL/min/kg.

In a series of fetuses with SCT and potential for high-output failure, we evaluated combined cardiac output measures and found that most fetuses tolerate increased combined cardiac output to levels that approach 750 to 800 mL/min/kg, nearly twice the normal. When values much above 800 mL/min/kg are reached, the likelihood of cardiovascular instability, heart failure, and hydrops increases (Figure 40-3). Serial evaluation of fetal echocardiographic parameters is part of a sound protocol for monitoring the fetus with SCT and determining the need for fetal intervention.

Prenatal Management

A number of therapies are available for treating SCT in the fetus. Amnioreduction in cases of polyhydramnios may improve maternal comfort and prevent premature labor. If the mass consists of sizable cystic structures, the tumor size can be reduced through cyst aspiration.[11] Percutaneous laparoscopic laser ablation and interruption of vascular supply to the SCT is feasible.[12,13] Alcohol sclerosis of the tumor mass has also been reported.[3]

Surgical debulking through the techniques of open fetal surgery is one possible form of therapy.[14,15] Fetal surgery for this anomaly is indicated only if the life of the fetus is threatened by the tumor and other options are not available. We performed fetal surgery in a series of four fetuses with giant SCT and evidence of high output failure at 21 to 26 weeks' gestation. The procedure included hysterotomy with manipulation of the fetus to bring the SCT up to the uterine incision for removal (Figure 40-4). Continuous intraoperative fetal echocardiography was performed to monitor the cardiovascular system during these procedures.[16] Figure 40-5 shows the Doppler-derived values for combined cardiac output before surgery (time #1) and at induction of anesthesia (time #2), after SCT removal (time #3), and after surgery (time #4). Before surgery, the mean combined cardiac output was markedly elevated at over 800 mL/kg/min. With induction of anesthesia for the surgery, there was a slight decrease in combined cardiac output likely related to the depressive effect of the agents administered; however, values still remained abnormally high. Immediately after removal of the mass, there was a dramatic drop in cardiac output to levels below normal, which persisted into the postoperative period.

Surgical removal of an SCT results in dramatic changes in cardiovascular physiology. The impetus for increased preload is suddenly removed from a heart that has been chronically volume loaded. In addition, the removal of the SCT eliminates a low vascular resistance circuit, resulting in an overall increase in afterload. The sudden imposition of increased afterload and acute removal of preload on an already fragile and unstable fetal heart can result in significant dysfunction. As myocardial mass is increased to match the chronic volume load, acute removal of the volume load leads to a mismatch between mass and volume, creating the echocardiographic image of a thickened, relatively hypertrophied heart.[16] This phenomenon results in diastolic dysfunction with difficulty in filling the heart and can complicate fetal surgery for this lesion. Of our four fetuses, three survived fetal surgery and one died a few days after birth due to this phenomenon with a very hypertrophied, stiff heart (Figure 40-6).

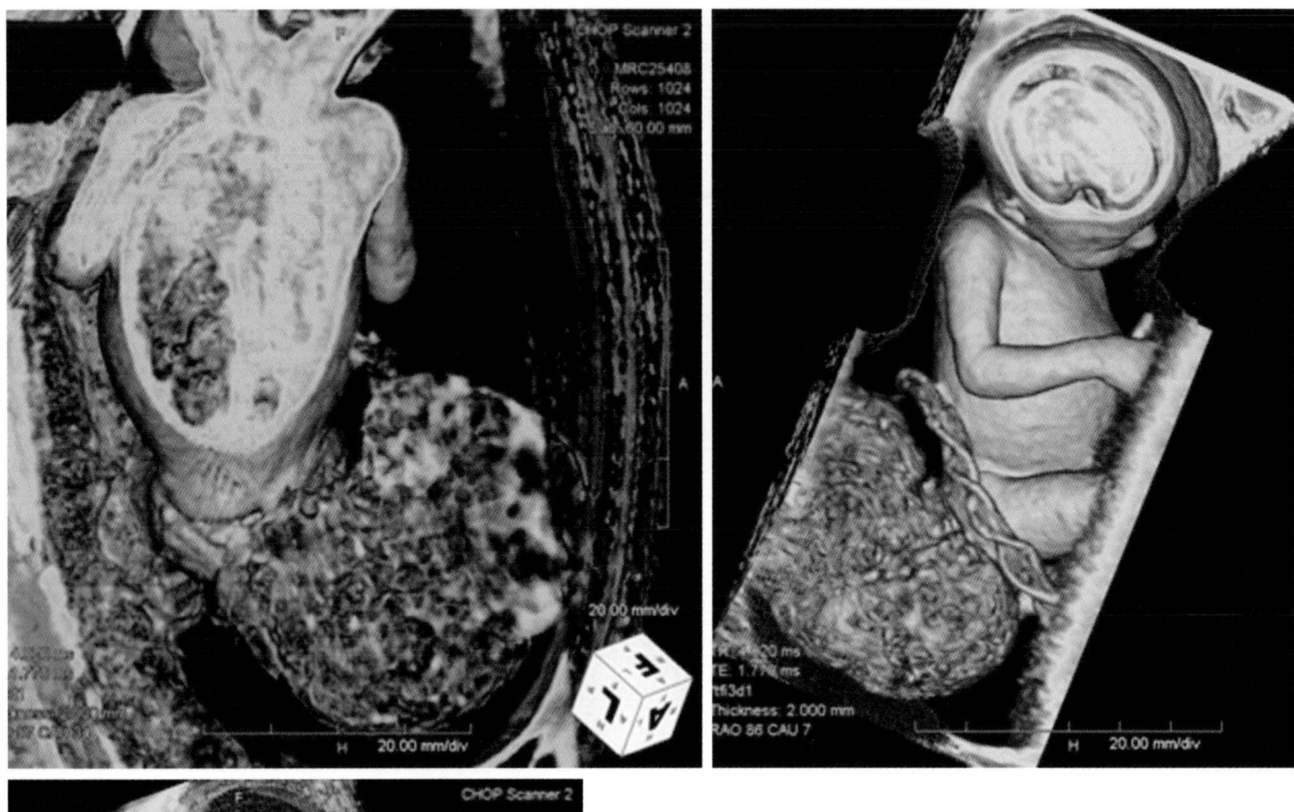

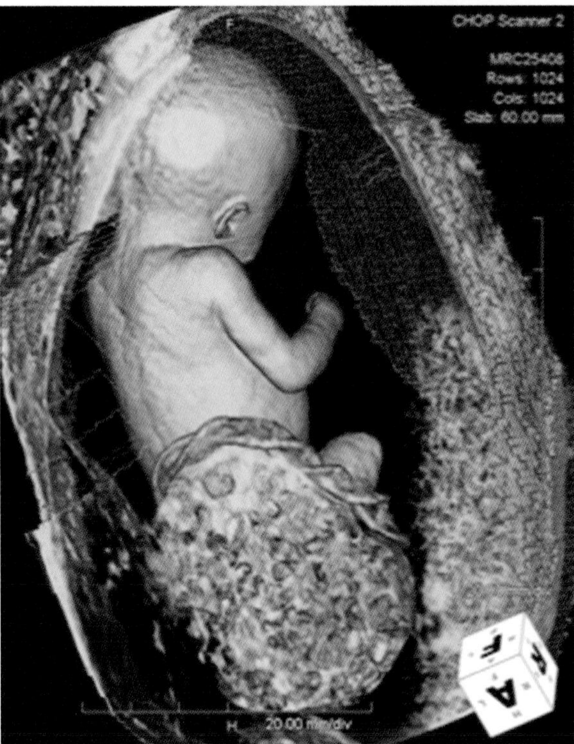

Figure 40-2. Magnetic resonance imaging can provide detailed prenatal information on the size, location, and extent of the tumor in relation to the spine and lower pelvic structures.

Postnatal Physiology, Management, and Outcome

Decision making for the fetus with giant SCT must strike a balance between the high-risk procedures of fetal intervention and the risk of non-intervention and ongoing heart failure, which may lead to fetal demise. Beyond 26 weeks' gestation, it is our view that delivery and postnatal care will likely offer a better chance for successful outcome in the ill fetus with SCT. Such infants may need to battle issues of prematurity; however, early delivery offers the opportunity for medical management of high-output

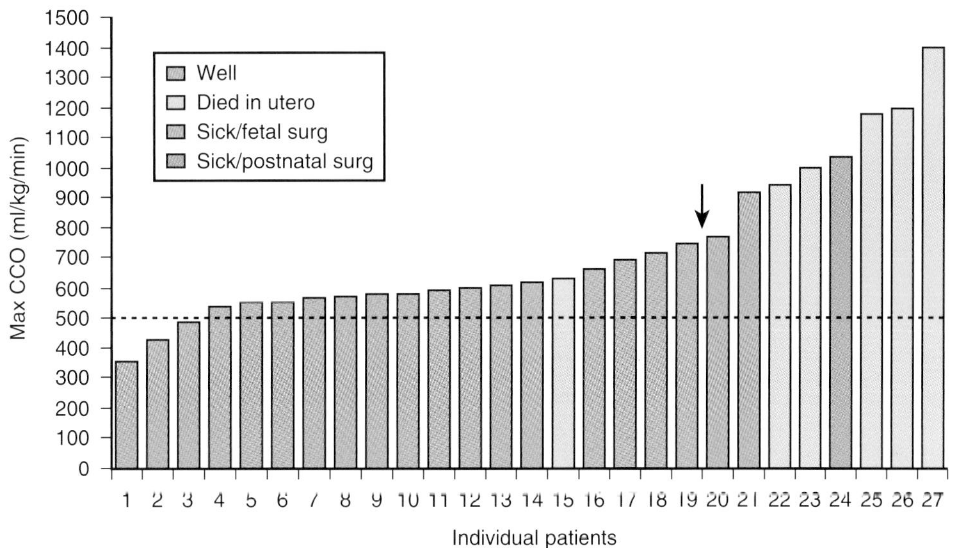

Figure 40-3. Bar graph of a series of 27 fetuses with SCT and their maximum calculated combined cardiac output (Max CCO). Subjects in *purple* are all fetuses who tolerated the SCT well without any hemodynamic compromise. In *green* are those who died in utero; in *orange*, those who underwent fetal surgical resection; and in *blue*, one subject who was delivered early and underwent urgent postnatal surgery. The *dashed line* designates the expected normal combined cardiac output of approximately 500 mL/kg/min. Most fetuses did well up until approximately 750 mL/kg/min, when either intervention or demise took place. There is one outlier case (Patient #15) who had only a moderately elevated CCO of over 600 mL/kg/min. At evaluation, this fetus also had reversal of diastolic flow upon Doppler assessment of the umbilical artery indicating a blood flow "steal" from the placenta into the SCT mass. Upon follow-up evaluation 1 week later, fetal demise was identified. The vascular steal away from the placenta likely resulted in anoxia. Hence, fetuses with CCO greater than 750 mL/kg/min or those with absent or reversed end-diastolic umbilical artery flow are at greatest risk.

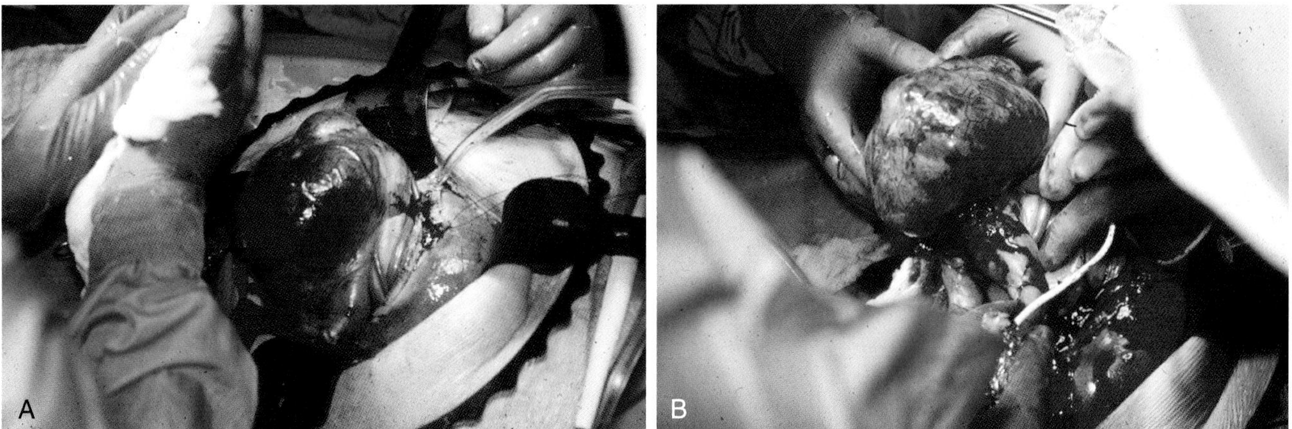

Figure 40-4. (A) Open fetal surgery for resection of a giant SCT. Through the hysterotomy, the mass and lower extremity are exposed, but the remainder of the fetal body remains in the uterus. (B) The mass is dissected and mobilized and the vascular supply is ligated as the teratoma is removed.

failure that cannot be effectively provided while in utero. Inotropic therapy and afterload reduction will help the volume-overloaded heart. Blood transfusion will optimize oxygen delivery. Such therapy will offer the opportunity to improve hemodynamics and optimize the neonatal condition for surgical resection.

Outcome for fetal SCT depends upon the degree of cardiovascular instability before birth. Those with high-output failure and hydrops do poorly; however, fetal therapy does offer hope for some. In a single large series of 39 fetuses with SCT, 12 had hydrops and underwent fetal intervention (not open surgery) and 17 did not have hydrops.[3] Of the 12 with hydrops, 3 died in utero and 3 died early in the neonatal period, providing 50% long-term survival. Median age at delivery was 33 weeks (range 27–37 wk). In the group without hydrops, 1 died of cardiovascular complications on day 1 of life, with 16 long-term survivors. Median age of delivery for these was 38 weeks (26–40 wk). Although outcome is clearly worse for those with hydrops, it is safe to say that perhaps all would

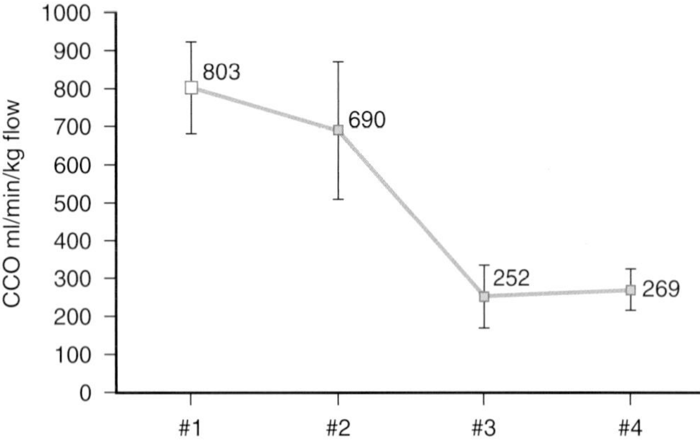

Figure 40-5. Graph of average combined cardiac output (CCO) for four patients who underwent fetal surgery for resection of SCT. Time #1 is before surgery; time #2 is with induction of anesthesia; time #3 is immediately after SCT removal; and time #4 is after surgery. Note the dramatic decrease in CCO after resection, from an exorbitantly high value (>800 mL/kg/min) to a level that is below expected normal (252 mL/kg/min). Acute volume removal after SCT resection influences cardiovascular function by severely reducing chronic preload and increasing afterload (removal of the low vascular resistance of the mass increases afterload on the heart).

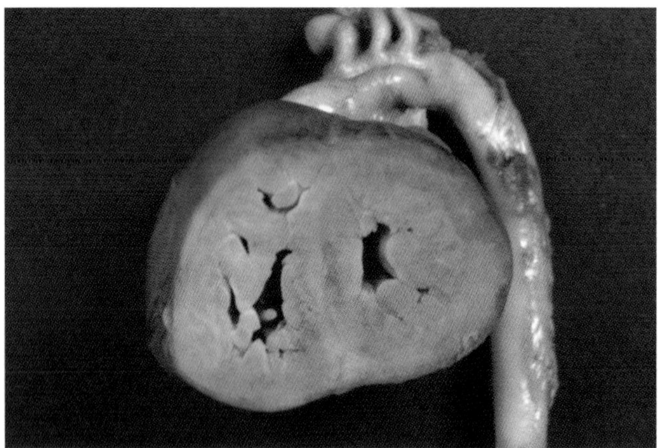

Figure 40-6. Autopsy appearance of a heart in a fetus that underwent SCT resection. Note the marked hypertrophy and small cavity volumes. The heart incurred a chronic volume load with increased compensatory hypertrophy. After acute removal of preload, hypertrophy remained, leading to a mismatch in mass to volume.

have died without fetal therapy. Further work is necessary to identify the optimal timing and type of therapy, which can best be tailored to specific characteristics in the fetus with SCT. Long-term functional outcome after resection of SCT can be problematic. In a questionnaire provided to survivors of surgical resection of SCT at a median age of 10 years of age, 46% reported impaired bowel function or urinary incontinence and 40% found the scar to be unacceptable, affecting their quality of life.[17] A small risk for recurrence of teratoma after resection exists.[18]

Imaging Essentials and Important Points

- Serial evaluation is key in the management of fetal SCT.
- Depending upon the degree of illness, we monitor such fetuses once or twice weekly because cardiac changes can take place quite rapidly. Rupture and/or bleeding within the tumor can lead to acute changes in loading conditions.
- Umbilical artery Doppler is very important. A sudden change in the diastolic component of umbilical arterial flow from forward flow to reverse flow may reflect a sudden change in tumor vascular resistance, heralding impending cardiovascular collapse.
- A general sense of the vascular nature of the SCT can be achieved by applying color Doppler over the tumor and lowering the scale. Oftentimes, circular or saccular regions of lucency may raise suspicion of high vascularity; however, in fact, these may be cystic, nonvascular structures. Application of color Doppler at low scale will not reveal any color in these structures, confirming that they are cysts.
- Careful surveillance is warranted after fetal therapy because a successful elimination or reduction in tumor mass will also reduce volume load and increase afterload. Such rapid changes can result in an acute change in ventricular geometry and the development of a stiff, noncompliant heart and diastolic dysfunction.

References

1. Danzer E, Hubbard AM, Hedrick HL, et al. Diagnosis and characterization of fetal sacrococcygeal teratoma with prenatal MRI. *AJR Am J Roentgenol.* 2006;187:W350-W356.
2. Wilson RD, Hedrick H, Flake AW, et al. Sacrococcygeal teratomas: prenatal surveillance, growth and pregnancy outcome. *Fetal Diagn Ther.* 2009;25:15-20.
3. Makin EC, Hyett J, Ade-Ajayi N, Patel S, Nicolaides K, Davenport M. Outcome of antenatally diagnosed sacrococcygeal teratomas: single-center experience (1993–2004). *J Pediatr Surg.* 2006;41:388-393.
4. Flake AW, Harrison MR, Adzick NS, Laberge JM, Warsof SL. Fetal sacrococcygeal teratoma. *J Pediatr Surg.* 1986;21:563-566.
5. Sy ED, Lee H, Ball R, et al. Spontaneous rupture of fetal sacrococcygeal teratoma. *Fetal Diagn Ther.* 2006;21:424-427.
6. Rychik J. Fetal cardiovascular physiology. *Pediatr Cardiol.* 2004;25:201-209.
7. Neubert S, Trautmann K, Tanner B, Steiner E, Linke F, Bahlmann F. Sonographic prognostic factors in prenatal diagnosis of SCT. *Fetal Diagn Ther.* 2004;19:319-326.
8. Olutoye OO, Johnson MP, Coleman BG, Crombleholme TM, Adzick NS, Flake AW. Abnormal umbilical cord Doppler sonograms may predict impending demise in fetuses with sacrococcygeal teratoma. A report of two cases. *Fetal Diagn Ther.* 2004;19:35-39.
9. Silverman NH, Schmidt KG. Ventricular volume overload in the human fetus: observations from fetal echocardiography. *J Am Soc Echocardiogr.* 1990;3:20-29.

10. Bond SJ, Harrison MR, Schmidt KG, et al. Death due to high-output cardiac failure in fetal sacrococcygeal teratoma. *J Pediatr Surg.* 1990;25:1287-1291.
11. Kay S, Khalife S, Laberge JM, Shaw K, Morin L, Flageole H. Prenatal percutaneous needle drainage of cystic sacrococcygeal teratomas. *J Pediatr Surg.* 1999;34:1148-1151.
12. Danzer E, Sydorak RM, Harrison MR, Albanese CT. Minimal access fetal surgery. *Eur J Obstet Gynecol Reprod Biol.* 2003;108:3-13.
13. Sydorak RM, Albanese CT. Minimal access techniques for fetal surgery. *World J Surg.* 2003;27:95-102.
14. Adzick NS. Open fetal surgery for life-threatening fetal anomalies. *Semin Fetal Neonatal Med* 2010;15:1-8.
15. Hedrick HL, Flake AW, Crombleholme TM, et al. Sacrococcygeal teratoma: prenatal assessment, fetal intervention, and outcome. *J Pediatr Surg.* 2004;39:430-438; discussion 430-438.
16. Rychik J, Tian Z, Cohen MS, et al. Acute cardiovascular effects of fetal surgery in the human. *Circulation.* 2004;110:1549-1556.
17. Derikx JP, De Backer A, van de Schoot L, et al. Long-term functional sequelae of sacrococcygeal teratoma: a national study in The Netherlands. *J Pediatr Surg.* 2007;42:1122-1126.
18. Derikx JP, De Backer A, van de Schoot L, et al. Factors associated with recurrence and metastasis in sacrococcygeal teratoma. *Br J Surg.* 2006;93:1543-1548.

CASES

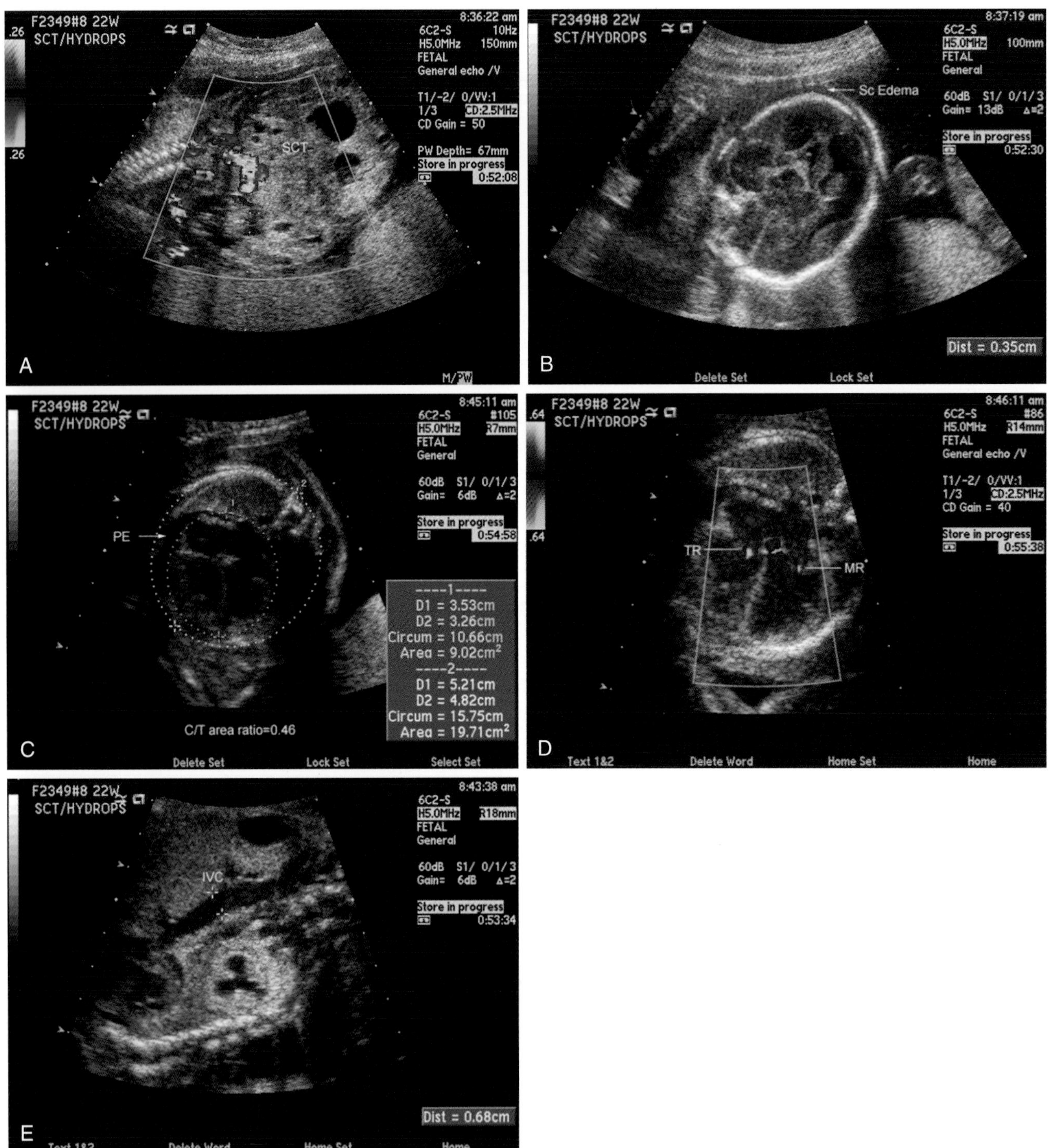

Case 40-1. **(A)** A fetus at 22 weeks' gestation with giant sacrococcygeal teratoma (SCT). The teratoma is partially intrapelvic because vascular aspects can be seen adjacent to the lower spine. **(B)** Because this SCT is quite vascular, there is a substantial volume load on the cardiovascular system with early development of hydrops. This image demonstrates the presence of scalp edema (Sc edema). **(C)** There is marked cardiomegaly with cardiothoracic area ratio of 0.46. PE, pleural effusion. **(D)** As a consequence of volume loading secondary to the SCT, there is dilation of the ventricles and annular dilation of the atrioventricular valves resulting in both mitral regurgitation (MR) and tricuspid regurgitation (TR). **(E)** Increased flow to the SCT causes increased venous return; hence, the inferior vena cava (IVC) is dilated.

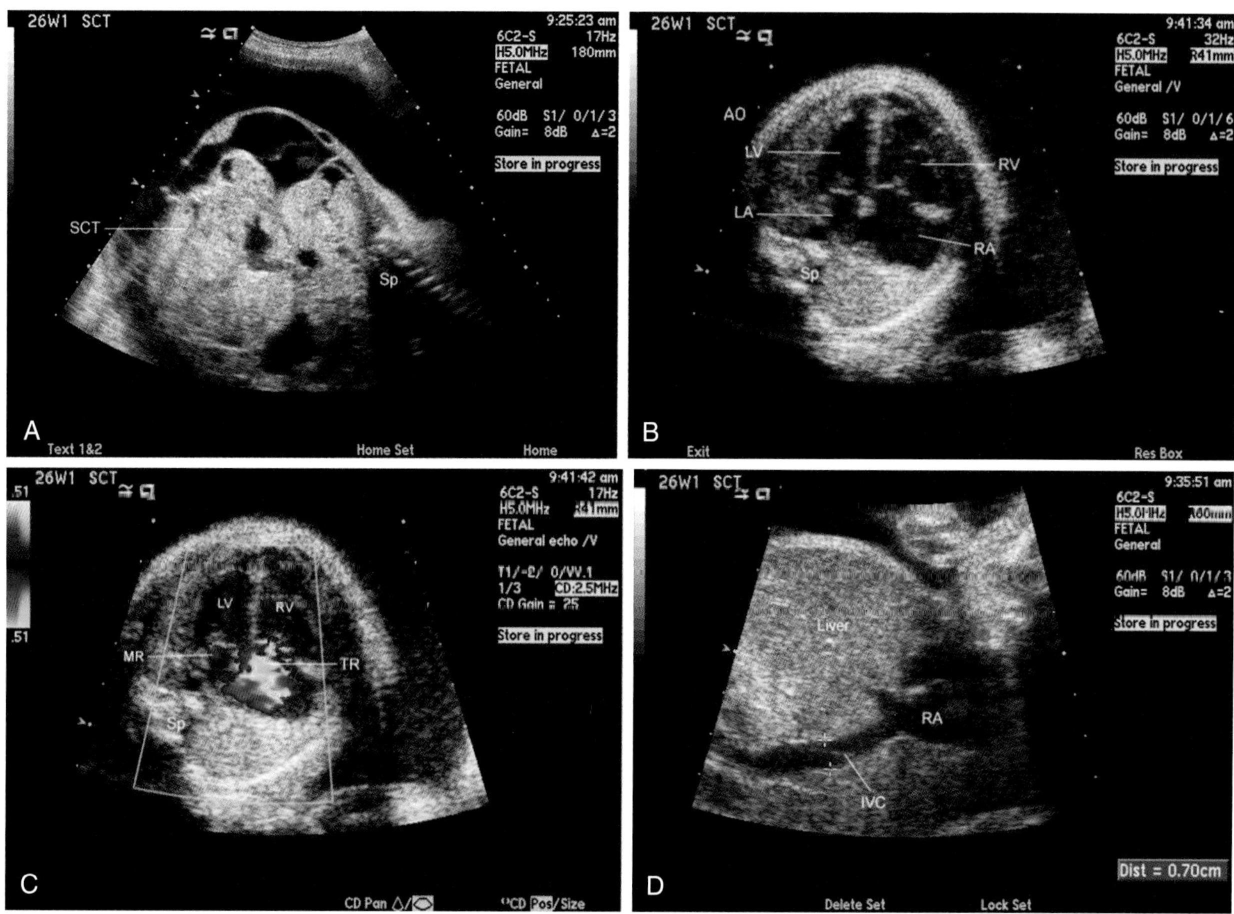

Case 40-2. **(A)** A fetus at 26 weeks' gestation with a large SCT. There is a substantial cystic component; however, the mass is also highly vascularized. Sp, spine. **(B)** There is significant cardiomegaly with enlargement of all chambers of the heart. LA, left atrium; LV, left ventricle; RA, right atrium; RV, right ventricle. **(C)** There is severe tricuspid regurgitation (TR) and mild mitral regurgitation (MR). **(D)** Secondary to increased venous return from the lower part of the body—the region of the SCT—the inferior vena cava (IVC) is dilated.

Continued

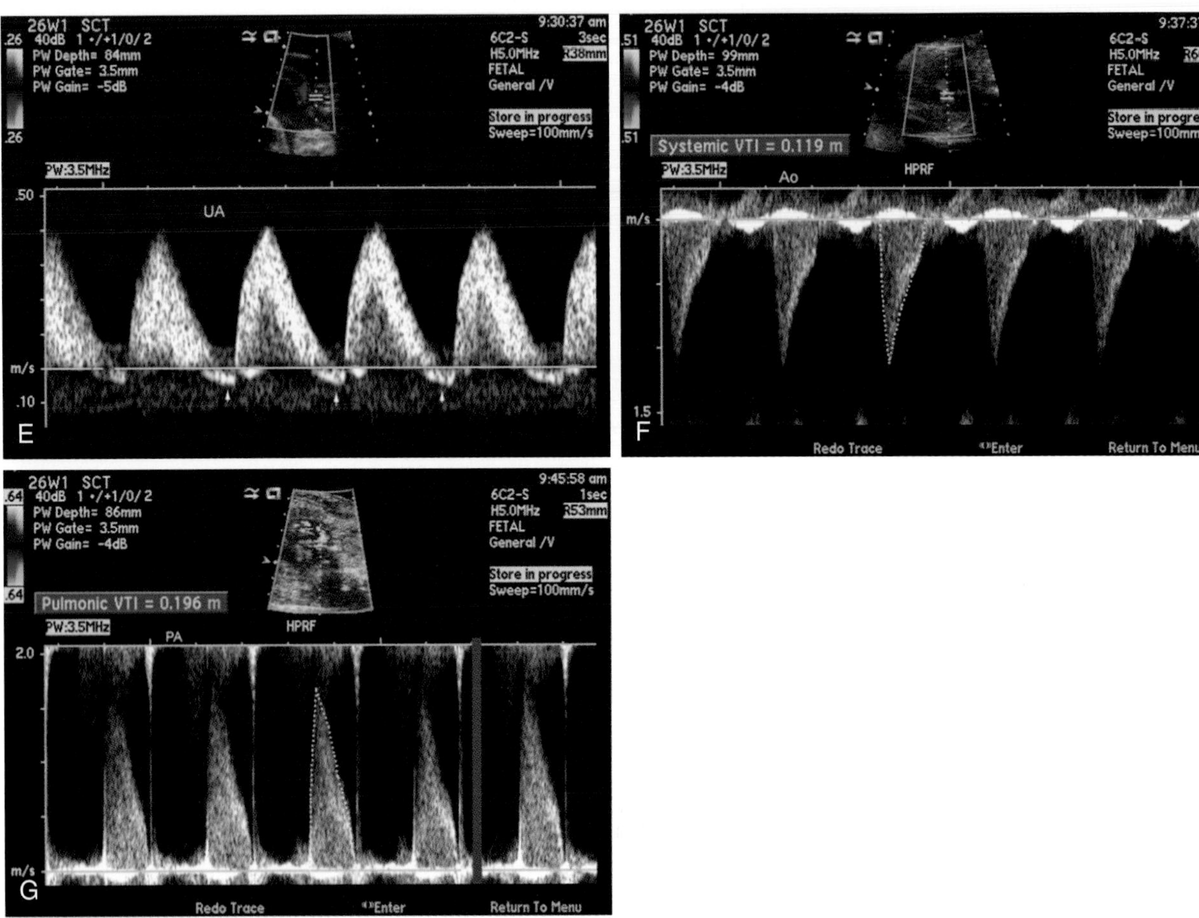

Case 40-2, cont'd (E) Doppler interrogation of the umbilical artery (UA). There is reversal of flow in diastole *(arrows)*. Because the SCT is highly vascularized and of very low resistance, blood is drawn away from the placenta to the lower resistance circuit of the SCT. This "steal" of flow away from the placenta is an ominous sign and may herald impending fetal demise. (F) Calculation of combined cardiac output is helpful in serial monitoring of the fetus with giant SCT. As cardiac output increases, so does the work and strain of the cardiovascular system. Doppler tracing of aortic flow reveals increased velocity, reflecting increased volume of blood flow. (G) Doppler tracing of flow across the pulmonic valve demonstrates markedly increased flow with peak velocity greater than 1.5 m/sec. The combined cardiac output of this fetus reached 900 mL/kg/min. PA, pulmonary artery.

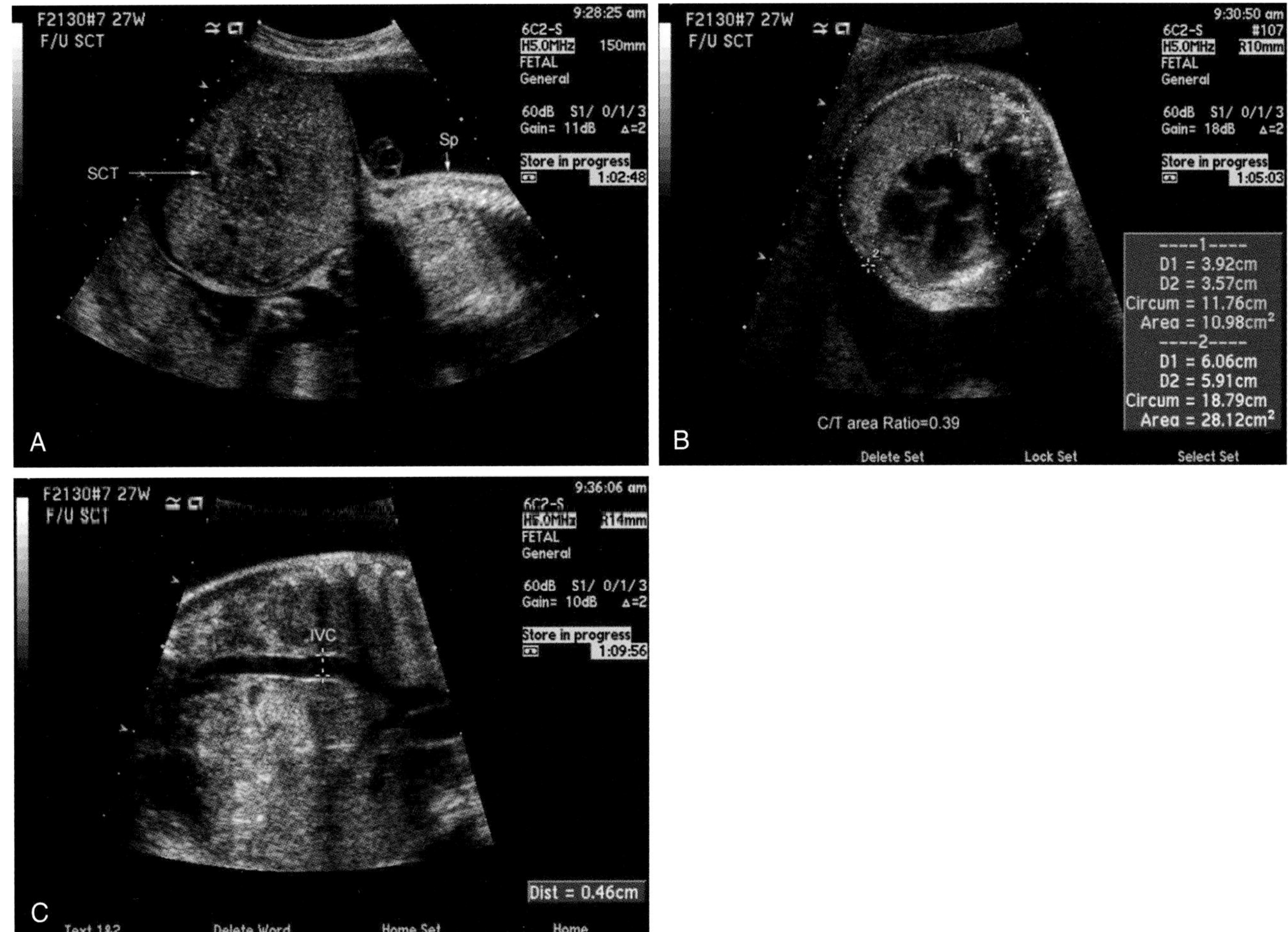

Case 40-3. **(A)** A fetus with SCT at 27 weeks' gestation. The SCT is large, pedunculated, and relatively solid in makeup. **(B)** There is only mild cardiomegaly, with cardiothoracic area ratio of 0.39. **(C)** The IVC is mildly dilated. Combined cardiac output was only mildly elevated at approximately 600 mL/min/kg. The physiology was tolerated well in utero and a postnatal resection was successfully undertaken with good outcome.

41

Cerebral Arteriovenous Malformation

Jack Rychik

Key Echocardiographic Features

- Enlarged heart, but with relatively preserved systolic function.
- No other obvious explanation as to why the heart is enlarged.
- Both right and left side of heart are enlarged.
- Dilated superior vena cava, out of proportion to the size of the inferior vena cava.
- Reversal of flow in the aortic arch in the absence of aortic insufficiency or other reason for aortic retrograde flow.
- Visualization of lucent, vascular structure in the brain.
- Increased middle cerebral artery systolic and diastolic flow.
- Mild or moderate tricuspid regurgitation.

Anatomy and Anatomical Associations

Cerebral arteriovenous malformations (AVMs) can occur as part of development of the cerebrovascular circulation and are generally quite rare. Although highly uncommon outside of prenatal life and infancy, the vein of Galen aneurysmal malformation is the most common type of cerebral AVM seen in the fetus.[1,2]

The vein of Galen aneurysmal malformation (VGAM) is a choroidal type of AVM involving the vein of Galen *forerunner* and is distinct from an AVM with venous drainage into a dilated, but already formed, vein of Galen. The congenital malformation develops relatively early in gestation during weeks 6 to 11 of fetal development as a persistent embryonic prosencephalic vein of Markowski; thus, VGAM is actually a misnomer. The vein of Markowski actually drains into the vein of Galen. Nevertheless, the effect is one in which arterial blood bypasses capillary beds and is shunted directly to the venous system. VGAM can result in marked dilation of the straight and sagittal sinuses as well as the venous system draining to the heart.

VGAM typically result in high-output congestive heart failure in the fetus.[3] The dilated venous structures may cause a mass effect leading to brain hypoplasia and altered cerebral development.[4] Cerebral hemorrhage can also occur, and thrombosis in the fetus has been reported.[5]

Interestingly, VGAM has been reported in association with two types of congenital heart disease—sinus venosus type atrial septal defect and coarctation of the aorta.[6,7] The association is hypothesized to be related to early alterations in blood flow patterns as a consequence of the AVM. Increased superior vena caval return in utero may interfere with absorption of the right horn of the sinus venosus into the right atrium, leading to development of the defect. In addition, preferential flow toward the low-resistance carotid arteries feeding the AVM and away from the aortic isthmus may lead to decreased isthmul growth. Size discrepancy with marked dilation of the ascending and transverse aorta and relatively small isthmus can result in postnatal coarctation of the aorta.

Frequency, Genetics, and Development

VGAM is rare, but it is the most common type of cerebral AVM. It is a developmental abnormality that is completed and present by the first trimester. The effects relate to volume of blood flow; hence, dilation, cerebral compression, and cardiac volume overload may not be seen until the second or third trimester. There is no known associated genetic basis to this malformation.

Prenatal Physiology

As cerebral blood volume increases with gestation, an increasing amount of blood is shunted from the arterial to the venous side resulting in increased volume load to the cerebral venous system and, ultimately, increased volume load to the heart.[8,9] The superior vena cava dilates as do the right ventricle and pulmonary artery. With volume loading of the right ventricle, the tricuspid annulus dilates, resulting in tricuspid regurgitation, which further adds volume load to the right heart. Blood ejected from the left side of the heart will take the pathway of least resistance up the ascending aorta and into the carotid arteries toward the low-resistance AVM connections. The head vessels will progressively enlarge. Blood flow in the isthmus of the aorta, or in the descending aorta, may flow retrograde in diastole as a "steal" phenomenon takes place, with blood being shunted into the fetal head, further increasing venous return.

Prenatal Management

Assessment of combined cardiac output can provide an overall measure of the potential degree of cardiovascular burden present in the VGAM. By measuring the diameter of the semilunar valves and sampling Doppler flow across the semilunar valves, one may calculate cardiac output for each ventricle. The normal combined cardiac output in the fetus is approximately 400 to 500 mL/kg/min of flow. In our experience, similar to what is seen in other volume-load lesions such as sacrococcygeal teratoma, the fetal cardiovascular system can tolerate volume loads as high as 700 to 800 mL/kg/min. However, values much higher than that typically lead to heart failure and hydrops.

The most common initial finding that prompts suspicion for VGAM is the identification of a large echolucent structure in the posterior aspect of the fetal head, midline behind the third ventricle.[10] Application of color Doppler flow onto the structure may reveal very low velocity swirling of blood. At times, feeder vessels into the dilated venous sac can be seen.

No fetal therapeutic maneuvers are currently available for VGAM. Progressive findings of increased cardiac output and worsening volume overload with impending hydrops may prompt decisions toward delivery, balanced against gestational age.

Postnatal Physiology, Management, and Outcomes

The neonate with VGAM will manifest signs and symptoms of volume overload and high-output heart failure. Seizures, hydrocephalus, and developmental delay may present in infancy.

Heart failure can be more effectively treated after birth using various oral or parenteral drugs than in the fetus. Definitive treatment of the source of the problem is available. Catheter-directed interventional treatment using coil embolization techniques is the current treatment for VGAM.[11] Such treatment is reported to be 50% to 80% effective in managing the heart failure.[12] However, developmental consequences such as altered brain structure or function may persist, and many patients require shunting procedures for hydrocephalus.

Imaging Essentials and Important Points

- Echolucent regions in the posterior aspect of the fetal head should raise suspicion of a VGAM. Doppler color flow evaluation in the region will reveal slow venous patterns of swirling blood flow.
- Serial assessment of combined cardiac output can provide a sense of the degree of cardiovascular burden and the potential for development of signs and symptoms of heart failure in advance of their clinical manifestation.
- Specific cardiovascular findings in VGAM include:
  - Cardiomegaly.
  - Superior vena cava dilation out of proportion to the inferior vena cava.
  - Right ventricular dilation and systolic dysfunction.
  - Tricuspid regurgitation.
  - Combined cardiac output greater than 500 mL/kg/min.
  - With progressive increase in cardiac output, left ventricular dilation and mitral regurgitation can be seen.
  - Head vessel dilation, in particular the carotid arteries.
  - Marked size discrepancy between the transverse aorta, which will appear larger than normal, and the aortic isthmus, which will appear smaller than normal.
  - Doppler interrogation of the aortic isthmus may reveal diastolic reversal of flow or retrograde flow in the descending aorta, suggesting a "steal" into the low-resistance VGAM
  - Decreased, absent, or reversed diastolic flow in the umbilical artery in severe cases, suggesting a "steal" away from the placenta toward the low-resistance VGAM

References

1. Paternoster DM, Manganelli F, Moroder W, Nicolini U. Prenatal diagnosis of vein of Galen aneurysmal malformations. *Fetal Diagn Ther*. 2003;18:408-411.
2. Sepulveda W, Platt CC, Fisk NM. Prenatal diagnosis of cerebral arteriovenous malformation using color Doppler ultrasonography: case report and review of the literature. *Ultrasound Obstet Gynecol*. 1995;6:282-286.
3. Chisholm CA, Kuller JA, Katz VL, McCoy MC. Aneurysm of the vein of Galen: prenatal diagnosis and perinatal management. *Am J Perinatol*. 1996;13:503-506.
4. Paladini D, Palmieri S, D'Angelo A, Martinelli P. Prenatal ultrasound diagnosis of cerebral arteriovenous fistula. *Obstet Gynecol*. 1996;88:678-681.
5. Vijayaraghavan SB, Vijay S, Kala MR, Neha D. Prenatal diagnosis of thrombosed aneurysm of vein of Galen. *Ultrasound Obstet Gynecol*. 2006;27:81-83.
6. Friedman DM, Rutkowski M, Madrid M, Berenstein A. Sinus venosus atrial septal defect associated with vein of Galen malformations: report of two cases. *Pediatr Cardiol*. 1994;15:50-52.
7. McElhinney DB, Halbach VV, Silverman NH, Dowd CF, Hanley FL. Congenital cardiac anomalies with vein of Galen malformations in infants. *Arch Dis Child*. 1998;78:548-551.
8. Yuval Y, Lerner A, Lipitz S, Rotstein Z, Hegesh J, Achiron R. Prenatal diagnosis of vein of Galen aneurysmal malformation: report of two cases with proposal for prognostic indices. *Prenat Diagn*. 1997;17:972-977.

9. Hartung J, Heling KS, Rake A, Zimmer C, Chaoui R. Detection of an aneurysm of the vein of Galen following signs of cardiac overload in a 22-week old fetus. *Prenat Diagn*. 2003;23: 901-903.
10. Comstock CH, Kirk JS. Arteriovenous malformations. Locations and evolution in the fetal brain. *J Ultrasound Med*. 1991;10: 361-365.
11. Kelly A, Rijhsinghani A. Antenatal course of a fetal intracranial arteriovenous fistula: a case report. *J Reprod Med*. 2005;50: 367-369.
12. Friedman DM, Verma R, Madrid M, Wisoff JH, Berenstein A. Recent improvement in outcome using transcatheter embolization techniques for neonatal aneurysmal malformations of the vein of Galen. *Pediatrics*. 1993;91:583-586.

CASES

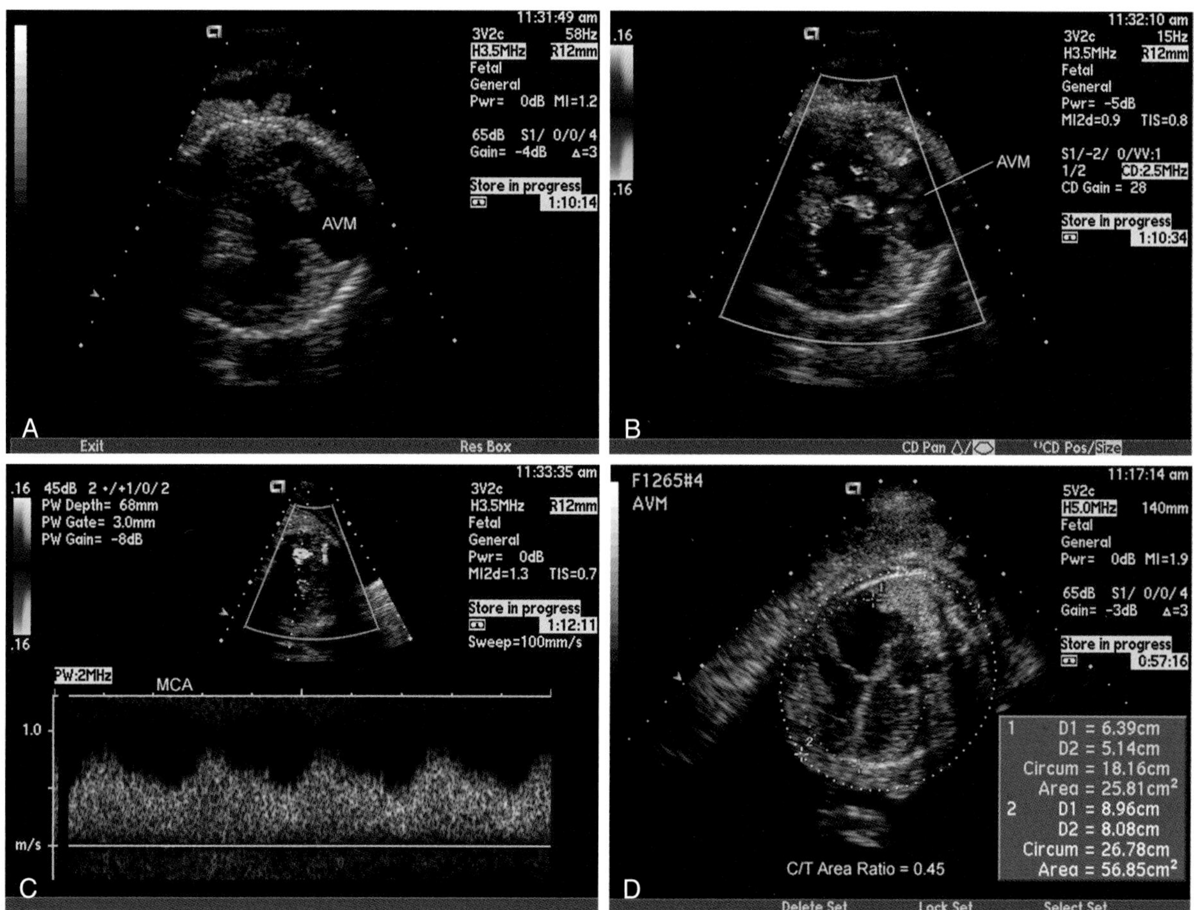

Case 41-1. **(A)** View of the head of a fetus with a large cerebral arteriovenous malformation (AVM). Note the lucency representing vascular space within the brain. **(B)** Color flow imaging at a very low scale (Nyquist limit set at 16 cm/sec). The lucency is filled with color suggesting very low velocity, swirling flow. This distinguishes a cerebral AVM from other nonvascular lucent abnormal structures of the brain. **(C)** Doppler sampling in the middle cerebral artery (MCA) reveals a high peak velocity and a markedly elevated diastolic flow velocity. This reflects the plethora of flow through the very low resistance vascular circuit of the AVM. **(D)** There is cardiomegaly due to increased venous return from the cerebral AVM.

Continued

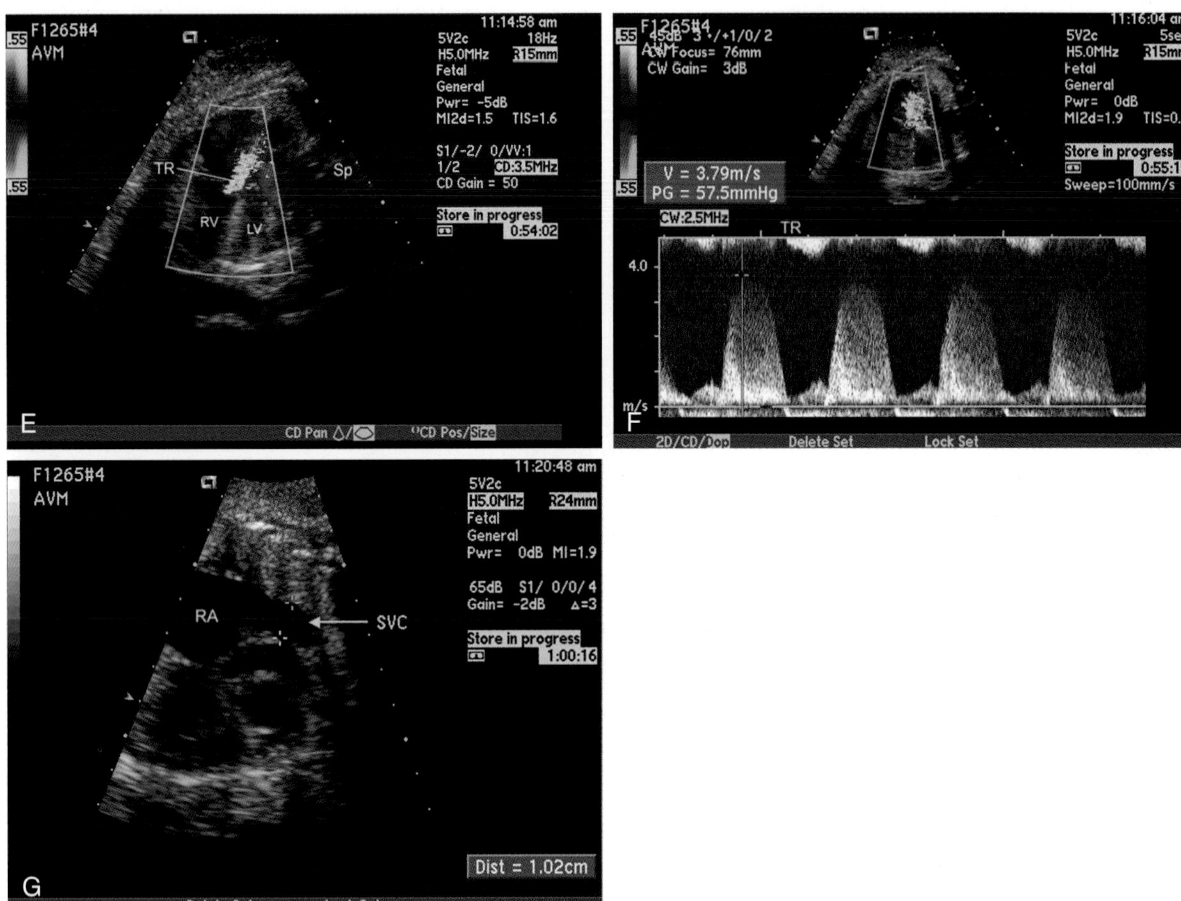

Case 41-1, cont'd **(E)** Color flow imaging demonstrates moderate tricuspid regurgitation (TR). Increased volume return to the right side of the heart can cause right ventricular dilation and tricuspid annular dilation leading to TR. LV, left ventricle; RV, right ventricle; Sp, spine. **(F)** The RV pressure estimate as determined by the peak velocity of the TR jet is 58 mm Hg higher than the right atrial V wave. There is relative systemic hypertension in this fetus as a consequence of the marked volume overload. **(G)** The distal superior vena cava (SVC) is severely dilated at greater than 1 cm due to the torrential superior venous return from the cerebral circulation. RA, right atrium.

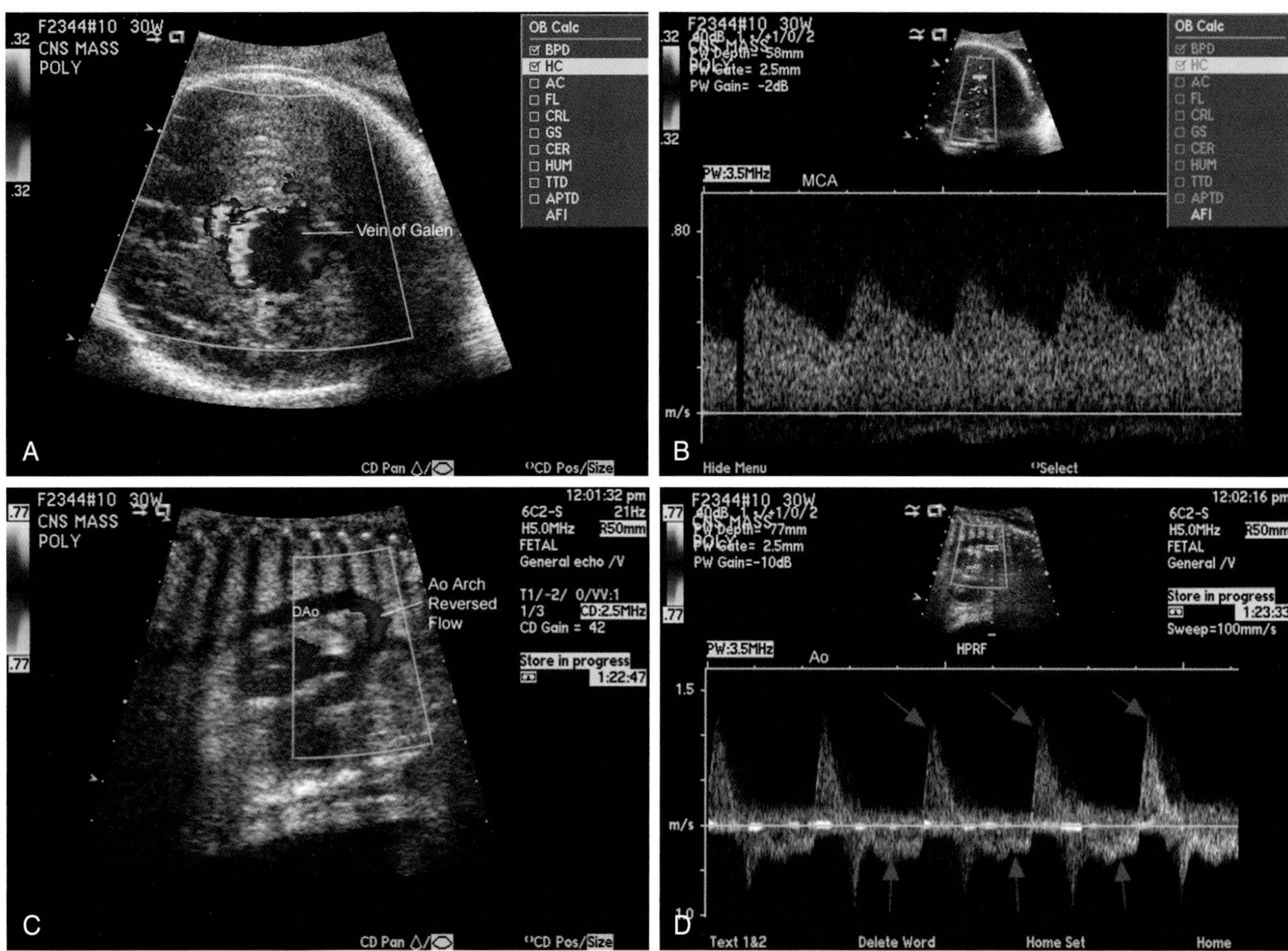

Case 41-2. **(A)** Vein of Galen malformation seen on color flow imaging in this fetus at 30 weeks' gestation. **(B)** Doppler interrogation in the middle cerebral artery (MCA). There is a "saw-tooth" pattern suggesting low distal vascular resistance, as the AVM draws blood forward during diastole. **(C)** Color flow imaging of the aortic arch at a relatively high color scale (Nyquist limit at 77 cm/sec). During diastole, there is reversal of flow seen in the transverse aortic arch (Ao Arch) as blood is drawn retrograde into the low-resistance cerebrovascular circulation due to the AVM. DAo, descending aorta. **(D)** Doppler sampling in the transverse aorta confirms antegrade flow in systole (above the baseline; *red arrows)* but retrograde flow (below the baseline; *blue arrows)* in diastole.

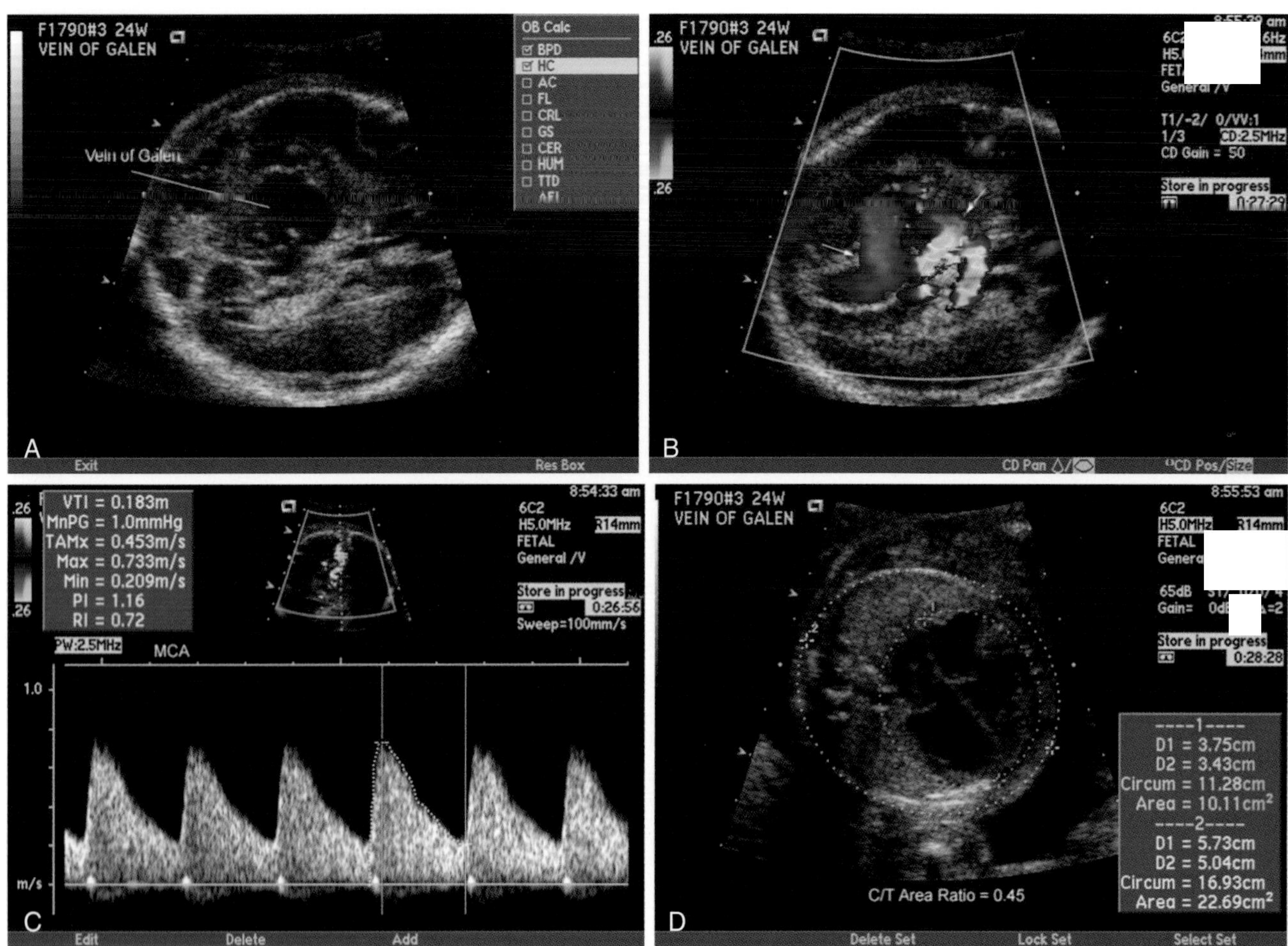

Case 41-3. **(A)** Vein of Galen malformation identified at 24 weeks' gestation. **(B)** Color flow imaging identifies the arterial limb in *multicolors* (high velocity) and the venous limb in *blue* (relative low velocity). **(C)** Doppler sampling in the MCA. The peak velocity is increased to over 70 cm/sec and the calculated pulsatility index is 1.16. **(D)** There is cardiomegaly with cardiothoracic area ratio of 0.45.

42

Pulmonary Arteriovenous Malformation

Jack Rychik

Key Echocardiographic Features

- Lucency in the lung with color flow imaging highlighting increased flow within the lucency.
- Dilated pulmonary veins and selective dilation of the left side of the heart.
- Enlarged heart, but with relatively preserved systolic function.
- Reversal of flow in the ductus arteriosus with flow from aorta to pulmonary artery, but in the absence of any right-sided obstruction.
- Inequity in size and flow between the branch pulmonary arteries.

Anatomy and Anatomical Associations

Pulmonary arteriovenous fistula or malformation (PAVM) is a direct connection between the pulmonary arterial system and the pulmonary veins, bypassing the capillaries. Its effect is to deliver pulmonary arterial blood to the pulmonary veins and left side of the heart, bypassing the gas exchange unit of the lung. In the postnatal state, this results in deoxygenated blood reaching the systemic circulation. In the fetus, it can lead to heart failure, hydrops, and altered lung development, resulting in profound postnatal hypoxemia.[1,2]

PAVMs are most typically seen in the adult patient with hereditary hemorrhagic telangiectasia (HHT), an autosomal dominant disorder in which multiple body telangiectasia are present.[3] These vascular abnormalities may be present in the lung, liver, kidney, or head, causing symptoms ranging from epistaxis to organ hemorrhage and infarction. When present in the lung, the fistulous connections may allow for right-to-left shunting with paradoxical embolism.

PAVM is rare in childhood, and rarer still in the fetus. When seen early in life, they may be isolated and not necessarily associated with HHT. PAVM appears to be an acquired phenomenon in some patients with single-ventricle type of congenital heart disease who have undergone a cavopulmonary connection.[4] When present in the fetus, PAVM is typically large and may adversely affect both heart and lung development.

Frequency, Genetics, and Development

PAVM in the fetus is extremely rare, with only a few case reports in the literature; however, it is a fascinating anomaly worthy of review and our attention. There are no known genetic associations beyond HHT, which is predominantly a disease that manifests in childhood with progression in adulthood. HHT does not typically manifest in the fetus.

There are interesting data to suggest that bypass connections between the pulmonary arterial system and the pulmonary venous system are normally present in the developing fetus. Animal work in the sheep using contrast echocardiography demonstrates significant right-to-left intrapulmonary shunting in the fetus, with persistence in the early newborn period, but disappearance at 4 weeks of life.[5] Development of PAVMs later in life, for example, after cavopulmonary connection, may be a return to an earlier primitive stage of development.

Hepatic venous flow may play a role in the development of PAVM. It has been observed in various forms of cavopulmonary connection that, if hepatic effluent is not directed toward the lungs, such patients are at highest risk for development of PAVM.[4] Furthermore, surgical connection and redirection of hepatic venous effluent into the lungs leads to resolution of PAVM.[6] It is plausible to speculate that a similar phenomenon is at hand in the fetus. In the fetal circulation, hepatic venous and portal venous flow are markedly different than in the postnatal state.[7] In addition, streaming patterns within the floor of the right atrium direct flow across the foramen ovale from right to left. It is conceivable that nature has created a natural pathway in which an "hepatic factor" is diverted away from the lungs during fetal life in order to allow for intentional intrapulmonary shunting through natural arterial-to-venous connections. With birth, the hepatic factor is redirected toward the lungs and these connections dissipate, except in unnatural cases such as various forms of congenital heart disease after palliation, in which the hepatic factor is once again denied entry into the lungs.

Prenatal Physiology

In the fetus, a large PAVM will act as a low vascular resistance "sink" and will drive blood to the region of the lung in which it is present. PAVM leads to an increased volume load, which may cause cardiac enlargement and lead to heart failure and hydrops. As blood is directed toward the PAVM, pulmonary venous return increases substantially because it is carrying both normal pulmonary venous effluent and the additional volume load that is being shunted into the PAVM. As a consequence, the pulmonary veins may become grossly enlarged and dilated and may appear as an echolucent region within the hilum of the lung. The volume load in PAVM is primarily carried by the left ventricle because it receives the increased pulmonary venous return. Left atrial pressure may be increased above normal due to torrential pulmonary venous return. Shunting at the foramen ovale may reverse from the normal right-to-left direction to left-to-right, as left atrial pressure exceeds right atrial pressure.

The low vascular sink of the PAVM may also drive blood into the lung via the ductus arteriosus. Blood flow in the fetal ductus arteriosus is normally directed from the pulmonary artery toward the descending aorta in an antegrade manner, diverting blood away from the normally high-resistance pulmonary vasculature. However, in the presence of a PAVM, the lung itself is now the pathway of least resistance and blood flow in the ductus arteriosus may be reversed, from the aorta into the main pulmonary artery, and further directed toward the lung and segments containing the PAVM. This can create a "steal" from the systemic circulation and further adds to the ventricular volume load.

Fetal PAVM can also inhibit normal lung development. The low vascular resistance sink of a PAVM will divert blood toward the region of the lung containing the PAVM and steal blood away from other regions. This creates a heterogeneous perfusion profile with some lung segments receiving excess flow and others receiving a paucity of flow. Such alterations in flow lead to histopathological changes in the pulmonary microvasculature.[2] PAVM can, therefore, lead to secondary changes in the pulmonary vasculature that may further contribute to difficulties at birth, such as pulmonary hypertension, once placental separation takes place.

Prenatal Management

No treatment strategies are available for fetal PAVM. When heart failure leads to early signs of hydrops, delivery should be considered depending upon gestational age.

We recently experienced a case of giant fetal PAVM detected at 28 weeks' gestation with evidence on echocardiography for marked cardiomegaly, left ventricular dilation, left-to-right shunting at the atrial level, and reversal of flow in the ductus arteriosus. Massively dilated pulmonary veins were seen, as was the actual site of connection between the right pulmonary artery and the right pulmonary veins, on color Doppler imaging. Qualitative ventricular dysfunction and progressive dilation was noted at 35 weeks, so the fetus was delivered by cesarean section in our hybrid cardiac surgery and catheterization suite using our IMPACT procedure (immediate postpartum access to cardiac therapy). This is an organizational endeavor in which a multidisciplinary team of obstetricians, maternal-fetal medicine specialists, pediatric cardiologists, cardiac anesthesiologists, and cardiac surgeons are all brought together as a team to optimize care for the mother and fetus. Care is offered in one facility, in a multidisciplinary manner, with focus on immediate rapid access to the newborn. Our fetus with PAVM was delivered in such a manner, with profound hypoxemia on initial blood gas assessment. Vascular access was achieved after placental separation and cardiac catheterization techniques were used to quickly deploy an Amplatzer occluder device into the PAVM.[8] Oxygenation improved within minutes of the occlusion because intrapulmonary shunting was essentially eliminated. Over the ensuing days, inotropic support for ventricular dysfunction was necessary because acute removal of volume load led to myocardial remodeling and the appearance of a thickened heart. At day 10 of life, the newborn was discharged to home with oxygen saturation in room air of 92%. At 3 years of follow-up, the child is asymptomatic with normal oxygenation and doing very well.

Postnatal Physiology and Management

Once a fetus with a large PAVM is separated from placental circulation, it is dependent upon its own lungs for oxygenation. Systemic venous return to the right side of the heart will take the pathway of least resistance, which will be through the PAVM, resulting in a massive shunt of deoxygenated blood to the arterial systemic side. Profound hypoxemia and acidosis will ensue unless the diagnosis is quickly made and the PAVM connection occluded. Even after successful occlusion, pulmonary histopathological changes may prevent normal lung function and pulmonary arterial hypertension and hypoxemia may persist with right-to-left shunting across the ductus arteriosus. Extracorporeal membrane oxygenation (ECMO) was used in a case of prenatally diagnosed PAVM; however, the pulmonary vasculature was markedly abnormal, leading to infant death.[2]

Large PAVMs will manifest with significant prenatal findings; however, small lesions may be detected in infancy. Elective catheter-based occlusion can take place based on the degree of hypoxemia or volume load and heart failure present. In our case of a large PAVM, an Amplatzer device was necessary to plug the connection. In smaller lesions, coils may be useful.

Outcomes

Overall prognosis for fetal PAVM is poor; however, outcome in the rare successful cases in which elimination of the connection is rapidly achieved appears to be good. Long-term functional outcome, in particular pulmonary function and exercise capacity, is of interest; however, currently, no data are available because there are so few survivors of this lethal and rare anomaly.

Imaging Essentials and Important Points

- Echolucency in the mediastinum, adjacent to and posterior to the heart, should raise suspicion of dilated pulmonary veins due to a PAVM.
- Color Doppler mapping within the lung parenchyma will reveal the pulmonary artery-to-venous connection as a high-velocity continuous flow.
- Dilation of the left ventricle, left-to-right atrial level shunting, and aorta-to-pulmonary artery shunting across the ductus arteriosus are unique findings seen in association with a large PAVM.
- Heart failure is the most concerning phenomenon in the fetus with PAVM; however, severe postnatal hypoxemia due to massive right-to-left intrapulmonary shunting is of greatest concern after birth.
- Persistent hypoxemia and pulmonary hypertension may be seen after PAVM occlusion if there is associated pulmonary vascular disease due to abnormal fetal perfusion patterns of the unaffected lung.
- Ventricular dysfunction may ensue after occlusion of a PAVM and acute removal of the volume load.

References

1. Heling KS, Tennstedt C, Goldner B, Bollmann R. Prenatal diagnosis of intrapulmonary arteriovenous malformation: sonographic and pathomorphological findings. *Ultrasound Obstet Gynecol.* 2002;19: 514-517.
2. Russell MW, Gomez C, Nugent C, Christiansen J. Large fetal pulmonary arteriovenous fistula: impact on pulmonary development. *Pediatr Cardiol.* 2002;23:454-457.
3. Shovlin CL, Guttmacher AE, Buscarini E, et al. Diagnostic criteria for hereditary hemorrhagic telangiectasia (Rendu-Osler-Weber syndrome). *Am J Med Genet.* 2000;91:66-67.
4. Duncan BW, Desai S. Pulmonary arteriovenous malformations after cavopulmonary anastomosis. *Ann Thorac Surg.* 2003;76: 1759-1766.
5. McMullan DM, Hanley FL, Cohen GA, Portman MA, Riemer RK. Pulmonary arteriovenous shunting in the normal fetal lung. *J Am Coll Cardiol.* 2004;44:1497-1500.
6. Shah MJ, Rychik J, Fogel MA, Murphy JD, Jacobs ML. Pulmonary AV malformations after superior cavopulmonary connection: resolution after inclusion of hepatic veins in the pulmonary circulation. *Ann Thorac Surg.* 1997;63:960-963.
7. Mavrides E, Moscoso G, Carvalho JS, Campbell S, Thilaganathan B. The anatomy of the umbilical, portal and hepatic venous systems in the human fetus at 14-19 weeks of gestation. *Ultrasound Obstet Gynecol.* 2001;18:598-604.
8. Boudjemline Y, Ladouceur M, Bonnet D. Neonatal transcatheter closure of a large pulmonary arteriovenous fistula. *Cardiol Young.* 2006;16:593-595.

CASE

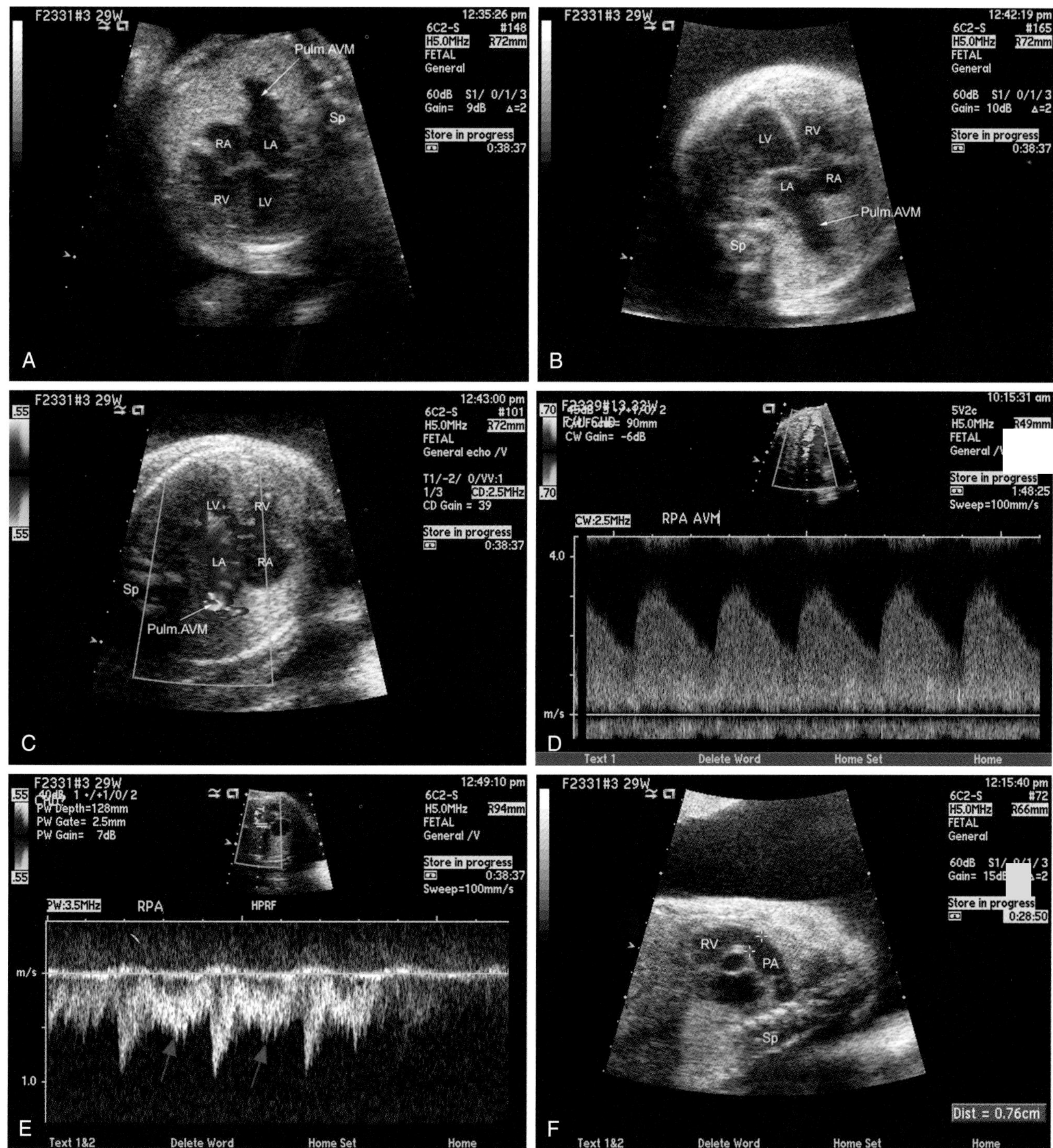

Case 42-1. **(A)** Four-chamber view demonstrates an enlarged heart with a markedly dilated vascular space just behind the left atrium (LA). This is the pulmonary arteriovenous malformation (Pulm AVM) and its venous limb of return to the dilated pulmonary veins. LV, left ventricle; RA, right atrium; RV, right ventricle; Sp, spine. **(B)** Image demonstrates the extent of the vascular lucency protruding into the lung parenchyma. **(C)** Color flow imaging demonstrates the turbulent high flow arterial connection to the dilated pulmonary vein, with increased preferential filling of the left side of the heart. **(D)** Doppler sampling at the arteriovenous malformation connection within the lung at the site of greatest turbulence. There is continuous very high velocity from the pulmonary artery to the pulmonary vein, with a pulsatile "saw-tooth" pattern, suggesting markedly increased flow during diastole as well as systole. The continuous high-volume intrauterine bypass of lung parenchymal tissue leads to a number of pathophysiological consequences including (1) increased volume load to the left ventricle, (2) bypass of lung vasculature altering lung development in the affected lung, and (3) postnatal potential for massive intrapulmonary shunt of desaturated blood away from the oxygen exchange unit, resulting in profound neonatal hypoxemia. RPA, right pulmonary artery. **(E)** Doppler sampling in the RPA at a site proximal to the AVM. The flow pattern suggests marked diastolic runoff *(arrows)* with very low distal vascular resistance secondary to the pulmonary AVM. **(F)** Short-axis view of right ventricular outflow tract and pulmonary artery. There is no right-sided outflow tract obstruction or pulmonic stenosis.

Continued

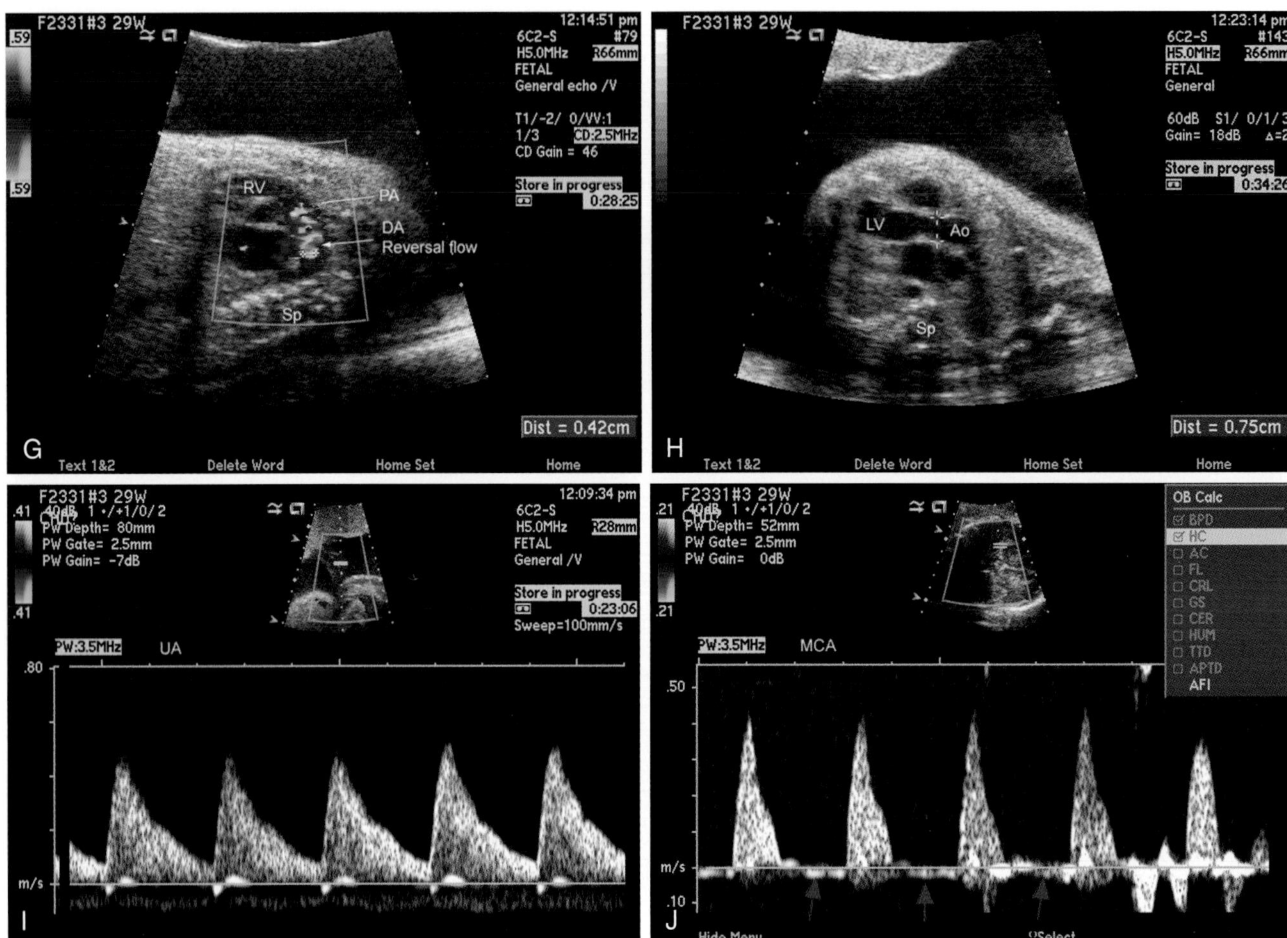

Case 42-1, cont'd (G) Short-axis view with ductal flow demonstrated. The ductus arteriosus (DA) is shunting in a retrograde manner from aorta to pulmonary artery, in the absence of any right ventricular outflow tract obstruction or pulmonic stenosis. This abnormal ductus arteriosus shunting is due to the extremely low intrapulmonary vascular resistance as dictated by the right pulmonary AVM. **(H)** Long-axis view of the left ventricular outflow tract. The aortic annulus is enlarged for gestational age (>7 mm at 29 wk' gestation), which is consistent with chronic increased left-sided flow. Ao, aorta. **(I)** Doppler examination of the umbilical cord reveals a relatively normal umbilical arterial and pulmonary venous flow pattern. UA, umbilical artery. **(J)** Doppler examination of the middle cerebral artery (MCA). Note the slight reversal in diastolic flow in the MCA. This is likely due to the markedly low pulmonary vascular sink causing retrograde flow in the DA, further pulling blood retrograde into the aortic arch and influencing diastolic retrograde head vessel flow, all due to the markedly low resistance pulmonary AVM.

43

Congenital Cystic Adenomatoid Malformation

Jack Rychik

Key Echocardiographic Features

- Compression of the heart, with small cardiothoracic ratio.
- Abnormal position of the heart within the chest.
- Distortion of the inferior vena cava as it enters the chest.
- Impaired filling of the heart can lead to findings on Doppler echocardiography of equilibration of peak E and A wave velocities and increased reversal of atrial contraction wave form in the inferior vena cava.
- Hydrops fetalis.

Anatomy and Anatomical Associations

Congenital cystic adenomatoid malformation (CCAM) is a rare developmental abnormality of the lungs.[1-3] It is characterized as a benign hamartoma or dysplastic lung tumor due to overgrowth of terminal bronchioles. The tumor can grow to be quite large, compressing adjacent lung tissue and impairing growth of normal pulmonary tissue. CCAM can grow to become a large and significant size intrathoracic space-occupying lesion. Cardiovascular compromise as a result of compression of the heart and vascular structures can occur. When a critical size is reached, hydrops may develop that heralds impending fetal demise in nearly all cases, unless intervened upon. The majority of fetuses with CCAM have a relatively good outcome, but appropriate identification and ongoing surveillance are required because growth patterns can be unpredictable, with significant and rapid growth potential noted between 18 and 26 weeks of gestation.

CCAM is typically unilateral and usually involves only one lobe of the lung. Cystic structures arise from overgrowth of the terminal bronchioles with a commensurate reduction in number of alveoli. A variety of classifications have been described based on the histopathology; however, our group at Children's Hospital of Philadelphia (CHOP) have found it most useful to characterize them in two ways based on gross anatomy and ultrasound findings. *Macrocystic* lesions contain single or multiple cysts that are 5 mm in diameter or larger on prenatal ultrasound, whereas *microcystic* lesions appear as a solid echogenic mass. In the macrocystic type, when multiple cysts are present, they typically communicate with one another.

CCAM is to be distinguished from other types of intrathoracic lung lesions in the fetus, in particular bronchopulmonary sequestration (BPS).[2] A BPS is a mass of nonfunctioning lung tissue that is supplied by an anomalous systemic artery and does not have a bronchial connection to the native tracheobronchial tree. On ultrasound, BPS appears as a well-defined echo-dense homogeneous mass and can be confused with a microcystic CCAM, except that the former has an arterial supply from the systemic arterial system. In CCAM, the arterial supply is from the pulmonary arterial tree and venous drainage is through the pulmonary veins. In BPS, the arterial supply is typically from a large artery emanating from the descending aorta and the venous drainage is through the pulmonary venous system. Hybrid lesions, with characteristics of both BPS and CCAM, have been described. Both can cause significant cardiovascular compromise when they grow to a large size. Other lesions to be distinguished include congenital lobar emphysema and peripheral bronchial atresia.[4,5] Occasionally, congenital diaphragmatic hernia can be confused with CCAM. Careful ultrasound or ultrafast magnetic resonance imaging (MRI) evaluation should be able to distinguish these very different anomalies with different management schema and outcome.

Frequency, Genetics, and Development

The incidence of CCAM in the general population is not known because small lesions may be subclinical and some lesions become smaller and resolve during in utero development or early childhood.

CCAM is believed to occur because of an abnormality of lung development.[1] The development of the mammalian vertebrate lung is divided into five distinct periods based on the anatomical changes that take place in lung architecture: embryonic (3-7 wk), pseudoglandular (7-17 wk), canalicular (17-29 wk), saccular (24-36 wk), and alveolar (36 wk to maturity). In the pseudoglandular period, there is rapid expansion of the conducting airways and peripheral lung tubules, which continue to branch and bud to form acinar tubules. The expansion of these small tubules in the periphery of the lung produces a glandular appearance. Uncontrolled growth and development of the macrocystic CCAM is believed to occur during the pseudoglandular phase, whereas microcystic CCAM is believed to develop later at the canalicular phase. Eight to 10 weeks of gestation is reported to be a particularly vulnerable period of time for teratogen impact on lung development leading to CCAM.[6]

Resected large CCAM specimens demonstrate increased cell proliferation and markedly decreased apoptosis when compared with gestational age–matched normal fetal lung tissue. Factors that enhance cell proliferation or down-regulate apoptosis have been studied including keratinocyte growth factor, platelet-derived growth factor, and fibroblast growth factor (FGF). Using a rat transgenic lung model, investigators have shown that FGF-10 overexpression in the proximal tracheobronchial tree during the pseudoglandular phase of lung development resulted in large cysts, whereas FGF-10 overexpression in the distal lung parenchyma during the canalicular phase resulted in small cysts, providing a possible developmental model for the anomaly.

We reported on the possible association of CCAM and congenital heart disease when in the presence of genetic abnormality.[7] Of 262 fetuses evaluated with CCAM at our center between 2000 and 2006, 4 (1.6%) had associated congenital heart disease consisting of 2 with ventricular septal defect, 1 with tetralogy of Fallot, and 1 with transposition of the great arteries. A review of the literature reveals that nearly two thirds of fetuses with CCAM and congenital heart disease have a known genetic/chromosomal abnormality.

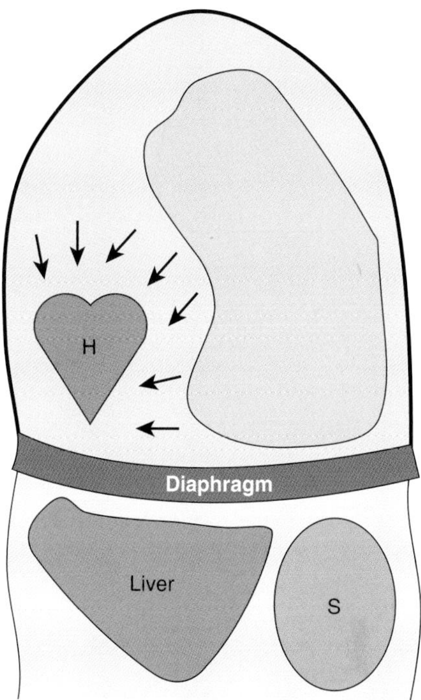

Figure 43-1. Effect of a large intrathoracic mass such as a congenital cystic adenomatoid malformation (CCAM) on the heart (H). Intrathoracic pressure is increased and there is cardiac compression impairing filling. The diaphragm is often inverted as the CCAM mass grows in size. S, stomach.

Prenatal Physiology

Large lung lesions such as CCAM have predictable pathophysiological effects on the fetus. Esophageal compression by the mass causes altered swallowing of amniotic fluid and results in polyhydramnios. Most important, a large mass can distort intrathoracic structures and compress the heart.

The fetal myocardium normally exists in a relatively noncompliant "stiff" state, with limited ability to increase preload or stroke volume. Extrinsic compression by a large intrathoracic, space-occupying lesion such as a CCAM can quickly lead to underfilling of the fetal heart, limiting cardiac output (Figure 43-1). Compression or tamponade of the fetal heart leads to increased atrial pressure and increased venous pressure, resulting in hydrops. The heart can appear "squeezed" within the chest cavity and is markedly distorted and deviated away from the side of the CCAM mass. While the heart is pushed over, the abdominal contents remain relatively fixed and the inferior vena cava can become distorted in its course through the abdomen, as it stretches to reach the abnormally positioned right atrium (Figure 43-2). Such inferior vena caval distortion may limit venous return, further contributing to the development of ascites. Interestingly, increased intrathoracic pressure and tension created by the CCAM mass inhibits the formation of pleural or pericardial effusion.

In order to obtain a clearer sense of the cardiovascular physiology in CCAM lesions, we investigated the echocardiographic and Doppler characteristics that distinguish the fetal CCAM with and without hydrops.[8] In a series of 41 fetuses with CCAM, hydrops was present in 15 (37%). Those that developed hydrops had a lower cardiothoracic ratio than those without hydrops, although in both, the heart size was smaller than normal (0.18 vs. 0.23, $P = 0.001$). The fetuses with hydrops also demonstrated increased early diastolic filling, with the ratio of early filling to atrial contraction (E/A ratio) significantly higher for both tricuspid and mitral valves. In addition, the degree of reversal of flow with atrial contraction in the inferior vena cava as well as frequency of presence of umbilical venous pulsation was higher in the hydrops group. Overall systolic performance of both the right and the left ventricle appeared to be normal or hyperdynamic. These findings are consistent with a picture of impaired filling and cardiac tamponade.

In another study, we looked at echocardiographic Doppler-derived parameters of ventricular performance in 36 fetuses with CCAM at 25 weeks' gestation and compared them with age-matched controls.[9] We studied the myocardial performance index (MPI), a global measure of systolic and diastolic performance, the ejection force, a preload-dependent measure of systolic performance, and cardiac output as an overall measure of cardiovascular productivity, because cardiac output/blood flow is the end result of cardiac performance (Table 43-1). For the fetuses with CCAM, MPI values were higher than normal, suggesting worse global dysfunction, and ejection force was lower than normal, suggesting a decrease in the volume of ejection. Combined cardiac output was approximately 17% lower in the CCAM group relative to normal.

Chronic cardiac tamponade in the mature heart creates an interesting situation in which the heart must accommodate to an environment of surrounding tension and increased intrathoracic pressure. In particular, coronary

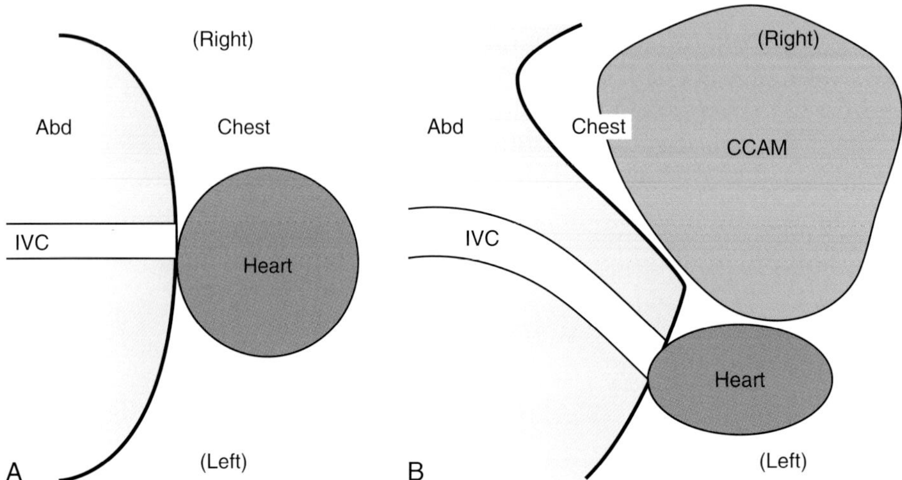

Figure 43-2. **(A)** Normal course of the inferior vena cava (IVC) as it punctures the diaphragm and enters the chest cavity and heart. Abd, abdomen. **(B)** In the presence of a large CCAM, the heart is pushed to one side and the course of the IVC can be distorted.

Table 43-1 Comparison of Parameters of Cardiac Function in Congenital Cystic Adenomatoid Malformation versus Normal Controls

VARIABLE	CCAM (N = 32)	NORMAL (N = 50)	P VALUE
GA (wk)	25.4 ± 4.0	25.5 ± 4.9	0.99
Fetal weight (kg)	1.03 ± 0.76	1.00 ± 0.69	0.84
RV MPI	0.48 ± 0.08	0.43 ± 0.05	<0.001*
LV MPI	0.39 ± 0.04	0.40 ± 0.05	0.32
RV Ej force (mN)	7.26 ± 6.24	8.44 ± 6.44	0.42
LV Ej force (mN)	6.03 ± 5.36	7.64 ± 6.76	0.24
CCO (mL/min/kg)	414 ± 87	496 ± 84	<0.001*

CCO, combined cardiac output; Ej force, ejection force; GA, gestational age; LV, left ventricle; MPI, myocardial performance index; RV, right ventricle.

*Statistically significant.

Data from Szwast A, Tian Z, McCann M, et al. Impact of altered loading conditions on ventricular performance in fetuses with congenital cystic adenomatoid malformation and twin-twin transfusion syndrome. *Ultrasound Obstet Gynecol.* 2007;30:40-46.

perfusion pressure, or the pressure necessary to fill the coronary bed, is lower than normal. Coronary blood flow predominates in diastole, and in the case of markedly increased intrathoracic pressure, intracavitary myocardial pressure is elevated; hence, there is less of a difference between the diastolic pressure of the aorta and the diastolic pressure of the myocardium. Less perfusion pressure is needed to fill the coronary circulatory bed. For the fetus with CCAM, this has important implications for treatment, either before or after birth. With sudden relief of chronic tamponade such as with removal of the CCAM or drainage of a large cyst, coronary perfusion pressure is suddenly increased. The surrounding diastolic myocardial pressure is acutely lowered and there is a need for a greater perfusion pressure to fill the coronary bed, this at a time of decreased preload because the heart is still likely to be underfilled. This phenomenon can create an acute mismatch between coronary circulatory demand and supply, resulting in myocardial ischemia. We have witnessed this acute decompensation with development of severe systolic dysfunction, marked bradycardia, and valvar regurgitation during treatment of CCAM, in particular, during fetal surgical resection.[10] Increasing preload through volume infusion can mitigate against this process.

Prenatal Management and Outcomes

Ultrasound and MRI can provide the information necessary to properly diagnose and manage fetal CCAM. The evaluation consists of assessment of the mass and its consequences on the cardiovascular system.

Location and size of the CCAM mass should be evaluated. A metric has been developed to assess mass size and aid in prognosis, the CCAM volume–to–head circumference ratio (CVR).[11] The CCAM volume (mL) is sonographically measured using the formula for an ellipse (length × height × width × 0.52) and is divided by the head circumference to correct for differences in fetal gestational age. High-risk CCAM lesions have a CVR greater than 1.6 or are lesions having a significant macrocystic component. The size of the defect measured in this manner has guided our degree of scrutiny and surveillance, because those with high-risk lesions are seen frequently with multiple visits per week for ultrasound and echocardiographic evaluation whereas those with CVR less than 1.2 can be evaluated once weekly. The greatest degree of potential change occurs between 18 and 26 weeks' gestation. This period demands the most frequent scrutiny and surveillance. The fastest growth in the CVR appears to occur between 20 and 25 weeks with a peak at 25 weeks' gestation.[1] Thereafter, there is a plateau, with actual regression in size with decreases in CVR commonly observed after 29 weeks. Microcystic lesions are more likely to regress than macrocystic CCAM lesions.

At serial fetal echocardiography, early signs of hydrops should be carefully looked for. Cardiothoracic ratio is measured, as is the degree of distortion of the inferior vena cava as it traverses the subdiaphragmatic region and enters the right side of the heart. The degree of diastolic reversal with atrial contraction in the inferior vena cava is measured just below the diaphragm and the umbilical vein is sampled for any evidence of pulsations. We have not found the patterns of ductus venosus flow to be of use in discriminating for prognosis. The region of insertion of the ductus venosus into the heart can be quite distorted, twisted, and narrowed due to inversion of the diaphragm and increased intrathoracic pressure. The ductus venosus may, therefore, not be a valid site for assessing cardiovascular hemodynamics as a reflection of atrial pressure in the fetus with CCAM.

If there is frank hydrops or signs of impending hydrops based on CVR, presence of large macrocystic lesions, and cardiovascular indicators such as umbilical venous pulsations, low cardiothoracic ratio, or low cardiac output, there may be an indication for fetal intervention. Expectant management without intervention in such cases is usually lethal because hydrops will not reverse without aggressive management, leading to fetal demise.

A number of options for fetal treatment of CCAM are at present available. If there are serious anomalies associated or chromosomal anomalies present, the fetus may not be a candidate for fetal intervention. If there are no other anomalies and the fetus is less than 32 weeks' gestation and has a single or multiple dominant cysts visible, fetal thoracoamniotic shunting is an appropriate approach. A shunt can be positioned through percutaneous techniques. Such a maneuver can reduce mass volume, ameliorate cardiac tamponade physiology, and improve filling of the heart leading to reduction or prevention of hydrops. At CHOP, we reviewed a series of 23 pregnancies with macrocystic CCAM in which ultrasound-guided thoracoamniotic shunting was performed.[1,12] Eleven were left-sided and 12 were right-sided lesions. Fetal hydrops was present in 18 and polyhydramnios in 11. Mean gestational age at shunt placement was 22 weeks. Mean CVR before shunt placement was 2.4, which was reduced to 0.7 after shunting. Prenatal outcome for these 23 shunted fetuses was 22 live-born and 1 intrauterine demise, but there was 5 subsequent neonatal deaths. Hence, overall survival was 17 of 23 or 74%.

If no dominant cyst is seen (microcystic CCAM) and the fetus is considered high risk for demise, open fetal surgery in order to remove the mass may be considered.[2,13] Removal of a fetal CCAM mass has been demonstrated to result in resolution of hydrops and to promote resumption of growth of normal lung tissue, allowing for adequate gas exchange at birth.

The techniques for fetal surgery are as follows. The uterus is incised and a small portion of the fetus is exposed in order to perform a thoracotomy and/or lobectomy of the mass containing the CCAM. Continuous echocardiographic monitoring of fetal heart function is performed because a sudden acute decrease in intrathoracic pressure may impair coronary perfusion (see "Prenatal Physiology," earlier). Intravenous access to the fetus is achieved and volume infused so as to maximize preload during mass extraction. Our group performed open fetal surgery for resection of giant intrathoracic mass in 24 cases at 21 to 31 weeks' gestation. There are currently 13 healthy survivors at 1 to 16 years of follow-up. In these 13 survivors, fetal CCAM resection led to resolution of hydrops within 1 to 2 weeks of surgery with return of the mediastinum to the midline and continued in utero lung growth. Follow-up neurodevelopmental testing has been normal in these survivors. Of the 11 fetal deaths after fetal surgery, 6 occurred intraoperatively with the previously described phenomenon of acute release of cardiac tamponade causing sudden visualization of the coronary arteries on continuous echocardiographic monitoring, a sign of coronary vasodilation in response to perfusion supply and demand mismatch. Marked bradycardia, perhaps due to sinus node ischemia, ventricular dysfunction, and severe tricuspid regurgitation followed with inability to successfully resuscitate.

If the fetus is greater than 32 weeks' gestation, delivery may be considered with performance of the EXIT procedure (ex utero intrapartum treatment).[14] The fetus is partially delivered via cesarean section and the chest exposed for thoracotomy. While still connected to maternal placental circulation, the CCAM mass can then be excised. This maximizes the potential for lung function and the neonate's own respiration once placental separation takes place. If respiratory insufficiency is present at birth, extracorporeal membrane oxygenation (ECMO) may be offered if the fetus is beyond 34 weeks' gestation and greater than 2000 g in weight. Our group at CHOP reported on nine fetuses with intrathoracic lung lesions that underwent EXIT procedure. The mean gestational age at EXIT delivery was 35 weeks. The lesions were large and remained large throughout gestation with CVR of 2.5 at initial evaluation and CVR of 2.2 at EXIT. Average time on placental bypass until separation was 65 minutes. Eight of the nine neonates survived. Postnatal complications included death from bleeding in one. ECMO was utilized successfully in four neonates for persistent pulmonary hypertension.

Another promising and intriguing therapy reported for fetal treatment of large CCAM is the use of high-dose steroids.[15] Maternal betamethasone administration has shown to improve survival in a series of fetuses with CCAM and CVR greater than 1.6, five of whom had early signs of hydrops. Although CCAM size was not significantly reduced, survival in a group that would have been expected to do poorly was possible in all. The mechanism of action is not clear but may involve improved tolerance to cardiac tamponade physiology.

Postnatal Physiology and Management and Outcomes

A majority of fetuses with prenatal identification of CCAM have regression of the mass in the third trimester. These fetuses may undergo vaginal delivery and have a postnatal elective resection of the mass at 5 to 8 weeks of life. In general, postnatal resection is performed at our center in order to reduce the risk of infection, pneumothorax, and malignant transformation, which may occur. Large CCAM lesions may impair respiratory function at birth by impairing proper lung growth, resulting in pulmonary hypoplasia. The EXIT procedure is an appropriate therapeutic strategy for these, as discussed previously.

Our understanding of the natural and "unnatural" treated history of fetal CCAM has expanded substantially. This anomaly can function as a model for how we should approach lethal congenital anomalies in the fetus in general. Through advances in fetal imaging and therapy, overall outcome based on appropriate prenatal stratification of care appears to be quite good for this heterogeneous and complex anomaly.

Imaging Essentials and Important Points

- Serial echocardiographic evaluation of the fetus with intrathoracic lung lesions such as CCAM should include assessment of cardiothoracic ratio, degree of distortion of trajectory and position of the inferior vena cava in relation to its entrance into the heart, degree of reversal of flow in the inferior vena cava, and presence of umbilical venous pulsations.
- Early signs of hydrops such as scalp edema and ascites should be evaluated. Pleural effusion or pericardial effusions are not seen in CCAM because of increased intrathoracic pressure.
- Measurement of combined cardiac output will reveal low flow as a reflection of decreased preload and poor ventricular filling
- Prominence of pulmonary veins on the same side as the lung mass may be seen. Pulmonary venous flow may be increased as a consequence of increased venous return from a well-vascularized lung mass or, alternatively, increased intrathoracic pressure may distort and twist the pulmonary veins, resulting in relative stenosis and the appearance of color aliasing upon color Doppler imaging.
- Echocardiography plays an essential role in stratifying disease severity and also in monitoring treatment effect, in particular during rapid reduction or elimination of lung mass size and acute elimination of tamponade physiology. Visualization of coronary arteries on two-dimensional or color Doppler imaging during treatment is an ominous sign suggesting coronary insufficiency.

References

1. Wilson RD, Hedrick HL, Liechty KW, et al. Cystic adenomatoid malformation of the lung: review of genetics, prenatal diagnosis, and in utero treatment. *Am J Med Genet A*. 2006;140: 151-155.
2. Adzick NS. Management of fetal lung lesions. *Clin Perinatol*. 2009;36:363-376, x.
3. Mann S, Wilson RD, Bebbington MW, Adzick NS, Johnson MP. Antenatal diagnosis and management of congenital cystic adenomatoid malformation. *Semin Fetal Neonatal Med*. 2007;12: 477-481.
4. Olutoye OO, Coleman BG, Hubbard AM, Adzick NS. Prenatal diagnosis and management of congenital lobar emphysema. *J Pediatr Surg*. 2000;35:792-795.
5. Peranteau WH, Merchant AM, Hedrick HL, et al. Prenatal course and postnatal management of peripheral bronchial atresia: association with congenital cystic adenomatoid malformation of the lung. *Fetal Diagn Ther*. 2008;24:190-196.
6. Kulwa E, Tharakan T, Baxi L. Congenital cystic adenomatoid malformation in the fetus: a hypothesis of its development. *Fetal Diagn Ther*. 2005;20:472-474.
7. Husler MR, Wilson RD, Rychik J, et al. Prenatally diagnosed fetal lung lesions with associated conotruncal heart defects: is there a genetic association? *Prenat Diagn*. 2007;27:1123-1128.
8. Mahle WT, Rychik J, Tian ZY, et al. Echocardiographic evaluation of the fetus with congenital cystic adenomatoid malformation. *Ultrasound Obstet Gynecol*. 2000;16:620-624.
9. Szwast A, Tian Z, McCann M, et al. Impact of altered loading conditions on ventricular performance in fetuses with congenital cystic adenomatoid malformation and twin-twin transfusion syndrome. *Ultrasound Obstet Gynecol*. 2007;30:40-46.
10. Rychik J, Tian Z, Cohen MS, et al. Acute cardiovascular effects of fetal surgery in the human. *Circulation*. 2004;110:1549-1556.
11. Crombleholme TM, Coleman B, Hedrick H, et al. Cystic adenomatoid malformation volume ratio predicts outcome in prenatally diagnosed cystic adenomatoid malformation of the lung. *J Pediatr Surg*. 2002;37:331-338.
12. Wilson RD, Baxter JK, Johnson MP, et al. Thoracoamniotic shunts: fetal treatment of pleural effusions and congenital cystic adenomatoid malformations. *Fetal Diagn Ther*. 2004;19:413-420.
13. Adzick NS. Open fetal surgery for life-threatening fetal anomalies. *Semin Fetal Neonatal Med*. 2010;15:1-8.
14. Hedrick HL, Flake AW, Crombleholme TM, et al. The ex utero intrapartum therapy procedure for high-risk fetal lung lesions. *J Pediatr Surg*. 2005;40:1038-1043; discussion 1044.
15. Peranteau WH, Wilson RD, Liechty KW, et al. Effect of maternal betamethasone administration on prenatal congenital cystic adenomatoid malformation growth and fetal survival. *Fetal Diagn Ther*. 2007;22:365-371.

CASES

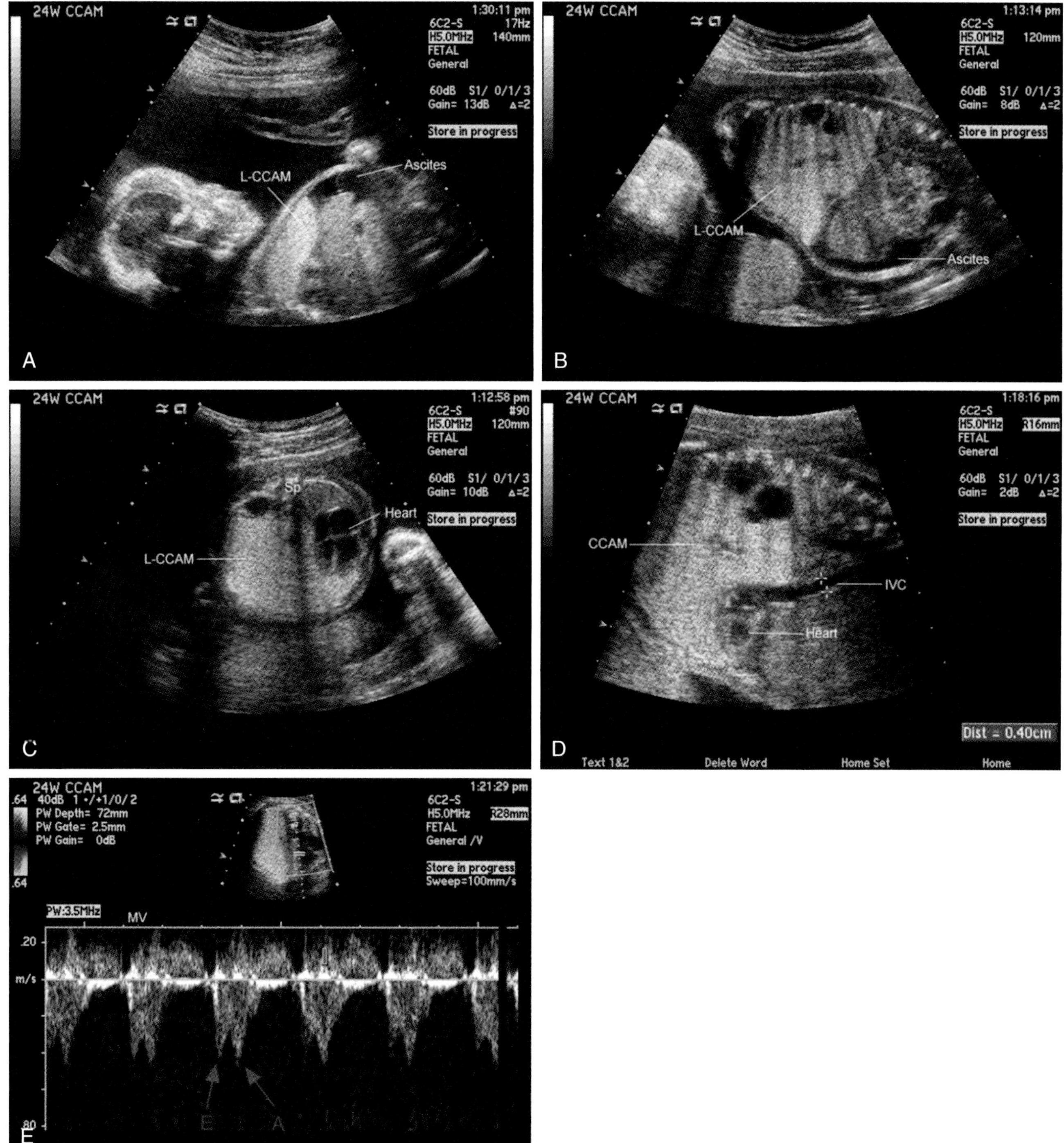

Case 43-1. **(A)** Fetus at 24 weeks' gestation with a large left congenital cystic adenomatoid malformation (CCAM). The CCAM is seen as an echo-bright dense mass within the chest, replacing normal lung tissue. There is ascites. **(B)** View of the abdomen and chest. Note the inverted diaphragm *(red arrow)*, suggesting increased intrathoracic pressure. **(C)** Cross-sectional view of the thorax. There is a large left-sided CCAM, which has shifted the heart to the right of the chest. The CCAM mass is echo-bright in comparison with the less bright small amount of normal lung tissue. **(D)** The CCAM has shifted the heart, and as a consequence, the inferior vena cava (IVC) is contorted in its course from the abdomen into the chest. **(E)** The heart is compressed and there is a tamponade physiology. As a result, the normal dominance of atrial filling with atrial contraction is blunted; hence, there is equal peak velocity for the E wave and A wave Doppler tracing across the mitral valve (MV).

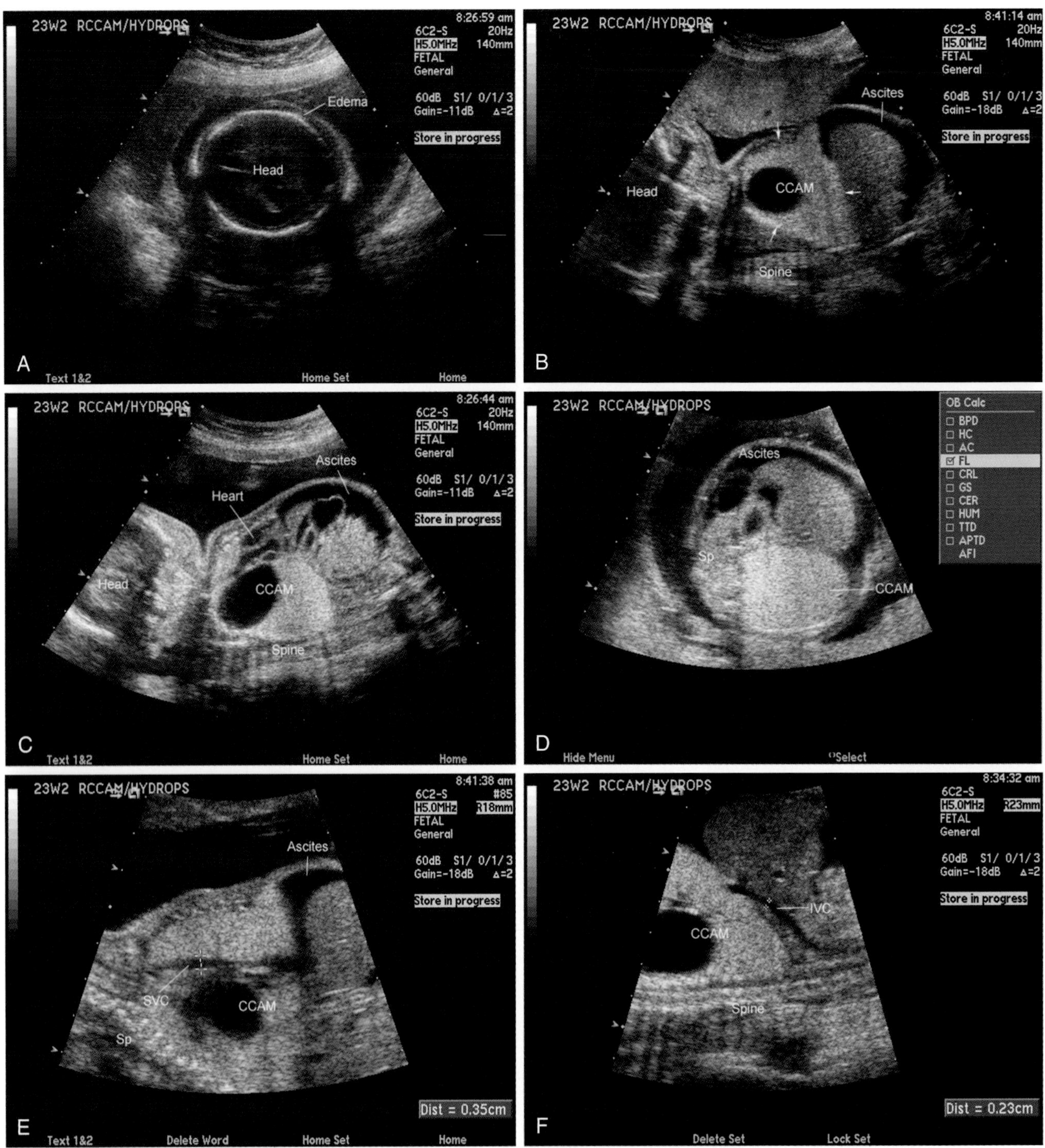

Case 43-2. (A) Fetus at 23 weeks' gestation with a large right CCAM and evidence of hydrops. Note the scalp edema. (B) The CCAM is demarcated by the *arrows*. It is echo-bright and there is a large cystic component. There is ascites. (C) The large CCAM is compressing the heart and shifting it anterior and leftward. (D) Note the difference in echo texture between the bright CCAM and the surrounding tissue. (E) The superior vena cava (SVC) is seen as it courses straight down into the heart in this horizontal view. Sp, spine. (F) The course of the IVC is distorted as it curves from posterior to anterior before entering the chest and heart.

44

Congenital Diaphragmatic Hernia

Jack Rychik

Key Echocardiographic Features

- Displacement of the cardiac position.
- Small left ventricle cavity volume.
- Assess mitral valve annulus and aortic annulus, which may be of normal size despite small left ventricle cavity volume.
- Assess aortic arch dimensions and direction of flow.
- Heart function is typically normal.

Anatomy and Anatomical Associations

Congenital diaphragmatic hernia (CDH) is a defect in the muscular diaphragm separating the chest and abdomen. Extrusion of abdominal contents into the thoracic cavity leads to pulmonary hypoplasia and pulmonary hypertension after birth.[1] CDH can be classified anatomically as Bochdalek or Morgagni type. Bochdalek hernia is most common and is a defect located in the posterolateral aspect of the diaphragm. The majority of Bochdalek hernias (85%) occur on the left side, some on the right side, and occasionally, it can be bilateral. Because the liver is situated on the right, it is deemed to be somewhat protective during development. Morgagni hernias are retrosternal or parasternal diaphragmatic defects and make up 2% of cases.

CDH is often associated with other anomalies and syndromes, congenital heart disease being quite common. Congenital heart disease occurs in 11% to 15% of CDH cases without a recognizable genetic syndrome, but the incidence may be even higher when syndromes are included.[2] The spectrum of heart disease mimics what is seen in the general population, ventricular septal defect being most common. There are some reports of a slightly increased frequency of conotruncal defects with CDH as well as left-sided obstructive disease; however, these descriptions do not separate out those in which CDH is present within the context of a syndrome that may also favor a particular type of heart defect.

CDH is associated with a number of structural abnormalities of the fetal heart.[3] Myocardial mass in CDH is smaller than normal. Left ventricular dimensions, in particular cavity size and wall thickness, are smaller than normal. Left ventricular "hypoplasia" has been described; however, left ventricular smallness in CDH is quite possibly a consequence of an underfilled ventricular cavity than true hypoplasia of the cavity due to abnormal development, because the mitral and aortic valve annulus diameters are typically within range of normal limits for gestational age or only slightly smaller. However, there are conflicting data on this matter.

The most important impact of CDH is on development of lung hypoplasia and pulmonary vascular disease. This feature dictates the clinical severity of the disease and its management.

Frequency, Genetics, and Development

CDH occurs in 1 of every 2000 to 4000 live births and makes up approximately 8% of all birth defects. Prenatal ultrasound has increased the prevalence of CDH, because it is now possible to capture many severe cases for which intensive perinatal management can be offered and in which survival would previously have been unlikely.

Formation of the diaphragm and separation between the chest and the abdomen takes place between the third and eighth week of gestation. CDH occurs as a defect in muscle formation, or fusion, of the various components that contribute to the diaphragm. If the diaphragm is incomplete, the intestines, stomach and liver can migrate into the chest cavity during critical times of lung development, leading to pulmonary hypoplasia. The effect is greatest on the side of the herniation; however, forces may impair normal development of the contralateral lung as well.

Bowel herniation into the chest cavity during critical periods of lung development results in inadequate formation of the bronchial tree, limiting airway divisions. Normally, airway development results in 23 to 35 generations of airway division, whereas in CDH only 12 to 14 develop on the affected side and 16 to 18 on the contralateral side. Alveolarization is reduced as well and there is functional deficiency in the surfactant and antioxidant systems. Pulmonary vascular development parallels airway development. CDH leads to abnormal formation of the pulmonary arterioles with increased muscularization, with far fewer arterial branches and truncated arborization.[4]

Although most of the structural abnormalities seen in CDH are presumed related to mechanical factors due to bowel contents in the thorax, some data suggest the presence of intrinsic abnormalities of the myocardium. A nitrofen-induced rat model for CDH has been extensively studied. Investigators have shown evidence for thinning of the myocardium and left ventricular smallness with down-regulation of various growth factors, independent of the degree of mechanical displacement.[5,6] Alterations in extracellular matrix and myocardial immaturity have also been described.[7] These studies suggest that an associated inherent developmental abnormality of the myocardium may exist in the fetus with CDH.

Whereas a number of syndromes are associated with CDH,[8] a few in particular are highly associated with congenital heart disease and are listed in Table 44-1.[2]

Table 44-1 Syndromes in which Congenital Diaphragmatic Hernia Is Associated with Congenital Heart Malformations

SYNDROME	FREQUENCY OF CONGENITAL HEART DISEASE	TYPE
Wolf-Hirschhorn syndrome (deletion 4p)	30-50%	ASD secundum, PS, VSD
Trisomy 18	95%	VSD, TOF, DORV, polyvalvar dysplasia
Brachmann-de Lange syndrome	25%	ASD, VSD, PS
Simpson-Golabi-Behmel syndrome	26%	No specific type
Fryns' syndrome	50%	ASD, VSD, conotruncal anomalies
Thoracoabdominal syndrome	50%	No specific type
Teratogen exposure—vitamin A	45%	VSD, defects of aorticopulmonary septation, aortic anomalies
Teratogen exposure—nitrofen (rats)	60%	Conotruncal anomalies, outflow tract anomalies, aortic arch anomalies

ASD, atrial septal defect; DORV, double-outlet right ventricle; PS, pulmonary stenosis; TOF, tetralogy of Fallot; VSD, ventricular septal defect.

Prenatal Physiology

CDH affects fetal cardiovascular physiology in a variety of important ways. Because the most common location for CDH is on the left, abdominal contents in the chest cavity enter the left chest and can cause mechanical compression of the heart, reducing the potential for ventricular filling. Distortion of the position of the entry site of the inferior vena cava (IVC) and ductus venosus (DV) into the floor of the right atrium due to cardiac compression can alter intracardiac flow patterns. Normally, IVC and DV flows are directed toward the foramen ovale which fill the left ventricle with relatively highly oxygenated blood in order to perfuse the essential organs of the heart and brain. In CDH, such streaming may be adversely affected owing to torsion of the heart and alteration in axis, with the IVC and DV angled away from the foramen ovale. This will limit the filling volume of the left ventricle but increase filling of the right ventricle. Enlargement of the right ventricle may further compress the left or give rise to the impression of relative size discrepancy between the two ventricles. Furthermore, pulmonary hypoplasia implies a decrease in pulmonary vascularity. Hence, pulmonary venous return is diminished in CDH because there is less lung to perfuse, further contributing to a decrease in left ventricular filling volume. Chronic underfilling and decreased preload to the left ventricle contribute to the relatively smaller left ventricular cavity size and thinner myocardial walls seen in CDH.

Chronic impaired filling probably plays a more important role in contributing to left ventricular smallness in CDH than actual pressure-induced mechanical compression. First, there is a general relationship between the degree of pulmonary hypoplasia and the degree of myocardial mass diminution in the animal model. Second, left ventricular hypoplasia is *not* seen in cases of congenital cystic adenomatoid malformation or bronchopulmonary sequestration, lesions in which intrathoracic tension is quite high. In fact, in these anomalies, pulmonary venous return is greater than normal, which further supports the notion that it is volume depletion and not increased pressure that is the predominant factor leading to left ventricular changes in CDH.

Prenatal Management

Ultrasound and magnetic resonance imaging (MRI) evaluation are helpful in planning a management strategy and in stratifying risk in the fetus with CDH.[9] Assessment of the location of the defect and identification of the position of the organs are important.[10] The position of the liver is critical, because those fetuses with the liver "up" in the chest have greater likelihood for pulmonary hypoplasia and have a poorer prognosis. Determination of the liver position can be made by ultrasound; however, fetal MRI provides a clearer image of the relationship of the liver to adjacent lung tissue, which may appear of similar echodensity on ultrasound.[11]

The "lung-head ratio" (LHR) is an index for measuring the degree of lung hypoplasia present and is determined by calculating the lung volume present on the side of the defect indexed to the head circumference. Controversy exists as to the best way to calculate the LHR and for its prognostic value; however, many have used it as a general way of gauging the severity of disease. The lower the LHR the worse the pulmonary hypoplasia and prognosis. A review of our experience at Children's Hospital of Philadelphia (CHOP) with 89 fetuses found that a low LHR of less than 1.0 predicted increased likelihood of needing extracorporeal membrane oxygenation (ECMO) support (75%) and poorer survival (35%); however, when LHR was measured at less than 24 weeks' gestation, it was much less predictive.[12] Liver position was a much better predictor of outcome. Whereas liver "up" fetuses required ECMO support in 80% of cases and survival was 45%, survival for those with liver "down" exceeded 90%.

Cardiovascular evaluation via fetal echocardiography is indicated in all fetuses with CDH, because the presence of significant congenital heart disease is common and seriously affects survival. When no congenital heart disease is present, echocardiography should focus on the degree of heart distortion within the chest and the change in cardiac axis. Left ventricular dimensions should be measured with particular attention to the mitral and aortic annulus diameters, because if these are normal, the left ventricular cavity size is likely to be normal as well (when there is an intact ventricular septum, as the mitral valve goes . . . so goes the ventricle!). The aortic arch can oftentimes appear slightly small in CDH and its course is distorted in the mediastinum, making it difficult to identify the presence of a coarctation of the aorta.[13,14] Measurements of the isthmus may be helpful; however, confident determination of arch anatomy in CDH, and ruling out a coarctation of the aorta when arch structures appear small, must oftentimes await postnatal evaluation.

Much effort has been exerted in finding an appropriate in utero treatment strategy for CDH. Early efforts at open fetal surgery with direct CDH repair yielded results that were no better than conventional postnatal management.[15] With improvements in postnatal care and neonatal outcome, fetal intervention for CDH is reserved for those with the worst prospects for good outcome.

The notion of increasing airway pressure to mechanically induce lung growth and development is currently of great interest. It has been argued that increased airway pressure can actually result in growth of normal lung tissue and vasculature. Initially, this was achieved through open techniques utilizing tracheal clips; however, currently, this can be achieved through a laparoscopic approach using a detachable balloon. The benefits of such a fetal endoscopic tracheal occlusion (FETO) procedure include (1) the lack of need for open uterine incision and its potential consequences of premature labor, (2) it is a relatively quick procedure performed under local anesthetic, and (3) there is the ability to percutaneously deflate the balloon before delivery. FETO has been demonstrated to be an effective strategy when undertaken by experienced hands in select cases.[16,17]

Investigators have looked at cardiac dimensions and measures of performance in CDH.[18] As expected, in comparison with normal matched controls, end-diastolic and end-systolic dimensions were smaller by 32% and 37%, respectively. However, measures of ventricular systolic and diastolic function including ejection fraction, shortening fraction, ratio of early filling (E wave) to atrial filling (A wave) velocities, and the myocardial performance index (MPI) were no different from normal.

Postnatal Physiology and Management

Following placental separation, the newborn with CDH is challenged to provide for adequate ventilation and oxygenation using its own lungs. If lung volume and pulmonary vasculature are abnormal, there will be substantially increased pulmonary vascular resistance with hypoxemia. If pulmonary vascular resistance exceeds systemic resistance, there will be right-to-left shunting at the level of the ductus arteriosus (DA).[19] Attempts to close the DA in such a scenario can result in severe right ventricular dysfunction and poor cardiac output because blood will have no easy way to exit the right side of the heart. Therefore, ductal patency is useful in the case of severe CDH. Other findings in the face of markedly elevated pulmonary vascular resistance and high right ventricular pressure will be right-to-left shunting at the atrial level and tricuspid regurgitation. A "pop-off" at the atrial level will allow for maintenance of cardiac output through left ventricular filling, although at the expense of oxygenation. One strategy to deal with this situation is to place the infant onto ECMO support until pulmonary vascular resistance can be lowered through pharmacological means and the passage of time.

Postnatal echocardiography plays an important role in the management of the infant with CDH. Assessment of overall heart function and, in particular, the degree of filling of the left ventricle cavity can provide a guide to management, for example, the need to increase volume delivery or the use of inotropes. Tricuspid regurgitation is commonly seen and can provide a means for measuring right ventricular pressure. If right ventricular pressure exceeds the blood pressure, there may be constriction of the DA, limiting right-to-left shunting and impairing systemic perfusion. We have found that, if there is severe tricuspid regurgitation, either the DA is constricted or there is myocardial ischemia causing the tricuspid valve to be incompetent. A careful assessment of the left side of the heart should be undertaken, in particular, the size and flow patterns within the aortic arch and isthmus. A relatively normal size mitral and aortic valve annulus will predict for an adequate size left ventricle, regardless of the appearance of the left ventricular cavity size. Marked right ventricular hypertension, dilation, and hypertrophy may further compress a slightly small and underfilled left ventricle. Reversal of flow in the isthmus in a retrograde manner from the DA is possible when the left ventricle is markedly underfilled and compressed and does not necessarily suggest for the presence of structural left ventricular inadequacy. We have found this finding to be present most commonly within the first few hours or days of birth. With better control of pulmonary hypertension and improved filling of the left ventricle, aortic flow will then revert back to a normal antegrade pattern in the isthmus and transverse arch. Serial evaluation of the neonate with CDH is of value in order to assess heart function, degree of tricuspid regurgitation, direction of flow within the DA, and direction of flow in the aortic isthmus and transverse aorta, all of which can paint a picture of overall disease status and response to treatment.

When prenatal evaluation predicts a poor prognosis such as in the case of a CDH with liver "up" and a low LHR, a planned "EXIT (ex utero intrapartum technique) to ECMO" strategy may be implemented.[20] The fetus can be partially delivered via cesarean section, and while still on placental bypass, neck cannulation for ECMO can be safely achieved, providing for a relatively smooth transition.

Outcomes

Management strategies and outcomes for CDH have improved substantially. With better understanding of prenatal risk factors and the use of ECMO has come improved selection of patient specific strategies, which have resulted in overall better survival. Newer strategies in neonatal ventilation have also contributed to better outcomes. Nevertheless, survival for the fetus with CDH and congenital heart disease remains relatively poor, but it is to a degree dependent upon the type of heart anomaly present.[21] If there is CDH and heart disease in association with a syndrome, outcome is extremely poor and families should be counseled appropriately. However, a fetus with the presence of CDH without evidence of a syndrome and with relatively good predictors such as liver "down" and an LHR greater than 1.4 may do quite well if associated with, for example, a large ventricular septal defect. More complex lesions such as conotruncal anomalies may become a greater challenge. Oftentimes, we are faced with the unfortunate situation of diagnosing a fetus with CDH and single-ventricle type of heart disease. The entire premise for a successful single-ventricle strategy greatly depends upon pristine lung function in order to accommodate passive venous flow at the cavopulmonary connection surgery. For this reason, the combination of CDH and single-ventricle type of heart disease is a lethal one because it is essentially impossible for such patients to have completely normal lung function, unless the CDH is small.

As success with early postnatal management CDH continues to improve, an increasing number of long-term survivors are presenting for follow-up. The outcomes are mixed and, as expected, depend upon the severity of disease and the nature of the immediate postnatal course. Many children continue to have evidence for residual pulmonary hypertension[22] or have neurodevelopmental impairment. Those with pulmonary hypertension may benefit from many of the new drugs available for treatment such as sildenafil or budesonide. The survivors of CDH will continue to require lifelong evaluation and care.

Imaging Essentials and Important Points

- Congenital heart disease is a relatively common finding associated with CDH. Inspect the septum carefully with two-dimensional color Doppler imaging in order to identify any muscular ventricular septal defects that may be present.
- Measurement of the mitral annulus and aortic annulus will provide a sense of the degree of left ventricular hypoplasia that may be present. Small, compressed-appearing left ventricles may in fact have a normal mitral valve annulus, suggesting adequacy of the left ventricular size for postnatal systemic perfusion.
- In CDH, the length of the left ventricle will commonly be normal and extend to the apex of the heart; however, the short-axis, midcavitary diameter may appear small, reflecting chronic underfilling.
- In CDH, flow across the foramen ovale may not appear as a "brisk" right-to-left flow, or in fact, the flap valve of the foramen may appear in a neutral position, because the internal geometry of the heart and patterns of streaming can be altered in the face of cardiac displacement within the chest.
- Attention should be paid to the aortic arch, its size, and flow patterns. With limited left ventricular filling and decreased aortic volumetric ejection, the amount of flow traversing the aortic isthmus is diminished in comparison with normal, which can be a setup for development of coarctation of the aorta. This can be a challenge to diagnose before birth, but it may also be a challenge after birth in the face of a wide-open DA and right-to-left shunting due to pulmonary hypertension.

References

1. Grisaru-Granovsky S, Rabinowitz R, Ioscovich A, Elstein D, Schimmel M. Congenital diaphragmatic hernia: review of the literature in reflection of unresolved dilemmas. *Acta Paediatr.* 2009;98: 1874-1881.
2. Lin AE, Pober BR, Adatia I. Congenital diaphragmatic hernia and associated cardiovascular malformations: type, frequency, and impact on management. *Am J Med Genet C Semin Med Genet.* 2007;145C:201-216.
3. Allan LD, Irish MS, Glick PL. The fetal heart in diaphragmatic hernia. *Clin Perinatol.* 1996;23:795-812.
4. Nobuhara KK, Wilson JM. Pathophysiology of congenital diaphragmatic hernia. *Semin Pediatr Surg.* 1996;5:234-242.
5. Correia-Pinto J, Baptista MJ, Pedrosa C, Estevao-Costa J, Flake AW, Leite-Moreira AF. Fetal heart development in the nitrofen-induced CDH rat model: the role of mechanical and nonmechanical factors. *J Pediatr Surg.* 2003;38:1444-1451.
6. Takayasu H, Sato H, Sugimoto K, Puri P. Downregulation of GATA4 and GATA6 in the heart of rats with nitrofen-induced diaphragmatic hernia. *J Pediatr Surg.* 2008;43:362-366.
7. Guarino N, Shima H, Puri P. Structural immaturity of the heart in congenital diaphragmatic hernia in rats. *J Pediatr Surg.* 2001;36: 770-773.

8. Pober BR. Genetic aspects of human congenital diaphragmatic hernia. *Clin Genet.* 2008;74:1-15.
9. Kitano Y. Prenatal intervention for congenital diaphragmatic hernia. *Semin Pediatr Surg.* 2007;16:101-108.
10. Hedrick HL. Management of prenatally diagnosed congenital diaphragmatic hernia. *Semin Fetal Neonatal Med.* 2010;15:21-27.
11. Walsh DS, Hubbard AM, Olutoye OO, et al. Assessment of fetal lung volumes and liver herniation with magnetic resonance imaging in congenital diaphragmatic hernia. *Am J Obstet Gynecol.* 2000;183:1067-1069.
12. Hedrick HL, Danzer E, Merchant A, et al. Liver position and lung-to-head ratio for prediction of extracorporeal membrane oxygenation and survival in isolated left congenital diaphragmatic hernia. *Am J Obstet Gynecol.* 2007;197:422.e1-422.e4.
13. Allan LD, Chita SK, Anderson RH, Fagg N, Crawford DC, Tynan MJ. Coarctation of the aorta in prenatal life: an echocardiographic, anatomical, and functional study. *Br Heart J.* 1988;59:356-360.
14. Quartermain MD, Cohen MS, Dominguez TE, Tian Z, Donaghue DD, Rychik J. Left ventricle to right ventricle size discrepancy in the fetus: the presence of critical congenital heart disease can be reliably predicted. *J Am Soc Echocardiogr.* 2009;22:1296-1301.
15. Harrison MR, Adzick NS, Flake AW, et al. Correction of congenital diaphragmatic hernia in utero: VI. Hard-earned lessons. *J Pediatr Surg.* 1993;28:1411-1417; discussion 1417-1418.
16. Deprest J, Jani J, Gratacos E, et al. Fetal intervention for congenital diaphragmatic hernia: the European experience. *Semin Perinatol.* 2005;29:94-103.
17. Jani JC, Nicolaides KH, Gratacos E, et al. Severe diaphragmatic hernia treated by fetal endoscopic tracheal occlusion. *Ultrasound Obstet Gynecol.* 2009;34:304-310.
18. Van Mieghem T, Gucciardo L, Done E, et al. Left ventricular cardiac function in fetuses with congenital diaphragmatic hernia and the effect of fetal endoscopic tracheal occlusion. *Ultrasound Obstet Gynecol.* 2009;34:424-429.
19. Tanabe M, Yoshida H, Iwai J, Takahashi H, Ohnuma N, Terai M. Doppler flow patterns through the ductus arteriosus in patients with congenital diaphragmatic hernia. *Eur J Pediatr Surg.* 2000;10:92-95.
20. Kunisaki SM, Fauza DO, Barnewolt CE, et al. Ex utero intrapartum treatment with placement on extracorporeal membrane oxygenation for fetal thoracic masses. *J Pediatr Surg.* 2007;42:420-425.
21. Cohen MS, Rychik J, Bush DM, et al. Influence of congenital heart disease on survival in children with congenital diaphragmatic hernia. *J Pediatr.* 2002;141:25-30.
22. Schwartz IP, Bernbaum JC, Rychik J, Grunstein M, D'Agostino J, Polin RA. Pulmonary hypertension in children following extracorporeal membrane oxygenation therapy and repair of congenital diaphragmatic hernia. *J Perinatol.* 1999;19:220-226.

CASES

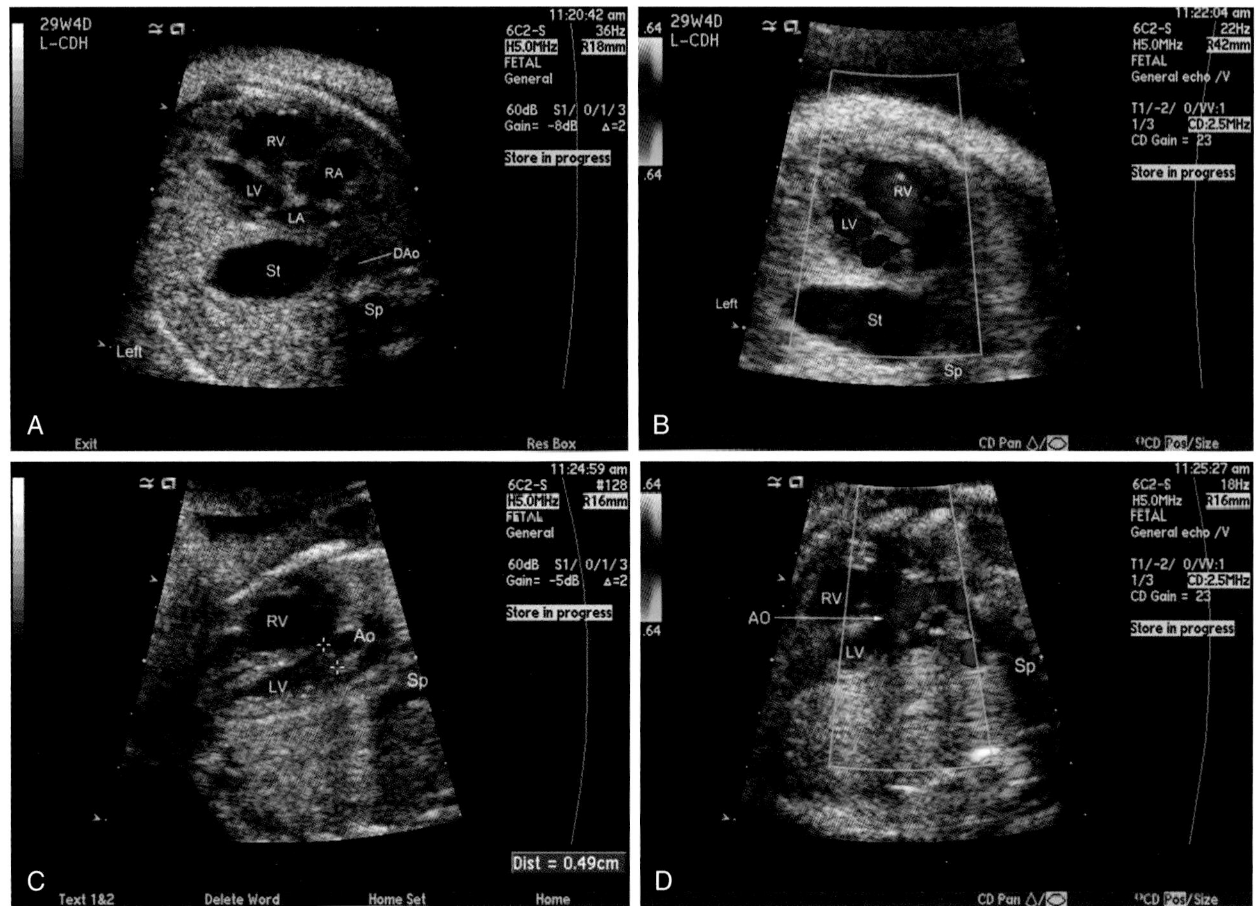

Case 44-1. **(A)** Left-sided congenital diaphragmatic hernia (CDH) in a fetus at 29 weeks' gestation. The stomach (St) is up in the chest and is positioned adjacent to the left side of the heart. Note the size discrepancy and disproportion between the left atrium (LA) and the left ventricle (LV), which appear smaller in cavity size in comparison with the right atrium (RA) and right ventricle (RV). DAo, descending aorta; Sp, spine. **(B)** Color flow imaging across the atrioventricular valves into the ventricles demonstrates limited flow into the LV. **(C)** Long-axis view of the left ventricular outflow tract. The aortic annulus measures nearly 5 mm in diameter, which is an appropriate size for a 29-week fetus. The LV appears underfilled with a small cavity volume. Nevertheless, the aorta (Ao) is well formed and of adequate size to support systemic perfusion. **(D)** Color flow imaging demonstrates a broad jet of flow across an unobstructed and good-sized aortic (AO) valve.

Continued

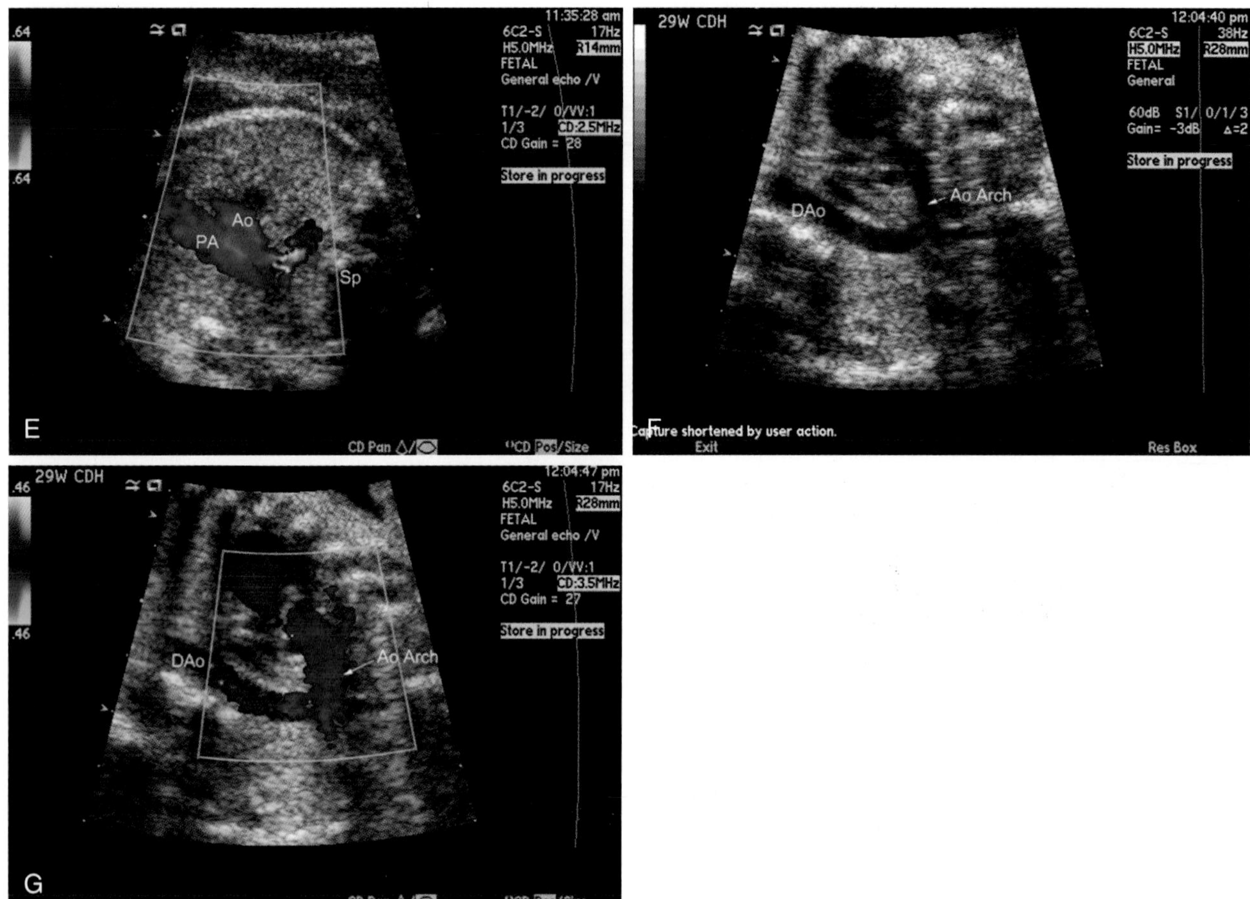

Case 44-1, cont'd **(E)** Color flow imaging in the mediastinum, modified three-vessel view. Antegrade flow, designated as a *blue color,* is seen in both the pulmonary artery (PA) and the Ao. **(F)** Two-dimensional image of the aortic arch (Ao Arch). The arch is of good size without hypoplasia. **(G)** Color flow imaging demonstrates antegrade flow around the arch, despite the limited filling of the ventricle. Based on the measures of the mitral valve, aortic valve, and aortic arch, the left-sided structures of this heart are deemed anatomically sufficient to handle the postnatal systemic perfusion.

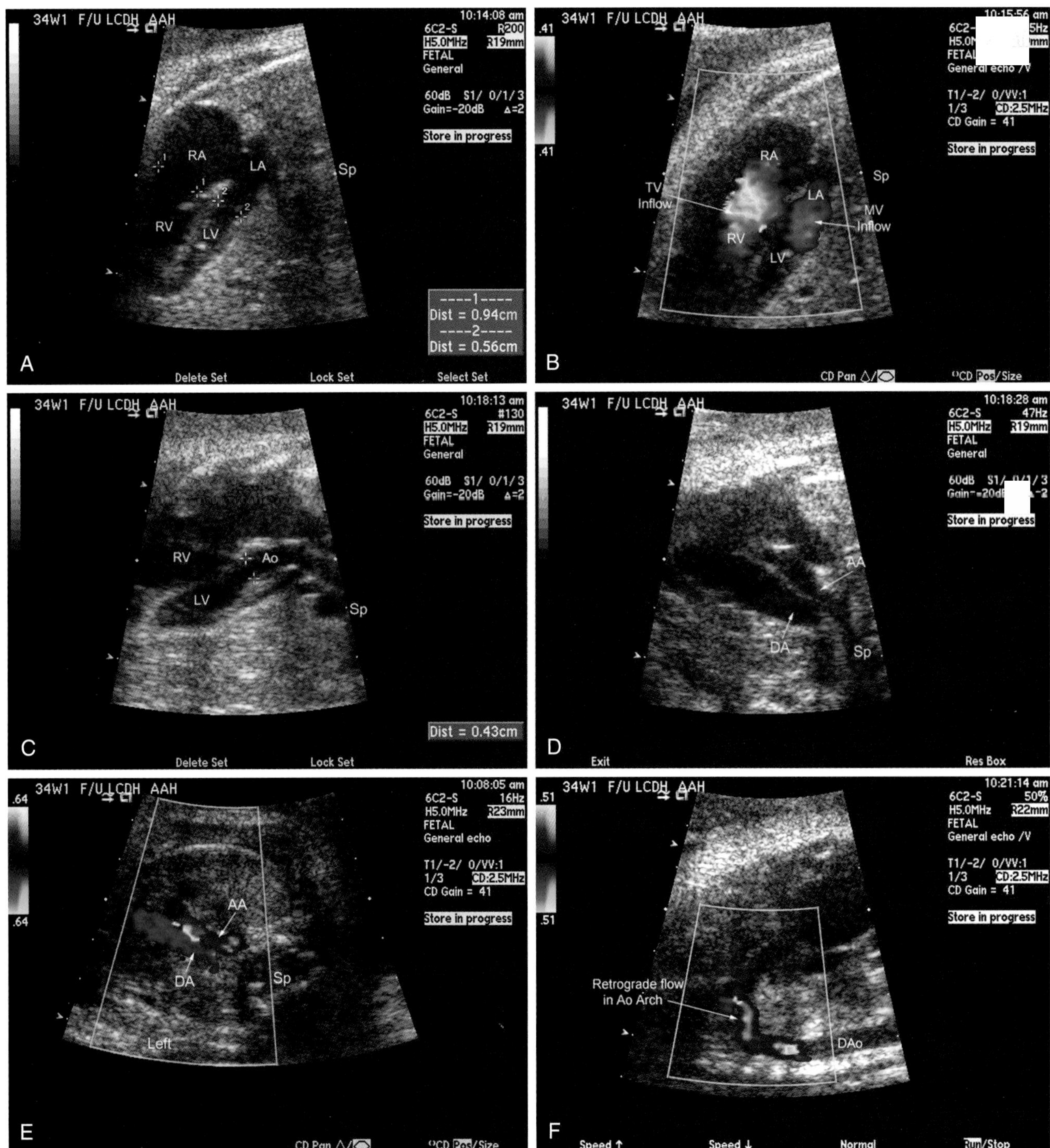

Case 44-2. **(A)** Fetus with left CDH at 34 weeks' gestation. The LV appears to reach near the apex of the heart, but the cavity is slender and underfilled. The mitral valve annulus measures 5 to 6 mm, and the tricuspid valve measures 9 to 10 mm. This suggests some element of mitral hypoplasia. LA, left atrium; RA, right atrium; RV, right ventricle; Sp, spine. **(B)** Color flow imaging demonstrates limited filling of the LV. MV, mitral valve; TV, tricuspid valve. **(C)** Long-axis view demonstrates an aortic annulus of 4 mm, which suggests mild hypoplasia at this gestational age. **(D)** Modified three-vessel view. There is marked discrepancy in size between the ductus arteriosus (DA) and the aortic arch (AA), with the aortic arch appearing smaller than normal. **(E)** Modified three-vessel view with color flow imaging. There is retrograde flow in the AA *(red)*. **(F)** Color flow imaging view of the Ao Arch demonstrates retrograde flow. The combined findings of a small left ventricular cavity volume, mild mitral and aortic valvar hypoplasia, and retrograde aortic flow raise suspicion for inadequacy of the left-sided structures to support the systemic circulation.

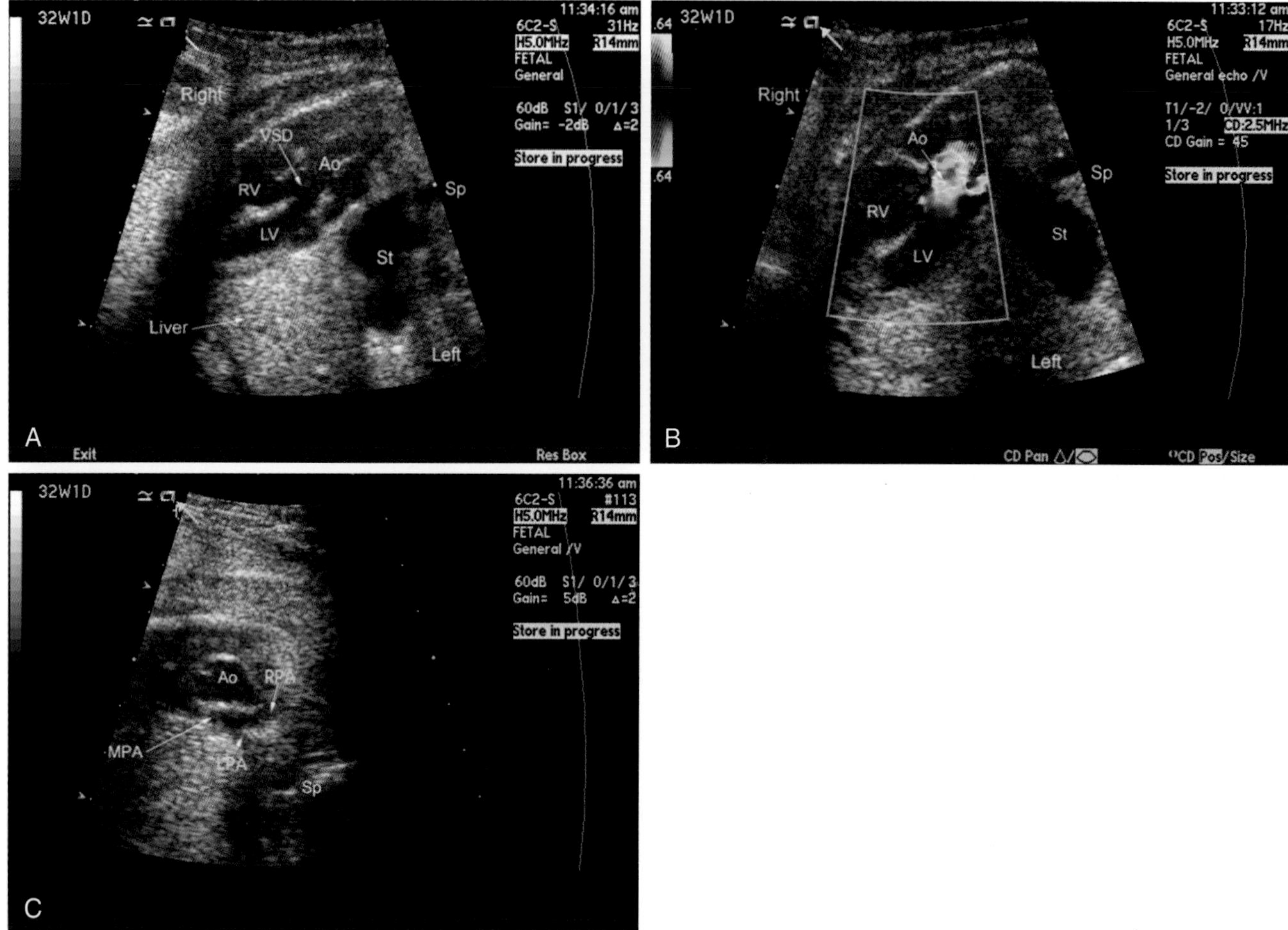

Case 44-3. **(A)** Fetus at 32 weeks' gestation with left-sided CDH and tetralogy of Fallot. Note the large ventricular septal defect (VSD) and overriding aorta (Ao). Both the stomach (St) and the liver are up in the left side of the chest and the heart is deviated to the right side of the chest. LV, left ventricle; RV, right ventricle; Sp, spine. **(B)** Color flow imaging demonstrates flow into the overriding Ao. **(C)** Short-axis view. The Ao is larger than the main pulmonary artery (MPA), as is typically seen in tetralogy of Fallot. The branch pulmonary arteries are seen arising from the MPA and narrowed right ventricular outflow tract. LPA, left pulmonary artery; RPA, right pulmonary artery.

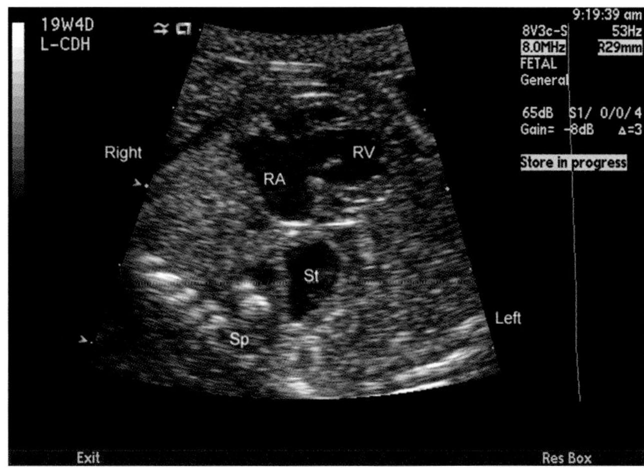

Case 44-4. A case of CDH at 19 weeks' gestation with hypoplastic left heart syndrome. A large right atrium (RA) and right ventricle (RV) are seen with the stomach (St) situated adjacent to the heart in the chest. Sp, spine.

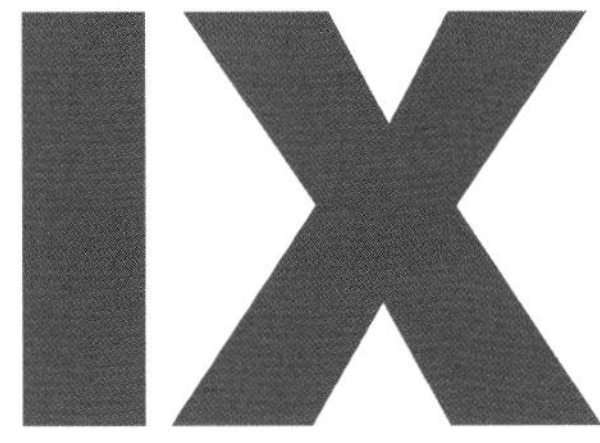

Abnormalities of the Conduction System

45 Arrhythmias in the Fetus

Matthew J. O'Connor and Maully J. Shah

Introduction

Disturbances of cardiac rhythm in the human fetus may come to clinical attention in a number of ways. First, an abnormally slow, fast, or irregular heart rate may be detected on fetal heart tone auscultation at routine prenatal visits. Second, fetal arrhythmia may manifest secondarily via its adverse hemodynamic effects; that is, nonimmune hydrops. Intrauterine fetal demise may also be the ultimate manifestation of fetal arrhythmia. Finally, arrhythmias detected in the early postnatal period are in fact continuations of previously unrecognized fetal arrhythmia.

A brief discussion of "normal" fetal electrophysiology aids the understanding of fetal arrhythmias. While the primitive heart tube begins organized contractions ("beats") by 12 days after conception, development of the fetal heart structure is not complete until 12 weeks' gestation, and development of the conduction system becomes mature at 16 weeks' gestation.[1] The developmental biology involving the generation and propagation has been reviewed,[2,3] with research concentrating on elucidating the specific mechanisms involved in differentiating specialized conduction tissues (i.e., those of the sinoatrial [SA] and atrioventricular [AV] nodes) from the primitive myocardium.

The fetal heart rate varies throughout gestation. During the first trimester, fetal heart rate ranges from approximately 110 to 180 bpm, with the maximum rate attained at about 9 weeks' gestation.[4] From this point onward in gestation, the average fetal heart rate falls to approximately 135 bpm near term, with an acceptable range of variability falling between 110 and 150 bpm.[5]

The true incidence of fetal arrhythmia remains unknown because many arrhythmias are transient, are of negligible hemodynamic significance, and therefore remain undetected. Other arrhythmias impart such a poor hemodynamic outcome (e.g., ventricular fibrillation) or are associated with major congenital abnormalities (e.g., complete heart block) that intrauterine fetal demise results. It is generally accepted that 1% to 3% of pregnancies manifest some disturbance of cardiac rhythm, with approximately 10% of these being regarded as life-threatening.[6] The remaining 90% are almost always transient, benign arrhythmia, typically as forms of atrial ectopy.

A large series of all fetal ultrasounds performed at a single center sheds some light on the proportion of fetuses with suspected arrhythmia ultimately diagnosed with a significant, potentially hemodynamically deleterious rhythm disturbance.[7] In this study, 12.3% of all referrals for fetal echocardiography were for perceived irregularities of heart rhythm, yet only 1.6% of these referrals were found to have significant arrhythmia. Isolated premature atrial contractions (PACs) were not considered "significant" in this study.[7]

The mainstay of diagnosis for fetal arrhythmia is the transabdominal fetal echocardiogram. The conceptual basis of diagnostic imaging of fetal arrhythmias is to visualize the mechanical or flow-related sequelae of electrical activity. This can be achieved through (1) careful visualization of the timing of motion of various portions of the myocardium through M-mode echocardiography or (2) the analysis of flow through various structures of the heart by Doppler echocardiography. M-mode or pulsed wave Doppler measurements taken via a sample volume encompassing both atrial and ventricular tissue allow for accurate assessment of cardiac rhythm.[8] Alternate sites of sampling may be used, for example, the superior vena cava and ascending aorta[9,10] and the pulmonary arteries and veins.[11,12]

In addition, tissue Doppler imaging has been described in the diagnosis of fetal arrhythmias.[13] The fetal electrocardiogram (ECG; electrodes placed on the mother's abdomen to detect fetal cardiac electrical activity) is unreliable at determining arrhythmias with acceptable accuracy or precision, on account of low-signal voltages. A newer, more specialized technique known as *magnetocardiography* has been utilized to gain further insights into fetal arrhythmias.[14,15] Fetal magnetocardiography creates an accurate representation of the fetal ECG, but it requires specialized equipment available at only a few referral centers.

This chapter is devoted to the definition, incidence, pathophysiology, and treatment of the most common fetal arrhythmias. These arrhythmias can be classified as follows: atrial and ventricular extrasystoles (PACs and premature ventricular contractions [PVCs]), supraventricular tachycardias (SVTs), ventricular tachycardias (VTs), and disturbances of AV conduction.

Premature Atrial and Premature Ventricular Contractions

As in children and adults, PACs and PVCs can be seen in the fetus. Such contractions will be followed by compensatory pauses in the ventricular rate. As a rule, PACs are much more common (~10 times more so) than PVCs.[6] An early study using echocardiography revealed an incidence of PACs and PVCs of 1.7% in all fetuses screened late in the third trimester.[16] In general, PACs are benign and, in isolation, are not associated with underlying disease. However, frequent PACs may herald the development of sustained tachyarrhythmia.[17] In addition, PACs are associated with structural congenital heart defects in between 1% and 10% of cases, depending on the study reviewed[18,19]; therefore, fetuses with PACs detected in utero may benefit from a complete echocardiographic assessment to rule out structural congenital heart disease (CHD). PACs commonly present in the late third trimester of pregnancy, and upon fetal echocardiographic imaging, a floppy, aneurysmal and

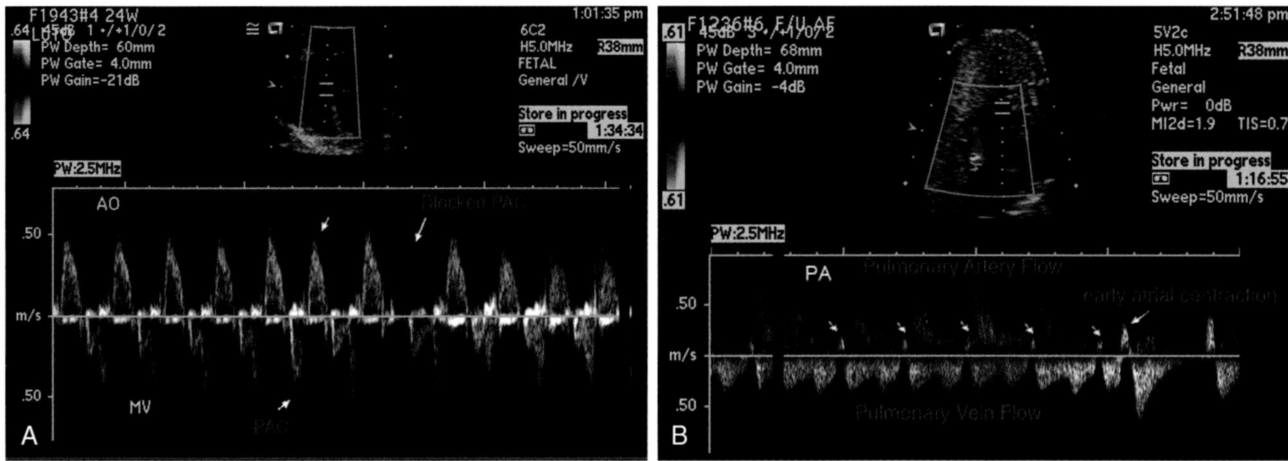

Figure 45-1. (A) Doppler sampling of simultaneous left ventricle inflow across the mitral valve (MV) and outflow across the aorta (AO). The recording sweep speed is set at 50 m/sec to maximize the number of beats in a frame in order to assess the relationship between the waveforms in multiple beats. Note the regularity of double-peak inflow across the MV for every aortic outflow waveform, up until a different waveform occurs, a premature atrial contraction (PAC; *bottom arrow*). This is a single-peak waveform because it corresponds to early atrial contraction only—there is no passive early diastolic filling. This is then followed by an associated early ventricular beat that completes the PAC *(top left arrow)*. Two beats later, there is another PAC that occurs early and is not conducted to the ventricle. This is a blocked PAC *(top right arrow)*. (B) Doppler sampling of a branch pulmonary artery (PA) and simultaneous pulmonary vein. Simultaneous sampling of arterial and venous structures can provide important insight into the timing and, hence, origin of fetal arrhythmias. The pulmonary arterial tracing is above the baseline and the pulmonary venous tracing is below the baseline. The *small arrows* point to the normal reversal of pulmonary venous flow seen with normal atrial contraction, which is identified as a small waveform above baseline. Fortunately, this can be superimposed upon the arterial waveform and provide a very nice tracing of the relationship of atrial activity to arterial systolic flow. There is a small atrial contraction waveform followed by an arterial waveform up until an early atrial contraction occurs, a PAC.

redundant atrial septum is often seen bouncing along the posterior atrial wall.

PACs may appear in a bigeminal pattern (i.e., every other beat is a PAC) (Figure 45-1). In this setting, the index of suspicion for anticipation of SVT should be higher and the fetus monitored more closely than if there are only isolated beats. PACs may also be blocked, in that the premature atrial depolarization reaches the AV node while it is still refractory (Figure 45-2). In this scenario, the resulting ventricular rate may be quite slow, on the order of 70 to 80 bpm (Figure 45-3). It is of paramount importance for diagnostic and therapeutic considerations to distinguish this entity from complete heart block.

PVCs similarly have a benign outcome in the fetus in the majority of cases. There is no association between PVCs and SVT. However, a full echocardiographic assessment is warranted to rule out structural and functional abnormalities because inflammatory processes such as myocarditis and intracardiac tumors may be associated with PVCs.

PVCs are identified when there are premature beats that occur early and originate in the ventricles (Figure 45-4). Whereas PACs originate from the atria and will "reset" the sinus node so that there is a pause in atrial activity after an early beat, PVCs are generally not conducted back to the atria and, hence, do not "reset" the sinus node. Sinus rhythm and atrial activity will continue in a regular manner, undisturbed in the presence of PVCs. Regularity of atrial activity with no disturbance in the cadence of the atrial beats is an important marker for distinguishing a premature contraction as being of ventricular, and not

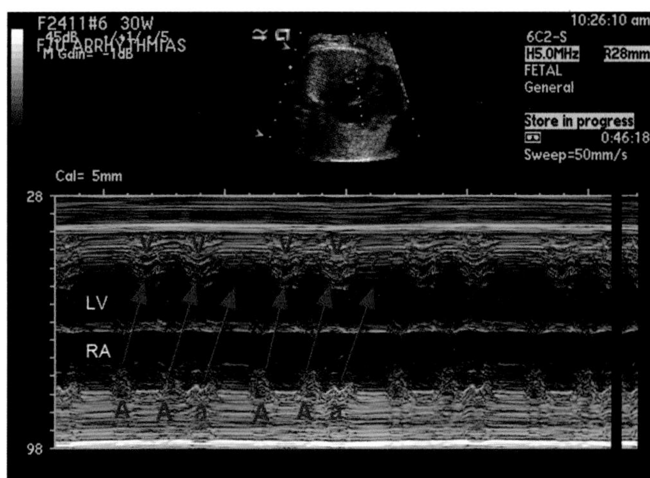

Figure 45-2. An example of blocked PACs. M-mode tracing across the left ventricle (LV; top of M-mode tracing) and the right atrium (RA; bottom of M-mode tracing). Large "A" represents a normal sinus atrial beat, small "a" represents the premature atrial contraction, and "V" is the movement of the left ventricle in response. The "A" contraction is always first in timing and is followed by a "V"; however, when an early "a" PAC occurs, there is no corresponding "V."

atrial, origin. Another way of looking at this is that in a PVC, because atrial activity and sinus node firing is not affected, the time interval between two sinus beats and the time interval between two beats that include the PVC will be identical. The sinus node continues to fire at the same cadence, despite the occurrence of a PVC (Figure 45-5). Because a PVC will occur without atrial activity, it will result in the ejection of blood without the benefit of

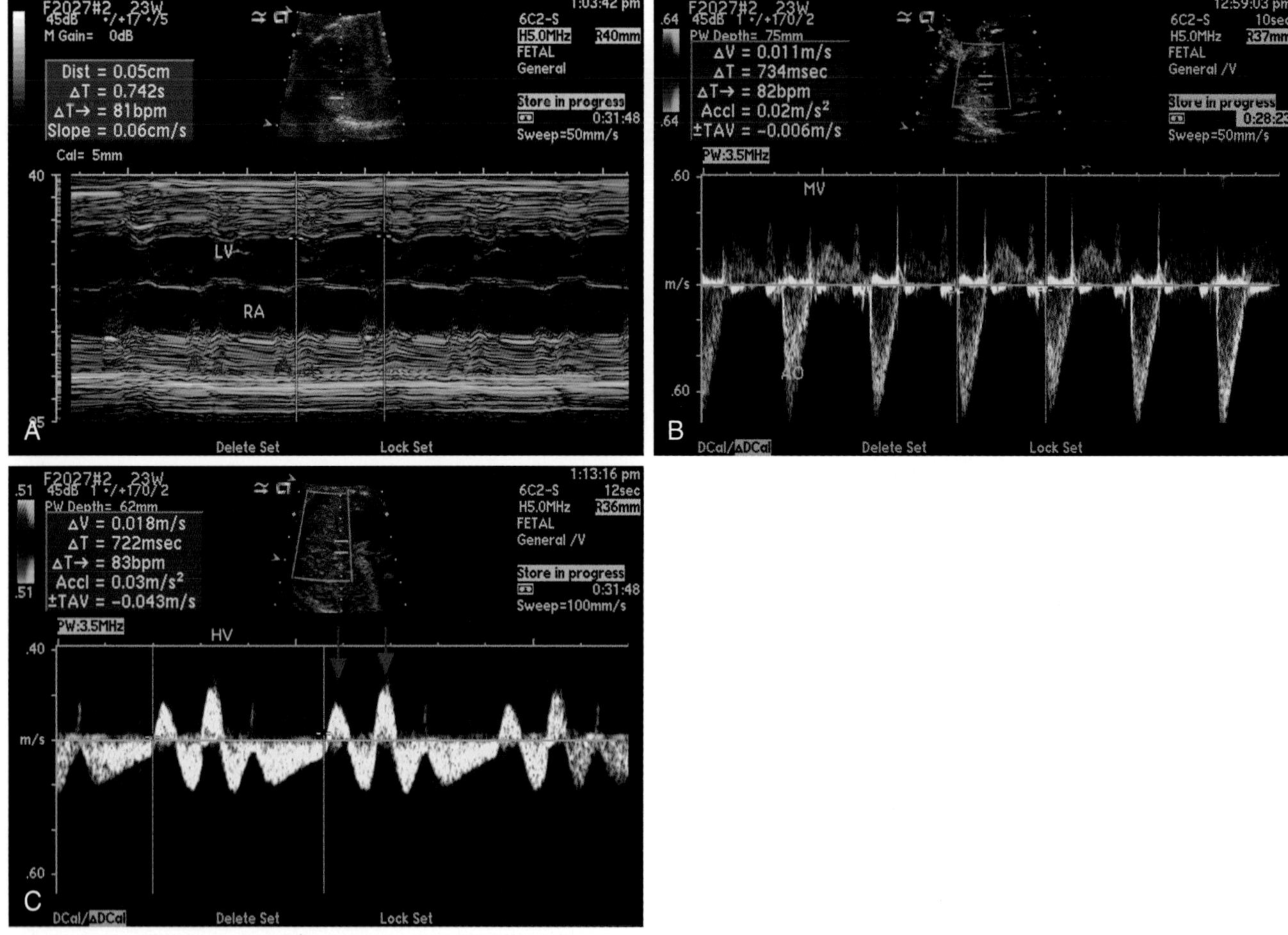

Figure 45-3. **(A)** M-mode tracing through the LV and RA of a fetus at 23 weeks' gestation with blocked PACs in an atrial bigeminy pattern. The normal sinus-related atrial contraction ("A") is quickly followed by an early PAC ("a"), which is not conducted. Hence, because only the sinus beats conduct and the PACs that are occurring in bigeminy are blocked, the overall ventricular rate is 81 bpm. **(B)** Doppler sampling of MV inflow and aortic outflow in this fetus with blocked PACs and atrial bigeminy. The ventricular outflow waveform is normal; however, early diastolic inflow waveform is augmented because it contains contribution from an early, nonconducted atrial premature beat. **(C)** Doppler sampling of a hepatic vein. There are two reversal waveforms *(arrows)* for each cardiac cycle, confirming the presence of a nonconducted premature atrial beat. The overall timing for a single cardiac cycle is equivalent to only 83 bpm.

having augmented filling through atrial contraction. Hence the stroke volume, or volume of blood ejected with a PVC, will be less than normal. This can be seen as an early beat with a lower peak velocity and smaller velocity-time integral relative to the prior sinus beats. Following the PVC, there is increased time for ventricular filling so the beat subsequent to a PVC may have augmented flow and will have an increased peak velocity and higher velocity-time integral relative to sinus beats (Figure 45-6).

Fetal Tachyarrhythmias

Supraventricular Tachycardia

SVT is the most common fetal arrhythmia having the potential for deleterious effects on fetal well-being. SVT is a nonspecific term that encompasses several arrhythmias originating above the AV node, all having different mechanisms of initiation and propagation. The prevalence of SVT in fetuses with tachycardia ranges from 66% to 90%.[20] In utero SVT has been associated with poor neonatal outcomes in a number of studies. Nonimmune hydrops is associated with SVT in 40% to 50% of cases[21]; furthermore, the response to therapy and mortality are markedly worse in hydropic fetuses.[17,18,22,23] The mechanism of hydrops in fetuses with SVT is complex, but likely relates to decreased diastolic filling time in the setting of the innately decreased ventricular compliance of the fetus during diastole relative to the adult. The adverse hemodynamics conferred by in utero tachycardia results in increased atrial and ventricular filling pressures. Such increased pressures are transmitted back through the venous system, which in turn elevates transudative forces, leading to cell and tissue edema.

In the fetus, SVT is largely (i.e., >90%) due to an orthidromic reciprocating tachycardia, in which an accessory pathway distinct from the AV node and bundle of His allows for electrical activation of the ventricle separately from typical nodal conduction.[22] Histopathology

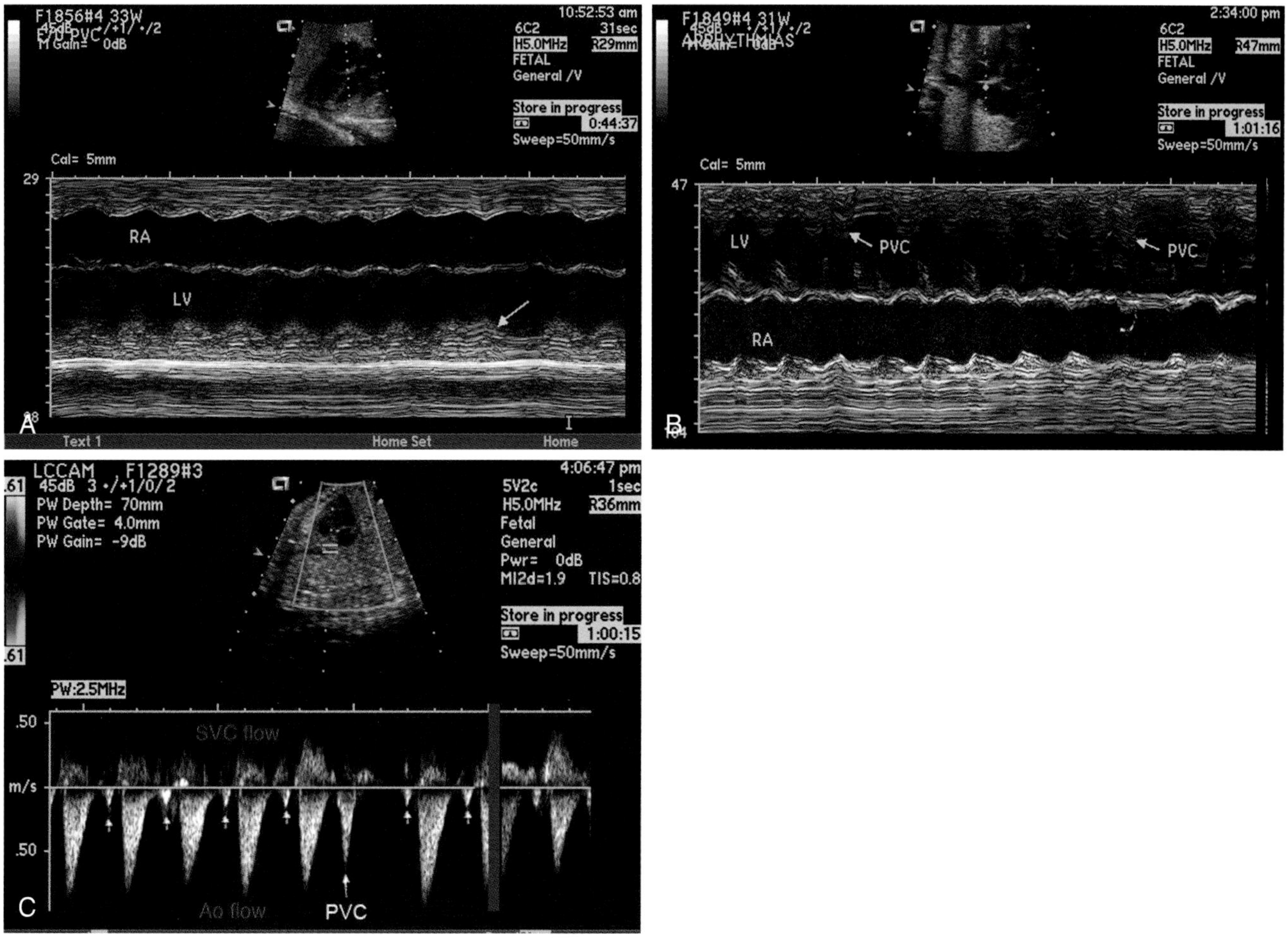

Figure 45-4. (A) M-mode tracing through the RA and the LV. There is an early beat *(arrow)*, which appears to originate from the ventricle, and does not in any way disturb the regular cadence of the atrial beats. This is a PVC. (B) M-mode tracing through the LV *(top)* and RA *(bottom)*. The ventricle appears to contract early, and there is no disturbance of the rate of atrial contraction; hence, these are premature ventricular contractions (PVCs). (C) Doppler sampling above the heart at the level of the aorta (Ao) and superior vena cava (SVC). Flow below the baseline is Ao flow and above the baseline is SVC flow. Normally, there is a small retrograde waveform of reversal in the SVC in conjunction with atrial contraction *(arrows)*. Note that there is an SVC-related atrial contraction waveform for every systolic aortic waveform up until an early beat disturbs this sequence and regularity. The early beat is a systolic aortic waveform that does not have a preceding atrial contraction associated. This is, therefore, a PVC.

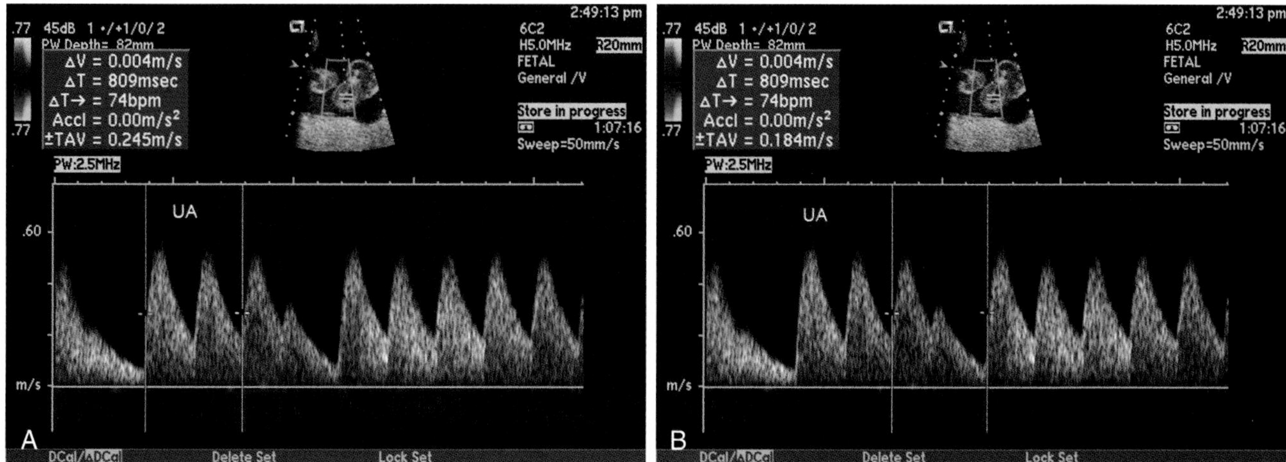

Figure 45-5. (A) Doppler sampling of the umbilical artery (UA) demonstrates an early beat. The timing between two normal beats is 809 msec. (B) The time measurement between two beats that includes the premature beat is 809 msec, precisely the same as when there are no premature beats. This suggests that there is no resetting of the sinus node; it is firing at its own pace, undisturbed by the premature beat. Hence, this is beat originating from the ventricle and not the atrium and is, therefore, a PVC.

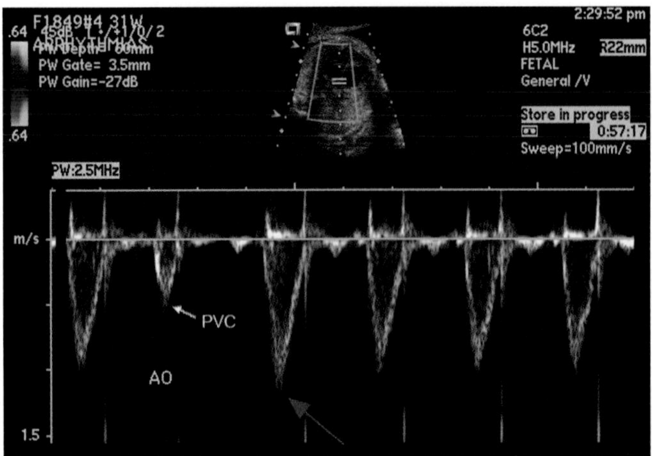

Figure 45-6. Doppler sampling of aortic flow. The peak velocity and overall appearance of the PVC waveform is smaller than the prior sinus beat; the following subsequent beat has a greater peak velocity than the normal sinus beat before the PVC *(red arrow)*. This reflects the augmentation of stroke volume that takes place in a beat following a PVC.

examination has shown parietal subendocardial accessory pathway fibers mostly composed of ordinary myocardium traversing through defects in the AV annulus fibrosus. In most cases of fetal SVT, a reentrant circuit utilizing antegrade conduction (orthidromic) through the AV node–bundle of His and retrograde conduction through the accessory pathway mediates the tachycardia. This is referred to as *atrioventricular reciprocating tachycardia (AVRT)*. The inciting events for AVRT are variable but typically involve appropriately timed PACs that allow for initiation and propagation of the reentrant circuit. A study using fetal magnetocardiography was able to precisely elucidate the mechanisms of AVRT initiation and termination in a series of fetuses with SVT.[24] A retrospective review of 23 fetuses at a single center with SVT used M-mode echocardiography to determine the ventriculoatrial (VA) time interval, via which the mechanism of SVT could be elucidated.[25] In 83% of the fetuses, the tachycardia was of the short VA type, thereby confirming an orthidromic AVRT.

A defining feature of AVRT is the 1 : 1 relationship between atrial and ventricular impulses (Figure 45-7); this distinguishes it from atrial flutter and atrial fibrillation, which are discussed later in this chapter. The ventricular rate in fetal AVRT is typically approximately 250 bpm, with this rate being relatively constant for each particular patient; that is, there is very little variability in the ventricular rate. Consistent with AVRT being a reentrant arrhythmia, the onset and termination of the arrhythmia are abrupt.

Atrial Flutter

Atrial flutter, as in the child and adult, can be differentiated from other types of SVT on the basis of a lack of 1 : 1 AV conduction and a variable ventricular rate (Figure 45-8). Rarely, 1 : 1 AV conduction may occur, in which case differentiation from AVRT becomes difficult. Typically, the ventricular rate will be slower than the atrial rate due to variable degrees of AV block. Experimental observations and the fact that atrial flutter occurs mainly during the third trimester support the hypothesis of atrial macroreentry as the underlying mechanism of fetal atrial flutter. The atrium probably reaches a critical size for establishing an intra-atrial macro-reentry circuit at approximately 27 to 30 weeks of gestation. Atrial flutter represents approximately 10% to 30% of all cases of fetal tachycardia.[20] A review of all published studies from 1990 onward comparing fetal AVRT and atrial flutter revealed several key distinguishing points: atrial flutter presents later in gestation, atrial flutter and AVRT have similar rates of hydrops and mortality; and there may be a slightly higher association of atrial flutter with structural heart disease than with SVT.[26] In some fetuses with atrial flutter, the presence of an accessory AV pathway has been demonstrated by postnatal transesophageal electrophysiological studies in the neonatal period.[27] The treatment for in utero atrial flutter is to a degree similar to AVRT and is described later.

Management of Fetal Atrial Tachyarrhythmias

Clear, established guidelines for treating fetal SVT are lacking owing to the absence of large, randomized, controlled trials.[28] In the absence of such trials, treatment is guided based on small case series, expert opinion, and institutional practice. Our approach to management starts with a diagnostic judgment of fetal hemodynamic status. At initial presentation, a comprehensive assessment of fetal well-being is indicated. Hydrops fetalis is an end-stage finding secondary to the sequelae of poor heart function, elevated venous pressure, and low cardiac output; its presence is related to poor outcome. In the past, hydrops has been used as the marker of severity and fetal impact; however, this is a very late event along a physiological spectrum of severity. Currently, a number of other measures can anticipate the onset of unwellness and instability prior to the onset of hydrops. These measures can be used to help decide upon initiation of therapy and monitor for response to therapy (Table 45-1). First, at initial presentation, it is important to determine whether the tachycardia is sustained (present for >50% of the time of observation) or nonsustained (present for <50%). Most nonsustained tachycardias and some sustained tachycardias can be monitored without intervention, so long as other measures of fetal wellness are present. The parameters of evaluation include cardiothoracic ratio, assessment of ventricular systolic function, presence or absence of tricuspid or mitral regurgitation, presence or absence of reversal of flow in the ductus venosus, presence or absence of umbilical venous pulsations, and the presence or absence of pericardial effusion. A comparative assessment of umbilical arterial flow and

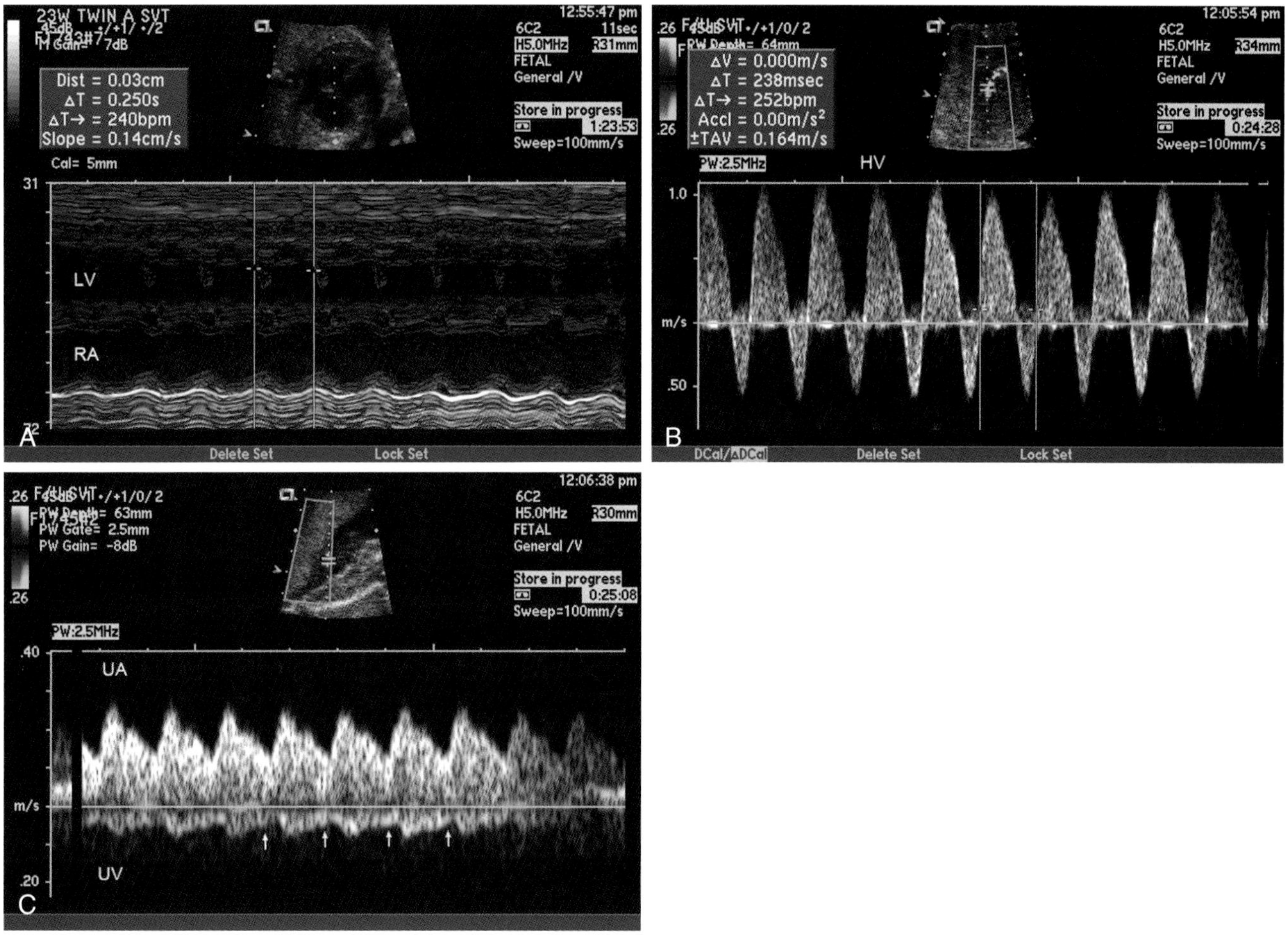

Figure 45-7. (A) M-mode tracing through the LV and RA. There is a 1:1 relationship between the atrial contractions *(bottom)* and the ventricular contractions *(top)*, both at a rate of 240 bpm. (B) Doppler sampling in the hepatic veins (HV). There is 1:1 reversal of flow waveform to forward flow waveform at a rate of over 250 bpm. As the atrium contracts against a stiff, noncompliant ventricle, the reversal waveform is quite prominent. (C) Doppler interrogation of the umbilical cord demonstrates venous pulsations consistent with atrial contraction during the tachyarrhythmia. This finding reflects elevated systemic venous pressure and may herald the onset of hydrops. UV, umbilical vein.

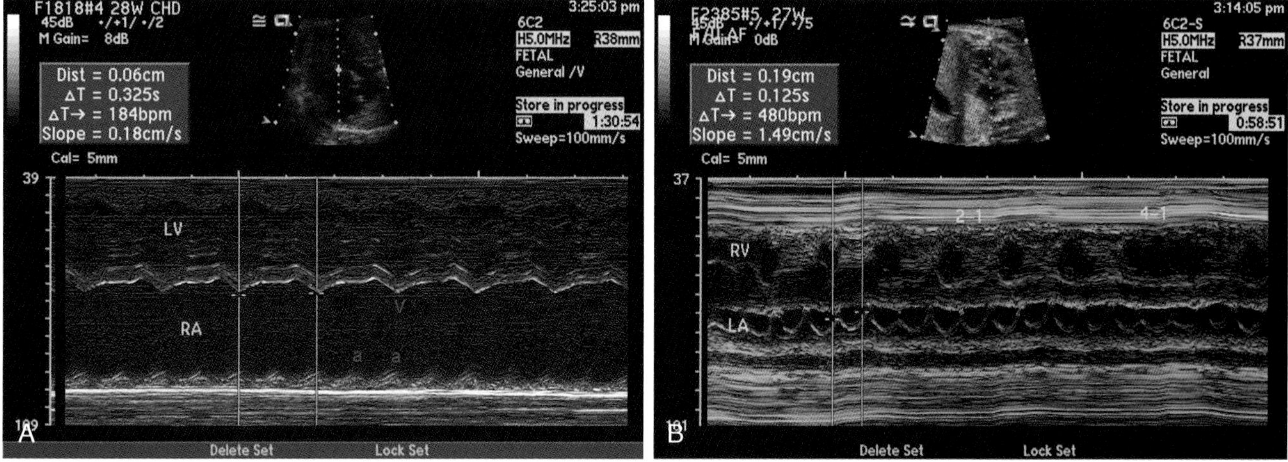

Figure 45-8. (A) M-mode tracing of a fetus at 28 weeks' gestation with atrial flutter. There is a 2:1 relationship between the atrial contractions ("a") and the ventricular contractions ("V"). (B) M-mode tracing of a fetus at 27 weeks' gestation with atrial flutter and variable conduction. The atrial rate is 480 bpm; in this tracing, there is evidence of 2:1 and 4:1 ventricular response.

middle cerebral artery flow provides for an indirect measure of cardiac output and perfusion. The ratio of vascular impedance as measured by the ratio of the pulsatility index (PI) between the placental circulation and the cerebrovascular circulation provides tremendous insight into the adequacy of perfusion. A middle cerebral artery PI that is lower than the umbilical artery PI suggests cerebrovascular vasodilation in an attempt to increase cerebral blood flow and reflects low cardiac output. Conversely, a high (normal) middle cerebral artery PI in comparison with the umbilical PI suggests adequate cardiac output (Figure 45-9). Serial imaging and close follow-up with evaluation of each of these parameters is essential at each assessment interval and provides for an overall picture of the hemodynamic status of the fetus with tachyarrhythmia.

Table 45-1 Parameters to Be Assessed at First Evaluation and at Serial Monitoring of the Fetus in a Tachyarrhythmia

SUGGESTIVE OF FETAL WELL-BEING AND ADEQUATE CARDIAC OUTPUT STATE	SUGGESTIVE OF POOR FETAL WELL-BEING AND LOW CARDIAC OUTPUT STATE
Normal cardiothoracic ratio (<0.4)	Increased cardiothoracic ratio (>0.4)
Qualitative good systolic ventricular function	Poor systolic ventricular function
No tricuspid regurgitation	Tricuspid regurgitation
No mitral regurgitation	Mitral regurgitation
Normal antegrade flow in the ductus venosus	Retrograde flow with atrial contraction in the ductus venosus
No umbilical venous pulsations	Umbilical venous pulsations
Umbilical artery/middle cerebral artery pulsatility index ratio <1	Umbilical artery/middle cerebral artery pulsatility index ratio >1
No pericardial effusion	Pericardial effusion
No hydrops fetalis	Hydrops fetalis (late event)

Treatment of fetal SVT can be grouped into several categories, starting with the least invasive and benign strategy, with escalation to more intensive therapy tailored to the status of the fetus: (1) observation only, (2) oral maternal transplacental therapy, (3) intravenous transplacental therapy, (4) so-called direct fetal therapy via the umbilical vein (cordocentesis), (5) fetal intraperitoneal or intramuscular routes, and finally, (6) delivery of the infant. The primary goal of treatment is restoration of sinus rhythm, although rate control alone may normalize hemodynamics sufficiently to resolve hydrops and improve fetal well-being.

Deciding upon a strategy of care depends upon the findings in relation to fetal hemodynamic wellness as described previously and the gestational age. Delivery of the premature infant with signs of compromise secondary to atrial tachycardia is fraught with untoward consequences and is best limited to the near-term infant in a center with a multidisciplinary team approach to the critically ill premature infant. Observation is warranted for fetuses with tachycardia that are near-term, have intermittent nonsustained bouts of tachycardia, and who display no signs of fetal unwellness as described previously, provided that frequent follow-up ultrasound assessments can be easily obtained. Many others will require some form of therapy with the objectives being to halt the arrhythmia and its consequences and provide for an optimal period of gestation to reach maturity.

The most commonly employed drugs for fetal atrial tachycardia include digoxin, sotalol, flecainide, and amiodarone. Digoxin is the most frequently used agent with the longest described experience in its use. Its antiarrhythmic effects are mediated by both decreasing the automaticity of the SA node and slowing conduction through the AV node. Digoxin may be administered to the mother orally, intravenously, or via direct intramuscular injection or to the fetus through the umbilical vein. Oral or parenteral maternal therapy is generally limited to nonhydropic fetuses; in hydropic infants, direct fetal therapy may be

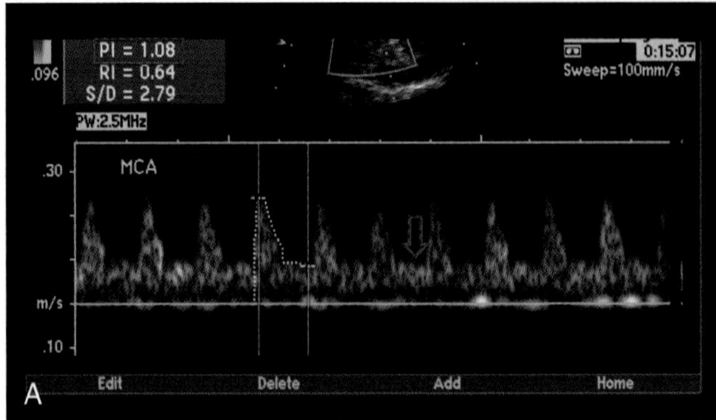

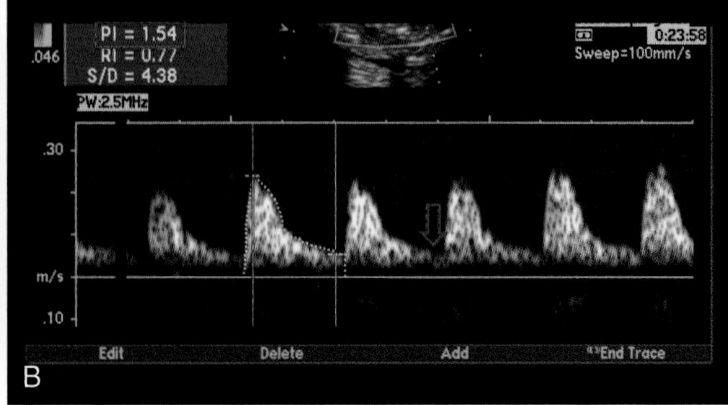

Figure 45-9. Fetus with supraventricular tachycardia (SVT) but with short periods of break into normal sinus rhythm such that sampling in the middle cerebral artery (MCA) could take place. **(A)** Doppler tracing of MCA flow while in SVT. Despite the fact that diastolic filling time is limited and short due to the tachycardia, there is still a significant amount of diastolic flow *(red arrow)* with a relatively low pulsatility index (PI) suggesting cerebral vasodilation in response to low cardiac output. The MCA PI is 1.08. **(B)** Same fetus now in sinus rhythm with less diastolic flow suggesting higher cerebrovascular resistance and an improved cardiac output. The MCA PI is now 1.54.

preferred secondary to impaired placental transfer of the drug. The maternal loading dose of digoxin is 1.0 to 1.5 mg/day divided into two or three doses, followed 24 hours later by a maintenance dose of 500 to 600 μg/day divided into two doses. Serum digoxin levels should be monitored with a therapeutic range of 1.5 to 2.5 ng/mL. The maternal ECG should be monitored for signs of AV block and maternal serum electrolytes should also be monitored. In the largest series of patients with fetal SVT to date, monotherapy with digoxin was able to reestablish sinus rhythm in 51.5%. Fetuses with hydrops had a significantly lower rate of conversion to sinus rhythm (24.6% vs. 65.4%).[26]

Flecainide, a class IC antiarrhythmic, has been used both as monotherapy and in conjunction with digoxin for the control of fetal tachycardia. In a study of this drug, consisting of 20 patients who had failed digoxin monotherapy, 75% were able to convert to sinus rhythm within 7 days of therapy, with nearly all the remainder converting to sinus rhythm within 14 days.[29] No deaths were reported. The maternal dose of flecainide is 300 to 400 mg/day aimed at maintaining maternal serum flecainide levels of 500 to 1000 μg/L. Maternal ECG monitoring for QRS prolongation should be performed. Flecainide has been reported to have good transplacental passage even in the setting of hydrops. Conversion to sinus rhythm may be expected in 72 hours of initiating therapy, but may occur up to 2 weeks afterward. Continuation of flecainide beyond 72 hours should be considered when there is a significant decrease in the fetal ventricular rate and establishment of fetal hemodynamic stability, because slowing of the fetal ventricular rate can be seen as an early therapeutic response, short of frank conversion to sinus rhythm.

Sotalol, a class III antiarrhythmic agent with beta-blocking properties, has been described in the treatment of fetal tachyarrhythmias. Its use in fetuses with SVT was previously associated with reports of excess fetal mortality[30]; however, a more recent investigation from the same group did not confirm this association.[31] Sotalol is typically started at a maternal dose of 80 mg twice a day and can be increased up to 160 mg three times a day. The maternal ECG should be monitored for significant QTc prolongation. The placental transfer of sotalol is excellent, even under conditions of hydrops. Sotalol accumulates in amniotic fluid but not in the fetus itself. Therefore, it appears that renal excretion in the fetus is efficient and is greater than the rate of oral absorption by fetal swallowing. The maternal blood level does not reliably predict successful therapy. Unlike other beta blockers, sotalol is not associated with fetal growth restriction.

Our own experience in treating fetal SVT favors the use of digoxin and sotalol dual therapy.[32] Mothers are admitted for inpatient surveillance. We commence with a loading dose of digoxin either oral or parenteral and within 24 hours will start sotalol at low dose of 80 mg twice daily. The sotalol dose is increased incrementally every 24 to 48 hours to a maximum of 160 mg three times a day, based on fetal hemodynamic parameters and response. Digoxin levels are monitored daily and dose adjusted, because we have found that relatively high doses of digoxin are necessary in order to reach therapeutic levels, considering the increased volume of distribution of pregnant women.

Amiodarone, another class III antiarrhythmic agent, is a potent oral or intravenous drug that has been investigated in the treatment of fetal tachycardia refractory to digoxin therapy. The transplacental transfer characteristics of amiodarone in the fetus have been controversial. In the single largest study to date, 26 fetuses with incessant tachycardia were treated with amiodarone.[33] Effective conversion to sinus rhythm in AVRT and junctional ectopic tachycardia was reported in 93%, without any fetal deaths. The conversion rate in atrial flutter was only 33%. The oral loading dose of amiodarone is 1800 to 2400 mg/day for 2 to 7 days, with single doses not exceeding 800 mg. Before amiodarone loading, the digoxin dose should be decreased by 50%. Serum chemistries and thyroid functions should be serially monitored in mothers and later in infants. Maternal ECGs (daily during loading and regularly during follow-up) should be monitored and the maternal QTc should not exceed 0.5 second.[33] Transient biochemical and rare clinical hypothyroidism and possible fetal growth retardation have been reported. These side effects may correlate with duration of amiodarone exposure.

Other forms of SVT in the fetus involve "automatic" foci within the atria or AV node and are much more uncommon than traditional reentrant SVT. Such forms can be difficult to treat and include entities such as ectopic atrial tachycardia, multifocal atrial tachycardia, and permanent junctional reciprocating tachycardia (PJRT).

The impact of antiarrhythmic drug therapy on the mother when treating for fetal indications should be considered. Most antiarrhythmic drugs are well tolerated in the pregnant patient; however, closer monitoring for the proarrhythmic effects of certain drugs should be employed owing to the physiological changes in cardiac output and first-pass hepatic metabolism during pregnancy.[34]

Ventricular Tachycardia

VT is quite rare in the fetus and is described mostly in case reports.[35,36] In a series of 127 patients evaluated and treated at a single center for fetal tachycardia, none had VT[17]; in another large single-center series of 356 patients, 1 had VT.[9] VT in the fetus is manifest by a ventricular rate of between 200 and 300 bpm; echocardiography will reveal the ventricular rate to be faster than the atrial rate (Figure 45-10). Using magnetocardiography, torsades de pointes, a form of polymorphic VT, was detected in a fetus in whom echocardiography revealed only sinus bradycardia, SVT, and 2:1 AV block. This fetus was later shown to have long QT syndrome.[37] Treatment of fetal VT

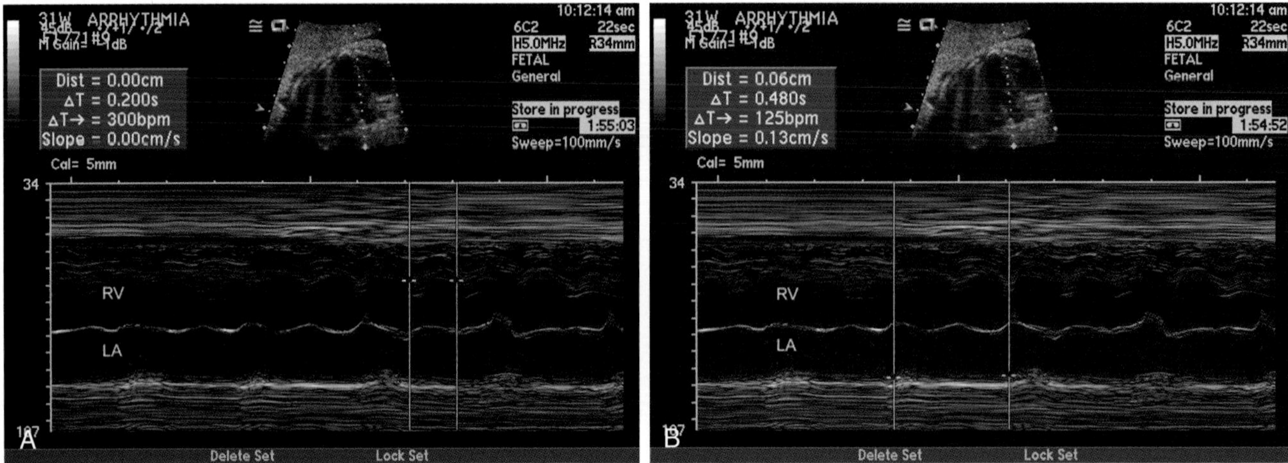

Figure 45-10. Fetus at 31 weeks' gestation with ventricular tachycardia as demonstrated by a ventricular rate that is faster than the atrial rate. **(A)** M-mode tracing through the right ventricle (RV; *top)* and through the left atrium (LA). The rate of RV contraction is at 300 bpm and is faster than the atrial rate below. **(B)** The atrial rate is 125 bpm, much slower than the ventricular rate.

is guided by anecdotal reports; successful use of transplacental amiodarone and lidocaine has been reported.

Sinus Bradycardia

Sustained sinus bradycardia in the fetus (<100-110 bpm) is an uncommon finding for which the etiology should be assiduously investigated. Transient bradycardia with documented resolution during the ultrasound examination is likely related to physiological alterations of vagal tone and is of no clinical consequence. This is a common phenomenon in the third trimester of pregnancy and is oftentimes related to excessive abdominal pressure during scanning, which can influence placental flow. Distinguishing complete heart block from sinus bradycardia is of the utmost importance. In general, persistent sinus bradycardia is a nonspecific marker of fetal distress, and treatment involves detection and therapy of the underlying cause. Certain structural abnormalities, particularly those associated with the heterotaxy syndrome, are associated with asymptomatic sinus bradycardia. Blocked PACs may also result in the appearance of fetal sinus bradycardia; in the absence of markers of fetal compromise, this finding requires no treatment, although a complete survey for structural CHD remains warranted.

The association of fetal sinus bradycardia and congenital forms of the long QT syndrome has been recognized.[37-40] Examination of the ECG of family members with measurement of the QTc may be informative. Fetal magnetocardiography is diagnostic but not always feasible given its limited availability.[36] Close observation is mandatory owing to the potential for malignant tachyarrhythmias in utero; the presence of VT or torsades de pointes portends a poor outcome. No treatment protocols currently exist. Successful use of lidocaine and magnesium has been reported for these malignant arrhythmias.[6] Infants confirmed to have long QT syndrome after birth require close surveillance, including careful inspection of the 12-lead ECG (and those of family members) and initiation of beta blocker therapy.

Congenital Complete Heart Block

Congenital complete heart block (CCHB) is a rare disorder of AV conduction affecting approximately 1 in 20,000 newborns. The overall incidence may be much higher given the high rate of fetal loss associated with CCHB. The hallmark of CCHB is AV dissociation, in which atrial impulses are not conducted to the ventricles and have no relationship to the slower ventricular rhythm. Cardiac output is thus dependent on the intrinsic ventricular "escape" rhythm, the rate of which may be as low as 30 to 40 bpm. The bradycardia associated with CCHB is easily detected on routine auscultation and is confirmed by fetal echocardiography (Figure 45-11).

CCHB typically presents in association with either immunological evidence of maternal connective disease or fetal structural CHD. Together, these account for approximately 90% of presentations; the remaining approximately 10% are regarded to have "idiopathic" CCHB.[41] In a study of 55 fetuses with CCHB, those found to have structural CHD were most commonly afflicted with heterotaxy syndrome. Disorders of AV alignment (e.g., congenitally corrected transposition of the great vessels) are the other structural congenital heart condition associated with CCHB. Heterotaxy syndrome encompasses an extensive variety of intracardiac lesions, with the common unifying theme relating to abnormal "sidedness" or laterality of the atria and intra-abdominal viscera.[42]

CCHB is a well-known manifestation of neonatal lupus, an autoimmune disease mediated by the transplacental transfer of the maternal autoantibodies anti-Ro (anti-SSA) and anti-La (anti-SSB) during gestation. The

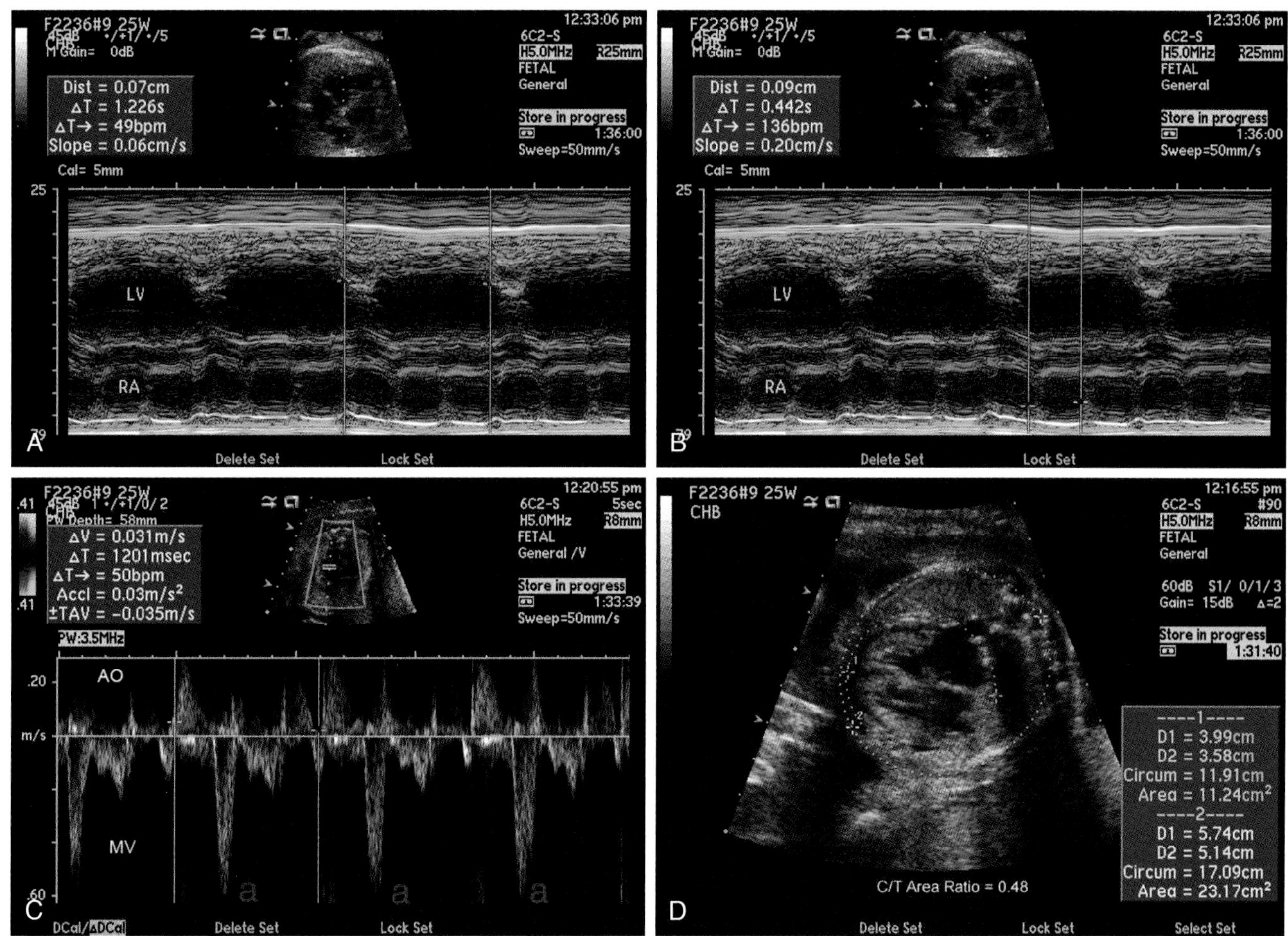

Figure 45-11. **(A)** M-mode tracing of a fetus at 25 weeks' gestation with maternal lupus–mediated complete heart block. The atrial rate is faster than, and not associated with, the ventricular rate. Ventricular rate is 49 bpm. **(B)** Atrial rate is 136 bpm. The atrial rate is a parameter to monitor in complete heart block (CHB), because a rapid atrial rate (>150 bpm) may reflect an attempt to increase cardiac output under conditions of poor perfusion. **(C)** Doppler interrogation of left ventricular MV inflow and aortic outflow. The cursor marker is placed at the onset of aortic flow and measures a heart rate of 50 bpm. There are occasional high-velocity "a" waveforms seen corresponding to atrial contraction under conditions of abnormal ventricular filling properties. **(D)** There is cardiomegaly in this fetus with CHB. Ventricular dilation in order to accommodate increased stroke volume is a compensatory response to a slower heart rate in CHB.

prevailing theory is that these antibodies have a particular predilection for the conduction tissue within the AV node and Purkinje fibers; however, the ability of these autoantibodies to induce a diffuse neonatal myocarditis has also been described.[43] The incidence of CCHB in mothers positive for anti-Ro or anti-La is quite low (~1-2%). A recent prospective, multicenter study evaluated the offspring of mothers positive for anti-Ro during pregnancy with ECG and Holter monitoring through the first year of life; CCHB developed in 1 child of the 62 women studied and 1 child developed second-degree AV block.[44] Therefore, whereas the incidence of CCHB is much larger in the fetuses of antibody-positive mothers, the individual risk for a mother positive for such antibodies is generally quite low. Moreover, the vast majority of mothers positive for anti-Ro and anti-La carrying infants with CCHB do not have any symptoms of a connective tissue disorder.[45]

CCHB typically presents in the late second or early third trimester (e.g., between 20 and 24 wk). Second-degree heart block may be the initial manifestation with progression to third-degree block noted as gestation progresses. A study employing fetal magnetocardiography in infants with second- and third-degree AV block revealed a number of other dysrhythmias in this group of fetuses, including junctional ectopic tachycardia (JET), VT, and atrial ectopy.[15] This study suggests that the underlying mechanisms of CCHB are diverse and more complex than can be appreciated with traditional two-dimensional ultrasound methods. CCHB is often associated with fetal hydrops and pleural effusions, although many fetuses may appear well by the usual biometric tests employed to assess fetal viability.

CCHB is widely regarded as an arrhythmia with high neonatal morbidity and mortality, and the discovery of CCHB frequently leads to pregnancy termination. Neonatal outcome is in large part determined by the etiology; the prognosis is much more sanguine for fetuses with CCHB associated with maternal autoantibodies; conversely, it is much bleaker for those affected by structural CHD. One of the largest studies to date reviewed the experience of CCHB not associated with structural CHD over a 33-year period at a single institution.[45] In this series, overall mortality of those infants diagnosed prenatally was 43%, despite the availability of newer treatment modalities such as pre- and postnatal corticosteroids, immediate postnatal pacing, and early neonatal pacemaker implantation. Fetal hydrops was most strongly associated with mortality, with 100% of these fetuses experiencing intrauterine demise or early postnatal death. A contemporaneous series with a similar number of cases reported 19% mortality, with 45% of the deaths occurring either in utero or within 3 months of birth.[46] The reasons for this discrepancy in mortality are unclear, but likely relate to differences in the populations studied, the fact that CCHB is not a uniform disease, and the absence of uniform treatment protocols for CCHB. It should also be mentioned that the morbidity of CCHB is not insignificant, with 60% to 90% of surviving patients in the two series discussed above requiring pacemaker implantation at some point during follow-up.

As mentioned previously, the outcome for fetal CCHB in the presence of CHD is significantly worse than antibody-associated CCHB. In a study of 24 fetuses diagnosed with CCHB in the setting of structural CHD between 1990 and 2003, 42% were terminated before 24 weeks' gestation.[47] Of those pregnancies intended to carry to term, the survival rates were quite poor, with only 56% resulting in live birth, 25% surviving beyond the neonatal period, and 19% surviving at 1 year. When compared with a comparable group of CCHB-affected fetuses without structural CHD, this 19% survival was markedly less than the approximately 80% 1-year survival seen in the non-CHD group.

The reasons for this marked difference in survival rates are not entirely clear. Many cases of structural CHD associated with CCHB are associated with so-called single-ventricle physiology, in which both cardiac outputs must by necessity cross one AV valve. It is speculated that the abnormal hemodynamics conferred by CCHB in the setting of already altered physiology may contribute to the increased rates of hydrops fetalis and other morbidity in this population. Surgical options for this group of patients are also limited and palliative in nature.

The treatment of CCHB can be divided into prenatal and postnatal stages. In the prenatal stage, detection and early therapy are paramount before signs of fetal compromise occur. Because CCHB is felt to evolve rather rapidly during the second trimester from first-degree AV block, through second-degree AV block, and culminating in CCHB, the ability to detect disturbances of AV conduction before the development of irreversible damage is appealing. A recent prospective study evaluated this hypothesis in 127 pregnant women positive for anti-Ro antibodies.[48] Serial fetal echocardiographic surveillance during the second and third trimester was performed,

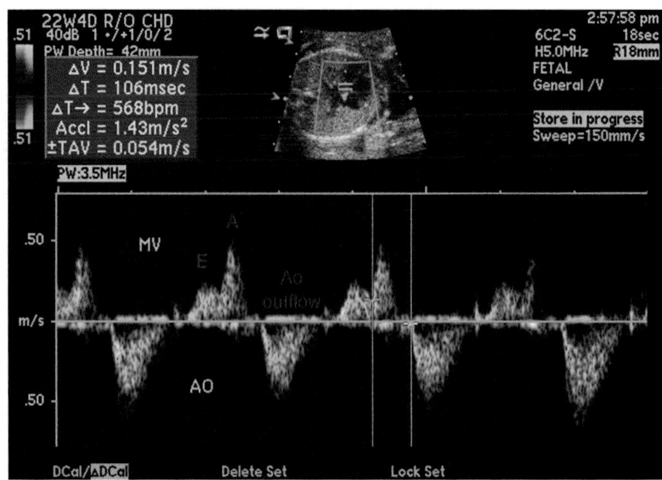

Figure 45-12. Doppler tracing of LV inflow across the MV and outflow across the AO in order to determine the timing of the "mechanical PR" interval. This is the time interval from onset of A wave flow, representing atrial contraction, to the onset of aortic outflow and systolic ejection. This flow-related time interval is the "mechanical" equivalent of the time interval of electrical activity from P wave to onset of QRS wave on the electrocardiogram (ECG). A, atrial contraction; E, early diastolic filling.

with the fetal PR interval measured via echocardiographic techniques (Figure 45-12). Three cases of CCHB were identified without preceding prolongations in the PR interval and, despite maternal therapy with dexamethasone, reversal of CCHB did not occur. However, in 2 of 3e fetuses noted to have prolonged PR intervals, maternal treatment with dexamethasone normalized the PR interval and CCHB did not occur in these 2 fetuses. The lack of a control group prevents proof of causality, but these preliminary results are encouraging.

Pharmacological management of CCHB, once diagnosed, is targeted toward halting any further immune-mediated damage to the AV conduction system and increasing fetal cardiac output via augmentation of the fetal heart rate. The mainstay of such therapy thus far has been maternal administration of dexamethasone and beta agonists. Given the initial role of inflammation, maternally administered corticosteroids, particularly fluorinated glucocorticoids such as dexamethasone (4-8 mg/day), have been used in an attempt to reduce the severity of myocardial inflammation and conduction tissue damage. Anti-inflammatory therapy may also have an impact on reducing the myocarditis and cardiomyopathic changes seen in maternal immune-mediated disease, thereby reducing myocardial damage and allowing for preservation of viable contractile tissue. Rare reports document the reversal of first- and second-degree AV block after starting corticosteroids. However, once third-degree heart block is established, it is irreversible. Myocardial dysfunction related to ongoing inflammation, however, may be reversible with steroid treatment. Only fluorinated corticosteroids cross the placenta and are thus appropriate for transplacental treatment. Despite the

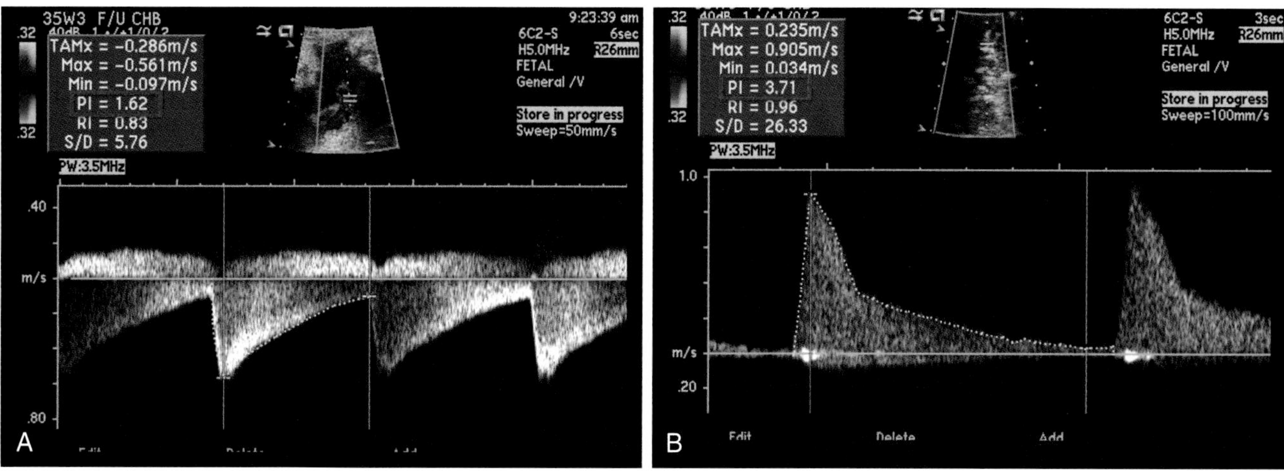

Figure 45-13. (A) Fetus at 35 weeks' gestation with ventricular heart rate of 45 bpm. Doppler tracing of the umbilical cord. There are umbilical venous pulsations that are typically seen in CHB. The UA PI is 1.62. (B) Doppler tracing of the MCA. The PI is 3.71. The higher MCA PI relative to the UA PI is a normal healthy relationship, which suggests adequate cardiac output and adequate perfusion despite the low heart rate. This parameter can be used to assess fetal wellness, gauge the hemodynamic impact of the bradycardia, and help guide timing of delivery.

widespread and accepted use of these agents in mothers with fetuses affected by CCHB, only one study has rigorously evaluated the effect of these therapies. In a nonrandomized trial with a historical control group, the routine prenatal use of dexamethasone and beta agonists increased fetal survival from 80% to 95%, although reversal of CCHB was not documented.[49] Oligohydramnios was noted as a potential adverse outcome of maternal dexamethasone therapy.

Beta sympathomimetics such as terbutaline, a $beta_2$ agonist, increase atrial and ventricular rates and have been used in the setting of CCHB. Maternal terbutaline administration of 2.5 to 7.5 mg orally every 4 to 6 hours (total daily dose 10-30 mg) is generally used when the fetal heart rate is less than 55 bpm. Terbutaline does not restore the normal coordinated response between atrial and ventricular accelerations but has been shown to increase the overall heart rate in fetal CCHB.[50] Improved ventricular rate and cardiac output from sympathomimetic effects may improve prognosis. However, in the study by Jaeggi and coworkers,[49] beta stimulation did not affect the fetal heart rate in 50% of their cohort. Other sympathomimetic drugs that have been used to augment fetal heart rate are salbutamol and ritodrine.

The successful use of maternal plasmapheresis and prednisolone therapy have been reported in anti-Ro mothers in preventing CCHB, but the success of this strategy has not been duplicated.[51] Because CCHB is irreversible, strategies aimed at preventing disease assume high priority. Although disease expression in the fetus requires additional factors to amplify the cascade to fibrosis, maternal anti-Ro/La antibodies are necessary. Accordingly, eliminating fetal exposure to these antibodies seems to be an important approach. The potential role for intravenous gamma globulin, either administered to the mother or directly administered through cordocentesis to the fetus in the treatment of the fetal AV block has been anecdotally reported.[21,52] A prospective trial is under way to determine whether treating the pregnant mother with intravenous immune globulin (IVIG) will prevent the development of fetal CCHB.[53] Finally, fetal pacing has been reported experimentally and in fetuses with impending demise from heart failure, but no survivors have been reported.[54,55]

The delivery of infants known to be affected by CCHB should ideally occur at a tertiary center with multidisciplinary expertise in perinatology, obstetrics, neonatology, and pediatric cardiology. The ability to rapidly provide heart rate support to the neonate is mandatory. At our institution, our consistent approach has been to perform close fetal surveillance, scheduled delivery, and more recently, immediate placement of temporary epicardial pacing wires in the delivery room itself in the very high risk neonate with AV block (Figure 45-13).

Summary

Disturbances of cardiac rhythm in the human fetus may manifest in a variety of ways, with the spectrum of clinical presentation ranging from incidentally detected PACs to fulminant arrhythmia resulting in fetal loss. The preponderance of fetal "arrhythmias," in fact, consist of benign atrial ectopy and do not require treatment. Close surveillance of fetuses utilizing serial ultrasound will, in most cases, distinguish these benign perturbations of rhythm from more serious arrhythmias. Careful inspection for associated structural heart disease is also warranted in all patients referred for rhythm disturbance. Even closer follow-up of fetuses with documented arrhythmia is mandatory for prognosis and to guide pre- and postnatal therapy.

References

1. Clark JM, Case CL. Fetal arrhythmias. In Gillette PC, Garson A, eds. *Clinical Pediatric Arrhythmias*. 2nd ed. Philadelphia: WB Saunders; 1999:293-302.
2. Mikawa T, Hurtado R. Development of the cardiac conduction system. *Semin Cell Dev Biol*. 2007;18:90-100.
3. Boullin J, Morgan JM. The development of cardiac rhythm. *Heart*. 2005;91:874-875.
4. Matias A, Montenegro N, Areias JC, Leite LP. Haemodynamic evaluation of the first trimester fetus with special emphasis on venous return. *Hum Reprod Update*. 2000;6:177-189.
5. Wheeler T, Murrills A. Patterns of fetal heart rate during normal pregnancy. *Br J Obstet Gynaecol*. 1978;85:18-27.
6. Strasburger JF, Cheulkar B, Wichman HJ. Perinatal arrhythmias: diagnosis and management. *Clin Perinatol*. 2007;34:627-652.
7. Copel JA, Liang RI, Demasio K, Ozeren S, Kleinman CS. The clinical significance of the irregular fetal heart rhythm. *Am J Obstet Gynecol*. 2000;182:813-817.
8. Fyfe DA, Meyer KB, Case CL. Sonographic assessment of fetal cardiac arrhythmias. *Semin Ultrasound CT MR*. 1993;14:286-297.
9. Fouron JC. Fetal arrhythmias: The Saint-Justine Hospital experience. *Prenat Diagn*. 2004;24:1068-1080.
10. Fouron JC, Fournier A, Proulx F, et al. Management of fetal tachyarrhythmia based on superior vena cava/aorta Doppler flow recordings. *Heart*. 2003;89:1211-1216.
11. Carvalho JS, Prefumo F, Ciardelli V, Sairam S, Bhide A, Shinebourne EA. Evaluation of fetal arrhythmias from simultaneous pulsed wave doppler in pulmonary artery and vein. *Heart*. 2007;93: 1448-1453.
12. DeVore GR, Horenstein J. Simultaneous Doppler recording of the pulmonary artery and vein: a new technique for the evaluation of a fetal arrhythmia. *J Ultrasound Med*. 1993;12:669-671.
13. Rein AJJT, O'Donnell C, Geva T, et al. Use of tissue velocity imaging in the diagnosis of fetal cardiac arrhythmias. *Circulation*. 2002;106: 1827-1833.
14. Hornberger LK, Collins K. New insights into fetal atrioventricular block using fetal magnetocardiography. *J Am Coll Cardiol*. 2008; 51:85-86.
15. Zhao H, Cuneo BF, Strasburger JF, Huhta JC, Gotteiner NL, Wakai RT. Electrophysiological characteristics of fetal atrioventricular block. *J Am Coll Cardiol*. 2008;51:77-84.
16. Southall DP, Richards J, Hardwick RA, et al. Prospective study of fetal heart rate and rhythm patterns. *Arch Dis Child*. 1980;55: 506-511.
17. Simpson JM, Sharland GK. Fetal tachycardias: management and outcome of 127 consecutive cases. *Heart*. 1998;79:576-581.
18. Boldt T, Eronen M, Andersson S. Long-term outcome in fetuses with cardiac arrhythmias. *Obstet Gynecol*. 2003;102:1372-1379.
19. Cuneo BF, Strasburger JF, Wakai RT, Ovadia M. Conduction system disease in fetuses evaluated for irregular cardiac rhythm. *Fetal Diagn Ther*. 2006;21:307-313.
20. Simpson J. Fetal arrhythmias. In Allan L, Hornberger L, Sharland G, eds. *Textbook of Fetal Cardiology*. 1st ed. Greenwich, England: Greenwich Medical Media; 2000:423-451.
21. Hornberger LK, Sahn DJ. Rhythm abnormalities of the fetus. *Heart*. 2007;93:1294-1300.
22. Kleinman CS, Nehgme RA. Cardiac arrhythmias in the human fetus. *Pediatr Cardiol*. 2004;25:234-21.
23. Simpson JM, Milburn A, Yates RW, Maxwell DJ, Sharland GK. Outcome of intermittent tachyarrhythmias in the fetus. *Pediatr Cardiol*. 1997;18:78-82.
24. Wakai RT, Strasburger JF, Li Z, Deal BJ, Gotteiner NL. Magnetocardiographic rhythm patterns at initiation and termination of fetal supraventricular tachycardia. *Circulation*. 2003;107:307-312.
25. Jaeggi E, Fouron JC, Fournier A, van Doesburg N, Drblik SP, Proulx F. Ventriculo-atrial time interval measured on M mode echocardiography: a determining element in diagnosis, treatment, and prognosis of fetal supraventricular tachycardia. *Heart*. 1998;79:582-587.
26. Krapp M, Kohl T, Simpson JM, Sharland GK, Katalinic A, Gembruch U. Review of diagnosis, treatment, and outcome of fetal atrial flutter compared with supraventricular tachycardia. *Heart*. 2003; 89:913-917.
27. Naheed ZJ, Strasburger JF, Deal BJ, Woodrow Benson D, Gidding SS. Fetal tachycardia: mechanisms and predictors of hydrops fetalis. *J Am Coll Cardiol*. 1996;27:1736-1740.
28. van den Heuvel F, Bink-Boelkens MT, du Marchie Sarvaas GJ, Berger RM. Drug management of fetal tachyarrhythmias: are we ready for a systematic and evidence-based approach? *Pacing Clin Electrophysiol*. 2008;31(suppl 1):S54-S57.
29. Krapp M, Baschat AA, Gembruch U, Geipel A, Germer U. Flecainide in the intrauterine treatment of fetal supraventricular tachycardia. *Ultrasound Obstet Gynecol*. 2002;19:158-164.
30. Oudijk MA, Michon MM, Kleinman CS, et al. Sotalol in the treatment of fetal dysrhythmias. *Circulation*. 2000;101:2721-2726.
31. Oudijk MA, Ruskamp JM, Ververs FFT, et al. Treatment of fetal tachycardia with sotalol: transplacental pharmacokinetics and pharmacodynamics. *J Am Coll Cardiol*. 2003;42:765-770.
32. Merriman JB, Gonzalez JM, Rychik J, Ural SH. Can digoxin and sotalol therapy for supraventricular tachycardia and hydrops be successful? *J Reprod Med*. 2008;53:357-359
33. Strasburger JF, Cuneo BF, Michon MM, et al. Amiodarone therapy for drug-refractory fetal tachycardia. *Circulation*. 2004;109: 375-379.
34. Joglar JA, Page RL. Antiarrhythmic drugs in pregnancy. *Curr Opin Cardiol*. 2001;16:40-45.
35. Rein AJ, Levine JC, Nir A. Use of high-frame rate imaging and Doppler tissue echocardiography in the diagnosis of fetal ventricular tachycardia. *J Am Soc Echocardiogr*. 2001;14:149-151.
36. Lopes LM, Cha SC, Scanavacca MI, Tuma-Calil VM, Zugaib M. Fetal idiopathic ventricular tachycardia with nonimmune hydrops: benign course. *Pediatr Cardiol*. 1996;17:192-193.
37. Horigome H, Iwashita H, Yoshinaga M, Shimizu W. Magnetocardiographic demonstration of torsade de pointes in a fetus with congenital long QT syndrome. *J Cardiovasc Electrophysiol*. 2008; 19:334-335.
38. Beinder E, Grancay T, Menendez T, Singer H, Hofbeck M. Fetal sinus bradycardia and the long QT syndrome. *Am J Obstet Gynecol*. 2001;185:743-747.
39. Hamada H, Horigome H, Asaka M, et al. Prenatal diagnosis of long QT syndrome using fetal magnetocardiography. *Prenat Diagn*. 1999;19:677-680.
40. Hofbeck M, Ulmer H, Beinder E, Sieber E, Singer H. Prenatal findings in patients with prolonged QT interval in the neonatal period. *Heart*. 1997;77:198-204.
41. Schmidt KG, Ulmer HE, Silverman NH, Kleinman CS, Copel JA. Perinatal outcome of fetal complete atrioventricular block: a multicenter experience. *J Am Coll Cardiol*. 1991;17:1360-1366.
42. Cohen MS, Anderson RH, Cohen MI, et al. Controversies, genetics, diagnostic assessment, and outcomes relating to the heterotaxy syndrome. *Cardiol Young*. 2007;17(suppl 2):29-43.
43. Costedoat-Chalumeau N, Georgin-Lavialle S, Amoura Z, Piette JC. Anti-SSA/Ro and anti-SSB/La antibody-mediated congenital heart block. *Lupus*. 2005;14:660-664.
44. Gerosa M, Cimaz R, Stramba-Badiale M, et al. Electrocardiographic abnormalities in infants born from mothers with autoimmune diseases–a multicentre prospective study. *Rheumatology*. 2007;46: 1285-1289.
45. Jaeggi ET, Hamilton RM, Silverman ED, Zamora SA, Hornberger LK. Outcome of children with fetal, neonatal or childhood diagnosis of isolated congenital atrioventricular block: a single institution's experience of 30 years. *J Am Coll Cardiol*. 2002;39:130-137.
46. Buyon J, Hiebert R, Copel J, et al. Autoimmune-associated congenital heart block: demographics, mortality, morbidity and recurrence rates obtained from a national neonatal lupus registry. *J Am Coll Cardiol*. 1998;31:1658-1666.
47. Jaeggi ET, Hornberger LK, Smallhorn JF, Fouron JC. Prenatal diagnosis of complete atrioventricular block associated with structural heart disease: combined experience of two tertiary care centers and review of the literature [see comment]. *Ultrasound Obstet Gynecol*. 2005;26:16-21.
48. Friedman DM, Kim MY, Copel JA, et al. Utility of cardiac monitoring in fetuses at risk for congenital heart block: the PR Interval and Dexamethasone Evaluation (PRIDE) prospective study. *Circulation*. 2008;117:485-493.
49. Jaeggi ET, Fouron J, Silverman ED, Ryan G, Smallhorn J, Hornberger LK. Transplacental fetal treatment improves the outcome of prenatally diagnosed complete atrioventricular block without structural heart disease. *Circulation*. 2004;110:1542-1548.
50. Cuneo BF, Zhao H, Strasburger JF, Ovadia M, Huhta JC, Wakai RT. Atrial and ventricular rate response and patterns of heart rate

acceleration during maternal–fetal terbutaline treatment of fetal complete heart block. *Am J Cardiol.* 2007;100:661-665.

51. Makino S, Yonemoto H, Itoh S, Takeda S. Effect of steroid administration and plasmapheresis to prevent fetal congenital heart block in patients with systemic lupus erythematosus and/or Sjögren's syndrome. *Acta Obstet Gynecol Scand.* 2007;86:1145-1146.
52. Kaaja R, Julkunen H, Ammälä P, Teppo AM, Kurki P. Congenital heart block: successful prophylactic treatment with intravenous gamma globulin and corticosteroid therapy. *Am J Obstet Gynecol.* 1991;165:1333-1334
53. Preventive IVIG therapy for congenital heart block (The PITCH Study). ClinicalTrials.gov identifier: NCT00460928.
54. Liddicoat JR, Klein JR, Reddy VM, Klautz RJM, Teitel DF, Hanley FL. Hemodynamic effects of chronic prenatal ventricular pacing for the treatment of complete atrioventricular block. *Circulation.* 1997; 96(3):1025-1030.
55. Carpenter R Jr, Strasburger J, Garson A Jr, Smith R, Deter R, Engelhardt H Jr. Fetal ventricular pacing for hydrops secondary to complete atrioventricular block. *J Am Coll Cardiol.* 1986;8: 1434-1436.

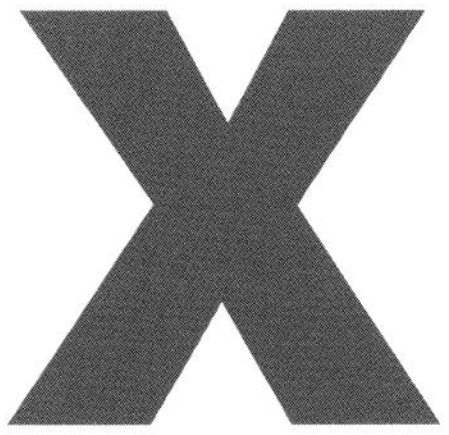

New Frontiers in Fetal Cardiovascular Imaging

46 Anatomical and Functional Fetal Cardiac Magnetic Resonance Imaging: An Emerging Technology

Mark A. Fogel

Why Apply Cardiac Magnetic Resonance Imaging to the Fetus: Is there a Need for Another Imaging Modality?

Assessment of fetal cardiac anatomy and function is an important component of the overall care of the newborn with cardiac disease.[1] Fetal echocardiography has been the mainstay of cardiac assessment in utero, and successful diagnoses and monitoring of fetal therapy have been well-documented in the literature.[1-5] Nevertheless, conventional fetal echocardiography is limited by the fact that it is not a technology that can readily offer three-dimensional (3D) visualization (which limits assessment of ventricular volumes and mass, for example), although recent advances over the past 10 years have enabled fetal echocardiography to provide for the reconstruction of two-dimensional (2D) images into 3D images through techniques such as spatiotemporal image correlation (STIC), and "real-time" 3D transducers and processing algorithms. Fetal echocardiography has a relatively limited field of view, can be constrained by acoustic windows and soft tissue characterization is lacking. Development of an alternative, noninvasive imaging modality to complement fetal echocardiography would be desirable and magnetic resonance imaging (MRI)—by virtue of its 3D capabilities to quantitatively assess morphology, ventricular volume, mass, and flow as well as its wide field of view—is uniquely suited to be this complementary imaging modality. MRI has been used for fetal extracardiac malformations for many years.[3,4] It has been stated from experts in the field that "[Fetal MRI is] firmly established as an excellent complementary tool [to fetal ultrasongraphy] capable of providing exquisite anatomic detail" and sonography and "MRI have played critical roles in the identification of those fetuses most likely to benefit from different treatment strategies."[4] With such a track record, it seems logical to extend this technique to fetal cardiovascular evaluation as well.

Clinical needs for the additional quantitative information can be obtained with a 3D imaging modality such as MRI. One of these needs is accurate measurement of ventricular volume and mass, which is illustrated in cases such as hypoplastic left heart syndrome or pulmonary atresia with intact ventricular septum, in which determination of ventricular adequacy is critically important in management. Quantitatively, fetal echocardiography relies on geometrical assumptions to determine ventricular volumes and mass that are invalid in the oddly shaped hearts (or a compressed heart as when a diaphragmatic hernia is present) found in congenital heart disease. Accurate functional data obtained by MRI can aid in the medical decision-making process when deciding, for example, whether a patient can undergo a one- or two-ventricle repair when born.[5] In addition, with the advent of fetal cardiac interventional techniques, accurate functional data obtained by MRI may be key in directing and evaluating the results of these interventions.[6]

Another functional 3D parameter that can be provided by MRI is quantitative blood flow.[7-9] When calculating blood flow by echocardiography, a sample volume is placed in the vessel of interest and the velocity-time integral is measured along with the diameter of the vessel. A number of assumptions are involved in this calculation including a circular cross-sectional area of the vessel and flat velocity profile. When cardiac MRI velocity mapping is utilized, velocity is measured "through-plane" across the cross-sectional area of the vessel, and when integrating this velocity across the cross-sectional area, blood flow (not solely velocity) can be obtained. This is a more direct measurement of blood flow and minimizes the assumptions made. In addition, blood flow measurements generally validate ventricular volume measurements made by MRI, confirming internal consistency. MRI velocity mapping has progressed to the stage at which now "instantaneous" or "real-time" flow measurements have been a reality ex utero since 2004[10]; the future holds promise for this to be applied in utero. Accurate fetal flow measurement would be useful in patients with poor ventricular performance such as twin-twin transfusion syndrome and fetal heart block.

Three-dimensional anatomic imaging in the fetus has obvious advantages in patients with structural heart disease. The malformed cardiovascular system can be visualized more easily in this manner rather than inferring the 3D structure from 2D imaging. The wide field-of-view of MRI affords a more global picture of the cardiovascular system as well as the syndromes associated with congenital heart disease such as heterotaxy. For example, because the trachea is filled with fluid, MRI can determine the branching of the tracheobronchial tree in utero and sidedness of the aortic arch (see Figure 46-2C later); this is a challenge for echocardiography. Because a number of patients with congenital heart disease have extracardiac malformations, MRI is poised to be a "one-stop shop" for fetal evaluation for both cardiac and extracardiac lesions.

MRI utilization in the fetus has other potential advantages. MRI has been used to determine blood oxygen levels ex utero using the "BOLD" (blood oxygen level dependent) technique, and recent reports suggest it can be used in the fetus as well.[11] MRI can also be used to assess myocardial metabolism and myocardial iron stores and holds the possibility of being used for interventions, in a manner similar to that of echocardiography. The applicability of MRI to the fetus can be utilized for research into the hemodynamic abnormalities that may cause or be a result of pathological heart defects. Fetuses may be followed over time to assess structure and hemodynamics after being identified with congenital heart disease.

The instances previously discussed are meant to convey that the development of fetal cardiac MRI is complementary to fetal echocardiography and is unlikely at this point in time to supplant it. For example, fetal echocardiography is limited to the acoustic windows available; MRI has no such limitation and can be used where windows are less than optimal. To assess soft tissues, ex vivo fetal imaging comparing MRI with echocardiography revealed that "MRI projections had better image quality and revealed more structural details than the sonographic views."[12] Finally, an important capability of cardiac MRI is that it can build images over multiple heartbeats, "averaging-out" or embedding ventricular performance over time into the image created, as opposed to the instantaneous ventricular performance obtained by echocardiography. The imager or clinician does not, therefore, have to evaluate multiple heartbeats and "average" the ventricular performance; it is embedded in the image created. This can complement the "instantaneous" temporal images and data derived from echocardiography.

The Development of Fetal Cardiac MRI for Visualizing Cardiovascular Morphology and Myocardial Motion

Although fetal MRI of extracardiac structures has played an important role in perinatal management for many years,[2,3] extension of these technique to anatomical and functional fetal heart imaging has been limited. To obtain high-quality MRI images of cardiac structure and hemodynamics, data acquisition typically must be segmented over multiple heartbeats, necessitating synchronization to the cardiac cycle. This synchronization is generally achieved with electrocardiographic (ECG) triggering. However, detection of a fetal ECG signal can be problematic, particularly within the bore of an MRI scanner. The fetal ECG recording is typically corrupted by the maternal ECG reading and movement, and the MRI scanner itself induces significant artifacts via rapidly switching magnetic field gradients. In addition, during segmented image acquisition, MRI relies on the subject remaining motionless in the scanner and, with active fetuses, this again poses problems that must be overcome.

The main approach to fetal cardiac MRI avoids cardiac synchronization entirely by using single-shot and real-time imaging techniques,[5] a method that can obtain bright blood anatomical and functional imaging in milliseconds. Considerable efforts have been devoted to the development of these rapid real-time imaging strategies including non-Cartesian k-space sampling,[13,14] parallel imaging,[15] and ultrafast MRI pulse sequence techniques.[16] Besides precluding the need for cardiac synchronization, real-time imaging offers other potential advantages in insensitivity to arrhythmia, gross fetal or maternal motion and potential for interactive control of scan plane and other parameters.[17]

An alternative approach to overcoming the problems associated with ECG measurement within the MRI system is to derive a physiological synchronization signal from the MRI data itself.[18,19] This strategy, dubbed "self-gating," offers the possibility of synchronizing MRI data acquisition with the motion of the fetal heart, providing the high spatial and temporal resolution benefits of segmented acquisition. This has already been demonstrated ex utero in adult and pediatric patients.[20] "Real-time" MRI can be used for cine imaging of vascular structures and ventricular function as well as quantitative flow measures using real-time phase encoded velocity mapping.[10]

Doppler ultrasound is commonly used to detect fetal heart rate and is a third approach to fetal cardiac imaging. The feasibility and safety of performing fetal ultrasound cardiotocography (CTG) in an MRI scanner have been evaluated independently in several studies.[21-24] Commercial ultrasound scanners were modified with electronic shielding and magnetically compatible components for use in the MRI scanner. The safety of performing fetal CTG in a 1.5-T MRI system was most recently evaluated by Michel and coworkers.[24] The monitoring of maternal and fetal heart rates, fetal movements before, during, and after MRI scanning for 10-minute periods showed no pathological accelerations, short-term or long-term changes in basal fetal heart rate, and no signs of fetal stress. An earlier attempt to use CTG monitoring to gate the MRI sequence[22] was hampered by severe artifacts in the MRI images created by the unshielded ultrasound device. This study, however, demonstrated the feasibility of using CTG signals to cardiac-gate MRI pulse sequences in adult subjects. Although the investigators have successfully shielded an ultrasound machine for use with MRI,[25,26] the same technology is yet to be optimized for fetal cardiac MRI.

Finally, a fourth approach leverages recent advances in ECG signal processing[27] and offers the possibility of noninvasively gating the MRI scan to the fetal heart rate via a fetal ECG signal. Modifications of the same vectorcardiogram technology that has been successful in adult cardiac MRI may make fetal ECG gating feasible.[28]

Safety of Fetal MRI

As with any imaging technique, safety should always be considered. Fetal MRI has been used as early as 1983, and to date, no negative side effects or delayed sequelae are known to be associated with fetal MRI.[29] Isolate cell, animal, and human studies have confirmed this finding.[30,31] Fetal MRI is considered by physicians working in the field as "firmly established as an excellent complementary tool to fetal ultrasongraphy capable of providing exquisite anatomic detail in many case."[4] In addition, these physicians have stated that sonography and "MRI have played critical roles in the identification of those fetuses most likely to benefit from different treatment strategies."[4]

Multiple animal research studies have been published with regard to the developing fetus and exposure to magnetic fields. Behr and colleagues.[32] exposed chick embryos to different static and time-varying gradient field strengths and found no influence from MRI on the embryo mortality, hatching rate, or the vitality of the chickens. In mice exposed to a magnetic field at 0.35 T in midgestation, Heinrichs and associates[33] found no gross effects of embryotoxicity and some "evidence" of reduction in crown-rump length. Yip and coworkers studied cell proliferation and migration effects at 1.5 T on chicks[34] as well as axonal outgrowth in the sympathetic nervous system[35] and found no effects. In pregnant mice exposed to 4.7 T (more than three times the field strength of a routine 1.5 T scanner) for 8 hours (more than eight times the exposure of a typical study) on day 9 or 12 of gestation, significant differences were found in biological endpoints such as fetal weight reduction, crown-rump length reduction, postpartum death rate increase, and a reduction in daily sperm production.[36] This is in contrast to the findings of Magin and colleagues,[37] who found no effects on fetal growth and postnatal development in mice as a result of long-term exposure to 4T. Chew and associates[38] reported no statistical effects in the rate of blastocyst formation between control groups and those exposed to 1.5 T with MRI clinical sequences.

A number of human studies also confirm the safety of fetal MRI. Baker and coworkers[39] performed a 3-year follow up study of children imaged in utero and no demonstrable increase in disease or disability could be related to the echo planar imaging (EPI) used at 0.5 T on 20 pregnant women. Similarly, Myers and colleagues[40] investigated the effects of EPI on 74 pregnant women exposed to 0.5 T, utilizing 148 women not exposed to MRI as a control group; no statistical difference was observed with regard to intrauterine growth retardation. There have also been a few studies on fetal heart rate (a measure of fetal distress) during MRI encompassing 34 pregnant patients exposed to 0.5 to 1.5 T, and none of the studies could detect any variance in fetal heart rate.[41-43] Although certainly not the same as undergoing a scan, a study by Kanal and associates[44] surveyed female MRI technologists to establish static fringe field effects and received 1915 responses covering 1421 pregnancies. They studied factors such as fertility, length of gestation, birth weight, pregnancy outcome, and offspring gender and found no statistical significant associations with working in an MRI. Shellock and Crues reviewed a number of studies on the safety of fetal MRI as part of an overall

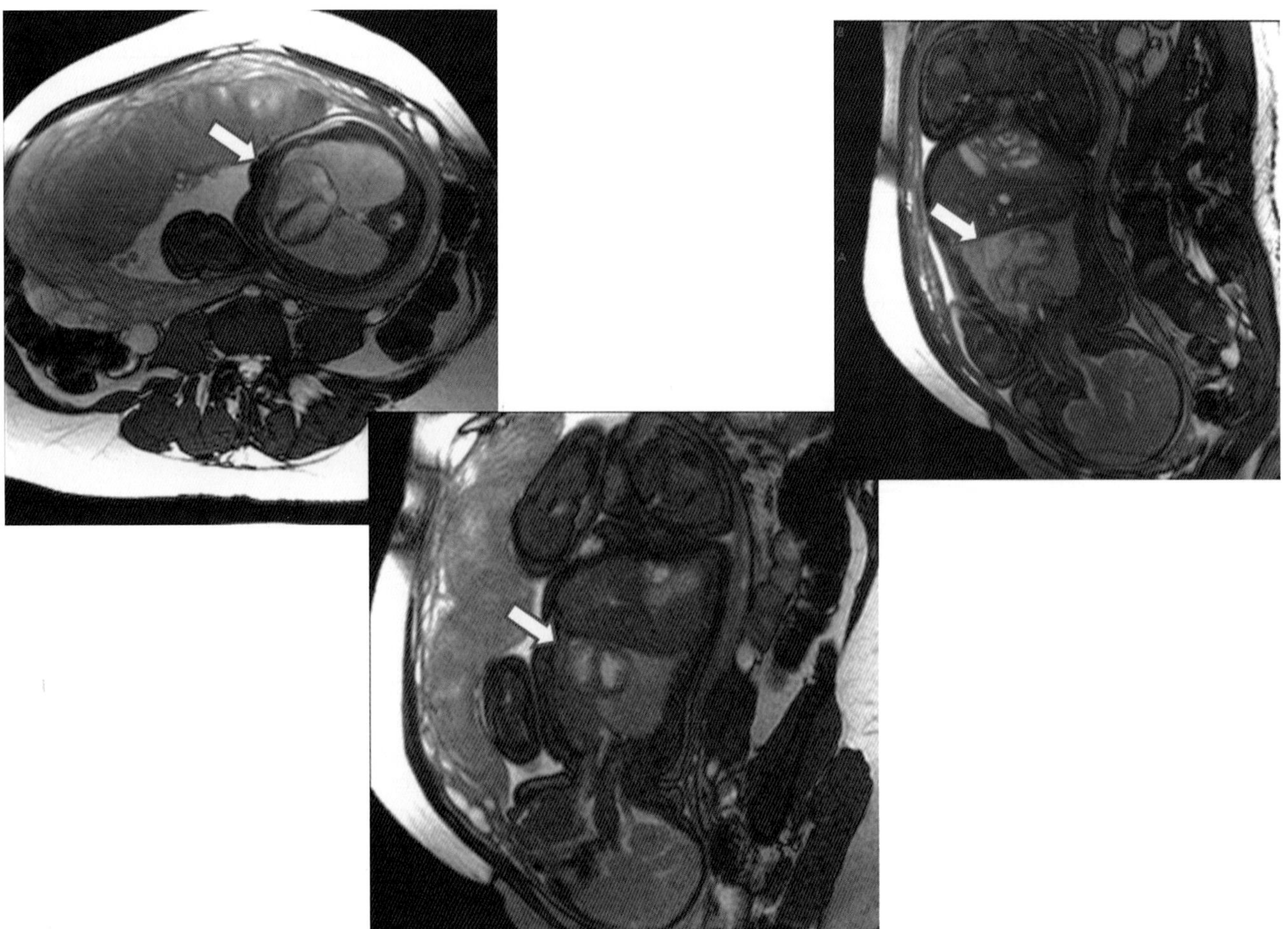

Figure 46-1. Fetal cardiac magnetic resonance imaging (MRI) of a patient with tetralogy of Fallot and pulmonary atresia. **Top right,** The left ventricular outflow tract in an off-axis coronal plane. **Bottom,** An off-axis sagittal view of the ventricular short axis. The *bottom* of each previously and referenced image is toward the head (brain can be seen) and the *top* of each image is toward the feet. **Top left,** A four-chamber view. *Arrows* point to the heart.

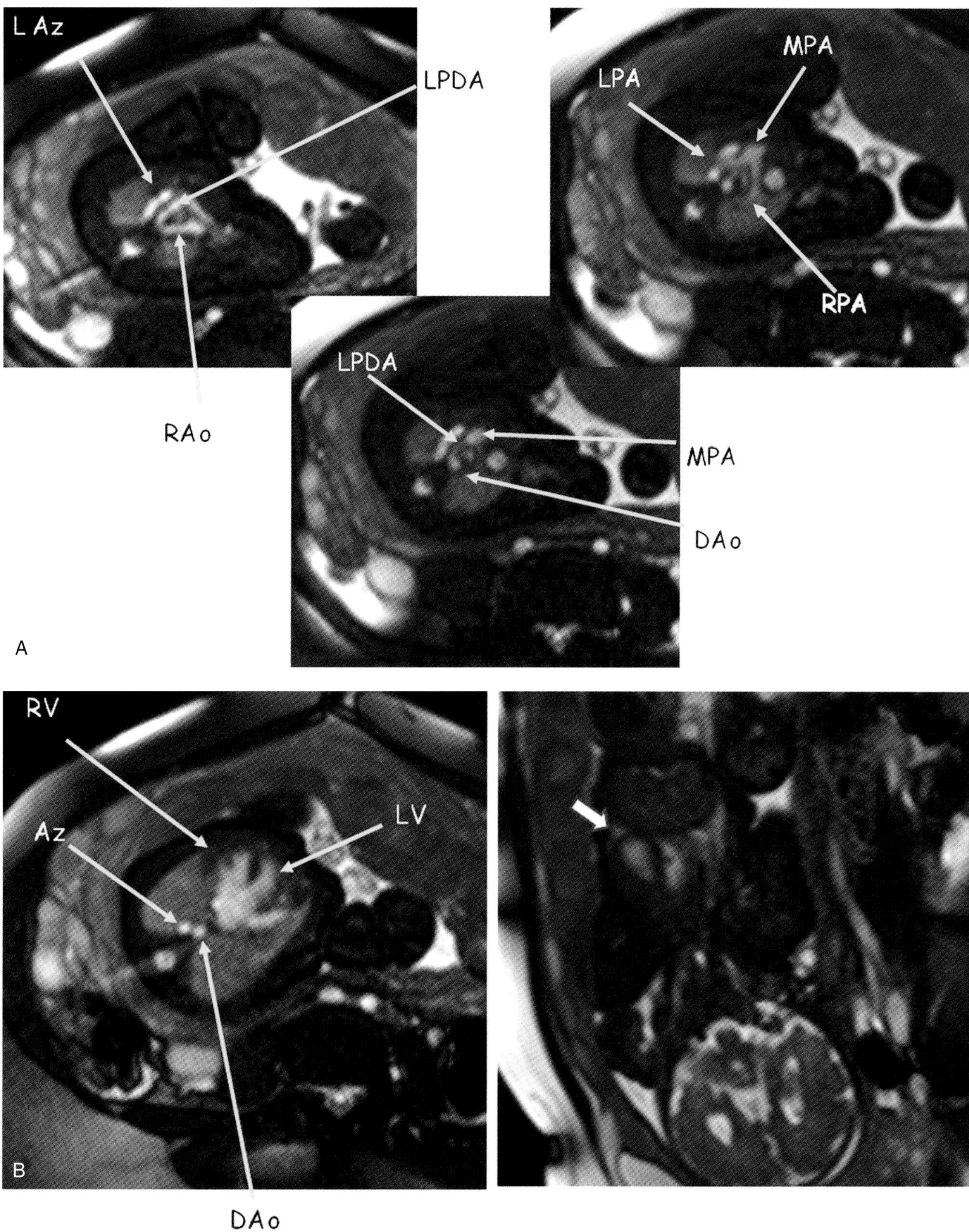

Figure 46-2. Fetal cardiac MRI of a patient with heterotaxy with an interrupted inferior vena cava with an azygos continuation to a left superior vena cava. **(A)** A series of axial bright blood images demonstrate various portions of the anatomy. **Top left,** The left azygos (LAz), left patent ductus arteriosus (LPDA), and right aortic arch (RAo). **Top right,** The right (RPA), left (LPA), and main pulmonary arteries (MPA). **Bottom,** An image at a level in between the upper two demonstrates the connection of the LPDA between the MPA and the descending aorta (DAo). **(B)** Ventricular function is evaluated in the four-chamber **(left)** and short-axis **(right)** views. Note how the patient has a complete common atrioventricular canal from the four-chamber view; positions of the DAo and left azygos vein (Az) can be seen in this image relative to the spine. LV, left ventricle; RV, right ventricle. **Right,** The head is toward the bottom of the image; the *arrow* points to the heart.

Continued

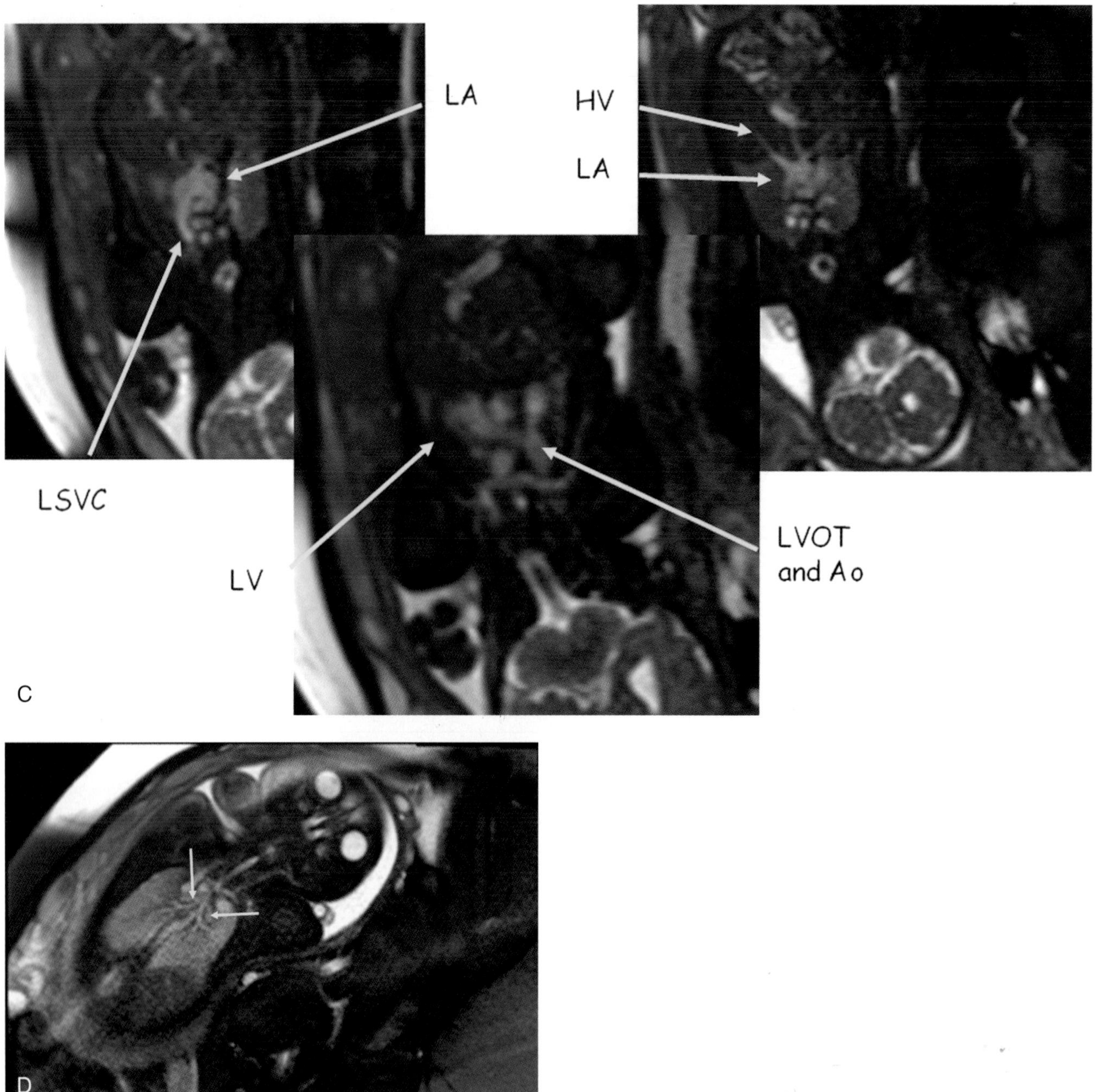

Figure 46-2, cont'd **(C)** Three off-axis coronal views at various levels with the head at the *bottom* of the images. **Left,** The left superior vena cava (LSVC) connects to the left atrium (LA). **Middle,** The left ventricular outflow tract (LVOT) and the aorta (Ao). The hepatic veins (HV) are seen connected to the LA on the **right panel.** **(D)** Off-axis coronal view demonstrates bilateral left-sided bronchi *(arrows)*; the head is toward the *top*.

review of MRI safety and concluded that the "overall findings from these studies indicate that there is no substantial evidence of injury or harm to the fetus, however, additional research on this topic in warranted."[45]

The Emerging Discipline of Fetal Cardiac MRI

As early as 1995, a case report on the anatomical delineation of hypoplastic left heart syndrome was published but nothing else was published in the subsequent 10 years.[46] The first use of MRI to visualize the heart beating in utero was published in 2005 and utilized real-time steady-state free precession.[5] In that report, "real-time" cine bright blood imaging was used to quantitate information regarding ventricular size and function in a patient with a borderline left ventricular size. Correlation with Doppler echocardiography was found, by "back calculation," to be consistent. Static bright blood imaging was also used for anatomy. A second patient in that manuscript was also reported with ductal constriction. In the years following, a number of other reports have surfaced on the use of MRI to visualize the fetal heart.[47-53] All have used either

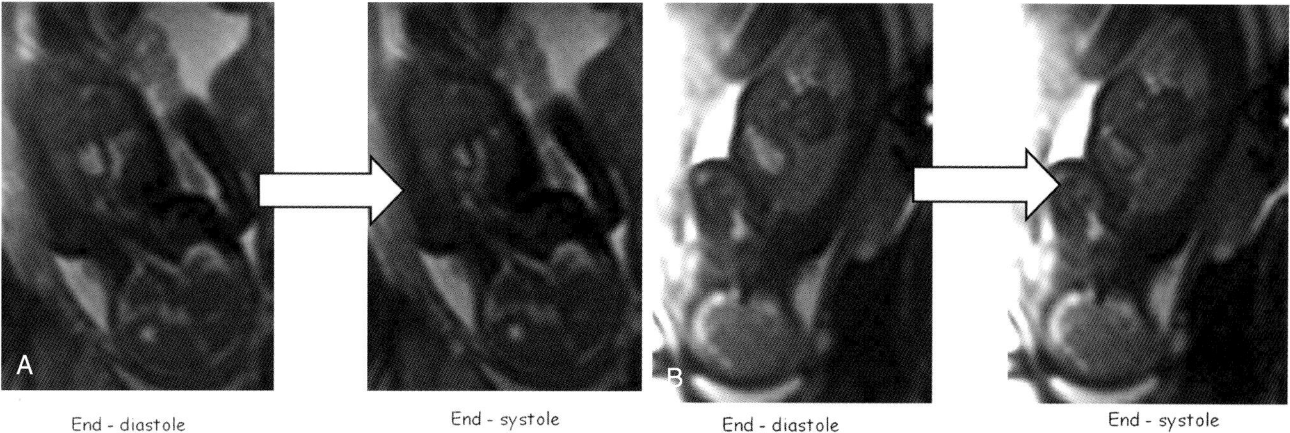

Figure 46-3. Ventricular shortening assessment utilizing fetal cardiac MRI. The short-axis **(A)** and long-axis **(B)** views of the ventricles at end-diastole **(left)** and end-systole **(right)** demonstrate ventricular shortening in the fetus.

static or real-time cine steady-state free precession bright blood imaging to visualize the fetus. Fetal cardiac MRI, however, has also been applied beyond just visualization of fetal cardiac anatomy or fetal ventricular function. Utilizing fetal cardiac MRI images, Pekkan and coworkers[54] applied computational fluid dynamic modeling to assess the flow fields in the normal embryonic arch as well as modeling various forms of congenital heart disease in the fetus.

Figure 46-1 includes images obtained from a patient with tetralogy of Fallot and pulmonary atresia and Figure 46-2 has images obtained from a patient with heterotaxy syndrome. Figure 46-3 demonstrates the evaluation of ventricular shortening in the fetus. These examples used bright blood steady-state free precession imaging. In the patient with heterotaxy syndrome, note that the trachea can be visualized because it is filled with fluid; hepatic venous drainage, important for later surgery with Fontan reconstruction, can also be seen.

The Future

Fetal cardiac MRI is truly in its fledgling stages of development. Many hurdles have been overcome and likely there are more to overcome before this technology is readily and widely utilized outside of major academic centers. Even with the great technological strides MRI has made, there is still a vast room for improvement in image quality and speed. MRI has numerous advantages as an imaging modality and is certainly worth exploring in the fetus. Time will tell whether these advantages can be exploited for advanced imaging of the fetal cardiovascular system and possibly contribute to the improved management and care of the unborn patient.

References

1. Cohen MS. Fetal diagnosis and management of congenital heart disease. *Clin Perinatol.* 2001;28:11-29.
2. Smith FW, Adam AH, Phillips WD. NMR imaging in pregnancy. *Lancet.* 1983;1:61-62.
3. Hubbard AM, Harty P. Prenatal magnetic resonance imaging of fetal anomalies. *Semin Roentgenol.* 1999;34:41-47.
4. Coleman BG, Adzick NS, Crombleholme TM, et al. Fetal therapy. State of the art. *J Ultrasound Med.* 2002;21:1257-1288.
5. Fogel MA, Wilson RD, Flake A, et al. Preliminary investigations into a new method of functional assessment of the fetal heart using a novel application of "real-time" cardiac magnetic resonance imaging. *Fetal Diagn Ther.* 2005;20:475-480.
6. Artz W, Tulzer G, Aigner M, et al. Invasive intrauterine treatment of pulmonary atresia/intact ventricular septum with heart failure. *Ultrasound Obstet Gynecol.* 2003;21:186.
7. Henk CB, Schlechta B, Grampp S, Gomischek G, Kelpetko W, Mostbeck GH. Pulmonary and aortic blood flow measurements in normal subjects and patients after single lung transplantation at 0.5 T using velocity encoded cine MRI. *Chest.* 1998;114:771-779.
8. Beerbaum P, Korperich H, Barth B, Esdorn H, Gieseke J, Meyer H. Non-invasive quantification of left-to-right shunt in pediatric patients. Phase-contrast cine magnetic resonance imaging compared with invasive oximetry. *Circulation.* 2001;103:2476-2482.
9. Fogel MA, Weinberg PM. Haselgrove J. Flow volume asymmetry in the right aortic arch in children utilizing magnetic resonance phase encoded velocity mapping. *Am Heart J.* 2003;145:154-161.
10. Korperich H, Gieseke J, Barth P, et al. Flow volume and shunt quantification in pediatric congenital heart disease by real-time magnetic resonance velocity mapping. A validation study. *Circulation.* 2004;109:1987-1993.
11. Wedegartner U. Kooijman H. Yamamura J. et al. In vivo MRI measurement of fetal blood oxygen saturation in cardiac ventricles of fetal sheep: a feasibility study. *Magn Reson Med.* 2010;64:32-41.
12. Meyer-Wittkopf M, Cook A, McLennan A, Summers P, Sharland GK, Maxwell DJ. Evaluation of three-dimensional and magnetic resonance imaging in assessment of congenital heart anomalies in fetal cardiac specimens. *Ultrasound Obstet Gynecol.* 1996;8:303-308.
13. Shankaranarayanan A, Simonetti OP, Laub G, Lewin JS, Duerk JL. Segmented k-space and real-time cardiac cine MR imaging with radial trajectories. *Radiology.* 2001;221:827-836.
14. Larson AC, Simonetti OP. Real-time cardiac cine imaging with SPIDER: steady-state projection imaging with dynamic echo-train readout. *Magn Reson Med.* 2001;46:10591066.
15. Guttman MA, Kellman P, Dick AJ, Lederman RJ, McVeigh ER. Real-time accelerated interactive MRI with adaptive TSENSE and UNFOLD. *Magn Reson Med.* 2003;50:315-321.
16. Lee VS, Resnick D, Bundy JM, Simonetti OP, Lee P, Weinreb JC. Cardiac function: MR evaluation in one breath hold with real-time true fast imaging with steady-state precession. *Radiology.* 2002; 222:835-842.
17. Guttman MA, Lederman RJ, Sorger JM, McVeigh ER. Real-time volume rendered MRI for interventional guidance. *J Cardiovasc Magn Reson.* 2002;4:431-442.

18. Larson AC, White RD, Laub G, McVeigh ER, Li D, Simonetti OP. Self-gated cardiac cine MRI. *Magn Reson Med.* 2004;51:93-102.
19. Crowe ME, Larson AC, Zhang Q, et al. Automated rectilinear self-gated cardiac cine imaging. *Magn Reson Med.* 2004;52:782-788.
20. Johnson TR, Simonetti O, Larson A, Fogel MA. Self gating in pediatric cardiac magnetic resonance imaging. Presented at: the 7th Annual Scientific Sessions of the Society for Cardiovascular Magnetic Resonance; February 13-15, 2004; Barcelona, Spain; and the 53rd Annual Scientific Sessions of the American College of Cardiology; March 7-10, 2004; New Orleans, La.
21. Shakespeare SA, Moore RJ, Crowe JA, et al. A method for foetal heart rate monitoring during magnetic resonance imaging using Doppler ultrasound. *Physiol Meas.* 1999;20:363-368.
22. Rubin JM, Fowlkes JB, Prince MR, et al. Doppler US gating of cardiac MR imaging. *Acad Radiol.* 2000;7:1116-1122.
23. Poutamo J, Partanen K, Vanninen R, et al. MRI does not change fetal cardiotocographic parameters. *Prenat Diagn.* 1998;18:1149-1154.
24. Michel SCA, Rake A, Keller TM, et al. Fetal cardiographic monitoring during 1.5-T MR imaging. *AJR Am J Roentgenol.* 2003;180:1159-1164.
25. Gunther M, Feinberg DA. Ultrasound-guided MRI: preliminary using a motion. *Magn Reson Med.* 2004;52: 27-32.
26. Feinberg DA, Günther M. Simultaneous MR and ultrasound imaging: towards US-navigated MRI. In *Book of Abstracts. International Society for Magnetic Resonance in Medicine (ISMRM)*. Toronto: ISMRM, 2003:381.
27. Khamene A, Negahdaripour S. A new method for the extraction of fetal ECG from the composite abdominal signal. *IEEE Trans Biomed Eng.* 2000;47:507-516.
28. Fischer SE, Wickline SA, Lorenz CH. Novel real-time R-wave detection algorithm based on the vectorcardiogram for accurate gated magnetic resonance acquisitions. *Magn Reson Med.* 1999;42:361-370.
29. Levine D, Barnes PD, Edelmann RR. Obstetric MR imaging. *Radiology.* 1999;211:609-617.
30. Schwartz J, Crooks L. NMR imaging produces no observable mutations or cytotoxicity in mammalian cells. *AJR Am J Roentgenol.* 1982;139:583-585.
31. Wolff S, Crooks L, Brown P, Howard R, Painter R. Tests for DNA and chromosomal damage induced by nuclear magnetic resonance imaging. *Radiology.* 1980;136:707-710.
32. Behr KP, Tiffe HW, Hinz KH, et al. Nuclear magnetic resonance (NMR) and the development of chick embryos. *Dtsche Tierarztl Wochenschr.* 1991;98:149-152.
33. Heinrichs WL, Fong P, Flannery M, et al. Midgestational exposure of pregnant Balb/C mice to magnetic resonance conditions. *Magn Reson Imaging.* 1988;6:305-313.
34. Yip YP, Capriotti C, Talagala SL, et al. Effects of MR exposure at 1.5T on early embryonic development of the chick. *J Magn Reson Imaging.* 1994;4:742-748.
35. Yip YP, Capriotti C, Yip JW, et al. Effects of MR exposure on cell-proliferation and migration of chick motoneurons. *J Magn Reson Imaging.* 1995;5:457-462.
36. Carnes KI, Magin RL. Effects of in-utero exposure to 4.7T MR imaging conditions on fetal growth and testicular development in the mouse. *Magn Reson Imaging.* 1996;14:263-274.
37. Magin RL, Lee JK, Klintsova A, et al. Biological effects of long duration, high field (4T) MRI on growth and development in the mouse. *J Magn Reson Imaging.* 2000;12:14-149.
38. Chew A, Ahmadi A, Goh PS, et al. The effects of 1.5T magnetic resonance imaging on early murine in-vitro embryo development. *J Magn Reson Imaging.* 2001;13:417-420.
39. Baker PN, Johnson IR, Harvey P, et al. A three year follow-up of children imaged in-utero with echo-planar magnetic resonance imaging. *Am J Obstet Gynecol.* 1994;170:32-33.
40. Myers C, Duncan KR, Gowland PA, et al. Failure to detect intrauterine growth restriction following in utero exposure to MRI. *Br J Radiol.* 1998;71:549-551.
41. Poutamo J, Partanen K, Vanninen R, et al. MRI does not change fetal cardiotocographic parameters. *Prenatal Diag.* 1998;18:1149-1154.
42. Vadeyar SH, Moore RJ, Strachen BK, et al. Effects of fetal magnetic resonance imaging on fetal heart rate patterns. *Am J Obstet Gynecol.* 2000;182:666-669.
43. Michel SCA, Rake A, Keller TM, et al. Fetal cardiographic monitoring during 1.5T MR imaging. *AJR Am J Roentgenol.* 2003;180:1159-1164.
44. Kanal E, Gillen J, Evans JA, et al. Survey on reproductive health among female MR workers. *Radiology.* 1993;187:395-399.
45. Shellock FG, Crues JV. MR procedures: Biologic effects, safety, and patient care. *Radiology.* 2004;232:635-652.
46. Hata K, Hata T, Manabe A, et al. Hypoplastic left heart syndrome: color Doppler sonographic and magnetic resonance imaging features in utero. *Gynecol Obstet Invest.* 1995;39:70-72.
47. Saleem SN. Feasibility of MRI of the fetal heart with balanced steady-state free precession sequence along fetal body and cardiac planes. *AJR.* 2008;191:1208-1215.
48. Gorincour G, Bourliere-Najean B, Bonello B, et al. Feasibility of fetal cardiac magnetic resonance imaging: preliminary experience. *Ultrasound Obstet Gynecol.* 2007;29:105-108.
49. McMahon CJ, Taylor MD, Cassady CI, Olutoye OO, Bezold LI. Diagnosis of pentalogy of cantrell in the fetus using magnetic resonance imaging and ultrasound. *Pediatr Cardiol.* 2007;28:172-175.
50. Moniotte S, Powell AJ, Barnewolt CE, et al. Prenatal diagnosis of thoracic ectopia cordis by real-time fetal cardiac magnetic resonance imaging and by echocardiography. *Congenit Heart Dis.* 2008;3:128-131.
51. Manganaro L, Savelli S, Di Maurizio M, et al. Fetal MRI of the cardiovascular system: role of steady-state free precession sequences for the evaluation of normal and pathological appearances. *Radiol Med.* 2009;114:852-870.
52. Manganaro L, Savelli S, Di Maurizio M, et al. Potential role of fetal cardiac evaluation with magnetic resonance imaging: preliminary experience. *Prenat Diagn.* 2008;28:148-156.
53. Manganaro L, Savelli S, Di Maurizio M, et al. Assessment of congenital heart disease (CHD): is there a role for fetal magnetic resonance imaging (MRI)? *Eur J Radiol.* 2009;72:172-180.
54. Pekkan K, Dasi LP, Nourparvar P, et al. In vitro hemodynamic investigation of the embryonic aortic arch at late gestation. *J Biomech.* 2008;41:1697-1706.

Index

Note: Page numbers followed by f refer to figures; page numbers followed by t refer to tables; page numbers followed by b refer to boxes.

D